Veterinary Forensics: Animal Cruelty Investigations

Second Edition

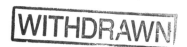

Veterinary Forensics: Animal Cruelty Investigations

Second Edition

Melinda D. Merck, DVM

Editor

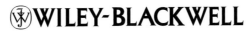
WILEY-BLACKWELL

A John Wiley & Sons, Inc., Publication

This edition first published 2013 © 2013 by John Wiley & Sons, Inc
First edition published 2007 © Blackwell Publishing

Wiley-Blackwell is an imprint of John Wiley & Sons, formed by the merger of Wiley's global Scientific, Technical and Medical business with Blackwell Publishing.

Editorial Offices

2121 State Avenue, Ames, Iowa 50014–8300, USA

The Atrium, Southern Gate, Chichester, West Sussex, PO19 8SQ, UK

9600 Garsington Road, Oxford, OX4 2DQ, UK

For details of our global editorial offices, for customer services and for information about how to apply for permission to reuse the copyright material in this book please see our website at www.wiley.com/wiley-blackwell.

Library of Congress Cataloging-in-Publication Data

Veterinary forensics : animal cruelty investigations / Melinda D. Merck, editor. – 2nd ed.
    p. ; cm.
   Includes bibliographical references and index.
   ISBN 978-0-470-96162-9 (pbk. : alk. paper)
   I. Merck, Melinda.
 [DNLM: 1. Animal Welfare.   2. Forensic Medicine.   3. Veterinary Medicine. SF 769.47]
   636.089′4–dc23

2012020845

A catalogue record for this book is available from the British Library.

Wiley also publishes its books in a variety of electronic formats. Some content that appears in print may not be available in electronic books.

Set in 9.5/12pt Times by SPi Publisher Services, Pondicherry, India
Printed and bound in Singapore by Markono Print Media Pte Ltd

Disclaimer

1   2013

Dedication

This book is dedicated to those who have risen above encumbrances and done the right thing. You are the true heroes.

Table of Contents

Companion Website

The book is accompanied by a companion website, accessible at

www.wiley.com/go/vetforensics

The website includes forms and checklists to download and use in forensics investigations.

List of Contributors

Gail S. Anderson, MPM, PhD, D-ABFE
Professor
Director, Undergraduate Programmes,
School of Criminology
Co-Director, Centre for Forensic Research
Diplomate, American Board of Forensic Entomology
Simon Fraser University
Vancouver, British Columbia

Diane E. Balkin, JD
Contract Attorney
Animal Legal Defense Fund
Denver, Colorado

Sharon M. Gwaltney-Brant, DVM, PhD, DABVT, DABT
Toxicology Consultant, Veterinary Information
Network, Davis, California
Adjunct faculty, College of Veterinary Medicine
University of Illinois
Urbana-Champaign, Illinois

Don J. Harris DVM
South Dade Avian & Exotic and Small Animal Hospital
Miami, Florida

Laura A. Janssen, JD
Former Senior Assistant District Attorney
Fulton County District Attorney's Office
Atlanta, Georgia

Richard A. LeCouteur, BVSc, PhD, Diplomate ACVIM (Neurology), Diplomate ECVN
Professor of Neurology & Neurosurgery
University of California
School of Veterinary Medicine
Davis, California

Melinda D. Merck, DVM
Veterinary Forensics Consulting, LLC
Atlanta, Georgia

Paulo C. Maiorka, DVM, MSc, PhD
Associate Professor of Veterinary Pathology and
Veterinary Forensics Department of Pathology
School of Veterinary Medicine and Animal Sciences
University of São Paulo
São Paulo, Brazil

Dana M. Miller DVM
Miller Veterinary Consulting
Spartanburg, South Carolina

Doris M. Miller DVM, PhD, DACVP
Professor
Associate Director of State Government Relations
Athens Veterinary Diagnostic Laboratory
College of Veterinary Medicine
University of Georgia
Athens, Georgia

Robert W. Reisman, DVM
Medical Coordinator of Animal Cruelty Cases
Forensic Sciences
Bergh Memorial Animal Hospital
American Society for the Prevention of Cruelty to Animals
New York, New York

Foreword

Of my 25 years as an attorney, I have spent just over 17 years in the trenches as a prosecutor. Then, and now in my work with the Animal Legal Defense Fund, I have always considered animal cruelty cases to be a top priority for any law enforcement agency or prosecutor's office. I recall a case I handled before I became the elected District Attorney in Benton County, Oregon, where a drunken man, without provocation, stabbed a puppy in the chest with a large knife, killing the little guy. After reading the incident report and looking at the photos of that innocent, limp body with a huge knife sticking out of his ribs, I recall experiencing a moment of profound anger directed at both the defendant for his unspeakably savage conduct and the state legislature for its lack of vision in classifying this conduct as a lowly misdemeanor (years later, this conduct is now a class C felony).

The fact is, in the early 1990s, there were only a handful of states that had a felony animal cruelty statute on the books. Now, as of this writing, only three states do not have a felony animal cruelty statute. Though on an accelerated timeline, the same trend is true with animal fighting cases. In the late 1970s it was still legal to fight dogs in some states and roosters in several others. But no more: animal fighting is now illegal in every state and a federal offense as well. There are even a handful of states that have elevated animal fighting to the level of a racketeering predicate offense (I am proud to note that Oregon took this step well in advance of a certain NFL player's highly-publicized foray into dogfighting).

With these increased criminal penalties comes an ever-greater need for quality investigations. Speaking from experience, when the State presents its case to a jury, a very common defense tactic is to "put the investigation on trial." This approach can be an effective one because jurors have come to expect the State to employ every technological advantage if it is to carry its heavy burden of proof. This is an impossible expectation to meet if the evidence at the crime scene was not collected properly, documented

accurately, or analyzed fully. When officers fail to recognize the reality that they have, in effect, two crime scenes (i.e. the physical location of the event and the victim animal's body) key evidence is overlooked, compromised or, sadly, affirmatively tossed in the trash.

If investigators fail to create a scene diagram noting the locations of where the evidence was found, the case is vulnerable. Likewise, if veterinarians fail to perform a full and accurate forensic exam or does not know how to properly document their findings, then the case is vulnerable. If prosecutors fail to properly prepare the State's expert witness (usually a veterinarian) for trial, then the expert will have a difficult time persuading the jury on direct examination and likely an even tougher time withstanding the rigors of cross-examination, and the case is vulnerable.

These very real dynamics are precisely why Dr. Merck's book is so important to the professionals working to ensure justice in animal cruelty cases. If every officer reads this book, one can safely conclude that gone are the days when a responding officer just tosses the body of the animal victim in the trash. Rather, the body will be treated like the critical piece of evidence that it is, seized and presented for necropsy, with investigators first measuring not just the body's core temperature (repeatedly, at fixed intervals), but also the ambient temperature where the body was recovered (a key piece of information necessary to any attempt to narrow the postmortem interval).

Veterinarians who read this book will come away with the expertise and confidence to conduct bomb-proof forensic examinations, render phlegmatic diagnoses of non-accidental injury cases, and accurately chart exam findings that holdup in court. They will be able to make discretionary (or mandated) reports of animal abuse without losing sleep over the decision. And ultimately testify at trial in a manner that not just communicates the facts of the case but also wins the trust and respect of the court.

Prosecutors who read this book will come away with not only a clear understanding of how to direct law enforcement to ensure that the crime scene investigation will withstand the rigors of trial, but also a full appreciation of the widely varied science one encounters in this line of work, be it a non-accidental injury case, a sexual assault case, or an animal fighting case. With this increased understanding of the underlying science comes a confidence and a credibility that attaches to the State's case and prosecutors will have little trouble dispensing with any effort by the defendant to put the investigation on trial.

This book is a seminal work and a vital tool to the men and women who work to ensure that those who abuse animals are held fully accountable for their conduct. Veterinary and criminal justice professionals who read Dr. Merck's work will, as a direct result, experience better outcomes in these important cases.

Scott A. Heiser
Sr. Attorney and Criminal Justice Program Director
Animal Legal Defense Fund

Preface

"The question is not can they reason, nor can they talk, but can they suffer?"

Jeremy Bentham, 1789
(Introduction to the Principles of Morals
and Legislation, Second Edition, 1823,
chapter 17, footnote.)

Since writing the first edition of this book, there have been significant world-wide changes in several areas that impact animal cruelty cases. In 2009, the Farm Animal Welfare Council recognized and defined the five freedoms of animals: freedom from hunger and thirst; freedom from discomfort; freedom from pain, injury, or disease; freedom from fear and distress, and freedom to express normal behavior. These freedoms succinctly summarize the core issues of animal abuse. Furthermore, they signal a shift in the perception of animals and acknowledge that animals suffer.

Animal cruelty laws have also changed internationally. The veterinary, legal, and animal welfare communities have worked together to pass stronger legislation with higher penalties. This has also created an even greater need for veterinary forensic science. Veterinary forensic medicine has been part of several international veterinary curriculums and it continues to grow in the United States. The passage of mandatory animal cruelty reporting laws for veterinarians places a responsibility on the veterinary schools to provide this as part of the student's education. National, state, and local veterinary organizations have taken up the cause, providing continuing education conferences for practicing veterinarians.

There has been a rise of interest in the field of veterinary forensic science and medicine from the veterinary, legal, law enforcement, and forensic science professionals. This book contains the latest in current knowledge and research as it applies to animals; it comes from both the human and veterinary fields. There continues to be ongoing and pertinent research and data collection from across the globe. This is reflected in the number and caliber of the professional contributors to this edition. There are new chapters in avian, poultry, and large animal cruelty in this book. The importance of forensic entomology and the valuable information that can be obtained from insects has prompted a stand-alone chapter on the subject. The first chapter has been enhanced to provide more information for those unfamiliar with the judicial process and reporting of abuse. The second and third chapters are greatly expanded with vast details to provide the formative basis for each subsequent chapter. Each of the following chapters is larger and has been augmented with new information. There is a new section on the pain and suffering of animals in an effort to provide a scientific basis for this issue. Of note are the significant additions regarding crime scene investigation, grave excavation, animal examination, evidence collection and packaging, forensic testing, forensic report writing, and large scale cruelty response. There are new photographs, tables, and figures throughout the textbook, along with new and improved appendices containing valuable forms, checklists, and resources. All of these additions are invaluable for law enforcement, legal, and veterinary professionals.

Animal cruelty investigations and prosecutions require a collaborative effort from all involved. It is important to recognize that knowledge is necessary for the greatest success. Treating an animal cruelty investigation the same as any criminal investigation will result in better outcomes and greater respect with positive changes in the laws and attitudes of those who can impact the animal world. This book will serve all parties in their work on animal cases by providing the requisite knowledge. My hope is that it prompts more interest and research into the field of veterinary forensics from the forensic science and veterinary communities.

Melinda D. Merck

Acknowledgments

I want to thank the contributors who have made this second edition possible. Their expertise, insight, and experience are invaluable. To those who have given me the honor of assisting with their cases, thank you. The knowledge in veterinary forensic science and medicine has greatly expanded through this work, so keep it coming. To my forensic colleagues, thank you for your insight and assistance with this book. Thanks to Dr. Julie Burge and Jim Crosby for granting the use of their forms. To the progressive and insightful veterinarians in Sao Paulo, you are an inspiration to us all. I want to express my deepest gratitude to those who investigate and prosecute animal cruelty with continued pursuit of excellence. It is your passion and dedication that has created the need for this textbook.

This book would not have been possible without the love and support of Theresa and my family on 6th Street in Gainesville. Your friendship surpasses all boundaries. I am grateful for the support and understanding from my friends and family, especially Asa and Tucker. I promise to be at the next sporting events.

Lastly, I want to thank my four-legged companions who suffered periodic neglect while writing this second edition, surrounding me with hopeful toys. I am eternally grateful they do not know how to post ads for "new home wanted" on the Internet.

Melinda D. Merck

1

The Legal System: The Veterinarian's Role and Responsibilities

Diane E. Balkin, Laura A. Janssen, and Melinda D. Merck

Without justice, there can be no peace. He who passively accepts evil is as much involved in it as he who helps to perpetrate it.

Martin Luther King

INTRODUCTION

There is a growing societal awareness about cruelty to animals. The veterinary community is no exception. There is an expectation that perpetrators of animal cruelty and neglect be held accountable. It has been long recognized that there is a link between cruelty to animals and violence toward humans, and that animal abuse is often one of the indicators of family violence and child abuse. The law enforcement community now recognizes that early and aggressive intervention in animal cruelty cases has a positive and proactive impact on public safety and human welfare.

To effectively prosecute those who harm animals there must be a collaborative effort among agencies and individuals. Animal cruelty cases are unique because none of the victims are able to tell the authorities what happened. Therefore, there is a need for the expertise of a veterinarian or other animal health care professional in nearly every case. According to Neumann (2005), society already sees veterinarians as animal welfare advocates, and there is an expectation that veterinarians will fully cooperate in the investigation and prosecution of a cruelty case. Veterinarians are perceived of as a caregiving profession and members of the public expect them to be at the forefront of setting the highest standards for animal welfare. "Research and

professional experience provide compelling evidence that the veterinarian is not only a public health authority, but a type of "family practitioner" with a potential for preventing several forms of family violence"(Arkow).

Most veterinarians have not received formal training in recognizing animal abuse as part of their primary education; rather, they have gained the knowledge through continuing education or textbooks. Veterinary forensic medicine has been part of the veterinary college curriculum in other countries, such as Scotland and Brazil, whereas in the United States it has only recently begun to be incorporated into the curriculum or offered as an elective course. Even with some training veterinarians tend to hesitate to act because they are concerned about being incorrect in their suspicions. There is an increasing trend in legislation regarding the veterinarian's role in reporting animal cruelty. Most of the provisions in the United States are found in either the state's Veterinary Practice Act or their animal cruelty statute. The laws address both the requirement to report and the civil and criminal immunity and protection given to the practitioner who does file a report. The Animal Legal Defense Fund (www.aldf.org) maintains a current list of the states with some type of duty to report and those that provide some type of immunity.

DEFINING ANIMAL CRUELTY

Cruelty to animals can involve anything from act to omission, from teasing to torture, and from intentional to negligent. It also includes animal fighting, animal hoarding,

Veterinary Forensics: Animal Cruelty Investigations, Second Edition. Edited by Melinda D. Merck.
© 2013 John Wiley & Sons, Inc. Published 2013 by John Wiley & Sons, Inc.

and animal neglect. A determination of whether or not a given instance constitutes animal cruelty is made on a case-by-case basis. This decision may be made by an animal control officer or law enforcement officer at the time of the incident or it may be made later by a prosecutor. It is important for the veterinary professional to familiarize him or herself with local statutes and ordinances. For example, the term 'animal' is not universally defined and varies from state to state and city to city. Some statutes and ordinances may exclude certain species.

"The diagnosis of non-accidental injury is not an exact science either in children or in the family dog or cat" (Munro and Thrusfield 2001) and is covered extensively in the following chapters. Several tools are available to assist the veterinarian in evaluating whether or not an animal (particularly a companion animal) has suffered non-accidental injury (NAI). One of the earliest studies on this topic was a 2001 series by Munro and Thrusfield, "Battered Pet Syndrome." Care should be taken to recognize cases in which a failure to act has resulted in an animal's pain and suffering. For example, veterinarians should check with their local animal cruelty investigator or prosecutor to determine if failing to seek timely veterinary care can constitute cruelty.

GOVERNING LAWS

Veterinarians should be mindful of the fact that numerous legal principles may be relevant to an incident involving an animal.

1. **Federal and State Constitutions**: A veterinarian who is employed by a law enforcement agency or humane society that has agents with law enforcement authority should be knowledgeable about constitutional protections afforded to all citizens. According to the Bill of Rights, for example, all individuals in the United States have the right to be free from unreasonable searches and seizures (Fourth Amendment). If at all possible, when seizing animals, it is preferable to have a search warrant signed by a judge. Veterinarians can play an important role in providing information for the affidavit, articulating why an animal(s) must be seized. They also can assist law enforcement by setting forth why certain items other than the animal(s) should also be collected during the execution of a warrant.

   One of the primary reasons a veterinarian must testify in a criminal case is due to the defendant's constitutional right to confront the witnesses against him or her (Sixth Amendment). The defendant has the right to subpoena witnesses and to cross-examine the prosecution witnesses in person and in the presence of the judge or jury.

2. **Federal Statutes, State Statutes, and Municipal Ordinances**: These are typically the laws that define animal cruelty, neglect, hoarding, and fighting. They also set forth the criteria for search warrants, arrest warrants, and restraining orders, and govern the practice of veterinary medicine.

3. **Federal and State Rules of Evidence**: These rules set forth the guidelines for the admissibility of evidence and testimony, including expert testimony. They also give the judge guidelines regarding relevancy, the admissibility of documentary evidence, and whether or not a statement is hearsay or if it is hearsay, whether or not it is admissible as an exception to the hearsay rule.

4. **Case Law**: Certain cases set a precedent and set forth guidelines for the admissibility of specific types of evidence.

HOW VETERINARIANS BECOME INVOLVED

Veterinarians can become involved in a case in a number of ways. Most commonly, an injured or deceased animal will be brought to the hospital, clinic, or shelter for evaluation and treatment. The animal can be brought in by an animal control officer, a good Samaritan, an established client, a stranger, etc. All animals should be treated in the same manner regardless of the circumstances. On occasion, a veterinarian may actually respond to the crime scene. This usually occurs if the veterinarian is an employee of a local law enforcement agency or has a contract with the local law enforcement agency. This is the optimum case scenario because the veterinarian becomes a "direct" witness to the crime scene and the animal(s) (see Chapter 2). Regardless of how veterinarians becomes involved it is critical to remain objective and to document their findings in an impartial and unbiased manner. It is important to be aware of the fact that it is as important or more important to exonerate the innocent suspect as it is to dispassionately substantiate the circumstances of a crime.

Reporting

Laws regarding the veterinarian's role in reporting animal cruelty and animal fighting vary state by state. Because there is an emerging trend toward mandatory reporting, the veterinarian is well advised to be prepared to act in the event the situation arises.

Factors that inhibit reporting

One of the primary concerns expressed by veterinarians regarding reporting is that they do not feel competent to recognize animal abuse. They feel a need to know and understand the exact provisions of the local cruelty laws. They mistakenly believe that it is their responsibility to apply that law to a particular set of circumstances. Most "reportable" cases will distinguish themselves and will be obvious to the veterinary professional. It is the responsibility of the law enforcement authority—animal control, the police, or the prosecutor—to make the ultimate determination as to whether or not criminal charges will be filed. It is *not* the responsibility of the veterinarian. A working knowledge of the law is all that is necessary.

For some veterinarians the hesitation to report is simply because they do not know where to report, what to say, and how to document their observations. These concerns can best be addressed by being proactive. The veterinarian should become familiar with the local cruelty laws and should cultivate a relationship with a local law enforcement agent before there is a need to contact them with an actual report (see Handling Suspected Abuse Cases and Developing an SOP). It is a common misperception that an animal abuser will not seek veterinary care for the injured animal, so it is far better to be prepared in the event the situation arises.

Another common misconception is that the veterinarian must be positive that an animal has been the victim of cruelty before reporting it to the authorities. All that is generally legally necessary is for the veterinarian to have a reasonable or good faith belief. Additionally, many veterinarians mistakenly believe that the cruel or neglectful act or omission must be deliberate or intentional. Many cruelty statutes cover reckless and negligent conduct as well. It is ultimately up to the law enforcement authorities to determine whether there is a provable mental state—it is only necessary for the veterinarian to report the suspected acts or omissions resulting in cruelty.

Many veterinarians are uncomfortable accusing another individual of what amounts to criminal conduct. In certain situations, the suspected perpetrator may be an established client. The client often does not look like a criminal or act like a criminal. The veterinarian must recognize the fact that like all other crimes, the offender may be of any socioeconomic, racial, ethnic, age, gender, or other category.

In rural and smaller communities there is a fear of the loss of the relationship with the client, the client's family, and the client's friends. There is also a fear of an adverse effect on the veterinarian's reputation in the community.

In actuality, the reverse may well be true. Veterinarians who demonstrates a willingness to report animal cruelty may experience an increase in their client base because this is perceived by existing or potential clients as an attractive altruistic aspect of the practice.

In some situations the veterinarian fears being sued by the client. In most, if not all, of the states that mandate reporting, there is built-in immunity from civil and criminal liability. There are some states without mandatory reporting that specifically provide this immunity. Civil and criminal immunity means that if veterinarians report a case of cruelty in good faith they should not be able to be sued. Additionally, veterinarians should be protected from allegations that they violated confidentiality requirements. Whether or not the veterinarian can release patient records varies state by state and is usually found under the Veterinary Practice Act. In some states the veterinarian must turn over the entire record and in others they are prohibited from turning over the records without a court order.

In states that require reporting, veterinarians who fail to report when they should have may be legally accountable under the law and may face serious consequences. Additionally, there may be circumstances when a veterinarian fails to report cruelty and the conduct may be perceived as aiding and abetting the perpetrator. If this is the case, the veterinarian could face criminal charges for being a complicitor to animal cruelty.

If the abuse was particularly heinous or was committed in the context of family violence, there may be a concern for the safety of the veterinarian, the employees, and other clients and patients. There also may be a concern that the situation will escalate. Law enforcement officers are equipped to handle these types of concerns and are able to afford protection to the reporting veterinarian. This is another example of why it is important to cultivate a relationship with local law enforcement agents before the actual need arises. If the veterinarian is concerned about safety during the pendency of a case, he or she should ask the prosecutor to get a restraining order against the defendant and list the veterinarian as a protected person, including the veterinarian's home and clinic as restricted places.

There are a number of veterinarians who simply do not want to get involved or invest the time. This is typically based on the lack of awareness of the importance of reporting. Some have concerns that law enforcement agents or the prosecuting authority will not advise them about what to expect, protect them, or prepare them for court. Some simply have a generalized fear or distrust of police, lawyers, and the court system.

Factors that support reporting

There are several compelling reasons to report. It is encouraged by the professional associations and it improves the welfare of the abused or neglected animal. Intervention in a particular case may break the cycle of violence, therefore preventing additional harm to other animals and humans. The veterinarian may well be making the community safer. Most importantly, it is the right thing to do. In 2010, The American Veterinary Medical Association's Executive Board took a bold step when it amended the Veterinarian's Oath to include animal welfare. The oath reads as follows: "Being admitted to the profession of veterinary medicine, I solemnly swear to use my scientific knowledge and skills for the benefit of society through the protection of animal health and welfare, the prevention and relief of animal suffering, the conservation of animal resources, the promotion of public health, and the advancement of medical knowledge" (AVMA).

Following is the American Veterinary Medical Association (AVMA) position statement regarding animal abuse and animal neglect: "The AVMA recognizes that veterinarians may observe cases of animal abuse or neglect as defined by federal or state laws, or local ordinances. The AVMA considers it the responsibility of the veterinarian to report such cases to appropriate authorities, whether or not reporting is mandated by law. Prompt disclosure of abuse is necessary to protect the health and welfare of animals and people. Veterinarians should be aware that accurate, timely record keeping and documentation of these cases are essential. The AVMA considers it the responsibility of the veterinarian to educate clients regarding humane care and treatment of animals" (AVMA). Regarding animal fighting: "The AVMA condemns events involving animals in which injury or death is intended. The AVMA supports the enforcement of laws against the use and transport of animals and equipment for fighting ventures. Further, the AVMA recommends that animal fighting be considered a felony offense. The AVMA encourages veterinarians to collaborate with law enforcement with respect to recognition, enforcement, and education" (AVMA).

In addition to their position statement regarding abuse and neglect, the AVMA has set forth eight integrated principles for developing and evaluating animal welfare policies, resolutions, and actions. Two of these principles may assist the veterinarian in determining whether an animal has been abused or neglected. First, "animals must be provided water, food, proper handling, health care, and an environment appropriate to their care and use, with thoughtful consideration for their species-typical biology and behavior," and second, "animals should be cared for in ways that minimize fear, pain, stress, and suffering" (AVMA).

Following is the American Animal Hospital Association (AAHA) position statement regarding animal abuse reporting: "The American Animal Hospital Association supports reporting of suspicions of animal abuse to the appropriate authorities when education is inappropriate or has failed. The association also supports the adoption of laws requiring veterinary professionals to report suspicions of animal abuse, provided such laws include provisions for immunity from civil, criminal or professional liability when filing such reports in good faith. Veterinary professionals are likely to encounter many forms of animal abuse, ranging from minor neglect and animal hoarding to intentional and malicious harm. While some acts can be addressed through education, other forms of animal abuse can be related to other forms of violence. Studies have shown there is a link between animal abuse and other forms of violence, including child, spousal and elder abuse. In order to encourage veterinarians and practice team members to be responsible leaders in their communities and to assist in the detection and reporting of animal abuse, the profession should educate its members to recognize, document and report animal abuse, develop forensic models, promote legislation concerning reporting by veterinarians and collaborate with other animal and human welfare groups and professionals within communities to eliminate the incidence of animal abuse" (AAHA).

Veterinary records

It is essential to realize that everything a veterinarian does, writes, and says will be disclosed to the police, the prosecutor, the defense attorney, and even perhaps the perpetrator. All documentation needs to be objective, honest, and thorough and will serve as the basis for the veterinarian's courtroom testimony. A veterinarian must not use any terminology that may be perceived as unprofessional. Although it is not necessary, it may be beneficial to consult with another veterinarian (or other witness) who may document their independent observations and assessments which may support or contradict the original findings. Either way, this process can help reach a well-documented, objective conclusion.

Each jurisdiction has rules that govern discovery. Most states require that the prosecutor turn over every statement, report, and record of an expert. Compliance must be timely and continue throughout the pendency of the case. Failure to comply may result in sanctions that may severely affect the case. Of particular significance is any evidence that is favorable to the defense. Such evidence is characterized as exculpatory (tends to negate the guilt of the defendant) and is governed by the U.S. Supreme Court case *Brady vs. Maryland*, 373 U.S. 83 (1963). If, after producing a report, the expert changes his or her view on any material matter, this change must be communicated to all the parties as soon as possible. Veterinary records include but are not limited to: written records (electronic and handwritten), photographs, radiographs, imaging, laboratory tests (raw data and results), and medication information.

It is particularly important that the veterinarian document what the client says when explaining the animal's condition. The veterinarian or staff member should note the client's relationship to the patient such as owner, neighbor, pet-sitter, good Samaritan, animal control officer, etc. What the client says is often as important as what is observed. In some situations, the person's behavior may be a factor for the veterinarian to consider and document, such as the appearance of genuine concern or apathy. Remember, however, that people may not act or react in an expected manner in any given situation, particularly a stressful situation. It is also significant to ask where the incident happened because this can affect which law enforcement agency has jurisdiction.

The client in the office or suspect at the scene may admit incriminating conduct. It is essential to write down exactly what is said and by whom. The client's account may change as the conversation proceeds. There may be more than one person accompanying the animal and it will be important later for law enforcement to note if one individual's account is inconsistent with another's. It may be apparent to the veterinarian that one or more than one account is at odds with the medical findings. It is important to be aware that a client may be fearful of telling the truth—he or she may simply want to avoid accountability or may be the victim of violence at home. The client may give the veterinarian a truthful account, embellish what happened, fabricate a story, or any combination of the above. If the patient is an established patient there should be a treatment history that will assist the veterinarian with the ultimate findings.

It is not uncommon for the veterinarian to be confronted with an instance in which a very young child is responsible for the act or acts which resulted in the injury. If the circumstance allows, the veterinarian may attempt to communicate concerns to the child's parent or guardian. However, one should not presume that the parent or guardian will follow up with appropriate intervention. On the contrary, the parent or guardian often minimizes or denies the seriousness of this type of conduct. The act of animal cruelty by a child, regardless of age, may be an indicator of problems within the home. Even if the

perpetrator is younger than the statute allows for criminal charges, veterinarians must abide by the laws governing reporting in their jurisdiction. It should be noted that some jurisdictions have mandatory cross-reporting laws for animal cruelty and child abuse or family violence.

It is essential for the veterinarian to conduct a thorough examination of the animal and perform appropriate laboratory and diagnostic tests. These findings should be fully documented, and chain of custody protocols followed (see Chapter 3). Diagrams are available for most species and are invaluable when recording the location and nature of all injuries, current, recent and older. In animal hoarding, animal fighting, and puppy mill investigations there may be seizures of several animals that will need to be examined. It is critical to prepare and maintain a separate and distinct identifying photograph and medical record for each individual animal. Concern for expenses should not be a consideration. The veterinarian may find that the money spent on exams and tests may be priceless in the long run. In many jurisdictions, if the individual responsible for the abuse is convicted, it is likely that the prosecutor can ask the court to order reimbursement as part of any restitution order (see compensation section below). If the case is unusual or peculiar, such as some types of poisonings, additional research or consultation with a specialist may be necessary. This is also true when the veterinarian is evaluating an animal species that he or she does not treat on a regular basis.

In nearly every cruelty case it is important for the veterinarian to note whether the animal was in pain or was suffering (see Chapter 4). It should be noted if the delay of seeking veterinary care resulted in additional pain, suffering, or the inability to successfully treat the animal. Although an individual animal's response to pain varies with many factors (age, sex, health status, species, breed), what is important is whether the animal experienced pain. "Unless the contrary is established, investigators should consider that procedures that cause pain or distress in human beings may cause pain or distress in other animals" (USDHH).

Any evidence of prior trauma or injury should be noted. Most states have a rule of evidence [Federal Rule 404(b)] that allows evidence of other acts and transactions. Similar acts, for example, may be introduced to show motive, intent, and absence of mistake or accident. That is why it is so important to note any previous healed or healing injuries to the abused animal. It is also important to note whether there are or were other animals in the household or under the control of the same suspect that may have been abused.

If an animal is euthanized the veterinarian must note the reason for euthanasia (see Chapter 3). For cruelty investigations, some states have guidelines that allow a veterinarian to euthanize an abused animal without a court order if the animal is experiencing "extreme pain and suffering" or is "injured past recovery." Alternately, the lead investigator or prosecutor may grant permission. After euthanasia, the body should be properly handled, including storage, transported for necropsy if indicated (usually by animal services), and the chain of custody procedures followed (see Chapter 3).

Where to report

In an emergency, dial 911. As stated earlier, it is important for the veterinarian to be proactive and establish a relationship with law enforcement before they are needed. It is advisable for the veterinarian to establish a protocol for his or her clinic or hospital (see Handling Suspected Abuse Cases and Developing an SOP). All associates and employees must be trained to use the protocol. Essential phone numbers should be posted in a place where they are readily available to staff members. In Colorado, a magnet was distributed to veterinarians shortly after reporting became mandatory.

Depending on the jurisdiction, a veterinarian should be able to report suspected cruelty to one of the following agencies: police; sheriff; animal control; humane societies or rescue agencies (if they have authorized cruelty investigators); district, county, or city attorney; and in some states, the state veterinarian, Department of Agriculture, or Bureau of Animal Protection.

Handling suspected abuse cases and developing an SOP

Numerous situations qualify as animal cruelty and it is important that veterinarians have an understanding of their animal cruelty laws and veterinary practice acts so they can respond appropriately and assist the investigators and prosecutors in a potential case. Reporting suspected abuse does not mean the alleged perpetrator will be arrested; it means that an investigation will be initiated.

It is very difficult for veterinarians to realize and accept the fact that animals who are victims of abuse will be brought into their practice. The Munro and Thrusfield 2001 article demonstrates how common this actually is. The person who brings in the animal may or may not be aware that the animal has been abused. That person, or a child, may also be a victim of abuse in the home. Often, the person bringing in the animal has a close relationship with the abuser. It is very important for veterinarians to realize that their discussions with the client may elicit important information, including possible confessions. Regardless of

whether a client's statement about the cause of an injury to or death of a patient is truthful or not, the statement is beneficial for a thorough evaluation of the case and a detailed investigation into what occurred.

The study by Munro and Thrusfield reported that in several cases a family member was implicated by the client. In twenty-five of the cases the client admitted to committing the abuse. It is of particular interest that in five of the cases, the admission came after the veterinarian had merely discussed the possibility of abuse as the cause of the injuries. Another common scenario is hoarders who bring animals into the hospital (see Chapter 11). Some of the veterinarians surveyed during the study reported that they were less likely to report abuse if the owner showed contrition (Munro and Thrusfield 2001). Such a determination based on the owner's behavior does not fall within the veterinarian's purview. It is important for veterinarians to understand that their duty is to report so that an investigation can be conducted.

It is important to have a standard operating procedure (SOP) for a veterinary hospital to handle and report suspected abuse cases. After mandatory reporting laws were enacted in Colorado, the Colorado Veterinary Medical Association in collaboration with the Denver District Attorney's Office, the Colorado Association of Certified Veterinary Technicians, and the Animal Assistance Foundation developed a guide for veterinarians to use in suspected cruelty case (see Appendix 1). Depending on the jurisdiction and the type of crime, the location of the crime, or the species involved, there may be one or more agencies responsible for investigating animal cruelty cases. The agencies may include, but are not limited to, law enforcement, animal services, and agents with the department of agriculture. The prosecutor responsible for animal cruelty cases should also be identified, which may vary depending on the level of crime. All staff should be trained on the SOP, the animal cruelty laws, and the veterinary practice act affecting the reporting of suspected abuse. Some areas have mandatory reporting requirements, liability protection, and/or clear rules for record confidentiality. These should be part of the staff training and SOP.

The SOP should include several key components:

- Agency(s) and individual(s) responsible for abuse investigations
- Contact information including after hours and emergencies
- Chain of command within the hospital, clinic, or shelter for authorization and approval to report suspected abuse
- Protocol for handling and treatment of the living or deceased animal after a report has been filed, including but not limited to documentation, chain of custody,

photographs, and records. Additionally, the investigating officer and prosecutor should provide input on legal protocol for retention and protection of the animal and for protection of the veterinary staff

• Protocol and secure area to maintain other evidence collected from the animal

The key is to establish a relationship early with the investigating agency/officers and the prosecutors. They should be invited to the hospital to provide training for the staff on the law, liability, reporting, and response.

SEARCH AND SEIZURE

The United States Constitution set forth guidance regarding search and seizure. The Fourth Amendment states that individuals have the right to be free from unreasonable searches and seizures. It further states that any search warrant must be based on probable cause. The warrant must be accompanied by a sworn affidavit setting forth the details about the place being searched and the items being searched for. An evaluation of whether or not a search or seizure is reasonable turns on whether or not the individual had an "expectation of privacy." This is most often claimed when the person's residence or place of business is the place to be searched. Only a law enforcement agent may apply for and execute a search warrant.

Under some narrowly defined circumstances no warrant is necessary. For example, if a person consents to a search of their premises no warrant is needed. Consent must be made freely and voluntarily. Another exception is "exigent circumstances." If there is an articulable emergency and an immediate need to seize property then the authorities do not need to get a warrant. However, care should be taken in cases involving numerous animals to only remove animals in dire need of immediate veterinary care. Other animals at that scene may be seized later pursuant to a search warrant. It is important for law enforcement authorities to secure the premises pending the issue of a search warrant to ensure that no evidence is lost or removed.

Often law enforcement authorities will rely on a veterinarian to articulate why an animal or animals should be seized. The veterinarian's statement and opinion become part of the affidavit supporting the search warrant. It is important for the veterinarians to be clear and accurate in their assessment of the circumstances. It is also necessary for the veterinarian, together with law enforcement authorities, to know the elements of the crime for which the animal evidence is being sought.

In animal cruelty cases, especially large scale seizures, it is essential to describe the property to be searched. It is important to include all aspects of the relevant property and include, for example: outbuildings, automobiles, curtilage, gardens, and fields. In some jurisdictions it may be important in cases involving animals that are likely to be pregnant to include unborn animals as part of the warrant. In cases involving animal fighting, puppy mills, or hoarding, a search warrant should also include searching for clandestine graves or other areas where deceased animals may be found.

HANDLING THE MEDIA IN ANIMAL CRUELTY CASES

Cruelty cases, especially violent or large scale cases, generate a tremendous amount of media attention. Once a case is reported and a criminal investigation has begun, it is important to resist the temptation to grant an interview with media representatives or to allow media personnel access to the crime scene or to the animals. It is advisable to have a media spokesperson that is trained to handle these matters. There will be ongoing pressure from the media for updates. The veterinary personnel should defer to law enforcement authorities to make any public statements or release any photographic or video footage. If law enforcement allows or directs the veterinarian to make a public statement, he or she should remain professional and objective. There should be clarification before the interview what prior media statements have been made or released by authorities and what can and cannot be discussed with the media. There should also be awareness that if the scene is outdoors the media may be videotaping the scene and activity via hand-held cameras or by helicopter with long-range lens and audio capabilities. There should be a presumption that everything that is said and done may be monitored by uninvited third parties, including by cell phone cameras, audio, or video recording. Everything that is done and said can and may be used in court. After a case is reported the best practice is for the veterinarian to refer all media inquiries to the law enforcement agency or prosecuting authority. Pre-trial publicity can have an impact on the successful prosecution of a case and can affect the jury selection process. Once a case is filed there are strict ethical rules that govern what a prosecutor or law enforcement agent can release to the media.

CONFIDENTIALITY

Regardless of whether the veterinarian is working for the prosecution or the defense, it is important to be aware of the confidential nature of the relationship. The veterinarian's photographs, videos, and records belong to the agency that brought them into the case. Only specifically assigned personnel may collect evidence or take still or video photo-graphs at the scene or of the animals. The use of private cameras (including cell phones) must be strictly prohibited. In addition, personnel associated with the case may not tweet, text, post, or in any other manner share information gained, and this includes family members and friends. Caution should be taken to communicate only with author-ized personnel. A careless mistake could result in sanctions against the veterinarian or against the inviting agency.

FILING CRIMINAL CHARGES AND HEARINGS

The filing of criminal charges is a decision made by law enforcement officers (including animal control officers) and prosecutors. The basic standard for arrest and for the filing of criminal charges is probable cause, which means that it is more probable than not that a crime was committed and it is more probable than not that the authorities have arrested the person or persons responsible.

After criminal charges are filed, there are often court hearings that take place in advance of the trial. A veterinarian may have to testify during a financial bonding or cost of care hearing, which is critical in a large scale case. During this type of hearing the veterinarian may be asked to state why it was necessary to remove the animals(s). He or she may also be asked to testify regarding how much money the defendant should have to pay for the cost of care of the animal(s) while the case is pending. It is helpful to use a case status form to keep a record of the legal proceedings including but not limited to: the names and contact information for the parties (including the attorneys); the assigned courtroom and judge; the dates of any depositions, hearings, or trials; and the ultimate outcome (see Appendix 2).

The defendant may also request a hearing for the court to order the prosecution to allow an independent examination of any seized animals or other evidence. If the defense requests an independent evaluation it should be allowed if at all possible with any necessary safeguards put in place. For example, the prosecutor may ask to be present or have another veterinarian present. As a safety measure, the defendant should not be allowed to be present during any independent evaluation of the animal. Depending on the exact nature of the request, a veterinarian may be needed to advise the court as to whether or not the requested testing could jeopardize the animal's health or if there is an inherent danger to the animal that overrides any possible benefit.

It should be noted that in cases in which animal abuse is associated with family violence, a growing number of jurisdictions now include animals in protective orders or restraining orders. In some states, the imposition of a protective order protecting a human victim is discretionary, and in other states it is mandatory. These types of orders are used in virtually all pending family violence and other victim-based cases. They are court-issued orders designed to protect victims from their alleged abusers while awaiting trial or other disposition of the case. The individual against whom the order is entered is commonly ordered to have no contact directly or indirectly with the victim. The intent is to protect victims from further injury or intimidation.

In many states animals are now recognized as protected property in a restraining order. These orders can exist in civil and divorce proceedings in addition to criminal proceedings. Veterinarians may be called upon as expert witnesses in various types of hearings. The addition of a no-contact-with-animals clause is a substantial step toward protection of animal victims in family violence cases. Several jurisdictions issue animal protective orders even when family violence is absent, thereby recognizing animal cruelty as an autonomous and serious crime. On occasion the testimony of a veterinarian may be key in seeking a court order to protect an animal.

Expert qualifications

If criminal charges are filed, it is likely that the veterinarian will be endorsed as an expert witness. All experts should prepare a curriculum vitae (C.V.), keep it current, and furnish a copy to the prosecutor. It does not have to be lengthy or detailed. It should contain information about the expert's educational background including but not limited to date and location of undergraduate degree, veterinary degree, licensure, any specialized degrees, or board certification; experience in the field and any special expertise; employment (present and past); any publications; and whether or not he or she has testified before as an expert witness.

Rules of evidence and laws regarding expert witnesses

The basic standards regarding the admissibility of expert testimony are as follows:

1. Is the testimony reliable?
2. Is the expert qualified?
3. Is the testimony relevant?

The Federal Rules of Evidence contain the general guidelines for expert testimony, which are followed by most courts in the United States.

Rule 702 states: "If scientific, technical, or other special-ized knowledge will assist the trier of fact to understand the evidence or to determine a fact in issue, a witness qualified as an expert by knowledge, skill, experience, training, or education may testify thereto in the form of an opinion or otherwise."

Rule 703 states: "The facts or data in the particular case upon which an expert bases an opinion or inference may be those perceived by or made known to the expert at or before the hearing. If of a type reasonably relied upon by experts in the particular field in forming opinions or inferences upon the subject, the facts or data need not be admissible in evidence in order for the opinion or inference to be admitted. Facts or data that are otherwise inadmissible shall not be disclosed to the jury by the proponent of the opinion or inference unless the court determines that their probative value in assisting the jury to evaluate the expert's opinion substantially outweighs their prejudicial effect."

Rule 704 states: "Testimony in the form of an opinion or inference otherwise admissible is not objectionable because it embraces an ultimate issue to be decided by the trier of fact."

Courts subject veterinarians to the same scrutiny as all other expert witnesses when deciding whether to allow their testimony. The United States Supreme Court and the Court of Appeals of the District of Columbia created formulas for measuring the admissibility of expert testimony in two significant cases: *Daubert v. Merrell Dow Pharmaceuticals, Inc.*, 509 U.S. 579 (1993) and *United States v. Frye*, 293 F. 1013 (D.C. Cir 1923). Because the standards in each case differ, most states either follow *Daubert* or *Frye* or portions of both in their determination of expertise. Following is a brief summary of each case.

Courts using *Daubert* hold that general acceptance of the underlying principle of the scientific evidence is not required. Instead, they consider:

1. Whether the theory or technique can be and has been tested
2. Whether the theory or technique has been subjected to peer review and publication
3. The known or potential rate of error
4. The existence and maintenance of standards controlling its operation
5. The degree to which the theory or technique has been generally accepted by the relevant scientific community

Courts using *Frye* require general acceptance of the principle underlying the scientific evidence for it to be admissible, stating: "Just when a scientific principle or discovery crosses the line between the experimental and demonstrable stages is difficult to define. Somewhere in this grey zone the evidential force of the principle must be recognized, and while courts will go a long way in admitting expert testimony deduced from a well-recognized scientific principle or discovery, the thing from which the deduction is made must be sufficiently established to have gained general acceptance in the particular field in which it belongs. Scientific publications, judicial precedent, practical applications, or testimony from scientists as the beliefs of their fellow scientists are suggested methods to prove this acceptance."

Types of experts

Fact witness

The veterinarian is a fact witness if she has personal, direct, first-hand knowledge of either the incident or the involved individuals. This knowledge is based on what she saw, touched, heard, smelled, read, felt, or did.

Opinion expert

All licensed veterinarians should be able to be qualified to testify as an expert based on their specialized training and experience. Following are the common areas of veterinary expert witness testimony: determining the cause of death; sequence of injuries and timing of premortem or postmortem wounds; distinguishing between death and injury resulting from human vs. non-human causes (for example predation) or intentional vs. accidental injury; identifying evidence that may link the injuries to a particular suspect or particular weapon; commenting on reasonably prudent actions that could have been taken to prevent disease, injury, or death; offering opinions regarding the speed of unconsciousness and/or death, including the degree of pain and suffering; and commenting on reports provided by other veterinarians or investigators.

Consulting expert

The veterinarian may also be a consulting expert. A consulting expert may also be a fact witness if he is able to make direct observations of the evidence, including the animal. The consultant may or may not testify in a case and may or may not be made known to the opposition. He has specialized knowledge, training, and experience that assists in analyzing and evaluating the evidence in a given case. Several types of situations give rise to this need. For example, a consultant may be contacted in a criminal case in which the animal was not evaluated or treated by a veterinarian, and in some instances where the animal itself was not or is not available for examination. In some cruelty cases the animal may have been cremated, may have been disposed of by one of the parties, or may have run away. The consultant's expertise is also valuable in complex veterinary medical cases or those involving exotic or rare species. Some cases require expertise in unique animal features, complex diseases of an animal, or cases that involve unusual issues related to the cause and manner of injury or death.

In some instances an attorney or law enforcement agent may seek an analysis of the records and findings of a veterinarian who has been hired by the opposition. It is critical for the consulting expert to be provided with every document and report attributable to the other veterinarian as well as relevant information, evidence, and photographs related to the case. The consulting veterinarian must have context to accurately evaluate the case.

The consulting expert may be asked to prepare a report regarding his or her analysis. As a result, the expert may be endorsed as an expert witness in the case. In a criminal case, if the expert (retained by the prosecution) reaches an opinion that the suspect was not involved, or that no crime was committed or that the suspect should otherwise be exonerated, then the prosecuting authority is under an affirmative obligation to disclose the information to the defendant or his or her defense attorney.

A consulting veterinarian also may be used in a different manner. An attorney may ask the veterinarian to attend a portion of a court proceeding to observe an expert testifying for the opposition. This type of consultant should also be familiar with the facts of the case and with any expert opinions that are already a part of the case file. In this scenario, the consultant is called upon to assist the attorney in the preparation of the cross-examination of the expert they are observing. On occasion these consultants may be asked to testify in rebuttal. In other words, they may be called to rebut what the observed expert said on the witness stand. This procedure is permitted under Rule 703 of the Federal Rules of Evidence which states that the expert may base his or her opinion or inference upon facts or data made known to the expert during a court hearing.

Social media

In the present electronic age all witnesses must be aware that the parties and lawyers in a pending case will do an Internet search about them, including their practice, clinic, or hospital. Like all expert witnesses, veterinarians need to be very careful about what they post on Facebook, MySpace, Twitter, or any other social media sites. Whatever is posted may be used against them when they testify. No one should have a false sense of security merely because they must "friend" someone before that person gains access to their information. Additionally, anything that is put on a C.V. will be investigated.

In addition to social media sites, veterinarians should be aware that attorneys have resources readily accessible that contain information about expert witnesses. Transcript banks contain prior testimony and prior depositions. If a veterinarian has testified on a previous occasion on a topic relevant to the current case, the opposing side will likely have a copy of the veterinarian's earlier testimony. Any conflicts may be used to impeach the veterinarian during the current case proceedings.

Credibility

The actual jurors who are sworn in to hear a case are the jurors who remain after both the prosecution and defense have excused the jurors that they believe cannot be fair and impartial to one or both sides. During the jury selection process (known as "*voir dire*") jurors may indicate that they simply are not able to sit on a case involving animal cruelty. The jury pool may also include some individuals who have never owned pets, do not like animals, and/or do not believe that animal cruelty should be treated the same as other types of crimes. During the jury selection process the prosecution and the defense will seek to elicit responses from the potential jurors that will assist the attorneys in determining who to excuse. Each side has a limited number of jurors that they can release from the case.

Prior to deliberating, the court will give the jury guidelines regarding the credibility of witnesses. The credibility of an expert is just like that of any other witness. The jury is told that they should carefully consider all of the testimony including each witness' knowledge, motive, state of mind, demeanor, and manner while on the stand. They are also instructed to take into account the witness' means of knowledge, ability to observe, and strength of memory. They are to reflect on any relationship each witness may have to either side of the case, the manner in which each witness might be affected by the verdict, and the extent to which, if at all, each witness is either supported or contradicted by other evidence in the case. They may believe all of the testimony of a witness, or part of it, or none of it.

NON-CRIMINAL CASES

There are several types of cases in which the veterinarian may be called upon as an expert. In some of these cases the veterinarian may have to testify in court proceedings.

- Animals in restraining orders
- Fatal dog attacks
- Accepted animal husbandry practices
- Animal custody disputes in divorce proceedings
- Disciplinary hearings against a veterinarian

- Administrative hearings regarding kennels and shelters
- Zoonotic diseases and other public health issues

TRIAL

When the case proceeds to trial, the jury is reminded that the defendant is presumed innocent and that the burden of proof is upon the prosecution to prove the case beyond a reasonable doubt. The jury is instructed that a reasonable doubt means a doubt based upon reason and common sense which arises from a fair and rational consideration of all of the evidence, or the lack of evidence, in the case. It is a doubt which is not a vague, speculative, or imaginary doubt, but such a doubt as would cause reasonable people to hesitate to act in matters of importance to themselves.

Subpoenas

A subpoena is a court order directing the witness to appear in a particular courtroom on a specific date at a specific time. There are two types of subpoenas: one is a subpoena to testify, and the other is a subpoena *duces tecum*, otherwise known as a subpoena to produce evidence and to testify. Both are official court orders and require compliance. The prosecution has the obligation to arrange for every one of their witnesses to testify in person during a trial. A trial is scheduled to begin on a certain date and may last from several hours to several weeks. Subpoenas are issued for a start date and starting time. Many if not most of the witnesses will be called to testify later that day or on a subsequent day. Testimony does not begin until the jury selection process has been completed. In complex cases, jury selection may take several hours or even days.

Often the prosecutor and the defense attorney subpoena every veterinarian to testify even if only one is necessary to prove their theory. This is a common practice and is designed to allow the attorneys some flexibility as the court date approaches. The attorney that subpoenas a witness should call that witness and let him or her know, in advance, if he or she will be called to testify. If the attorney does not initiate a call, the veterinarian should call the attorney and arrange a meeting in advance to go over any expected testimony and anticipated cross-examination.

Most witnesses are subpoenaed by mail. If the prosecution is dealing with a "hostile" witness or a witness that they fear will not show up in court, then that witness will be personally served with a subpoena. Remember that a subpoena is a lawful court order and the veterinarian must appear in court at the time and place on the subpoena. Often cases do not proceed as originally scheduled. The case may be postponed or may be continued by the defense, the pros-

ecution, or the judge. Additionally, it is not uncommon for more than one case to be set on the same date in the same courtroom and only one can proceed to hearing, resulting in delays for the other cases. Most prosecutors have victim/witness coordinators to advise the witnesses of any scheduling changes. The attorneys should try to accommodate the veterinarian and consider the witness' schedule and commitments. The lawyers are routinely able to place the witness "on call" and give him or her enough notice to travel to the courthouse, find a place to park, and get to the courtroom.

If a veterinarian is subpoenaed by the defense, he or she must comply with the subpoena and understand that the prosecutor has no authority to release him or her from that subpoena or place him or her on call for that subpoena. The veterinarian should let the prosecutor know that the defense has subpoenaed him or her so that perhaps the lawyers can work on scheduling the testimony to be most convenient for the witness.

If a veterinarian receives a subpoena and realizes that he or she will not be able to appear on the date set in the subpoena, the veterinarian must let the attorney know as soon as possible. The attorney may be able to rearrange witnesses to allow for some flexibility and, if it is essential, the attorney may be able to ask for a postponement or to reschedule the case. If it is not possible to reschedule the case, the expert may have to work with the lawyers to facilitate his appearance in court during the time required.

When the witness arrives at the courthouse it is important to be aware that there will be numerous individuals in the building that are or may be involved with the case. There will be other witnesses (including other experts), possible co-workers of the witness, law enforcement, attorneys, friends and relatives of the parties, courtroom observers, media, and jurors. It is critical to be professional, respectful, and courteous at all times. It is advisable to turn off cell phones.

In most court hearings and trials, the judge will impose a sequestration order. That means that there can be no conversations about the case with other witnesses who are waiting to testify or with witnesses who have already testified. If a sequestration order has been entered, witnesses may not watch the proceedings before they testify and most likely after they testify. The exception to the sequestration order is that the witness may talk to the lawyers or the lawyers' advisory witness. An advisory witness is a witness that assists the prosecution or the defense during the trial. He or she usually sits at the attorney's table throughout the trial. In most cases the assigned investigating detective is the advisory witness.

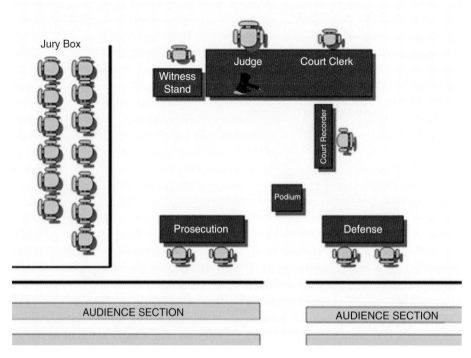

Figure 1.1 Courtroom diagram. (Photo courtesy of Diane Balkin.)

If the veterinarian is unfamiliar with the courthouse it is advisable to arrive early to survey the landscape and the parties (Figure 1.1). It is advisable to use the restroom prior to testifying. It is best to use a restroom on a floor other than the floor with the courtroom in order to avoid any interaction with potential jurors or other witnesses. It is important for the witness to follow courtroom decorum and avoid behavior that can be distracting or perceived as unprofessional including chewing gum, overtly sighing, or making facial expressions such as rolling one's eyes.

If a veterinarian receives a subpoena to produce, it also must be honored. On occasion an attorney may already have the basic information relevant to a case but may choose to serve a subpoena to seek additional information that may or may not be relevant. The veterinarian should contact the party who sent the subpoena to clarify the matter if there is any confusion. Be aware that these subpoenas are a court order directing the witness to appear in court with the requested documents. The witness should take care not to simply turn over the requested documents to the party who has subpoenaed them. Also, if the subpoena directs the veterinarian to produce items over which he or she has

no custody or control the veterinarian needs to so advise the attorneys.

Preparing for court

A veterinarian who is expected to testify should be contacted by the prosecutor prior to testifying. Additionally, the veterinarian may be contacted by opposing counsel. All witnesses have the right to speak to or to refuse to speak to either or both. Prior to any pretrial or pre-deposition interviews the veterinarian should review all of the information he or she has about the case to refresh his or her recollection. The veterinarian should be aware of exactly who he or she is talking to and which side they represent. It is perfectly proper to ask for photo identification. It is also important to ask whether or not the interview is going to be recorded. The witness may also request that a representative from the prosecutor's office attend the interview. A deposition is recorded and typically attorneys from both sides are present. If an interview or a deposition is recorded, it is important for the witness to demand to be provided with an unredacted copy of the recording immediately after the interview or deposition has concluded. This request should be reflected on the recording itself. All interviews and depositions should be reviewed prior to testifying at any court proceeding.

Testifying

First and foremost it is imperative for any witness to tell the truth. Veterinarians as a profession are respected, liked, and trusted. It is important for the veterinarian to listen closely to the questions and answer only what is asked. The jurors are not scientists so the expert must explain his or her observations and opinions in a manner that is easily understood and that relates to the elements of the charge. The veterinarian should be respectful to all parties and should not argue and should not interrupt. He or she should avoid saying "I believe" or "I think" or "I imagine" or "I guess." And if the veterinarian does not know an answer he or she should say they do not know.

The veterinarian should bring all notes, medical documents, and C.V. to any pretrial meetings to make sure that the attorney has everything. He or she may bring these notes and documents to court but it is not necessary to do so if the attorney has a copy readily available. It is important to be aware that anything that is used by the veterinarian to prepare for trial is discoverable.

During the testimony phase it is critical to listen closely to the question and to have it rephrased if the veterinarian is unable to answer it as it was stated. If an attorney raises an objection after a question is asked, the veterinarian should wait for the judge to rule on the objection before answering. If the objection is sustained the question may not be answered. If it is overruled it must be answered.

It is not necessary for the veterinarian to memorize all of the records ahead of time. He or she may refer to such documents in court to refresh recollection so long as the documents have been provided to opposing counsel. In cases involving several animals it is not unusual for the veterinarian to refresh his or her memory by looking at the records of a particular animal. This is a perfectly proper and understandable procedure.

Be aware that if the prosecutor writes some or all of his or her expected questions for the veterinarian during pre-trial preparation, and if the veterinarian responds to the prosecutor with written responses, then the document is considered discoverable and must be provided to the defense attorney. In some jurisdictions all communications authored by an expert, including e-mails, must also be turned over during the discovery process.

Qualifying the expert witness

Before the expert is allowed to give an opinion, he or she must first be accepted by the court as an expert. The parties may stipulate that a given witness is qualified as an expert. If there is no agreement then the party offering the expert must lay a foundation for the judge. The opposing party may *voir dire* (or question) the witness's qualifications during this phase of the proceeding.

What sets one veterinarian expert witness apart from another can be a combination of factors including experience, training, specialty areas, and academic achievement. Aside from providing the prosecutor their C.V. as part of case preparation, veterinarians should explain their credentials in terms of the minimum requirements it takes to be a licensed veterinarian and what features they possess that are above and beyond minimum standards. The veterinarian should also point out any specialized training and experience. The expert's qualifications should be discussed with the prosecutor before testifying.

When the expert veterinarian finally takes the witness stand and is sworn in, the first order of business is to qualify him or her as an expert. Prosecutors lay the foundation by having the veterinarian describe his or her background including training and experience. Veterinarians typically have expertise in several aspects of medicine, including but not limited to anatomy, surgery, radiology, infectious diseases, and emergency medicine. This is not often the case for their human medical counterparts, who have subspecialties of expertise (board certification). The prosecutor should go through all the areas of the veterinarian's expertise that are relevant to the trial or hearing.

The following is a typical line of questions asked of the expert:

- Please state your name.
- What is your current occupation and where are you currently employed?
- Are you licensed to practice veterinary medicine? In what state(s)? For how long? What were the licensure requirements?
- Do you have any special certifications?
- What is your title and what are your responsibilities in general and specifically related to the field of _____?
- Briefly describe your educational background.
- Briefly describe any special training and continuing education you have received related to the field of _____.
- Describe any previous employment and experience you have had in the field of _____.
- Can you estimate how many cases you have handled involving _____?

- During your training and while on the job has your testing and findings been subject to administrative review? What's the purpose for this type of review?
- Do you belong to any professional organizations?
- Have you written any articles on topics related to _____ ?
- Have you delivered any presentations on the topic of _____ at professional meetings?
- Have you ever been qualified as an expert witness before? How many times and in what courts?
- Offer Dr. _____ as an expert in (veterinary medicine, veterinary forensics, veterinary radiology, etc.)

Depending on the field of expertise and the nature of the case, the prosecutor may ask that the witness be qualified as an expert in the general area of veterinary medicine or a specific area or areas such as veterinary forensic medicine, animal fighting, animal cruelty, or possibly a subspecialty such as radiology.

As soon as the witness is offered as an expert the judge will ask the defense attorney if they object. If they state that they have no objection, the witness will be accepted as an expert. If they object then they can simply object or they can *voir dire* the witness.

At this stage of the proceeding the *voir dire* is limited to the veterinarian's qualifications—it has nothing to do with the actual facts of the case. *Voir dire* may include but is not limited to questions about how long the witness has been licensed, whether or not he or she is board certified, if the witness has ever testified as an expert on any previous occasion, how many necropsies he or she has performed, or whether or not he or she actually has examined or treated a certain species.

At the conclusion of the attorney's *voir dire* the judge will decide whether or not the witness has been qualified as an expert and if so, in what area(s).

Demonstrative evidence

Most jurors and judges are visual learners. It is always advisable to use demonstrative evidence to assist them. Demonstrative evidence can be used in any type of a court proceeding. It includes actual evidence, such as a chain, knife, or bottle of poison as well as illustrative evidence such as photographs, charts, or diagrams. A courtroom is like a classroom and demonstrative evidence is a tool that can help educate the jurors and judge. The veterinarian may assist the prosecutor in selecting photographs that are most demonstrative and appropriate to illustrate relevant evidence (Chapter 3). In a case of self defense, it may be relevant that the animal was shot while retreating rather than advancing. Demonstrative evidence in the form of a diagram showing the wound path can assist the jury in evaluating the case. In a case in which canine DNA is a critical piece of evidence, a chart showing the unknown canine DNA profile side by side with a known canine DNA profile that matches is a common type of demonstrative evidence.

Crime shows such as "C.S.I." have had an incredible impact on jurors. They expect forensic, state-of-the-art evidence and expert crime scene technicians in every case. Prosecutors typically discuss this during the jury selection process. Veterinarians should be aware that jurors may have these unrealistic expectations of them as well.

If the animal was cremated, or was never found, a photograph of the animal can be introduced. If the weapon is missing, a weapon similar to the weapon or a photograph of the weapon that was used may be introduced. Body condition charts are valuable tools for both the clinic and the courtroom and are objective standards that the judge and jury can appreciate and accept. Sometimes the prosecutors need to be educated by veterinarians about the educational tools available for the courtroom. Admissibility, resources, and use in the courtroom may vary greatly among prosecutors and jurisdictions.

It is common for photographs depicting deceased or mutilated animals to draw vigorous objections from the defense. Defense attorneys argue that these images are more prejudicial than probative and will likely inflame the jury. Prosecutors should anticipate such objections during trial preparation. The key to overcoming these objections is to honestly ask the veterinarian whether or not he or she needs the exhibit to assist him or her in explaining what happened to the animal or to explain the basis of his or her expert opinion. The prosecutor should argue that there is a legitimate purpose for showing the photograph because it will assist the expert in explaining a certain theory or finding to the jury.

Cross-examination and attacking the expert

Before testifying, the veterinarian should prepare for cross-examination. One of the most common attacks on the expert is that he or she is biased and that he or she always testifies for one side rather than the other. The opposition may also try to expose the expert's bias based on the fact that he or she received some type of compensation for his or her opinion. There may be cross-examination regarding postings on the expert's social media sites or questions about memberships in groups and organizations.

They may attack the veterinarian regarding the basis of his or her opinion. For example, they will try to suggest that critical facts exist that the veterinarian failed to consider or that the veterinarian assumed the truth of facts that were not verified. Additionally, they may argue that the veterinarian's examination was incomplete, substandard, or defies common sense. Another common technique is to make the veterinarian agree that there is room for varying opinions.

Anticipating the defense

There is accuracy to the statement that "a chain is only as strong as the weakest link." The same is true with any criminal case. If the veterinarian is a witness for the prosecution, the best way to face this issue is to anticipate any potential defenses. Although this is the prosecutor's job it is prudent for the veterinarian to also be prepared.

Assuming identification of the perpetrator is not an issue, perhaps the most common defense in a cruelty or neglect case is that it was an accident and the defendant had nothing to do with the resulting injury. In some cases it may be difficult to definitively state one way or the other but the veterinarian must remain objective and unbiased. In many jurisdictions it is a recognized defense to animal cruelty that the acts or omissions were part of accepted animal husbandry which means practices generally recognized as appropriate in the care of animals consistent with the species breed and type of animal. The veterinarian needs to be aware of the accepted standards in the community if this defense is raised.

There is another group of defenses that are called confession and avoidance, meaning the defendant admits the act but tries to avoid accountability due to some type of recognized legal excuse. What they are saying is "I did it, but I was justified or I am legally entitled to be excused." Among these defenses are self-defense, defense of others, defense of property, and training or discipline. Also included in this group are the mental defenses, for example, intoxication, insanity, and impaired mental condition.

Prosecutors must also be aware that the defense may simply argue that an element or significant aspect of the case has not been proven beyond a reasonable doubt. This includes failing to prove the defendant's mental state; failing to rule out natural causes, predation, or accident; and failing to disprove a recognized defense. Another tactic that may be used by the defense is to hire an expert whose opinion is at odds with the prosecution expert's opinion. In this way the defense may argue that the jury simply cannot decide who to believe, thus establishing a reasonable doubt.

The veterinarian's opinion should not be affected whatsoever by who hires him or her or who subpoenas them to testify. A veterinarian's report and subsequent testimony should be based on facts and accepted scientific principles.

The simple fact is that all the expert needs to remember to do on the witness stand is tell the truth.

Sentencing recommendations

After a defendant is convicted by a jury or pleads guilty or pleads no contest, he or she will be sentenced. Often there is a stipulated sentence that is agreed upon with the prosecution as part of a negotiated disposition. Sentencing for a crime against an animal can range from probation to incarceration. The crime may be a municipal code violation, a misdemeanor, a felony, or a federal offense. If sentenced to probation, many states require a mental health evaluation and treatment. Depending on the facts of the case, family violence counseling or sex offender counseling may be required. Some courts impose a fine or some type of community or public service. In some cases when probation is ordered, the prosecutor should ask that the judge enter an order banning the defendant from any animal ownership and ordering that the defendant have no contact with animals. On occasion a veterinarian may be called upon to testify during the sentencing phase to assist the judge in understanding the dangerousness of allowing a particular defendant to own or be in contact with an animal.

COMPENSATION FOR THE VETERINARIAN

In many jurisdictions, if the individual responsible for the abuse is convicted, it is likely that the prosecutor can ask the court to order reimbursement to the veterinary hospital, clinic, or shelter as part of any restitution order. There is variation regarding whether or not and how much a veterinarian may charge as a fee for his or her services. Working with cruelty cases can be labor intensive and may include having to review voluminous records and then generate a report. Some cases require depositions, courtroom testimony, or out-of-state travel. Veterinarians should keep a record of time spent on a case and any attendant expenses. They can charge by the hour, half day, or full day for their time and may consider a minimum charge. Charging for their time may include travel time, casework (crime scene and/or examination time), report writing, depositions, interview, phone consults, courtroom preparation, and actual testimony. They can also charge by the case or procedure. In cases where the animal-investigating agency has a laboratory account for submission of diagnostic testing, the veterinarian may charge for his or her time for reviewing the test results. Consideration should be made for any out-of-pocket expenses such as supplies, diagnostics, etc. If there is a test or procedure that should be conducted for the veterinarian to better evaluate the case, and if circumstances permit, the test or procedure should be conducted without regard to cost. The investigating and/or prosecuting agency that requested the veterinarian's assistance should be responsible for payment to the veterinarian. Ideally a fee structure and payment agreement should be established at the beginning with the responsible party. There may be situations where the veterinarian incurred expenses for the animal prior to the investigation which may be recovered from the defendant after conviction in the form of restitution. Some veterinarians do not charge for their time or services rendered. Others may have received public or private donations to offset the cost of care for the animal.

Veterinarians should be aware that if they are paid for their services this must be disclosed by the prosecution in a criminal case. This fact may be used in cross-examination of the veterinarian and the defense may argue that the veterinarian was paid for their testimony. The defense does not have to disclose this fact to the prosecution; however, most prosecutors will simply ask the expert in advance of their testifying.

CONCLUSION

The veterinarian's role is essential in the investigation, evaluation, and prosecution of suspected crimes against animals. His or her expertise is also invaluable to exonerate those individuals who should not be prosecuted. The forensic veterinarian needs to be part of a collaborative effort to reach a fair and just resolution to a case of animal cruelty.

REFERENCES

American Animal Hospital Association (AAHA). www.aahanet.org. Positions and Endorsements.

Arkow, P. The Veterinarian's Role in Preventing Family Violence: The Experience of the Human Medical Profession. http://www.animaltherapy.net/Vets-abuse.html.

American Veterinary Medical Association (AVMA). www.avma.org. AVMA Policy.

Munro, H.M.C. and M.V. Thrusfield. 2001. Battered Pets: Non-Accidental Physical Injuries Found in Dogs and Cats. *Journal of Small Animal Practice.* 42:279–290.

Neumann, S. 2005. Animal Welfare—the Need for a United Veterinary Voice. *Canadian Veterinary Journal.* 46(9): 834–836.

U.S. Department of Health and Human Services (USDHHS). U.S. Government Principles for the Utilization and Care of Vertebrate Animals Used in Testing, Research, and Training. In: *Public Health Service Policy on Humane Care and Use of Laboratory Animals.* http://grants.nih.gov/grants/olaw/references/phspol.htm#principle.

2
Crime Scene Investigation

Melinda D. Merck

Actions taken at the outset of an investigation at a crime scene can play a pivotal role in the resolution of a case. Careful, thorough investigation is key to ensure that potential physical evidence is not tainted or destroyed or potential witnesses overlooked.

Janet Reno

INTRODUCTION

Crime scene investigation is the first and most critical step in any investigation. The three most important actions at a crime scene are recognition, proper collection, and preservation of evidence. Due to the unique aspects of animals, important evidence may be overlooked or the value misinterpreted or underestimated. Involving the veterinarian at the very beginning of the investigation helps ensure that all the evidence is recognized and analyzed. Similar to medicolegal death investigators for human cases, it is important for animal case investigators to gather all information needed for the veterinarian to examine any live or deceased animal. Having a veterinarian at the scene, functioning similar to a medical examiner or coroner, helps ensure that all necessary information and documentation is completed. The veterinarian must rely on the crime scene evidence (or lack thereof) to help determine proximate cause of death/injury, mechanism of death, and manner of death/injury.

Forensic science begins at the crime scene. The crime scene speaks a silent language, providing information about the victim, suspect, and crime that took place. Processing a scene requires time, attention to detail, and thorough documentation. The goal of any criminal investigation is to solve the forensic triad: Link the victim to a suspect and connect them to a crime scene. Important principles in crime scene investigation include "Every contact leaves a trace" (Locard's Exchange Principle) and the absence of evidence is not evidence of absence. Forensic evidence may be used to support or refute examination or investigation findings such as an alibi or witness statements, assist with reconstruction of the crime scene, or develop important investigative leads. There are actually two crime scenes to process: the macro crime scene, which is the physical area, victim, or suspect's body located where the alleged crime took place (also called peri-necropsy in death cases) and the micro crime scene, which is the body itself. To better assist investigators, veterinarians should become familiar with crime scene procedures and protocols for handling evidence.

There are five methods for documenting a crime scene:

- Sketching/mapping
- Photography/videography
- Measuring
- Note-taking
- Collection of evidence

Physical evidence is non-biological evidence and most commonly refers to objects found. Biological evidence includes blood, saliva, sperm, hair, tissue, bones, teeth, or other bodily fluids. Many types of biological evidence may be present at a crime scene. Each type of biological evidence has a unique importance and its own probative value. Evidence may be further classified as transient, conditional, pattern, transfer, or associative. Transient refers to

Veterinary Forensics: Animal Cruelty Investigations, Second Edition. Edited by Melinda D. Merck.
© 2013 John Wiley & Sons, Inc. Published 2013 by John Wiley & Sons, Inc.

evidence that is easily lost or changed over time, such as body temperature and decomposition. Conditional refers to evidence resulting from an action or event that can be transient as well, such as rigor, weather conditions, entomology, and stomach contents. Pattern refer to evidence with imprints, markings, or other patterns such as bite marks, blood spatter, wound patterns, and weapon patterns. Transfer evidence is the physical exchange of material between objects after contact, such as fibers, hair, or plant matter. Associative evidence is anything that can link items together such as a suspect or victim to the scene or each other (Ladd and Lee 2005).

All evidence must be preserved for potential testing and use at trial. In addition to testing performed for the prosecution side, the defense has the right to perform independent tests and analysis. Every reasonable effort should be made to preserve evidence and make it available for opposing counsel, with consideration that this may not occur for an extended period of time.

THE VETERINARIAN'S ROLE AND HANDLING OF ANIMALS AT THE CRIME SCENE

The veterinarian's role and responsibility at a crime scene may include assisting investigators with identification, collection, examination, and assessment of evidence; assisting with crime scene investigation; coordinating medical teams; handling of zoonotic issues; emergency triage; and euthanasia. A veterinarian may be requested to inspect a property and give an opinion on whether the care of the animals is adequate in suspected abuse or neglect investigations. The expert opinion of the veterinarian is often the deciding factor on whether the condition of the animals constitutes a violation of state law. The lead law enforcement or investigative unit is in charge of the scene. The personnel responsible for crime scene investigation should include people who have received training on crime scene processing, documentation, and evidence handling. There are several textbooks available devoted exclusively to the subject of crime scene processing procedures. This chapter will cover general considerations and highlight important aspects of analyzing a crime scene involving animals.

The veterinarian should meet with the lead investigator, discuss the case, and develop a plan for investigating the scene and handling evidence and the animals as evidence. It is important to record all observations of the scene and the animals. A checklist may be used to ensure everything is recorded and evaluated depending on the type of case and the veterinarian's role (Appendix 7). This checklist should be used as a general guideline because each case is

unique and the issues and questions of the investigation dictate what needs to be done for each scene. Several things usually need to be addressed simultaneously upon arrival to the scene, and the veterinarian can be of invaluable assistance. The situation often requires working under time pressures due to limited personnel available, warrant time limits, or weather or other environmental conditions that could alter or destroy potential physical evidence. Some types of evidence on live and deceased animals may be lost or altered during transport such as loosely adhered trace evidence, saliva from bite marks, and bloodstain patterns. This evidence is better preserved if documented and collected at the scene. The use of e-collars should be considered to prevent the animal from removing evidence during transport through grooming, especially in sexual abuse cases.

There may be sick or critical animals that must be triaged for transport to veterinary hospitals. The status of each animal at the scene should be recorded because it may negatively or positively change after arrival at a veterinary facility.

There may be deceased and decomposing animals that should be examined to preserve potential evidence. Certain on-scene tasks can be performed to assist with time of death determination. The veterinarian should obtain from the investigator information pertaining to when the animal was last seen alive. Ideally, a rectal temperature should be taken of deceased animals at the scene with the exception of suspected sexual abuse cases with potential rectal penetration. This can aid in the time of death determination or support findings in suspected heat stroke deaths. Rectal temperatures should be taken hourly over a three- to six-hour period to establish the rate of cooling or heating for the environmental conditions (Chapter 14). Any entomological evidence related to the body or the scene should be collected (Chapter 15). It should be noted if the animal was in direct sunlight, shade, under any cover, or exposed, and if the conditions would change at different times during the day. A determination of the state of rigor and lividity should be made and recorded (Chapter 14). Paper bags should be placed on the feet of all deceased animals at the scene and secured with rubber bands or zip-ties. Plastic bags should not be used on the feet, especially if the body is placed in a cooler prior to examination because of the formation of water condensation, which can destroy potential evidence.

Consideration should be given to protect fluid leakage from the head and contaminating the body during transport, and precautions taken by wrapping the head in a cloth and/ or plastic bag, securing it with a zip-tie, string/rope, or tape around the plastic (Figure 2.1). Ideally, the body should be wrapped in a clean white sheet and then placed in a clean

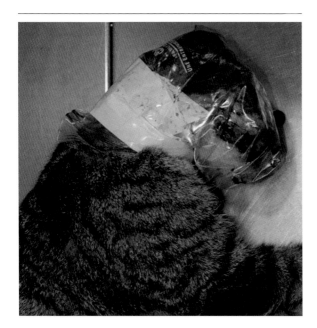

Figure 2.1. Example of how to wrap the head for transport to protect the rest of the body from fluid (blood, purge fluid) contamination.

body bag or thick plastic bag with an evidence ID tag for transport. Decisions for postmortem handling of the body should be based on the best method to slow down the decomposition process and maximize the potential gross pathology and histopathology findings.

Refrigeration is preferred for bodies that will be examined within a few days to a week. Depending on the nature of the case, freezing may be preferred if the exam will be delayed for longer than a week. For facilities that only have a freezer for holding, placing the body within an insulated cooler may help delay freezing for a short period of time until the exam. With advanced decomposition cases, freezing may be preferred if the examination will not take place within a short time in order to preserve any viable evidence. For cases of suspected heat stroke or when the body temperature has increased postmortem due to environmental conditions, temporary storage in a freezer may be needed to speed cooling with transferral to refrigeration. It is advisable to consult with a veterinarian for recommendations of handling on cases other than fresh bodies.

GENERAL CONSIDERATIONS FOR CRIME SCENE PROCESSING

Appropriate protective equipment should be worn when entering the crime scene. This includes equipment to protect the personnel as well as prevent contamination of the scene.

The use of masks, boots, and protective clothing, such as Tyvek® suits, may be used depending on the case. Clean gloves should be worn to collect evidence (see Evidence Collection and Packaging, below). Secure protected areas should be designed for trash and equipment with a separate area for evidence collection and packaging.

ENVIRONMENT: WEATHER DATA

The most important information to initially document at the scene is the ambient temperature and weather conditions. For indoor and outdoor scenes, the environmental temperature of the general area should be recorded, noting the time it was taken, along with the location of live or deceased animals; the temperature should also be recorded at the level of the deceased. This information is important for entomology analysis and time of death determination. It can be a factor in neglect cases and provide valuable information for the veterinary assessment of the animal. For enclosed structures, first responders may open doors or windows which can alter the interior temperature; however, the original ambient temperature information can be determined by checking the heating and air conditioning thermostat settings and determining if they were set to on or off (Figure 2.2). If the unit is turned off or power was disconnected, the temperature gradient between the indoor and outdoor environment can be determined by taking temperatures indoors and outdoors. If power is on, the unit can be turned on and a photograph taken of the temperature setting. An investigation into the power usage for the building can help determine the last time the heating and a/c unit was in use.

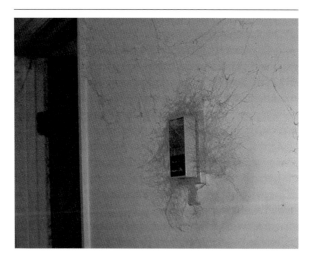

Figure 2.2. Cobwebs covering a thermostat, indicating that it had not been touched for an extended period of time.

PHOTOGRAPHY AND VIDEOGRAPHY

Photography is the most important documentation of a crime scene. The purpose of scene photography is to create a permanent record of the scene and the evidence collected. Animal cruelty crime scenes, especially large scale cases, can be chaotic and the evidence is often overwhelming and may be overlooked. The photographic preservation provides a record that can be examined after the scene processing is complete to identify additional evidence or reassess crime scene findings. The photographic process should be done in such a manner as to capture the scene, place the evidence in context, and show relationships of evidence to the scene (see below). The photos should be taken systematically without jumping from one picture to another. In cases where a crime scene unit is called in to take general photographs and video, there should be someone else assigned to take additional evidence photographs.

The type of camera used is important, and with the prevalence of inexpensive digital cameras Polaroid and film cameras should no longer be used. Digital cameras are ideal because the quality of the photograph can be immediately evaluated, the photographs are digitally preserved, and if necessary, may be enhanced for further evaluation. Digital SLR cameras with interchangeable lenses are ideal, allowing the flexibility for long-range and macro photography. The photographer should be familiar with the camera and make any adjustments needed based on the quality of the photograph. Camera manuals often have good information about photographic techniques and there are several books on forensic photography available. Lighting is a consideration for all photographs. Natural light, camera automatic flash, or the use of external lighting such as flashlights or portable flood lights may be required. Efforts should be made to avoid shadows over the area of interest. Diffused light can be used when surface reflections obscure important information. There are several photography lighting accessories available that can assist with correcting these issues.

For digital cameras, the pictures may be downloaded to a computer and preserved on a CD for later authentication in court, and the digital card may be cleared and re-used. A minimum of three CDs should be made: one for the veterinarian, one for the lead investigator, and one for the prosecutor. Each disc should be labeled with the case number, date, a description of the contents, and the person responsible for the photographs (photographer or lead investigator). A reference number should be assigned, noting if there are multiple copies (e.g., the first CD of six designated "1 of 6") and the copy number (e.g., "Copy 1").

The number of CDs and copies made can be recorded in the evidence log. A copy of the photo log should be included with any copies provided.

There are some general guidelines regarding photography for legal cases. A separate digital card should be used for each scene. After taking a photograph using a digital camera, the image should be checked for quality and adjustments made as needed. No photographs should ever be deleted. This is to prevent the appearance that exculpatory evidence was deleted. A photo may be altered only after the original is preserved and any enhancements or alterations documented. Several photography software programs automatically record the alteration steps. Photographs should only be of items related to the case and no personal photos should be on the digital card. The photos should be professional because they are evidence in a legal case and may be presented in court. Care should be taken to avoid including personnel in the photographs if possible. The use of hands should be avoided to hold or point to the area of interest; instruments or pointer labels may be used instead. Whenever possible, all photographs should be taken at a 90° angle to the area of interest.

The photography process begins with the most general and progresses to more detailed. The scene photography starts with panoramic photographs of the area and buildings, including a picture of the address. For all photography it is important to capture perspectives of the scene starting with overall views, then medium views, and finally close-ups. Taking only close-up views fails to provide the reference or context needed for analysis or presentation in court. This process of narrowing down the focus and showing perspective may take several photographs to achieve.

When photographing evidence at a scene the evidence marker should be in the photo, including the close-ups views. Crime scene evidence markers come in a variety of colors, shapes, and sizes using number or letter systems. The letter or number assigned by the marker is carried over as the evidence ID. There are adhesive markers, scales, and pointers for small evidence and vertical surface evidence such as bloodstains. Disposable evidence markers, scales, and pointers can be made on the computer and templates are available online (Appendix 37). The evidence marker used may be changed during the narrowing down process, reducing the size, e.g. using a small piece of paper to accommodate close-up photos. Photo scales should be used in the photo series when size of the evidence is important to document, such as for weapons and injuries. The photo scale contains a measuring scale, in centimeters or inches, and should be placed in the same plane as the area of interest. There are special photography scales, such as

ABFO (American Board of Forensic Odontology) no. 2 scales, that also have symbols and a gray scale to allow correction for size distortion (elongation) and photographic color alterations. If a photo scale is not available, other items may be used with known established sizes such as a coin or dollar bill. Close-up photographs should be taken with and without a photo scale to show no evidence was obscured by the scale. When taking pictures of the animals, there should be a card or dry erase board with case and animal information placed next to the animal for at minimum the first photograph. This information should contain the case number, animal ID, and the date (Chapter 3). All photographs should be recorded on a photo log (Appendix 4), which may be performed as photographs are taken or filled out after all photography is completed.

Videography of the scene may be of value, especially to show certain conditions of the animal, such as weakness, limping, injuries, or vocalizing. The person handling the video equipment should be familiar with how to operate the camera and know how to video a crime scene, including viewpoints and evidence to capture, and be able to do so with minimal movement. When taking video it is important to inform the others at the scene so they can minimize noise and refrain from talking. The audio mute button may be used, or the volume turned down, if capturing audio is not desired. Copies of the video should be labeled and recorded in the evidence log in the same manner for photograph CDs.

The use of 3-D scanners in crime scene documentation has become more popular with human crime scene investigations. There are several models and styles that provide panoramic photographic documentation from a single viewpoint. Most models use a computer-controlled laser range-finder that can measure millions of points at a crime scene in minutes. The images are put in computer graphics software that varies from a computer-aided design (CAD) model to more advanced graphics with animation. Evidence may be measured within the images using the software and examined from different viewpoints. The use of 3-D scanners could prove most valuable for use in large scale scenes, such as hoarding and animal fighting, and with complex trauma scenes with blood evidence. It also has a distinct advantage of capturing a 3-D image of ephemeral or transient evidence at a scene and during live animal or necropsy examination.

EVIDENCE RECOGNITION AND DOCUMENTATION

Crime scenes are complex and chaotic, requiring systematic evaluation to interpret what the evidence is saying. The entire scene should first be carefully observed to avoid developing tunnel vision and focusing only where the crime occurred. Depending on the type of scene, it may be searched using several methods: spiral, grid, strip (line), or zone (quadrants). For large scenes the strip or line search is preferred, though it requires a larger number of personnel (see Search Techniques under Burial Scenes section). The recognition of evidence involves the ability to identify probative evidence that is among irrelevant or unrelated evidence at the scene. It is especially important to recognize evidence that warrants further testing. Some evidence may become more significant later based on further investigation findings.

Note-taking is an important part of scene and evidence documentation. The notes should be a detailed record of everything observed and what was done. It should include time of arrival, a description of the scene, and a chronological order of everything done. The names of personnel present at the scene should be recorded, including their affiliations. The narrative should include a description of the victim, species, identifiers, and any wounds observed. The environment should be described, including sizes of rooms or areas.

After photographing the scene a map diagramming the scene should be sketched describing and assigning a label to the different areas within the crime scene. Sketching helps eliminate the clutter and confusion of photographs when later analyzing the scene. It should include essential elements of the scene and their relationship. It should also include the location of the animals, live and deceased, and assignment of identification numbers which serve as their evidence IDs. A sketch is not drawn to scale and measurements of distances and dimensions for areas of interest may also be included for reconstruction purposes. To make a sketch, a minimum of two people are usually required to take measurements. A rough sketch is made at the scene and a finished sketch can be made later. The sketch starts with a rough outline of the area, recording pertinent information such as doorways and windows, including a scale for north. A measurement system for locating items and bloodstain areas within the sketch should be established. The choice of measurement methods usually depends on the type of scene; this is extensively covered in human crime scene investigation textbooks and manuals. Objects located in the sketch may be measured using triangulation or baseline techniques. Triangulation takes measurements from the two closest fixed points, designated A and B. The baseline method involves establishing two axes, X and Y. For indoor environments this can be along two walls. For large open areas, this requires establishing a north-south (N-S) and east-west (E-W) axis (see Burial Site Mapping). Measurements are taken from each axis and recorded as inches or centimeters along X and Y. For a deceased animal, measurements should be taken to multiple points on the body. The sketch should include a completed measurement chart, a legend, a "not drawn to scale" disclaimer, and the sketcher's name and signature.

All evidence should be identified with a labeled evidence marker (see Photography). Different markers and systems may be used depending on the preference of the investigating agency. It is important to determine ahead of time how the evidence will be marked, especially when there are multiple processing teams, including those responsible for animal exams. To prevent duplication of letters or numbers, one option is to designate a letter (or number if the markers are letters) for each team based on the type of area to be searched, i.e., animals versus the scene, which is used as part of the evidence ID. This can be as simple as "A" for evidence found on the animals to be used by the veterinarian (A1, A2, etc.) and "P" for all other physical evidence. Alternatively, the scene may be divided into physical areas to be processed by separate teams with a letter designation assigned to each area (when using numerical evidence markers) to be used with each evidence ID number. Depending on the type of evidence, measurements may be taken to locate the item within the scene. This information should be recorded on the crime scene map listing the evidence and their measurements. There are special mapping and identification procedures for large scale animal cases (Chapter 4).

The purpose of the scene investigation is to identify evidence related to the crime, including probative and exculpatory evidence. Depending on the nature of the crime, search considerations for evidence items include evidence that can prove timelines for living conditions or injuries; any evidence that shows ownership or how the animal(s) was obtained; medications and supplies; deceased animals/burial sites; weapons; animal medical records; supply/animal purchase records; biological evidence; bloodstains; evidence that can prove time of injury or death; and food, water, and housing conditions. Each of the following chapters discusses evidence that may be associated with different types of cruelty. Veterinarians can provide invaluable assistance to investigators in evidence recognition and the assessment of the significance. They can also assist with the identification of medical evidence, correct documentation on the investigator's evidence receipt, and provide explanation of the medical evidence found which could result in additional charges or prompt further investigation. The veterinarian should make a list of any medications or supplies found at the scene including

quantities, form of medication (injectable, oral, topical), and pertinent details on the label such as expiration date and prescription information.

The animal housing and the condition of the food and water should be documented. The location of the food/water container, container size, and food/water level should be evaluated to determine if the animal could access it. The area should be searched for food supplies, noting the expiration date on the package. The appropriateness of the food for the species and life stage should be evaluated. It is important to know what food was normally fed for comparison of vomit or stomach contents, especially in suspected poisoning cases. If the animal was confined using a tether, the length of the tether should be measured and collected leaving any knots intact. If a chain was used as a tether it should be collected and weighed. Any housing should be evaluated for appropriateness including size, bedding, and protection from weather conditions. The bedding and underneath the dog house should be searched for hidden evidence such as illegal narcotics.

The scene should be examined for bodily fluids, such as blood, saliva, urine, vomit, or feces. The use of an alternate light source (ALS) can assist with the detection of biological evidence or trace evidence that would otherwise go undetected under standard lighting or daylight. ALS uses light that has been separated into its basic components. ALS using visible light ranges, wavelengths between 400 nm (blue) and 720 nm (red), are used in conjunction with different filters to remove backgrounds and highlight objects. Another important light source, ultraviolet light (UV; 190 nm–400 nm), while not visible itself, can often make hidden objects visible. Semen, urine, saliva, and trace evidence can be identified through their natural fluorescent properties using UV light. Blood will not fluoresce, appearing black, unless treated with chemical enhancements (see Blood Evidence). Items such as bone fragments and teeth can be exposed with blue light (455 nm) through the use of an orange barrier filter and can be separated from the background for easy recovery. Blue light can also identify semen, urine, and saliva.

The lack of animal feces present at the scene can be due to failure to feed the animal, inappetance, copraphagia, or an indicator that the caregiver had removed the feces. The appearance of the feces should be noted, such as diarrhea, formed, soft, hard, fresh, dried, or moldy. The lack of urine can be indicative of dehydration, medical conditions, or recent environmental cleaning. For violent crimes, consideration should be given to the fact that animals often lose bladder and bowel control under extreme fear or distress. Samples of any bodily fluids may need to be collected. With starvation cases, animals may ingest inanimate objects and the scene should be inspected for items the animal could access to chew on. The feces from the animal should be inspected at the scene and for the following twenty-four hours for any evidence of foreign material (Chapter 11).

Any physical evidence that could be associated with the cause of injury or death should be collected for potential analysis. Projectiles that pass through the victim's body may have traces of DNA. Weapons may be a source of fingerprints or DNA from the victim or perpetrator. The scene should be searched for blood evidence, documenting the location and taking samples (see Blood Evidence). Blood-soaked items may be weighed and compared with a clean similar item as a control. The difference in weight provides the estimated blood loss volume (1 kg = 1 L).

EVIDENCE COLLECTION AND PACKAGING

An important consideration for evidence collection is that the person performing the collection should be prepared to testify to the method of collection. Appropriate equipment is needed for evidence collection and packaging (Appendix 5). Proper protocol to prevent contamination should be followed when collecting and packaging evidence. Gloves should be changed between handling different evidence items to prevent cross-contamination. If the gloves were stored in such a manner as they could have been contaminated, the gloves may be rolled with a fresh lint roller tape to remove any trace evidence contamination prior to touching the evidence. Caution should be exercised to avoid touching one's face, hair, or body prior to handling the evidence. A mask may be worn to prevent contamination of DNA through coughing or sneezing. The item should be picked up or touched at areas where the suspect would not normally grab the item to protect fingerprint evidence. Sterile cotton-tipped swabs should be used for swabbing evidence. Disposable or thoroughly cleaned tools should be used and cleaned between handling each piece of evidence. Tools may be cleaned by rinsing with clean water and then drying with a clean tissue, repeating the process twice prior to sampling. Bleach should not be used when collecting DNA evidence (Chapter 4).

An evidence log is used to document all collected items and track chain of custody (Appendix 3 and Chapter 3). Different types of evidence require different types of packaging and storing. The type of packaging should be appropriate in size and material for the particular item and should be clean or new to avoid contamination. The goal is to preserve the integrity of the evidence. Clean paper evidence bags and envelopes are preferred over plastic, which may allow moisture to build up over time,

which can damage the evidence. However, plastic storage has been shown not to degrade DNA for up to three months (Wilson and Adams 2010). Each item of evidence should be packaged separately and in an appropriately sized envelope or container to prevent loss or damage. Evidence that is wet or moist needs to properly dry. For wet items, a piece of clean paper can be placed over the top of the item and the item can be folded so that the paper helps to prevent direct contact between separate stains, then placed in a paper bag. Depending upon the stained item, more than one sheet of paper may be required. Sharp objects should be packaged to prevent puncturing to prevent contamination and injury while handling.

Special evidence boxes and tubes are available from criminal investigation supply companies. Fragile items should be packaged carefully to prevent damage in handling and transport. Gunshot projectiles should be packaged in a manner to prevent damage or causing surface marks; a cardboard box is appropriate. Small items such as hair or fibers should be placed in coin envelopes or pharmaceutical folds and then placed in a larger envelope. To create a pharmaceutical fold, also called a paper bindle, a piece of clean paper is tri-folded from top to bottom then tri-folded again from side to side. The item collected is placed in the center of the unfolded paper and the paper refolded, securing the evidence. Tape or other similarly tacky evidence or other sticky material should be placed in a box lined with wax or slick paper (e.g., magazine). Arson evidence requires special packaging to prevent vapors from escaping or being absorbed, such as can occur with plastic containers. Clean, unused metal paint cans may be used, or special arson packaging containers are available from evidence collection supply companies.

The standard recommendation for collecting biological evidence is not to remove the stain from an object but rather to collect the object with the stain. The advantages of this method are that the entire stain is obtained, collection of an unstained control sample is not necessary, and no further manipulations are required that might negatively impact the sample. If the stain is on a smooth, non-porous surface that can be easily flaked off, it will be necessary to package the item to protect the stain from contact with other objects. This can be done by immobilizing the item in a cardboard box or by taping a piece of paper over the stain if the tape will not destroy other evidence such as fingerprints (Spear).

For stains found on immovable objects, samples will need to be collected in the field. If the entire object cannot be collected, then the next best way to collect biological evidence is to remove the stain by cutting it out, such as from a piece of carpet, using clean scissors. An unstained controlled sample must also be cut out (Spear).

There are occasions when it is not possible to collect a stain by cutting it from an object. The two methods traditionally used to collect these stains are: (1) to use a dampened cotton swab, thread, or piece of gauze to collect the stain, or (2) to use a clean tool, such as a scalpel, to scrape the stain into a clean paper bindle. With either method it is usually necessary to take an unstained control sample. The scraping method can be used only when the stain is in the form of a dried crust which can be lifted from a smooth, non-porous surface. The most significant problem encountered while scraping stains is that samples tend to turn to powder when scraped and it may be difficult to control the retrieval of the entire sample. The powdered stain, which is not retrieved, may contaminate adjacent stains. Therefore, the scraping method is not appropriate for most samples (Spear).

The best method for swabbing a dried stain is to use a minimum amount of distilled water to dampen an appropriate, clean substrate (e.g., cotton swab or cotton gauze without any additive) and then absorb the stain onto the slightly dampened substrate. Ideally a minimum of two swabs should be collected if the stain is large enough. After the first swabbing the area may be moistened and a dry swab may be used to collect more material. An unstained control swab is taken in the same manner as the stain from an unstained area as close as possible to the biological evidence sample. It may be useful to test the apparent unstained area with an appropriate presumptive test to see if it contains a biological sample. The stain should be as concentrated as possible so the size of the collection substrate should be as small as possible. For 1- to 2-mm stains a small piece of gauze may be used and handled with clean tweezers to swab the stain (Spear). If DNA testing is a consideration, known samples from other humans or animals, called standards, should be collected.

After a stain is collected the sample should be allowed to dry to preserve it because moisture can cause degradation. The longer the time required for drying, the greater the risk for degradation. This is a potentially significant problem in small samples. Swabs placed in plastic swab containers with air holes can take more than twenty-four hours to dry. Moist swab samples may be placed directly into paper envelopes. Cardboard swab boxes with air holes may be used and the entire swab box placed inside a paper envelope or bag to protect it from contamination while drying. Ideally, samples should be left open to the atmosphere and allowed to air dry before they are packaged in paper envelopes. Depending on the swab moisture and the environmental

humidity, swabs are usually dry enough to package in two hours or less (Spear).

All evidence needs to be properly sealed with tape to protect it and to visually show that the integrity of the evidence has been maintained. Staples should not be used to prevent damage or loss of evidence. Evidence tape is made to easily tear and is not meant to hold bags closed or boxes together. Packing tape may be used to seal the container and then evidence tape placed over it. The person who packaged the evidence then signs their initials and the date across the tape using a permanent marker. In lieu of evidence tape, other tape may be used as long as it can be written on and visibly show if it has been compromised, such as duct tape or waterproof medical tape. A sealed evidence package should be opened in a different area than where the evidence tape is located and then resealed using evidence packaging protocol.

The package should be properly labeled with the evidence number, case number, date, collection location, description of the item, time collected, and the collector's name and signature. If the evidence contains biological fluids or tissue and/or poses a potential human health hazard it should be marked with a biohazard label. Each item of evidence is assigned an evidence identification number and all evidence is recorded on the evidence log. Certain evidence will change or degrade if not handled properly, such as refrigeration of certain blood tubes. Chain of custody procedures should be followed documenting any transfer, storing, and transport of the evidence (Chapter 3).

EXCLUSIONARY BIOLOGICAL TESTING

When evaluating biological stains at a crime scene or on an animal it may be necessary to exclude the source as human. A negative human test can serve as a presumptive positive test that the sample is from an animal source. This can help with decisions on further testing of evidence samples. IFI Independent Forensics created a human urine confirmation test kit for use in the field or a lab called Rapid Stain Identification Urine (RSID™). This test detects tamm-horsfall protein and reacts with dog urine but does not cross react with horse, cat, gorilla, or turtle urine. It does not cross react with human saliva, semen, blood, vaginal secretions, or menstrual blood. IFI also created a human saliva confirmation test kit called Rapid Stain Identification Saliva (RSID™). This is the first specific test for human α-amylase and it does not cross react with animal saliva— dog, cat, horse, sheep, goat, cow, pig, opossum, guinea pig, rabbit, llama, ferret, woodchuck, hedgehog, mongoose, skunk, lion, tiger, rhinoceros, tokay gecko, chameleon, marsh snake, tamarin, marmoset, grey gull, cuckoo, Sykes monkey, and Capuchin monkey were tested. It does not cross react with human urine, blood, semen, vaginal secretions, or menstrual blood. IFI provides a similar test for semen (Chapter 12). There are several tests for blood available to help exclude human sources (see below).

BLOOD EVIDENCE

Overview

Blood evidence can provide valuable information regarding the victim, perpetrator, and scene events. Interpretation of bloodstains can reveal the position of the victim, attacker(s), presence of a witness, type of weapon used, number of blows, movement of the victim and/or attacker, height of the attacker, and sequence of events. This evidence can determine the events, what did not occur, and the presence of other individuals at the time of the event. In addition, older bloodstains may be analyzed to determine their age (Chapter 14). It is possible to use mRNA to determine the age of bloodstains. A study found mRNA could be used to differentiate between fresh bloodstains and those more than two years old but not between fresh blood stains and those one year old (Connolly 2012).

The analysis and interpretation of bloodstain patterns requires training and experience. The bloodstain patterns in animal cases may differ from human cases based on the species and the animal behavior. The amount of bleeding from wounds in an animal is greatly different than from humans. To properly interpret bloodstain patterns in animal cases, the human bloodstain analysis expert should work with a veterinary medical expert who can provide information regarding the species physiology, expected hemorrhage, and animal behavioral considerations. Veterinary medical professionals who are trained in bloodstain analysis may offer valuable assistance at the crime scene, including proper documentation. The purpose of this section is not to replace the needed training for bloodstain analysis but to provide general information to facilitate the recognition of important blood evidence and ensure the proper documentation for later analysis.

Presumptive blood testing

The purpose of presumptive blood testing is to determine whether the substance tested is likely blood. Depending on the case and the test used, positive presumptive blood tests may be followed with a confirmation test at a laboratory. Several commercial blood test kits are available through evidence collection supply companies. For all presumptive testing, a photograph of the visible test outcome, including the sample ID, should be taken for each test.

The presumptive and hidden blood detecting products (see below) may vary in their sensitivity, specificity, and effects on DNA recovery. A study was conducted on diluted blood, common household substances (saliva, semen, potato, tomato, tomato sauce, tomato sauce with meat, red onion, red kidney bean, horseradish), and chemicals (5% bleach, 10% cupric sulfate, 10% ferric sulfate, 10% nickel chloride, 0.1 M ascorbic acid) using phenolphthalein, Bluestar©, luminol, Hemastix®, Hemident™, and leuchomalachite green as presumptive blood tests. All were able to detect blood diluted to 1:100,000 except leuchomalachite green, which had a sensitivity of 1:10,000. None of the tests reacted with the common household substances but all had some reaction to the chemicals. DNA was recovered and amplified from all testing products except Hemident™ and leuchomalachite green (Tobe, Watson, and Daéid 2007).

The Kastle-Meyer test, also known as the phenolphthalein test, is a catalytic blood test that detects the possible presence of hemoglobin. It tests positive for any blood containing heme and therefore reacts to animal and human blood. It uses a chemical indicator, phenolphthalein, which turns bright pink as a positive reaction. Easy-to-use, self-contained individual test pouches are available. Phenolphthalein also may react to other oxidizing chemicals and compounds such as rust, copper, nickel, and vegetable peroxidases, though the reaction is not typically as bright as with blood. Leghemoglobin is produced by some plants that have a similar structure as hemoglobin. *Pisum sativum*, a class of plants that is widely prevalent in U.S. gardens, gives phenolphthalein false-positive reactions. In addition, these plants can cause staining on surfaces that mimic aged bloodstains (brown to red-brown). These false-positive reactions can occur for more than four years (Petersen 2011).

The Hexagon OBTI® test was originally designed for detection of fecal occult blood in humans and is commonly used as a field presumptive blood test. It tests positive for human, primate, and ferret blood. It does not test positive for orangutan, donkey, camel, pigeon, chicken, cat, dog, goat, sheep, cow, turkey, horse, ostrich, rabbit, trout, mountain gazelle, lemur, and squirrel monkey (Hermon et al. 2003). IFI Independent Forensics created a human blood confirmation test kit for use in the field or lab called Rapid Stain Identification Blood (RSID™). This test detects glycophorin A instead of hemoglobin. The RSID™ blood test does not cross-react to ferret or primate blood. It has no cross-reactivity to human semen, urine, saliva, or breast milk.

Detection of hidden blood evidence

Hidden blood evidence and patterns may be detected even after there have been attempts to remove the visible blood. Bluestar® Forensic is a popular product used to detect latent blood by a chemical reaction that creates a visible blue luminescence. This product is easy to use and does not degrade DNA, and the area may be sprayed repeatedly without a required wait time. The blue luminescence does not require complete darkness to be visible. Bluestar® is extremely sensitive, detecting blood after cleaning with several commercial products (Thurston, Sebetan, and Stein 2011).

Bloodstain pattern recognition, documentation, and analysis

It is important to recognize basic bloodstain patterns and understand pattern interpretation. Bloodstain evidence can provide valuable information for reconstruction and may lead to discovery of additional evidence at the scene. Bloodstain patterns should be properly documented for accurate analysis. Precautions should be taken to preserve any bloodstains which may be easily disturbed or destroyed. The function of bloodstain pattern analysis is to reconstruct the event and includes determining the bloodstain origin; distance between impact areas of blood spatter and point of origin; type and direction of impact which produced the spatter or pattern; object that produced the pattern; number of blows or gunshots; position of the victim, assailant, or object at the scene during bloodshed; and movement or direction of travel of the victim, assailant, or object at the scene. Bloodstain information may be used to confirm or refute witness or suspect statements, assist with time of death determination, and correlate the pattern with the necropsy findings (Johnson 2010). Bloodstain pattern analysis is conducted through the evaluation of the bloodstain size, shape, and target surface. Although proper bloodstain pattern analysis requires special training, there are some basic generalities of bloodstain patterns that an investigator may be able to interpret at the scene.

The fall distance and target surface have notable effects on the size and edge characteristics (smooth vs. spines) of the blood drop and the extent of its spatter. This often requires blood drop distance experiments using the same target surface. In general, the harder and less porous the surface, the less spatter will result (MacDonell 2005). When a drop of blood lands on a rough surface or falls from a great height, it may appear star shaped with spines surrounding the primary stain. Rough, irregular surfaces have protuberances which can rupture a drop's surface and result in spatter (MacDonell 2005).

The blood drop shape is also affected by the angle of impact. Measurements of blood drops determine the angle of impacts which may be used to calculate the height or

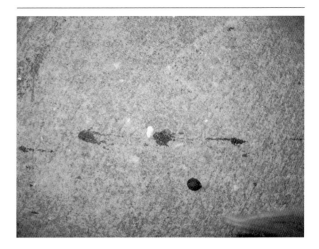

Figure 2.3. Bloodstains with directionality. Notice the irregular shape due to the concrete surfaces.

point of origin of the blood source. Using bloodstain width and length ratios, the blood drop flight pattern may be extrapolated back on an X-Y-Z axis. Directionality can be determined by the shape of the blood drop. If the blood strikes the wall at a 90° angle, it will be circular. Blood drops that impact at angles less than 90° will be more elongated and narrow, with the narrower part indicating the direction of travel with some exceptions. At less acute angles, the directionality may be noted by the predominance of spines toward one side of the blood drop. At more acute angles, a portion of the drop may break off on surface impact, creating a wave cast-off drop which is similar in appearance to an exclamation mark. The location of the smaller drop of blood indicates the direction of travel. Larger blood drop volumes may have several wave cast-offs (Figure 2.3). In contrast, for cast-off droplets, or spatter, that originate from a primary blood drop, these tadpole shaped stains point back toward the blood drop origin (MacDonell 2005).

Passive bloodstain patterns are drops formed by the force of gravity alone. Transfer or contact stains are formed when something comes into contact with the blood and transfers it onto another surface. Projected bloodstains are created when an exposed blood source is subjected to a force greater than the force of gravity. These may be externally or internally produced, such as with an arterial spurt. A flow pattern may be seen whenever there is a change in the shape and direction of a bloodstain caused by the influence of gravity or movement of the object. A drip pattern is the result of blood dripping into blood, usually creating satellite spatter. A perimeter stain consists of only its outer periphery, the central area having been removed by wiping or flaking off after the blood has partially or completely dried. A swipe pattern is caused by the transfer of blood from a moving source onto an unstained surface. The direction of travel may be determined by a feathered edge depending on how the bloodstain was created. A wipe pattern is created when an object moves through an existing stain, removing and/or altering the bloodstain's appearance.

It is important to keep in mind that an injured animal may be mobile and shake the head or body, causing spatter from a blood source. Expirated blood (i.e., from mouth, nose, or lungs) may be diluted or have air bubbles, producing characteristic stains called ghost drops, ghost-centered drops, or bubble drops. These stains are hollow-centered blood drops created when blood mixes with air, creating an air bubble which eventually pops, leaving a hollow center. Ghost drops are associated with coughing, sneezing, or open chest wounds and can be a mixture of sizes.

Insects can cause blood artifacts by moving through the blood and creating a false blood trail. Flies may cause bloodstain pattern artifacts from landing, feeding, defecating, or regurgitating blood, making careful analysis by a trained bloodstain pattern analyst essential. Different species of flies may create different types of stains by feeding from bloodstains located on walls and hard surfaces but seemingly avoiding carpet bloodstains. The blow fly *Calliphora vicina* may alter the shape of bloodstains through feeding and depositing insect stains randomly, but the stains seldom show directionality. The blow fly *Lucilia sericata* feeds on pooled bloodstains without altering the shape or chemistry but deposits stains through regurgitation or defecation. The defecation stains may show directionality, making impact bloodstain pattern analysis difficult. It was found that the defecation stains fluoresced when viewed at 465 nm with an orange filter in contrast to blood, which does not fluoresce (Fujikawa et al. 2011).

Blood spatter size analysis

Blood spatter can be categorized based on the size of the blood drops, which is directly related to the force that caused the spatter. The velocities of blood spatter refer to the force that caused the blood to move and is measured in feet per second (fps). The analysis of these blood drops requires interpretation of events such as weapon acceleration (Akin 2005). When comparing circular bloodstains on the same crime scene surface, three general trends have been identified regarding velocity (Hulse-Smith and Illes 2007):

- A larger bloodstain with fewer spines is derived from a larger droplet impacting at a lower velocity

- A larger bloodstain with greater spines is derived from a larger droplet impacting at a higher velocity
- Bloodstains without spines or on different surfaces cannot be compared in this manner .

It should be noted that smaller volume drops travel less distance than larger volume drops subjected to the same force due to air friction.

High-velocity blood spatter

High-velocity blood spatter (HVBS) is due to drops of blood propelled by an explosive force greater than 25 fps (MacDonell 2005). The blood spatter droplets are less than 1 mm in size and may travel several feet from the impact site. A large number of smaller droplets may create a mist pattern, primarily caused by gunshots, which rarely travels a horizontal distance over three–four feet due to the small mass and air friction (MacDonell 2005). Tissue fragments may be propelled farther because of their larger mass. Backspatter also may be seen with gunshot cases (Chapter 8). In addition to gunshots, HVBS may be seen with explosives, machinery, and expirated blood (Akin 2005).

Medium-velocity blood spatter

Medium-velocity blood spatter (MVBS) is due to blood propelled by an external force of greater than five fps and less than 25 fps. The drops are typically 1–3 mm in size. Usually they are caused by blunt- or sharp-force trauma, such as stabbing, weapons, punches, arterial spurts, and weapon cast-off (Akin 2005). Arterial spurts create a large amount of blood that can be confusing to interpret. The victim may have continued to be assaulted while bleeding, creating overlying bloodstain patterns. There may be swipe patterns caused by transfer from the assailant or victim, or wipe patterns from assailant or victim contact with the arterial spurt pattern (Akin 2005). The arterial spurt pattern is created by the contraction and relaxation of the left ventricle of the heart resulting in an arcing pattern due to the cyclical high-low pressures (Akin 2005).

Weapon cast-off blood spatter, also known as cast-off, is caused by blood flung off a weapon when the weapon is swung upward or backward. These bloodstains are usually circular at the beginning and more elongated at the end of the motion, deposited in a somewhat linear pattern. A wide blood-soaked weapon may create two simultaneous cast-off patterns from each side. When the body is struck with a weapon, there is no cast-off blood spatter from the weapon unless it strikes an existing blood source. Usually, the first strike produces the blood source and subsequent strikes result in cast-off blood spatter. This cast-off pattern can be

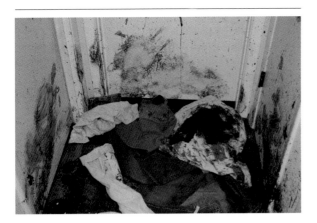

Figure 2.4. Complicated bloodstain patterns including swipes, wipes, weapon cast-off, impact spatter, and blood clot spatter.

very small and easily missed at a crime scene. Weapon cast-off can also be classified as low velocity blood spatter if the drops measure 8 mm or larger (Akin 2005). Impact spatter can occur when an existing blood source is struck (Figure 2.4). For chainsaw dismemberment, the associated blood and tissue spatter is primarily deposited directly beneath the saw and bar when the chainsaw bar is held parallel to the ground. When the discharge chute is not oriented directly to the ground the blood and tissue may be spread on lateral surfaces or areas some distance from the chainsaw (Randall 2009).

Low-velocity blood spatter

Low-velocity blood spatter (LVBS) is caused by a force less than 5 fps, equivalent to the force of normal gravity. These drops usually measure 3 mm or higher. They are most often caused by blood dripping from a stationary blood source or are associated with the movement of walking or running (Akin 2005). Blood dripping from a body or object usually falls at a 90° angle, and is circular when it hits a flat perpendicular surface. The stain edges are usually smooth if the target surface is smooth.

Spines, or crenations, may be caused by surface textures if several blood drops repeatedly land in the same spot, or if the blood falls from a distance. When blood falls passively during walking or running, depending on the speed of movement, the blood stain may be more elliptical or angular with a narrower end or produce a wave cast-off. As discussed above, the shape can indicate the direction of travel. Larger pools of blood may be seen with active bleeding and the blood source is stationary for a period of time in one area. Splashed blood occurs when the volume

is greater than 0.1 ml and it is subjected to either a minor impact or allowed to fall at least four inches. Spattering may occur with large volumes of blood impacting a flat perpendicular surface (MacDonell 2005).

Bloodstain documentation

Bloodstains should be documented in a manner that provides the location and accurate size of each pattern to enable proper analysis. This is achieved through the use of scales in photography and videography, note-taking, and sketching. In addition to the standard supplies for scene photography, the supplies needed for documentation include: photo metric scales; tape measures (metal and/or wooden) for vertical and horizontal use; adhesive scale labels, metric labels, letters, numbers, and arrows; glue sticks for adhesive difficulties; graph paper and pencils for sketching; a color variety of reinforcement circles to place around small bloodstains; and permanent marking pens.

Photography should be performed in the same manner as with all crime scenes (long range, mid-range, close-up) with particular attention to documenting the orientation of the bloodstain pattern to provide perspective. After the initial photo sequence without scales, photo scales are placed on the surface (wall, floor, ceiling, object) adjacent to the selected bloodstain, within the same plane, and the photo sequence repeated. Every effort should be made to take the photograph at 90° to minimize distortion problems for later analysis. An arrow is placed pointing toward the bloodstain that is to be collected for DNA testing. All blood evidence that is sampled for DNA should be photographed. For pattern directionality, labels showing direction (north, south, east, west, and direction of travel) should be used in addition to a vertical and horizontal photo scale. The placement of a colored reinforcement circle, available from office supply stores, may be used to document high velocity patterns that are difficult to see (Johnson 2010). Oblique light sources may be used to enhance areas for photographic capture.

Videography is important to provide orientation references for bloodstain patterns when analyzing photographic documentation. It is expected that there will be some angle distortion with videography. The same photography protocol should be followed for videography, that is, taking video before and after placement of markers. Ideally, video should be conducted without audio recording.

In addition to standard crime scene note-taking, certain data and observations should be recorded. The environmental conditions data should include information regarding air flow and anything that may affect it such as open windows or fans. Note the condition of the bloodstains such as wet, coagulated, drying, dried, thick, pooled, spattered, or disturbed. Record if any items were moved prior to bloodstain documentation, which may affect pattern analysis. Note the time of body removal and the presence or void of bloodstains underneath the body (Johnson 2010).

The purpose of sketching is to supplement photographs by recording the exact location and relationship of pieces of evidence and the surroundings, which is essential to reconstruct the point of origins of bloodstains. Photographs supply detail and sketches eliminate unnecessary details. The sketch is for illustration purposes and is not drawn to scale. It should only contain items relevant to the scene, and a red pencil should be used to depict bloodstain patterns. Depending on the size of the scene and complexity of bloodstain patterns, there may be several sketches, including an overall view and individual rooms or areas (see Evidence Recognition and Documentation).

Fire exposure and bloodstain patterns

Bloodstain patterns remain visible and intact unless the surface that held the blood was burned completely away. Soot can form a physical barrier that interferes with chemical enhancement of blood; it may be removed using distilled water or 70% isopropyl alcohol prior to application of the chemical. Collection of samples for DNA should include both cutting and scraping the blood stain (see Evidence Collection). DNA recovery is unaffected by the heat until the temperature reaches 800°C (1472°F) or higher. Presumptive blood tests may produce a false negative reaction and should not be used as a screening test to eliminate samples for DNA testing (Tontarski et al. 2009).

Analysis of animal fighting blood evidence

A dog fighting pit or cockfighting ring is often covered in blood spatter on the walls and flooring. If the flooring is made of absorbent material it may be possible to estimate the amount of blood loss (see Evidence Recognition and Documentation). Because the bloodstains are often mixed from multiple animal sources, it is important to look for isolated blood drops to decrease the risk of getting a mixed DNA profile. Expirated bloodstains are commonly found. Bloodstains may be found in the surrounding areas (including the ceiling), along pathways where the dogs were carried or walked, in dog holding areas (including vehicles), or "medical treatment" areas. Presumptive blood tests may be performed on suspected bloodstains, including exclusionary testing. A positive phenolphthalein reaction is followed with a human confirmation test (Hexagon OBTI or IFA Rapid test), where a negative reaction, i.e., exclusion of human (see above), is a positive indicator that the phenolphthalein reaction was to animal blood. Bloodstains should be collected as discussed in Evidence Collection and Packaging. Submission to the U.S. Canine CODIS Dogfighting database should be considered (Chapter 13). Additional sources of animal DNA, such as urine, may be discovered through the use of ALS (see Evidence Recognition and Documentation).

The bloodstains should be documented as discussed above. It may be useful for bloodstain analysis to have length and height measurements of the suspected fighting dogs, including from the end of the muzzle to the caudal pelvis; from the end of the muzzle to end of the tail; and from the floor the top of the head, the shoulders, and pelvis.

BURIAL SCENES: GRAVE DETECTION, MAPPING, AND EXCAVATION

The possibility of burial sites on the crime scene should be considered in every cruelty case, especially in large scale cases (Chapter 4). Burial sites may be detected using a variety of methods. Once a burial site is detected, proper mapping and excavation procedures should be followed to fully document the evidence and increase the recovery percentage of any evidence contained within the grave (Appendix 6). The assistance of forensic experts, such as forensic anthropologists, archeologists, and entomologists, can be invaluable. In addition, these experts may have students who can provide additional help on-scene.

Search techniques

Several search techniques may be employed at a crime scene to detect hidden remains or burial sites. The search technique chosen is based on the terrain conditions, the size of the scene, the type of evidence being sought, and the number of people available for the search team(s). These techniques include grid, quadrant (zone), line (strip), and spiral, which are covered in detail in crime scene investigation textbooks.

The most common search technique used is the line (strip) search. The search team should be briefed on what they are searching for including a recent or older burial and evidence related to human or animal presence within the search area. Each team member should have flags or markers to place on any area or items of interest. A flag color system may be used to identify physical evidence, biological evidence, and possible burial markers, with color assignment based on the flag/marker colors available.

The team forms and maintains a line for the entire search. Spacing between team members should be such that the entire area around each individual can be thoroughly searched. The person on each end of the line is responsible for monitoring the line to ensure it stays in formation throughout the search. A third, middle designee may be needed depending on the search line length. Clear verbal commands are used to advance the search line, maintain the formation, and communicate between the searchers such as: "stop," "advance", or "go," avoiding easily misinterpreted words such as "okay." After the area is searched in one direction, the search is repeated in the opposite direction; then the same two-direction search is conducted perpendicular to the initial search. Evidence can be partially hidden and burial markers can be subtle; they may be more visible from one direction. While searching, it is important to look for evidence of previous human presence such as depressed or broken vegetation, track marks (transport method), or foot prints. These may be found at the ground surface or above, indicating a pathway or proximity to the burial site. In addition, there may be evidence caught in foliage from human passage and body transport such as hair, torn clothing, or fibers.

Burial features

General

Burial features and indicators differ for recent and older burials. For more recent burials there may be soil indicators including disturbed soil and/or ground cover, soil displacement by the decomposition of the body (see below), adjacent leftover fill dirt, clumps of sod or clods of soil, and a visible surface soil mix of wilted vegetation, leaves, and cut roots. It should be noted that displaced soil from nearby animal burrows may be mistaken for leftover fill dirt. Foliage indicators include depressed foliage due to trampling or fill dirt, dead foliage around the burial site due to decomposition or damage during the burial, and evidence of intentional concealment with other foliage.

For older burials the indicators may be more difficult to detect and investigation information may be required to locate the general area. Depending on the length of time since burial, the soil indicators may be similar to recent burials but more difficult to detect. Foliage indicators include voids where the vegetation failed to regrow, more lush foliage (compared to surrounding foliage) due to retention of nutrients and water in the burial area, different types of foliage than adjacent areas, and different ages of foliage (younger) than surrounding areas (see Bioturbation).

Burial features are affected by water. The pooling, evaporation, drying, and fine sedimentation in an open and filled burial pit create patterns of cracking (Hochrein 2002). Surface cracks may occur at the edges of the grave which helps identify the boundaries for excavation. The cracks may disappear with rainfall but consistently reappear along the same margins. In contrast, sedimentation

over shallow or flat surfaces causes patterns of cracking in irregular, spider-web–like fashion (Hochrein 2002). The width of the cracks should be measured: in dry conditions, the crack widens at a rate of approximately 1 mm per day. Heavy rainfalls cause rapid closure of these cracks. By using the soil type and historical weather information, it may be possible to determine the post-burial interval to the last rainfall (Hochrein 2002).

Compression and depression of the burial site change the surface contours in and around the pit. These changes may be seen through aerial or pedestrian observations. Primary depressions occur as the fresh fill dirt settles. Secondary depressions are caused by the body bloating because of putrefaction and then collapsing as the gases and fluid are released. Within the grave, the body must be positioned in such a way that the bloating and subsequent collapse causes the change within the burial pit and enough time has elapsed for the putrefaction process to have occurred (Hochrein 2002). If a body has been placed in a container, the secondary depressions may be created as the container deteriorates. Holes dug by scavengers may be misinterpreted as secondary depressions. As time goes on, the evidence of both primary and secondary surface depressions becomes more subtle and harder to detect. Eventually, all evidence may be obliterated by bioturbation, sedimentation, and other changes to the landscape.

Bioturbation: plant and animal

Bioturbation refers to the environmental factors that turbate or naturally churn, displace, or modify the position and nature of the remains (Hochrein 2002). These can include plant (flora turbation) and animal (fauna turbation). The animal factors include rodent burrows, which are often at the upper edge of the burial pit. The species of animal and the behavior of burrowing related to season may be used to determine timelines related to the burial. These burrow routes also may be examined for scavenged evidence.

Disruption of the soil in burials will cause alteration in surface plant growth. The plants may be younger and smaller than the surrounding vegetation or contain completely different plants (Chapter 4). There are certain ammonia and postputrefaction fungi that may provide visible indication of a hidden burial. These fungi also may be analyzed by specialists to provide a post-burial interval (Carter and Tibbett 2003). The roots inside a grave also may provide evidence of the instrument used to dig the grave. Large, broad-bladed tools, such as shovels, tend to tear and slice the roots at the edges of the walls. Thinner-profile tools, such as pitchforks and crowbars, tend to preserve root networks within the grave, usually located beneath the body.

Stratigraphy

Stratigraphy refers to the study of the soil layers. Within a burial, these soil layers are different than the surrounding natural and undisturbed area. One cannot dig a grave and then fill it back in without causing disruption and mixing of the original soil layers. A hole may be dug near the burial site to document the normal soil stratigraphy which can be used during excavation to identify the burial walls.

Tool mark evidence

Tool mark evidence may be present at a burial site on the surface or along the boundary walls. These marks are of forensic importance in that they indicate the tool or tools used to dig the grave. They may provide insight to the burial planning if the tool used was one of opportunity and readily available at the grave site. If more than one tool was used it may indicate there was an accomplice. Subterranean tool marks have been found many years later and under different environmental conditions (Hochrein 2002). The tool mark impression may be smaller than the actual tool size due to the soil springing back (Hanson and Cheetham 2009). The type of soil affects the retention of tool marks, with gravel or dry sandy soils being the least conducive. Handle tool marks may be at or near the surface edges of the grave. As the grave is dug deeper with a long tool, such as a shovel, the edges of the grave may be used as a fulcrum for the handle, which can indicate the position of the person digging the grave. The back fill dirt may hold tool marks such as in clumps of sod or clods of soil.

The surface of the grave and the surrounding area often contain hand, shoe, or knee impressions. These impressions are unavoidable in digging a grave regardless of the instrument used. When using small digging tools, the person must kneel or sit around the edges, possibly leaving fabric impressions. When using a shovel, the person must put his foot on the top of the blade, often leaving heel impressions. These may be misinterpreted as two different instruments used instead of the heel of the foot in conjunction with a shovel blade tool mark. Often the digger stomps or tamps the surface to pack the fill, leaving shoe or foot impressions (Hochrein 2002).

Ground penetrating radar and remote sensing

Ground penetrating radar (GPR) may be used to detect buried remains. It has limitations of use depending on the terrain, and requires training on the equipment. It works best on level terrain and in soils with minimal artifacts such

as rocks. The small size of animals can make detection of remains difficult. A study was conducted in Florida using small pig cadavers (57–74 lbs.) buried in sand, with shallow and deep burials. Detection of the remains became difficult soon after they were mostly or completely skeletonized. This was due to the lack of strong contrasting area of the body and surrounding soil from the lack of soft tissue when compared to the surrounding undisturbed soil. Deeper burials were detected for a longer period of time due to reduced decomposition rates (Schultz 2008).

Remote sensing technologies may be used to record and process reflected electromagnetic radiation in the visible to shortwave infrared wavelengths to detect mass graves (defined as two or more associated bodies). This can be conducted *in situ* using a field portable spectroradiometer with which the data is collected from point measurements of reflected radiation. It can also be obtained from a satellite platform in which the data is in an image form or from an aircraft with an imaging spectroradiometer. A study of an animal mass grave in Costa Rica, comprised of eight juvenile cattle with estimated total weight of 750–800 lbs., found the reflectance spectra was easily distinguishable from soil disturbance in a false grave starting one month after burial and continuing for a total of sixteen months using both *in situ* spectrometry and airborne hyperspectral imagery. The study also found the vegetation regeneration was severely inhibited over the grave for up to sixteen months (Kalacska et al. 2009).

Odors of decomposition

There has been research and development of equipment to detect and measure volatile chemical components of burial decomposition. These surface compounds may not be detected for up to 17 days post-burial. When referring to burial conditions, the measurements are reported in burial accumulated degree days (BADD), which refers to the accumulated average daily temperature (°C) in the burial vault. The compounds detected can be segregated into three distinct groups. The first group is surface compounds, which are detected throughout the burial decomposition process (both soft tissue decomposition and breakdown of mineral and collagen in bone known, as diagenesis). The compounds include benzene derivatives, the most prominent halogen compounds and aldehydes. These tend to be non-cyclic and may be found in burials more than sixteen years old.

The second group are compounds that only appear in the early decomposition process and include esters, certain benzene derivatives, and some halogen compounds. They are usually only detected for slightly more than one year.

The third group are surface compounds which persist until all soft tissue is gone, including mummified tissue. This can last up to 18,000 BADD (note: Eastern Tennessee, U.S.A, averages 5,234 BADDs/year). The compounds include sulfur and halogenated compounds where the majority tend to peak in the first year. The value of these measurements lies in knowing what compounds will be present at what time during the decompositional process, their relative abundance, and their relative ratios compared to other compounds.

The odor of bone for different species is unique in terms of ratios of the compound classes of aldehydes, ketones, alcohols and amides. When comparing dogs, pigs, deer, and human bones, there are distinctive features. For alcohols: dogs 44%, pigs 42%, deer 9%, and humans 5%. For aldehydes: dogs 7%, pigs 50%, deer 39%, and humans 4%. For amides: dogs 46%, pigs 31%, deer 23%, and humans 0%. For ketones: dogs 3%, pigs 27%, deer 42%, and humans 28% (Vass et al. 2008).

Burial scene processing

After the burial site is located it is processed like any other crime scene including photography, note taking, and sketching. The area is secured and the site searched for surface evidence including metal detector survey. Botany and entomology evidence is collected (Chapters 4 and 15). Areas outside the site boundaries should be designated for sifting, equipment, and evidence packaging (Appendix 5 for excavation and mapping equipment list). The team composition should include a team leader, photographer, scribe (note-taking and sketching), excavator(s), soil mover/sifter(s), and evidence custodian. Depending on the number of team members, some may be assigned more than one duty. The team members may rotate through the different roles and responsibilities during the excavation, although ideally the scribe, photographer, and evidence custodian should remain the same.

Burial site mapping

The mapping of the burial site is important to document the evidence found in the adjacent areas and within the burial sites (Appendix 6). This is achieved by establishing a grid from which measurements are recorded in north-south (N-S) and east-west (E-W) directions. A marker should be used for true north and included in photography. After establishing true north, the first step is to establish the datum point that is a reference point. The datum point should something permanent that can be located later and the GPS coordinates recorded. If the area is remote without a permanent point available, a very large tree may be used, GPS coordinates recorded, and triangulation measurements

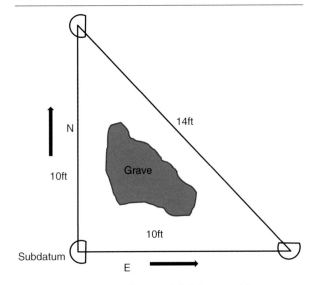

Figure 2.5. Diagram for establishing a grid.

(with distance and direction) taken to a nearby location, e.g. road).

Next, the subdatum point is established at the southwest corner of the grid that will be constructed around the burial site. When selecting this point, the grave site should be located within the center of the final grid and it should be the highest corner within the grid to allow depth measurements. If this is not possible, additional soil may be added to build the corner elevation. A linear measurement from the datum point and subdatum GPS coordinates are recorded. A piece of rebar should be driven into the subdatum point for later detection.

To construct the grid, it is preferable to use wooden stakes. The stakes are "D" shaped and the flat surface should be oriented toward the interior of the grid. The grid is constructed on an N-S and E-W axis with the establishment of two lines of measurement. The size of the grid is determined by the size of the grave. It is important that the axes are at 90° at the subdatum point. This is accomplished by creating a right-angle triangle using the Pythagorean theorem: $A^2 + B^2 = C^2$, where A is the N-S axis, B is the E-W axis, and C is the diagonal connection. Commonly used measurements for the grid are: 8 feet each for A and B, 11 feet for C; 10 feet each for A and B, 14 feet for C. To establish the north and east axis, a stake is placed in either direction at the appropriate distance, using a compass at the subdatum, string, and a measuring tape, and the position adjusted based on the required diagonal measurement to establish the right angle triangle (Figure 2.5). A measuring tape is left in place from the SW stake to the NW stake, i.e., the north (N) wall, from which evidence measurements will be taken. Next, string is tied starting at the SE corner with the string coming off the interior face, wrapped counter-clockwise once around the SW stake, and then tied off at the NW interior face. The 90° angle at the SW corner should be verified with a builders or T-square. A second string is tied at the SW stake for depth measurements, keeping the spool attached for use. The location of this string should be measured from the surface and marked on the stake to establish the elevation.

This grid is used to measure any evidence found at the burial site and within the burial. The scribe should create a table for recording the N and E measurements and depth measurements. When taking measurements from the N wall, it is important to use a T-square, or something square shaped, to verify that the tape measure extending from the grid is 90° to the wall. A line level is attached to the depth string to establish that the line is horizontal, and a plumb-bob used alongside a wooden or measuring tape to establish true vertical for depth measurements. For evidence located outside the interior of the grid, measurements may be recorded in S and W directions. Once the body is uncovered, measurements should be taken at multiple points of the body. A sketch of the body denoting the position should be made.

Excavation of the grave

The excavation process begins after the grid is established, the area searched, and the surface evidence documented and collected. There should be photographic documentation throughout this process. To visualize the burial surface, the vegetation over the burial site is removed by clipping it down but preserving any botany evidence that needs to be collected with the roots intact during the excavation. Entomology evidence should be considered throughout the search, surface clearing, and excavation processes. Leaf litter is removed by hand or light raking and thoroughly searched in the designated area. Small amounts of soil from the top surface may be removed to identify the grave outline by skimming or shining. This is done by using a flat-bladed shovel, keeping the back of the blade in contact with the ground, and scraping the top soil layers. This skimming process smoothes the soil surface and highlights color changes indicating soil disturbance and mixing, which will appear different than the adjacent undisturbed soil area. In some cases the grave outline will be difficult to visualize clearly. Probes may be used to help define this outline by detecting differences in soil resistance. Disturbed soil, i.e., the burial area, will have less resistance than undisturbed soil. Probing is conducted by applying consistent pressure to the probe starting outside the suspected grave area to

determine the undisturbed soil resistance, progressively moving toward the grave area until the resistance decreases. Care should be taken when applying pressure to prevent damage to evidence within the grave.

After the burial outline is identified, the excavation of soil can begin. Using trowels, the soil is removed from the surface in 1-cm layers, moving from the interior of the grave toward the grave walls, and the soil lifted up without scraping the side walls and placed in a bucket. This methodical stratigraphic 1-cm soil removal, or spits, will recover 95% of the evidence *in situ* vs. arbitrary spits, which recovers 50% (Hanson and Cheetham 2009). The fill is removed at even levels over the entire surface, noting any cut roots or sticks in the wall or fill that could have been cut in the digging process.

Any roots, including new root growth, within the grave and around the body should be noted, and the position of the roots and the penetration in and around bones should be documented. These roots should be collected for analysis by a forensic botanist who may be able to provide a time line for the date of interment of the body based on the rate of root growth.

The grave sidewalls may show tool mark remnants or ballistic evidence, which can be used to reconstruct events and corroborate witness statements. Soil immediately against the sidewall surface should be left until after 10 cm of fill is removed so it can be levered away and have room to fall away from the grave wall. All soil cleared from the site and removed from the grave should be carefully sifted and examined for evidence. For sifting, nylon mesh is preferred over metal to minimize potential evidence damage; it should be small enough to prevent loss of small bones. Hair and fibers are shed by the human perpetrators in the soil and grave. Approximately 40%–60% of small objects or trace evidence may be found during excavation, and the rest will be recovered during sifting. A tarp should be placed under the sifter and a separate sifting site designated for each burial site. Wet sifting may be required for hard compact or wet soil. A metal detector may be used on the removed soil prior to sifting or performed periodically within the burial site throughout the excavation. By removing the soil in 1-cm spits or layers and sifting, 98% of the evidence will be recovered (Hanson and Cheetham 2009).

Once the excavation gets close to the body, it may be necessary to switch to brushes and plastic or wooden tools to prevent damage to the body. Smaller or loose bones that may be easily lost during the excavation may be removed separately. The body should be completely exposed, leaving a supporting pedestal of soil underneath. The body is then carefully removed and placed on a tarp adjacent to the

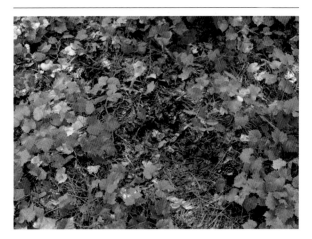

Figure 2.6. Darkened area from decomposition where most of the skeletal remains have been removed by scavenging.

grave. Skeletal remains are inventoried to ensure all bones are accounted for and no additional bones are present, indicating additional bodies within the grave (Appendix 19). The remains are properly packaged for transport, keeping the body in the original burial position. For skeletonized remains, the bones may be packaged in groups such as individual legs and feet. Excavation is continued after the body removal until the bottom of the original grave is identified, continuing metal detector surveys, to collect any additional evidence and verify there are no additional bodies within the grave.

Live vs. Deceased burial

An important consideration is whether or not the animal was alive when buried (Chapter 9). Evidence of soil compaction within the grave has been found in cases of humans buried alive where the victim pressed on the sides with body area movement such as bound legs, shoulders, knees, or hands. Evidence of scratching and biting may be found in the soil or on the inside surfaces of any bag or wrapping. The animals may have frayed or broken nails on their feet with embedded soil.

Surface remains

Surface remains are often scattered due to animal scavenging and the search area should be appropriately broadened. Depending on the species of scavenger and the size of bone, remains can be found within a few feet or over 50 feet. The core area, which is where the body was located when decomposition began, should first be determined. This may be identified by the dark decompositional fluid

staining in the area and/or the location of the highest concentration of skeletal remains, usually the torso (Figure 2.6). Due to the weathering effects on bones, they may be difficult to detect in the outdoor environment. With a longer postmortem interval, small bones may be lost due to scavengers or dissolution by soil acidity. The topography can affect where items may be found. The skull may naturally disarticulate and roll downhill. Any potential physical barriers for scavengers should be searched thoroughly for skeletal remains. Small scavengers may not be able to carry bones across small physical barriers, such as fallen trees, and drop or feed on the bone in that area. Animal burrows should be inspected for physical and skeletal evidence potentially carried away from the original body. The same mapping techniques described for burial sites are used for surface remains.

REFERENCES

Akin, L.L. 2005. Blood Spatter Interpretation at Crime Scenes. *The Forensic Examiner*. 14(2):6–10.
Carter, D. and M. Tibbett. 2003. Taphonic Mycota: Fungi with Forensic Potential. *Journal of Forensic Science*. 48(1):1–4.
Fujikawa, A., L. Barksdale, L.G. Higley, and D.O. Carter. 2011. Changes in the Morphology and Presumptive Chemistry of Impact and Pooled Bloodstain Patterns by *Lucilia sericata* (Meigen) (Diptera: Calliphoridae). *Journal of Forensic Sciences*. 56(5):1315–1318.
Connolly, J.-A. C. 2012. The Use of Forensic Messenger RNA (mRNA) Analysis to Determine Stain Age. Presented at the American Academy of Forensic Sciences Annual Scientific Meeting, 20–25 February, Atlanta, Georgia.
Hanson, I. and P. Cheetham. 2009. Advances in Archeological Approaches to Crime Scene Investigation. Presented at the American Academy of Forensic Sciences Annual Meeting, 17 February, Denver, Colorado.
Hermon, D., M. Shpitzen, C. Oz, B. Glattstein, M. Azoury, and R. Gafney. 2003. The Use of the Hexagon OBTI Test for Detection of Human Blood at Crime Scenes and on Items of Evidence, Part I: Validation Studies and Implementation. *Journal of Forensic Identification*. 53(5):566–75.
Hochrein, M.J. 2002. An Autopsy of the Grave: Recognizing, Collecting, and Preserving Forensic Geotaphonomic Evidence. In: *Advances in Forensic Taphonomy*, W.D. Haglund and M.H. Sorg, eds. pp. 45–70. Boca Raton: CRC Press.
Hulse-Smith, L. and M. Illes. 2007. A Blind Trial Evaluation of a Crime Scene Methodology for Deducing Impact Velocity and Droplet Size from Circular Bloodstains. *Journal of Forensic Sciences*. 52(1):65–69.
Johnson, J. 2010. Basic Bloodstain Pattern Analysis for Veterinarians with Concepts for Animal Abuse Cases. Bloodstain Pattern Analysis Workshop, 9–10 November, University of Florida Maples Center, Gainesville, Florida.

Kalacska, M.E., L.S. Bell, G. Arturo Sanchez-Azofeifa, and T. Caelli. 2009. The Application of Remote Sensing for Detecting Mass Graves: An Experimental Animal Case Study from Costa Rica. *Journal of Forensic Sciences.* 54(1):159–166.

Ladd, C. and H.C. Lee. 2005. The Use of Biological and Botanical Evidence in Criminal Investigations. In *Forensic Botany: Principles and Applications to Criminal Casework*, H.M. Coyle, ed. pp. 97–115. Boca Raton: CRC Press.

MacDonell, H.L. 2005. *Bloodstain Patterns, Second Edition.* Elmira Heights: Golos Printing.

Petersen, D.J. 2011. Phenolphthalein False-Positives: What's Buried in Your Garden? Presented at 63rd Annual Scientific Meeting of the American Academy of Forensic Sciences, 21–26 February, Chicago, Illinois.

Randall, B. 2009. Blood and Tissue Spatter Associated with Chainsaw Dismemberment. *Journal of Forensic Sciences.* 54(6):1310–1314.

Schultz, J.J. 2008. Sequential Monitoring of Burials Containing Small Pig Cadavers Using Ground Penetrating Radar. *Journal of Forensic Sciences.* 53(2):279–287.

Spear, T.F. Sample Handling Considerations for Biological Evidence and DNA Extracts. California Department of Justice and California Criminalistics Institute.

Thurston, C., I.M. Sebetan, and P. Stein. 2011. Detection of Altered Bloodstains with Bluestar®. National University. Abstract presented at American Academy of Forensic Sciences Annual Scientific Meeting, 21–26 February, Chicago, Illinois.

Tobe, S.S., N. Watson, and N.N Daéid. 2007. Evaluation of Six Presumptive Tests for Blood, Their Specificity, Sensitivity, and Effect on High Molecular-Weight DNA. *Journal of Forensic Sciences.* 52(1):102–109.

Tontarski, K.L., K.A. Hoskins, T.G. Watkins, L. Brun-Conti, and A.L. Michaud. 2009. Chemical Enhancement Techniques of Bloodstain Patterns and DNA Recovery After Fire Exposure. *Journal of Forensic Sciences.* 54(1):37–48.

Vass, A.A., R.R. Smith, C.V. Thompson, M.N. Burnett, N. Dulgerian, and B.A. Eckenrode. 2008. Odor Analysis of Decomposing Buried Human Remains. *Journal of Forensic Sciences.* 53(2):384–391.

Wilson, A. and E. Adams. 2010. Studying the Effects of Plastic Storage Systems on DNA Degradation of Blood Evidence. Presented at the 62nd Annual Scientific Meeting of the American Academy of Forensic Sciences, 22–27 February, Seattle, Washington.

3

CSI: Examination of the Animal

Melinda D. Merck, Doris M. Miller, and Paulo C. Maiorka

Doubt, indulged and cherished, is in danger of becoming denial; but if honest, and bent on thorough investigation, it may soon lead to full establishment of the truth.

Ambrose Bierce

GENERAL CONSIDERATIONS

Veterinary forensic medicine is unique in that there are many different species that may be part of an investigation. It is important that the animal is examined by a veterinarian with the knowledge and experience in that species or group of animals. Veterinarians should follow the cardinal rule of staying within their boundary of expertise and professional competence. It should be determined if a specialist in a particular area or discipline should be involved. The veterinarian should disclose to the investigating agency if there are any potential conflict of interest issues such as personal knowledge of one of the involved parties.

Certain key details should be recorded when the veterinarian is first contacted regarding a case, by phone or upon presentation of the animal (Appendices 8–11). This is the beginning documentation for the case and it is continued throughout the case (see Documentation sections). These notes should be factual and will be used to complete a forensic report. The veterinarian may need to rely upon them if called to testify and the notes may eventually be requested by the attorneys or the court. The date, time, agency, case number, and name and contact information of the person who contacted the veterinarian should be recorded. Information should be obtained regarding the type of animal(s) to be examined, how it is being transported, general details of the alleged crime, what is expected of the veterinarian, and a time frame for which the findings are required. The veterinarian should request from the investigator certain documents to be examined including incident reports, witness statements, photographs, and videos. The number, condition, and quality of the documents should be noted and each item recorded in the evidence log (Appendix 3).

It is important that the veterinarian guard against biases and provide a clear, objective analysis of the findings. With information overload there is a tendency to use mental shortcuts, heuristics, which may or may not be subject to biases. There is a tendency to prefer less complex information instead of relying on thinking and analyzing. There may be a tendency to believe witness accounts instead of carefully considering their statements. There may be a tendency to have confirmation bias, which refers to believing more positive information than negative. This can result in giving negative information less weight, possibly making it insignificant. There can be the anchor effect in which there is a tendency to rely heavily on one piece of information, usually the first information encountered. Theory development and formation of judgments start at the beginning.

Investigations done in a confirmatory manner may have the effect of making judgments to increase confidence of a theory instead of maintaining objectivity and considering all information. There are several things a veterinarian can do to guard against biases. The information from the case and photographs should be reviewed several times. Alternate theories should be examined and ways to

Veterinary Forensics: Animal Cruelty Investigations, Second Edition. Edited by Melinda D. Merck.
© 2013 John Wiley & Sons, Inc. Published 2013 by John Wiley & Sons, Inc.

disprove the manner of death or injury considered. All negative evidence should be confirmed as documented. Peers should be encouraged to review and discuss theories and findings. With awareness of what can create bias on a subconscious level, steps can be taken to form impartial and objective conclusions.

DETERMINING NON-ACCIDENTAL INJURY

Overview

Determining accidental vs. non-accidental injury (i.e., abuse) begins with an index of suspicion when the exam findings are not supportive by the presenting history. It is important to have all of the available crime scene and investigation information prior to examining a suspected victim of animal cruelty. The veterinarian must analyze all of the examination findings in context with the history, crime scene, and investigation findings. A conclusive determination may not be possible without this information or it may require further investigation by the investigating agency.

Certain types of injury and conditions raise suspicion of abuse in and of themselves. The pathognomonic features for child abuse include fingertip bruising, cigarette burns, and lash marks. Features that are highly suggestive of child abuse are retinal hemorrhages, unexplained subdural hematomas, and torn lingual frenula. A triad of injuries has been described in infants: subdural hemorrhage, brain edema, and retinal hemorrhages. Additional indicators of child abuse include inconsistent history and delay in treatment, with the latter being the biggest indicator (Gilliland 2011). Fracture distribution patterns have been described in child abuse: 77% affecting the extremities, 34% in the skull, and 19% involving the ribs (Platt, Spitz, and Spitz 2006).

The most pathognomonic feature of abuse in animals is repetitive injuries. This may present as multiple injuries in different stages of healing, indicating that they occurred at different times, or the animal may have a medical history of repeated injuries. The Munro and Thrusfield study revealed repetitive injury in sixteen dogs out of 243 reported cases of non-accidental injury and in thirteen cats out of 182 cases (Munro and Thrusfield 2001b). Another consideration for suspected abuse is households in which the patient or other animals have suffered similar injuries, unexplained death, or disappearance. The patient may have a pattern of unexplained symptoms or injuries. The owner may have several animals listed that the veterinarian has only seen once, or they may adopt frequently from their local shelter because their pets never live long or always "run away."

Extensive data published on child abuse parallel findings in animal abuse, which may be used for identification and classification of animal injuries (Munro and Thrusfield 2001a). Child abuse can be categorized as physical abuse (non-accidental injury), psychological abuse, sexual abuse, and neglect. A study of non-accidental injury in animals was conducted by Munro and Thrusfield of 1,000 veterinarians in the United Kingdom. The study found that certain things either raised suspicion or caused recognition of non-accidental injury, which included something indicative in the history, behavior of the animal and/or owner, type of injury, implication of a particular person, or involvement of the police or animal control in the case. These are very similar to diagnostic pointers to non-accidental injury in children (Munro and Thrusfield 2001a).

It is interesting to note that the study found age, gender, and breed factors in the reported cases of non-accidental injury. Abuse was found in a higher number of dogs (63%) and cats (71%) less than two years of age when compared to the general population. This may result from the fact that younger animals are harder to manage, are possibly more aggravating to the owner, and are more likely to incite aggressive acts by the owner (Munro and Thrusfield 2001b). Juvenile animals may be more susceptible to abuse by people other than their owners because this category is more prone to explore new environments and become victims of neighbors. It may be that older animals are less likely to be abused due to the time for the human–animal bond to strengthen. The study also found that male dogs were abused in a higher proportion to female dogs. This may be because violent offenders tend to prefer male dogs or that male dogs may be more aggressive and less manageable than female dogs (Munro and Thrusfield 2001b). No statistical gender difference was found in the cases involving cats. The study also considered dog breed differences and compared those with the general population in the United Kingdom. They found that the Staffordshire bull terrier, Staffordshire bull terrier cross, and mixed breed dogs were at increased risk of abuse. The study suggested possible explanations for the breed risk may include the nature of the person who seeks to own the Staffordshire bull terrier, and that more cross- or mixed-breed dogs are owned by people of lower socioeconomic status. They also found that the Labrador retriever showed a lower risk of abuse (Munro and Thrusfield 2001b).

Feline cruelty appears to be different than with dogs in terms of type and severity of injuries and outcome. Abused cats also have a higher likelihood of death than dogs. Cats have the greatest variety of cruelty inflicted using different methods. They are the most frequent target in all forms of abuse and the predominant victim in cases of burning, bone fractures, and being thrown from a height (Lockwood 2010). When compared to dogs, cats are overrepresented in cases of torture, beating, throwing, mutilation, suffocation, and drowning. With hoarding cases, dogs and cats were equally represented but cat deaths were twice as high as dogs (Lockwood 2004). A study in Brazil of 644 cats that presented to the veterinary school for necropsy found 29.66% (191) had lesions highly suggestive of cruelty: evidence of trauma, fractures, organ rupture, and carbamate poison. The average age was 23.66 months (range 1–144 months) of which 62.3% were one to twenty-four months old (119/191 cats). They also found that cats were three times more likely than dogs to be poisoned with carbamate (Maiorka and de Siqueira 2011).

Feline cruelty is likely to be significantly underreported. This may be due to negative societal attitudes towards cats, where cruelty goes unreported or prosecuted. In addition, the behavior of cats and the human-cat relationship may be contributing factors. Cat owners may not pursue looking for their missing cat, relying that it will come home eventually or believing that it has found a new home. They may also assume the cat was the victim of a motor vehicle accident or predator. The most common behavior of an injured or fearful cat is to hide as opposed to seeking human interaction, even with fatal wounds. This behavior contributes to the lack of detection of injured or deceased cats that have been victims of abuse.

The psychology of animal cruelty

It is important for veterinary professionals to understand the psychology of animal cruelty and the forms it can take to increase their recognition of abuse. Animal abusers come from all socioeconomic classes. There may be parallels to those found in child abuse, which is more common in the lower socioeconomic class where there is more social deprivation and family dysfunction (Munro and Thrusfield 2001a). Animal cruelty can be part of a cycle of abuse associated with interpersonal violence.

There can be several motives for cruelty to animals. The motive may be to demonstrate power and control over others; a tool for emotional abuse; to secure silence or compliance; or as revenge, retaliation, or blackmail. Other motives may be curiosity and exploration; ignorance of the animal's needs, abilities, or signals; boredom; as a method for mood alteration; deviant sexual arousal; or non-specific sadism. There may be reactive motives which include imitation of others, identification with an aggressor, as a means of avoiding or denying attachment, post-traumatic play, to induce self-injury, or rehearsal of

suicide. Social motives may be seen, including peer reinforcement, forced participation, gang or cult activity, to establish autonomy or reject societal norms, or to shock and offend (Lockwood 2011).

For juvenile offenders, the suggested typologies include a child who is developmentally immature and lacks cognitive and/or social skills (e.g., sees something on TV), a child who is a victim of abuse and whose abusive behavior is reactive to his/her own victimization, and a child whose maliciousness is consistent with an overall pattern of conduct disordered behavior. It should be noted that one-third of mothers who were physically abused reported their child for animal abuse. It has also been found that most juvenile offenders are six to seven years old when diagnosed with conduct disorder and commit animal cruelty (Lewchanin and Zimmerman 2000).

The psychology of animal cruelty can be characterized based on the type of abuse. In neglect cases, it may include ignorance, laziness, apathy, underlying physical or psychological barriers to providing proper care, caregiver stress, poverty, or passive aggression such as denying care to get at or control a human. In hoarding cases, it may include attachment disorder (possibly due to parental abuse or neglect), obsessive-compulsive disorder, borderline personality disorder, addictive behavior, dementia, and others such as paraphilias or psychoses. In dog fighting, it may include power and control, greed, social status, the possible absence of empathy (though some claim to love their dogs), and non-specific sadism in which the types of killing are vengeful (such as electrocution, drowning, hanging) incited by the dog fighter living vicariously through his or her dog's performance (Lockwood 2011).

Abused animals in the veterinary practice setting

Animal abuse is commonly seen in veterinary practices. It is important to consider developing a standard operating procedure (SOP) for handling suspected abuse cases within the hospital and provide training to all staff (Chapter 1). The veterinarian must have knowledge of the laws regarding what procedures or treatments may be performed and under what authority. These may be in the veterinary practice act, animal welfare act, or elsewhere under the criminal code.

Every case is unique in presentation and how it should be handled. In some cases, permission of the owner may be obtained. Under some laws, the veterinarian can take samples without owner consent when abuse is suspected or the animal is suffering or likely to suffer (Newberry and Munro 2011). Under most laws the veterinarian does not have the legal authority to seize an animal. In every case in which abuse is suspected, the investigating authority should be called immediately. That agency can take possession of the animal and direct or authorize procedures and treatment. If the investigator cannot be on-site at the hospital or his or her arrival will be delayed, there may alternative solutions. The investigator can contact the local law enforcement agency, who also has jurisdiction under the criminal code to investigate cruelty, and direct them to take custody of the animal. This form of taking custody can be to direct that the animal remain at the veterinary hospital. Then the authorities can direct the veterinarian to perform the necessary exam, procedures, and treatments for the animal. This can be done verbally but should also be recorded in a written form, which can be faxed or e-mailed, and which is signed and dated by the agency granting permission. An injured or neglected stray animal brought in by a good Samaritan may be a victim of cruelty, and euthanasia should not be performed unless medically necessary and local enforcement authorities called.

Taking a history in suspected abuse cases

Taking a history in suspected abuse cases requires special consideration of several factors that can influence the accuracy of the information obtained. One important consideration is that the owner or someone familiar with the owner may be responsible for the abuse. It is important to avoid accusations when taking a history, especially if the suspected abuser is present. The caregiver (and the family) may be a victim of ongoing interpersonal violence. This can result in reluctance to be forthcoming of details of the causes of injury out of fear for their personal safety. The abuser may accompany his or her partner to the veterinarian. A recommended practice is to have literature for domestic violence shelters in the bathroom, including animal organizations that can shelter the animals, which is often the only place the victim can separate from the abuser.

It is important to get a more thorough history in animal abuse cases than what is normally obtained in routine examinations. In abuse cases, certain questions need to be answered to better interpret exam findings. Questions should be asked to determine who had access to the animal (including other animals), what the animal had access to, when and where the event occurred, how it happened, and why it happened. Details are needed about the environment, including if the animal had access to the outdoors and if it was allowed outside unattended. If the animal was confined outside, it is necessary to know how it was confined, if a gate is present on the fence, and if so, if is it locked. If the animal lives strictly indoors, then the layout of the home is needed, including the presence and location of stairs.

Specific information is needed regarding where the animal was found, what was present around the animal (e.g., blood or other bodily fluids), and the initial symptoms observed. The history should include information regarding the food fed to the animal (including brand, dry or can), the frequency of feeding, the last known time when the animal ate or drank, and when the animal last had access to food or water.

The suspicion of non-accidental injury should be raised when there is a significant discrepancy between the history provided and the clinical findings. Suspicion also should be raised when explanations are vague, inconsistent, or contradictory. Common sense and experience are needed to analyze all the information to determine if the injury is due to non-accidental causes. A common explanation offered is the animal fell off something within the home or outside. The veterinarian must consider the height of the fall, the species involved, and the known injuries associated with falls (Chapter 5), and compare those with the exam findings to determine if that scenario is plausible. Another common explanation given is that the animal was hit by a motor vehicle. There are characteristic injuries associated with motor vehicle accidents (Chapter 5).

The behavior of the owner may raise suspicion of non-accidental injury. The owner may be apathetic, uneasy, angry, or defensive with routine history questions; embarrassed; or generally respond inappropriately to the situation, especially when apprised of the gravity of the situation. If the behavior of the owner becomes an issue, it may be advisable to have someone else in the room for safety.

Hearsay

Hearsay is an extremely complex subject. Veterinarians often make the incorrect assumption that what a client tells them is admissible in court. In a court hearing or trial the defendant has the right to confront and cross examine the witnesses called against him or her. During cross-examination, the defense attorney is able to test the reliability, believability, and accuracy of the witness. An out-of-court statement made by someone other than the witness who is actually testifying is presumed to be inadmissible because the defendant is not able to test the statement's truthfulness in front of the judge or jury. There are several exceptions to the hearsay rule. One exception is that the prosecutor may introduce out-of-court statements made by the defendant. It is the prosecutor's decision. The defense attorney cannot introduce out-of-court statements made by the defendant. Whether or not the prosecutor elects to offer the out-of-court statement of the defendant is a tactical move (Balkin 2012).

A veterinarian should pay close attention to what the client tells him or her and should try to record what is said verbatim to the best of his or her ability. If the veterinarian believes that he or she has written down exactly what the client said, then quotation marks should be placed around the statement. If there is more than one client present, it is important for the veterinarian to note who says what. A client may be truthful, embellish, or fabricate an explanation for an animal's injury, illness, or death. The veterinarian needs to write down what is said by the client regardless of whether or not the veterinarian believes it to be truthful or accurate. If a client makes a statement against his or her interest it is technically not hearsay and is admissible as outlined above (Balkin 2012). An example would be if a person makes a statement implicating him or herself in the crime.

BEHAVIORAL CONSIDERATIONS OF ANIMALS

The behavior of animals in response to a threat or injury can determine what evidence is found on examination and at the crime scene. Behavior may be influenced by the animal species, breed, age, gender, and neuter status. Animals often lick at the area of injury, potentially removing critical evidence. When in pain, the animal may roll, hide, and/or vocalize. When experiencing extreme fear, animals typically involuntarily urinate and/or defecate. This knowledge is an important consideration when examining the animal and evaluating a crime scene to determine the sequence of events and where to look for evidence.

It is important to consider what the animal's behavior might have been in response to the assault to determine what evidence may be found on a suspect. Defensive reactions to an assault are highly variable in animals including avoidance, submission, or defense aggression which may or may not result in injuries to the assailant. Avoidance or submission may result in injuries to the rear or exposed areas of the body. There may be additional injuries caused by the assailant grabbing or restraining the animal. Defense wounds on an animal may not be present or may be difficult to interpret. It is also highly likely that there was a transfer of evidence from the assailant to the victim and from the victim to the assailant.

The animal's behavior may raise suspicion of abuse, such as fear toward the owner, dullness, depression, or anxiety. The fear and anxiety reactions of the animal may be so severe as to cause the animal to vocalize, urinate, or defecate when the owner is present. It is important to note if fear/anxiety behavior goes away when the person leaves and if it returns when he or she reappears. It should be documented if notable fear anxiety is associated with a person of a specific gender, certain clothing or accessories (e.g., baseball caps, eyeglasses), or physical items that may have been used as a weapon such as a shovel. These behavior manifestations may not be admissible in court but may provide possible clues that can be valuable to the investigator. It should be noted that animals may have seemingly positive responses to their abuser, including tail wagging and licking, which can be mistaken for an indicator that the animal has not been abused.

EVIDENCE DOCUMENTATION, COLLECTION, AND PACKAGING

Evidence documentation and collection from the animal follows the same protocols as in crime scene investigation and is covered in detail in Chapter 2. The veterinarian or person who collects evidence should be prepared to testify to the method of collection. All evidence should be photographed *in situ* prior to collection and packaging. Precautions should be taken to minimize contamination of evidence by wearing cap, mask, gloves, and a clean gown. It is important to consider that the significance of a piece of evidence may change later based on crime scene findings, additional investigation, witness statements, or the suspect's statement. A suspect or defendant is free to change his or her statement and the veterinarian should try to anticipate all possible defenses in their forensic evaluation and collect potential evidence.

It is important to have the proper tools to detect and collect evidence from the animal (Appendix 5). The body should be inspected with a UV light source to detect fluids and trace evidence (Chapter 2). A flashlight may be used for indirect lighting, holding it at an angle to detect trace evidence such as foreign hairs and fibers (Chapter 4). A magnifying glass is helpful when examining the body for small pieces of evidence. Plastic tweezers are needed to retrieve fine pieces of evidence without causing damage. Swabs and/or gauze are needed to collect biological evidence. It is helpful to have a foam block to hold the swabs while they dry. Supplies are needed to package evidence, and protocols for packaging are covered in detail in Chapter 2.

CHAIN OF CUSTODY

Any evidence related to a crime must follow a chain of custody. This refers to a process of continuous, chronological documentation of evidence collection/seizure, custody, control, transfer, analysis, and disposition. This serves as a record that the evidence submitted in court is the same evidence collected at the scene and documents any alteration of the evidence. Evidence includes anything collected from the animal: all samples, photographs, video, radiographs, test results, and the animal itself. Ideally it should be the police or animal control that transports the body to the veterinarian to maintain the chain of custody. When selecting what personnel will be assisting in the examination and evidence handling, especially in a hospital environment, it is important to consider that all people who are part of the chain of custody may be subject to subpoena to court for trial.

All evidence must be properly collected, packaged, and labeled, with each item recorded in the evidence log (Chapter 2, Appendix 3). All evidence should be kept in a locked area with restricted access. If the evidence must be kept in an unlocked refrigerator or freezer, it should be located in an area with limited personnel access. A restricted access box may be placed inside the refrigerator or freezer, such as a metal lockbox, that will allow the evidence to be maintained under acceptable conditions. If the evidence, including the body, is transferred to another person, location, or laboratory, it must be noted in the evidence log with the time and date, obtaining a signature from the sender and recipient.

Whenever evidence needs to be transferred, including laboratory samples, chain of custody procedures should be followed. A separate evidence log should be sent along with the evidence with instructions for the receiving agency/person to fill out the chain of custody section and fax it back. For laboratory submissions, it should be noted on the test form that the samples are "evidence," "forensic samples," and/or "criminal investigation." This may assist the receiving lab to institute proper handling protocols and assign the appropriate person to perform the analysis.

If evidence is removed from storage it should be documented in the evidence log, including the purpose, if opened, and any testing or alteration. When opening a sealed evidence package it should be opened in a separate area and the original seal preserved. This will later provide proof that the original seal was not broken. After the examination is complete, the item is placed back in the original package, sealed with evidence tape, and signed and dated. Evidence must be held until the legal case is over. Because additional legal avenues may be pursued after a case is closed, the prosecuting authority should be consulted prior to disposing of any evidence.

PHOTOGRAPHY AND VIDEOGRAPHY

Photographic documentation, and possibly videography, should be performed on all live and deceased animal examinations. Forensic photography and videography protocols, documentation, and techniques are covered in Chapter 2. As with crime scene photography, the photographs should begin with the case information including the case number,

date, and animal ID written on a card or dry erase board. This first picture with the case and animal information may be taken with or without the animal in the photo and all photographs following this initial picture should only be of that animal. When working with cases involving multiple animals, this protocol will ensure consistency of the photographs and reduce the chance of errors. If additional photographs are needed of an animal that has already been examined and photographed, the sequence starts again with the case and animal ID information card. Small identification labels may be used for closer views and should contain at minimum the animal ID. Other markers such as arrows also may be helpful in close-up photos.

General photos should be taken showing the entire body of the animal: right and left sides, front (facial), hind (rear), dorsal, and ventral (if possible or appropriate) views. Photographs, with and without scale, should be taken of any obvious lesions, abnormal physical findings, and any evidence found on the body. It is important to take photographs showing the absence of injury, or "negative" photographs. Clear close-up views should be taken of any pertinent findings. The resolution of the photographs should be high enough to prevent loss of detail with photo enlargement for court. Digital SLR cameras with interchangeable lenses are preferred and a macro lens can be used to obtain clear close-up views of small lesions. Because of the sensitivity of fine detail lenses to movement, a mini-tripod may be used for stability.

For cases involving large numbers of animals, the photographs should first be downloaded in the original sequence to correspond to the photo logs. Folders may then be created for each animal ID and the photos from the scene and any examinations may be copied into that folder. This organization is extremely useful for the investigator, veterinarian, and prosecutor to refer to a particular animal.

Ultraviolet (UV) or infrared (IR) photography has been used extensively in humans to document underlying injuries when the skin is unbroken. UV light penetrates into the superficial tissue layers, whereas IR photography penetrates into the deeper tissue but fails to capture the more superficial injuries. The camera manufacturer should be contacted because not all digital cameras can be used for UV or IR photography. Handheld digital polarizing microscopes allow subdermal imaging. These units connect to a computer through a USB cable to enable viewing and image capture.

Video may be taken of the live animal exam. The video should begin with a shot of the case and animal ID number. Videography is most valuable when an animal shows obvious difficulty performing certain functions, such as neurological or ambulation problems. It is also helpful to show certain behaviors, such as vocalizing, because of pain or severe brain injury. In starvation cases, it is useful to video the animal's response when first given water and food. It is best to videotape anything that can be better appreciated through live recording.

EXAMINATION AND DOCUMENTATION OF THE LIVE ANIMAL

General

The examination of the animal involves looking for evidence that either supports or refutes the suspect's statement, investigation findings, or circumstances surrounding the crime. The veterinarian is working on behalf of the court and all findings should be recorded. Ideally, no examination should be conducted without all the information from the investigators and/or owner, including photographs and any reports or statements. This information provides the proper context from which the veterinarian can more accurately interpret the exam findings. In addition, it is important to understand the dynamics and potential movement of the victim and the assailant during the event when analyzing injuries, especially for reconstruction purposes. Using a live animal intake questionnaire (Appendix 9) can ensure that all pertinent information is obtained from the investigator.

When examining an animal, there must be full documentation of all the findings, including the positive and negative. From a legal standpoint, if it is not documented it was not done and what is not done in a case is more important that what is done. The exam should include written and photographic documentation. There are exam forms and diagrams that are useful for documenting exam findings and ensure that all pertinent information is collected (Appendices 10, 15–18). In addition, the exam form correlates to the report form (Appendix 20). It may be helpful to have a recording device when examining the animal to dictate findings. All notes, recordings, photographs, and reports are considered evidence and will be reviewed by the investigator, prosecutor, defense attorney, and judge or jury. There are some general considerations when documenting findings. Avoid leaving blanks when using forms; instead use "N/A" or strike through the item if no entry is required. Avoid editorial remarks on the record. Correct errors by drawing a single line through the entry and marking it "error" with the date and initials.

Upon arrival of the animal, any general impressions should be noted. This includes level of consciousness, behavior, posture, locomotion, body shape, nutritional condition, coat, abnormal sounds, and any notable abnormalities (Newberry and Munro 2011). The animal's strength, activity level, and any interaction with people and animals should also be documented. The record should contain the date and time of the animal arrival, method of transport, information on the person who brought the animal in, and date and time of exam. The animal identification should be recorded: species, breed or breed-type, sex (intact or not), age, weight, coat length, color, markings, tattoos, evidence or previous surgery and microchip information.

An age estimate should be made and a specific age only used if there is documentation provided and there is a notation in the record for the basis for the definitive age (e.g., verbally from the owner, medical records, dentition, growth plate closures; Table 3.1). There are numerous factors that can lead to erroneous determination of an animal's age. A broader category system may be used such as "juvenile," "adult," and "geriatric." Any medical history information should be obtained, including veterinary care, current medications or supplements, diet, and owner treatment.

EXTERNAL EXAMINATION

It is important to do a complete physical exam on a victim of animal cruelty. Depending on the nature of the case, additional diagnostics may be indicated. Radiographs are recommended for suspected cruelty cases to detect hidden trauma and evidence of historical abuse. The animal should be processed as a micro crime scene as discussed above and in Chapter 2. Every effort should be made to collect evidence prior to treatment to prevent contamination or loss of evidence, as long as the health of the animal is not placed at risk. One exception is with the presence of a penetrating object, where removal must be performed in a manner to protect the animal with effort to preserve associated evidence (Chapter 6). The following chapters discuss in detail the findings, examination considerations, and documentation of specific types of abuse.

The examination should be conducted with consideration to avoid transfer of evidence while handling the animal. The body should be inspected using a UV light source or ALS to detect biological and trace evidence (Figure 3.1). Trace evidence may be found on the surface or embedded deeper in the fur. Detection and collection of foreign trace evidence as well as the collection of fur exemplars are covered in Chapter 4. Any trace of biological evidence should be collected prior to proceeding with the exam.

The exam should include the weight, temperature, pulse, respiration, mucous membrane color, capillary refill time, and assessment of hydration status. In cases of sexual abuse, the temperature should be taken after appropriate

Table 3.1. Appearance of ossification centers and growth plate closures in dogs and cats.

Anatomic site	Dog	Cat
Vertebral column		
Vertebrae (except C1 and C2)	7–14 m	
Atlas	4 m	
Axis		
Apex of dens	3–4 m	
Dens and cranial articular surface	7–9 m	
Intercentrum	4 m	
Caudal epiphysis	7–9 m	
Two sides of arch	3 m	
Forelimb skeleton		
Scapula		
Coracoid process	5–8 m	5–8 m
Supraglenoid tubercle	3–7 m	3.5–4 m
Tuber of scapular spine	4–7 m	3.7 m
Humerus		
Proximal epiphysis (head and tubercles)	10–15 m	18–24 m
Distal epiphysis	5–8 m	4 m
Lateral condyle	5 m	3.5 m
Medial condyle	5 m	3.5 m
Lateral epicondyle	At birth	3.5 m
Medial epicondyle	5–6 m	4 m
Radius		
Proximal epiphysis	5–11 m	5–7 m
Distal epiphysis	6–12 m	14–22 m
Ulna		
Olecranon tubercle	5–10 m	9–13 m
Anconeal process	3–5 m	
Distal epiphysis	6–12 m	14–25 m
Carpus		
Radial carpus	3–4 m	
Other carpal bones	3–6 m	4 m
Metacarpus		
Metacarpal I (proximal epiphysis)	6–7 m	
Metacarpal II–V (distal epiphysis)	5–7 m	7–10 m
Phalanges I–V (proximal epiphysis)	4.5–7.5 m	4–5.5 m
Sesamoids		4–5 m
Carpal and dorsal sesamoids	4 m	
Volar sesamoids	2 m	
Hindlimb skeleton		
Pelvis		
Ilium	4–6 m	6 m
Ischium	4–6 m	6 m
Pubis	4–6 m	6 m
Acetabulum bone	4–6 m	
Iliac crest	1–2 y	
Tuber ischia	8–14 m	
Ischial arch	12 m	
Caudal pelvic symphysis, interischiadic bone	15 m–5 y	
Pubic symphysis	2.5–6 y	
Femur		
Lesser trochanter	8–13 m	8–11 m
Greater trochanter	6–9 m	7–10 m
Proximal epiphysis (head)	6–11 m	7–10 m
Distal epiphysis	6–12 m	13–19 m
Trochlea	3 m	
Patella	9 w	
Tibia		
Tibial tuberosity	8–10 m	12–18 m
Proximal epiphysis	6–15 m	12–18 m
Distal epiphysis	5–11 m	10–13 m
Medial malleolus	4–5 m	
Fibula		
Proximal epiphysis	6–12 m	13–18
Distal epiphysis	5–13 m	10–14 m
Tarsus		
Calcaneus (tuber)	3–8 m	7–13 m
Fibular	3–8 m	7–12 m
Metatarsus (distal epiphysis)	5–7 m	7–10 m
Phalanges: same as above		
Sesamoids		
Gastrocnemius	3 m	2–4 m
Popliteal	3 m	4–5 m
Metatarsophalangeal		2–4 m
Plantar phalangeal	2 m	
Dorsal phalangeal	5 m	

Source: Dyce, K.M., W.O. Sack, and C.J.G. Wensing, editors. 1996. *The Textbook of Veterinary Anatomy, Second edition*, pp. 395, 456, 471. Philadelphia: W.B. Saunders Company.

Liebich, H.-G. and H.E. König, editors. 2009. In: *Veterinary Anatomy of Domestic Mammals, Textbook and Colour Atlas*, Fourth edition, pp. 148, 224. Stuttgart: Schattauer.

Newton, C.D. and D.M. Nunamaker, editors. 1985. Canine and Feline Epiphyseal Plate Closure and Appearance of Ossification Centers, Appendix C. In: *Textbook of Small Animal Orthopaedics*, p. 1107–1113. Philadelphia: Lippincott.

Ticer, J. W., editor. 1975. Age of Appearance of Ossification Centers and of Bone Fusion in the Immature Canine. In *Radiographic Technique in Small Animal Practice*, First edition, p. 101. Philadelphia: W.B. Saunders Company.

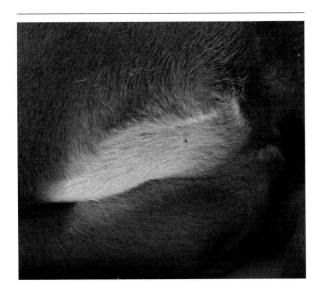

Figure 3.1. Use of UV light on a dog to detect foreign hair and fibers.

evidence collection (Chapter 12). The mentation and behavior should be noted, including interactions with people. The response to the offering of food or water should be recorded, especially in neglect cases, in which videography can be of value. All animals should be scanned for the presence of a microchip.

A general assessment of the animal's overall condition should be performed, including haircoat, skin, nails, and body condition score. The forms, including diagrams, provided in the Appendices may be useful (Appendices 15–16).

Body condition scoring (BCS) refers to a system of scoring the animal's body fat and muscle mass (Chapter 11). In animal cruelty cases it is primarily used in cases of starvation. It also may be used with large animal seizures such as hoarding or puppy mill cases. In these cases the animals may range in condition from emaciated to overweight. There are several BCS systems that may be used, depending on the species and nature of the case. The most commonly used system for dogs and cats is the Purina scale, which is a 9-point scale, and is available at their website: www.purina.com (Appendices 13–14). Tufts University has developed a system called the Tufts Animal Care and Condition (TACC) scales for dogs (Appendix 29). This system is a 5-point scale which is assigned in reverse order of the Purina scale (i.e., 1 = ideal). It should be noted on the report which BCS system is being used and a reference scale provided. The TACC also has a scoring system for weather safety, environmental health, and physical care scale, with detailed descriptions that may be useful in neglect cases.

The body should be inspected for any bruises, wounds, lesions, or evidence of older injuries. The fur should be shaved to show the extent of any injury found. Casting of penetrating wounds may be considered for analysis of bite wounds and weapon characteristics (Forensic Necropsy, below). The injuries should be documented by their location, distribution, and size. An estimate of the age of injury should be given, as is discussed in the following chapters. A time of injury can be estimated by the amount of granulation tissue (see Embedded Collars, Chapter 11).

The head should be examined for evidence of trauma including a fundic, oral, and otoscopic exam (Chapter 5). The head should be palpated for fractures and swellings. The mouth should be inspected for injury and foreign material. Depending on the nature of the case, swabs may be taken of the teeth for potential human DNA testing. The oral structures should be closely examined for evidence of trauma or neglect.

The animal should be evaluated for any signs of pain, especially related to a specific area. The presence and degree of pain play an important role in animal abuse cases (Chapter 4). Pain is indicative of the amount of suffering and severity of injury, which should be conveyed in the forensic report. Every animal is different in how it presents pain, which may be subtle, depending on the species, breed, and personality. It is important to describe the degree of pain and document any pain treatment and the response. The body should be palpated for swellings, area of tenderness, and other signs of injury. The tail is often injured in animal cruelty situations and the animal may present with the tail down. This subtle sign of injury may often go unnoticed because fearful animals usually tuck in their tails, which is a routine observation in the veterinary practice. The most common tail injuries are vertebral separation and fractures. Separation near the base of the tail may present as dissecting subcutaneous hemorrhage in the perineal region.

The examination of the feet is a crucial part of the physical exam. Extremely long nails may be an indicator of animal neglect. Nail growth rate can be variable in animals and negatively impacted by malnutrition. In young dogs, nails grow 1.9 mm/week, then slow to 0.8 mm/week (Muller et al. 2001). The feet may hold valuable trace evidence embedded in the fur or nails. Frayed nails, more commonly found in cats, are indicative of frantic movement of the feet against a rough surface that is associated with dragging, struggling to escape, or motor vehicle accidents. The nails may be slightly frayed, worn down to the base of the claw, or completely avulsed. Location descriptions of axial and abaxial can be used to identify the sides of the toes (Newberry and Munro 2011). The foot pads may show evidence of injury such as abrasions, lacerations, or punctures. Feet injuries are commonly found in severe, accidental trauma cases such as motor vehicle accidents. The feet may appear completely unremarkable, which, when placed in context with the rest of the exam findings and the case information, may be the key to what happened to the animal. It should be noted that the absence of findings may provide the most important clue to the cause of injury.

Measurements of the body may be taken and recorded to provide a baseline of information regarding the animal's condition to assess progress on follow-up examinations. Circumference measurements of the thorax (at the elbow), abdomen, neck, and thighs should be documented (Newberry and Munro 2011). If any blood stains or blood spatter are found at the crime scene, certain measurements of the body may be needed for the bloodstain analysis (Chapter 2). Whenever there is a wound on the body that could have created blood spatter at the crime scene, measurements are be taken from the wound to the muzzle, tail, and floor. Additional measurements may be taken of any area of interest based on circumstances surrounding the death or injury, crime scene findings, or the initial exam.

After examination and any treatments, it is important to document the progress of the animal's recovery, including weight gain, and repeat appropriate tests. The plan for monitoring the animal's progress depends on the type of case and the medical issues. When the animal does not remain under the direct care of the examining veterinarian, a protocol is needed ensure communication and documentation of the animal's progress. The timelines, treatments, and response should be documented. The reasons for the animal's negative or positive progress or recovery should be addressed in the final report.

Radiographs

A common finding in victims of animal cruelty is evidence of historical or repetitive abuse. In cases of interpersonal violence, blunt force trauma is the most common type of injury found in animals. It is important to take radiographs of suspected victims of cruelty, regardless of the physical exam findings. Full body radiographs can detect hidden injuries as well as previous fractures.

Fractures seen on radiographs without bony callus may be due to acute or non-acute fractures. Palpation may reveal evidence of non–bony callus indicative of a healing fracture. Some fractures cannot be palpated and the callus may be detected only on necropsy exam. The time for healing of a fracture is variable depending largely on the degree of displacement, stability of the fracture, and nutritional

status and age of the animal. With rib fractures, the surrounding rib cage serves to stabilize the site to promote healing despite respiration movement. A minimally displaced rib fracture can be expected to heal in eight to 16 weeks in adults, though healing can occur more rapidly with juvenile animals.

Radiographs also can be useful in poisoning cases, especially when a food source different than the animal's normal diet has been used. Depending on the food, there may be radiographic evidence of bony fragments within the gastrointestinal tract, or in early digestion the form of food may be identified such as dry kibble.

Sample considerations

With any cruelty case, consideration should be given to the potential of evidence transfer between the animal, the scene, and the abuser, which may become important as the investigation progresses. Samples should be collected as discussed in Chapter 4. A fecal sample may be needed for DNA testing (Chapter 4). In starvation cases, the feces should be examined for evidence of foreign material the animal had ingested (Chapter 11). Any vomitus, blood, and urine should be collected for possible testing in suspected poisoning cases (Chapter 10). Additional samples and analysis may be indicated based on the examination findings and case information. Consideration should be given to collecting and holding samples, such as blood and urine, until a decision is made regarding any testing.

Clinical pathology

Consideration should be given to performing blood work to establish a minimum database and to detect underlying problems and contributing causes of injury or illness as well as confirm physical exam findings. It may be important to rule out infectious diseases such as parvovirus or feline leukemia. Common conditions seen in animal cruelty cases, including stress, inflammation, dehydration, and fasting (starvation), can all affect laboratory values.

Markers of stress may be found in clinical pathology tests. Stress is a common cause of mature neutrophilia along with lymphopenia and eosinopenia. However, expected stress-induced changes may not be found on every laboratory result. In dogs, mild to moderate monocytosis may be seen with stress. In cats, it is common to see neutrophilic leukocytosis in response to fear or excitement such as with struggling or exercise. This is because of the marginal pool of neutrophils that are shifted to the circulating pool. Cats have a much larger marginal pool than dogs, which can cause a significant physiological leukocytosis (three marginal neutrophils to every one circulating neutrophil). Cats also can have pronounced transient lymphocytosis in response to the same stimuli because of the lymphocytes' ability to divide and recirculate between blood and tissues (Latimer and Tvedten 1999).

In hospitalized animals, monocytosis is found in approximately 11% of cats and 30% of dogs. Monocytes serve to replenish macrophages in tissues. In addition to stress causes, monocytosis may be seen in acute and chronic disease processes, although they are considered a later component of the inflammatory response. Severe stress is normally the cause of lymphopenia and eosinopenia. With monocytosis in the absence of lymphopenia and eosinopenia, inflammation or tissue destruction should be suspected (Latimer and Tvedten 1999).

Inflammation can cause leukocytosis, neutrophilia with or without a left shift, and toxic neutrophils (Burkhard and Meyer 1995). Acute inflammation (septic and nonseptic) usually causes neutrophilia. Chronic inflammation typically has monocytosis with minimal to absent leukocytosis or left shift. The leukogram may be normal with mild, chronic, or surface inflammation, such as with cystitis (Latimer and Tvedten 1999).

Dehydration causes decreased glomerular filtration and the urine specific gravity may be increased. The animal may be azotemic because of dehydration. Total protein, sodium, chloride, and potassium may be increased as a result of dehydration (Chapter 11).

Elevated creatine kinase may be an indicator of muscle trauma, inflammation, or increased catabolism seen with starvation (Chapter 11). Myoglobinuria may be seen with muscle disease or trauma. The urine occult blood test may be positive with hematuria, hemoglobinuria, or myoglobinuria.

Blood loss calculation

The amount of blood lost by an animal because of injury is an important measurement for a criminal investigation (Chapter 5). This can be calculated from the animal's hematocrit or the environment (Chapter 2). In response to acute blood loss, the body draws fluid into the blood vessels over time to maintain the blood pressure which in early evaluation may present as a reduced hematocrit and normal total protein. The accuracy of the initial hematocrit depends on the time elapsed and the administration of resuscitative fluids. A calculation of the blood loss volume may be made using the presenting hematocrit, the normal blood volume (8%–9% of body weight (kg) for dogs and 5%–6% of body weight (kg) for cats), and the average normal hematocrit for the species.

$$(\text{Normal Ave. Hct} - \text{Current Hct}) \div \text{Normal Ave. Hct} = \text{Fractional Blood Loss}$$

$$\text{Fractional Blood Loss} \times \text{Normal Blood Volume} = \text{Blood Volume Loss}$$

Parasites

When conducting an exam on a live or deceased animal, it is important to look for, identify, and address heartworm infection, intestinal parasites, or ectoparasites. Parasites are typically easily prevented and treated. They are normally addressed during routine veterinary visits, especially in young animals. They can cause stunted growth and disease, which may become life threatening. Several parasites have zoonotic potential, posing a significant health risk. It is important to document the treatment and standard prevention protocols for each parasite. The medical history should be reviewed for any prior documented recommendations regarding parasite treatment or prevention.

FORENSIC NECROPSY

Docimasia is a word that derives from the ancient Greek "*dokimasia*," which means "examination" or "test." In the medicolegal context it is used as "proof." It was first applied in the determination of whether a fetus was born alive or dead. It is one of the tests performed at necropsy, called Hydrostatic Docimasia of Galeno, which consists of placing the lungs of the fetus in the water: if lungs float, it indicates that the lungs contain air and that the newborn was born alive and breathed. It is also a useful test for cases of drowning. Nowadays docimasia is also applied to the tests that help forensic scientists prove causes of death and time of death. With respect to veterinary forensic pathology there are vast areas of investigation and comparative methods that can be very important in forensic pathology for human and veterinary medicine. Both areas can benefit with joint efforts made by the two professions working together to promote forensic science.

Overview

The difference between a necropsy and a forensic necropsy is in its objectives and relevance. In addition to determining the cause of death, the goal is to establish the manner of death (non-accidental, accidental, natural, undetermined), any contributory causes, and the time of death. Because of the medicolegal implications of the forensic necropsy, all positive and negative findings must be documented. The forensic necropsy exam is a process of documentation and interpretation of findings, the determination or exclusion of other contributory or causative factors, and a final determination of the cause and manner of injury and death. It is important to obtain information about the circumstances leading up to and surrounding the death prior to performing a necropsy.

Information should be obtained regarding any medical exam prior to death including photographs, diagnostics, test results, treatments, procedures, any resuscitative measures, and if the animal was euthanized, including the route of administration because it could affect the necropsy finding (enlarged spleen, euthanasia solution, and hemorrhage in the chest). Prior procedures may have created wounds that may be misinterpreted as injuries or altered original injuries. Any medical devices should not be removed until a necropsy is performed. The case information should be provided, including the investigator's report, crime scene findings, and photographs. Using a deceased animal intake questionnaire can ensure all pertinent information is obtained (Appendix 8). If the body is being submitted to a veterinary diagnostic laboratory it is important to make them aware that this is a potential legal/forensic/abuse case and discuss their protocols and lab policies concerning such cases.

The forensic necropsy actually begins at the scene, known as peri-necropsy in medicolegal terminology. The documentation and handling of deceased animals at the crime scene is discussed in Chapter 2. Although it has been recommended that the body should not be frozen prior to examination, in some cases it may not be possible due to limited facilities or the body was found frozen. If the animal is found in a frozen state, the body temperature and condition should be recorded and the body kept frozen until the necropsy is performed. The veterinarian or veterinary pathologist can then thaw the body in a controlled environment to prevent further decomposition artifacts. For forensic purposes histopathological examination should be performed even in a body that was previously frozen. Freezing can preserve evidence of injury within the tissue such as hemorrhage, neglect such as bone marrow fat, and evidence of poisonings such as oxalate crystals associated with ethylene glycol.

Gross necropsy

A complete necropsy should be performed in cases in which the cause of death is unknown, with full photographic documentation (Photography and Videography, above). Submission forms and case information should be reviewed prior to the necropsy to verify the identity of the animal, determine imaging needed, and ensure that appropriate precautions are taken to prevent human and animal health risks such as suspected rabies or cyanide poisonings. It is advisable to have protocols or standard operating procedures for handling and performing forensic necropsies. This helps establish consistency, thoroughness, and objectivity (Munro and Munro 2011). A necropsy exam form (which correlates to the necropsy report template), diagrams, and a fixed tissue checklist are provided in the Appendices (Appendices 11, 12–18, 21).

The condition and method of the body arrival should be documented, including courier information and retaining the shipping label. The packaging should be recorded, including bags and wrapping, noting any fluid leakage. Information about the prior body storage should be recorded. The photographs begin with the case and animal ID information, are followed by photographs of the unopened body package, and continue with documentation of the removal of each layer of packaging or wrapping around the body. Depending on the case, consideration should be given to retaining all material immediately surrounding the body, bag, or other wrapping for possible evidence analysis such as trace or biological evidence. Any additional evidence associated with the animal may have become detached or was placed inside the bag by investigators such as dog collars, tie-outs, or dog toys. This evidence should be collected and packaged separately. The feet or head may have been covered and secured with bags to prevent evidence loss and contamination. These bags should be carefully removed and examined for loose evidence inside. The bags may need to be held for further evidence examination and packaged appropriately.

External exam

The external exam is conducted in the same manner and with the same considerations as covered in the Live Animal section above. Any identifying tattoos, ear tags, or brand marks (large animals) should be photographed and recorded. The body should be scanned for microchips if possible. The sex of the animal should be verified. The findings and documentation associated with different types of injuries and abuse are discussed in detail in the following chapters. For necropsies, the presence and location of rigor and lividity should be recorded. The level of decomposition should be assessed. Any odors from the body (decomposition, smoke, motor oil, insecticides, feces, etc.) should be described. Any entomology evidence should be collected and preserved according to the instructions in Chapter 15.

Casts may be taken of penetrating wounds and bite marks to capture weapon characteristics and preserve bite mark patterns. Mikrosil™ is an easy-to-use and inexpensive casting material available from evidence collection supply companies. It comes in a variety of colors, but brown is the preferred color by tool mark examiners. It is a two-part substance with two speeds of hardeners in the kit. The slow hardener is appropriate for normal casting and the fast hardener used for very cold climates. The casting material and hardener must be completely mixed and the material is workable for approximately one to two minutes with the cast properly hardened in approximately 10 minutes. The cast cannot be permanently marked with a pen so it must be placed in a suitable marked container.

In human forensic medicine the use of computed tomography (CT) and magnetic resonance imaging (MRI) has gained favor to complement the forensic autopsy and is being used more frequently in animal forensic necropsies. The images produced allow better visualization of injuries and assessment of impact forces. They can aide in the detection of evidence not easily seen on routine radiographs. In addition, they are more aesthetically acceptable in court.

Necropsy technique

Because any necropsy may potentially involve infectious agents, appropriate protective clothing should be worn such as coveralls or scrubs, plastic apron, boots, and gloves. Goggles and masks should be available. The location for performing a necropsy should be a designated area for necropsies in the veterinary practice or a veterinary diagnostic laboratory. If a field or on-site farm necropsy must be performed there should be a readily available water source to help remove blood and ingesta from instruments and organs as needed.

Instrumentation needed to perform necropsies on either large animals, avian, or small animals includes knives, knife steel, scissors, forceps, scalpel with blades, cutting board, rib-cutters, cleaver or hacksaw, Stryker saw (if electricity is available), large-mouth glass or plastic containers, sterile Whirl-pak® bags, plastic bags, string, rubber gloves, culture swabs, paper bags, glass microscope slides, labels, formalin, centimeter rulers, sterile syringes and needles, glass blood collection tubes and insulated containers with ice packs or other coolants for chilling specimens. The primary fixative needed is 10% buffered neutral formalin. Remember that samples for histopathology should be no more than 0.5 cm–1 cm thick and 3×4 cm (length and width) to fix properly. The exceptions are brain, spinal cord, and eye. The ratio of tissue to formalin is 1:10 in the wide mouth containers.

The necropsy should include an examination of all the internal organs and consideration given to sample collection for histopathology, microbiology, virology (fluorescent antibody testing), parasitology, clinical pathology, and toxicology. Histopathology should always be considered when there are no significant findings on gross necropsy. It should also be considered to determine or eliminate contributing causes of illness or death.

Before starting the procedure it is important to consider shaving the entire body of the animal to allow observation of skin lesions that are hidden by fur. Shaving of specific areas can be done after skin reflection if evidence of injury is detected in the subcutaneous or deeper tissues. Unless prohibited by the history and trauma/evidence, the body of reptiles, birds, and very small mammals (rodents, pocket pets) are placed on their backs. Horses are placed on their right side. Cattle, sheep, goats, pigs, dogs, cats, etc. are placed with their left side down. An incision is made through the skin on the midline from the tip of the chin to the rectum, avoiding the penis. The skin is dissected away from the body, exposing the underlying subcutaneous tissue and muscle. The muscle layers are dissected and reflected to expose deeper tissue areas. These are critical steps in the necropsy procedure, allowing visualization of the extent of obvious external injury and detection of hidden injuries (Figure 3.2).

The necropsy procedure should be adjusted based on the crime scene information, the alleged events, and the exam findings. The following process of cutting limbs should only be conducted when those areas are not involved with injury. The right front leg should be grasped and lifted. All muscles should be cut between the subscapular area and the rib cage to free the limb; the leg should be laid back on the table or removed entirely from the body. The prescapular and axillary lymph nodes should be examined for location, size, and color. The hind limbs can be cut at the coxofemoral articulations to allow them to lie flat on the table. When deflecting the coxofemoral joint the articular surfaces of the acetabulum and femur should be evaluated. The skeletal muscles of the limbs should be evaluated at this point. The body should be examined for hemorrhages, fractures, body condition, fat atrophy, and amount of autolysis. Fractures, lacerations, puncture wounds, and any lesions should be photographed and measured using scales and appropriate markers. For areas of trauma with vascular injury, a catheter guide wire may be useful for the detection of the vascular injury site. The vessel may be collapsed and be hidden by clots or surrounding tissue. The guide wire may be inserted in the site of injury or from a nearby vessel to determine the branch from which it originated (Takahashi, Kinoshita, and Funayama 2011). Another method is to use a syringe filled with water which can be inserted into a portion of the

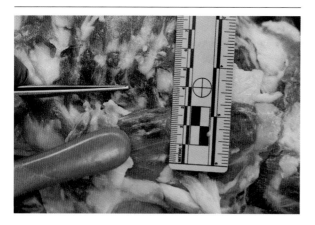

Figure 3.2. Deep tissue bruising over the thorax, revealed with muscle reflection.

blood vessel proximal to the area of concern using a soft IV catheter. A relatively tight seal must be made around the catheter end using fingers, sutures, or a clamp. As the water is injected into the vessel water can be visualized escaping from the area of injury.

A routine necropsy procedure should be followed. To open the abdomen, a shallow incision should be made through the abdominal muscles and peritoneum adjacent to the last rib. The opening should be lifted and then enlarged to the xiphoid cartilage of the sternum. The opening should continue to be enlarged dorsally and then caudally. Any fluid, blood, or foreign objects in the abdomen should be noted. The amount of fluids or blood should be measured, especially when cases of blunt trauma and rupture of internal organs are suspected. The abdominal cavity is examined for any abnormalities such as organ displacements, torsions, color of internal organs, and size of organs. A note should be made about whether the diaphragm is intact. The diaphragm is punctured and one should listen for the presence of negative pressure.

Next, one should cut deeply into the submandibular muscles close to the inner rims of the mandibles, then dissect around the tongue and retract the tongue and disarticulate the hyoid bones. The tonsils, palate, and mouth should be examined. The tongue should be lifted backward toward the chest and the trachea and esophagus dissected back to the thoracic inlet. In cases of suspected trauma to the neck the tissue around the esophagus, trachea, and neck in general is examined thoroughly prior to removal of the tongue/trachea/esophagus, as just described. It is recommended to remove the chest and abdominal organs prior to removal of congested neck organs to prevent producing artifactual hemorrhages in the neck muscles.

The ribs are removed using pruning shears or rib cutters and cutting along the costochondral junctions from the last to the first rib. The wall of the rib cage is detached by cutting along the base of the ribs to expose the internal thoracic organs. The presence and amount of any fluids or blood should be measured. Samples for culture of fluid or organ surfaces should be taken at this time. The position, color, texture, and size of the lungs and thoracic tissues should be noted. The lungs should be palpated for any nodules or firmness.

Next, samples can be taken or the organs can be removed to a necropsy table for individual examination. For cases of lung injury, especially with decomposed tissue, the lungs can be placed in water and then inflated to better visualize the damaged areas. A tracheal intubation tube is inserted into the trachea, a blower attached (such as a shop vac), and the lesions detected with bubble formation (Gerdin 2011). The esophagus and trachea should be opened and the mucosal surface examined. White foam (edema fluid), fluid, or aspirated food should be documented and sampled. The intestinal tract should be opened and any parasites noted, including a description of the estimated parasite burden. Any heartworms found should be described, including the amount.

Sample collection is important for potential testing and/ or histopathology evaluation to document any abuse and any underlying conditions which may have contributed to antemortem illness, disease, or death. Samples of all organs (trachea, esophagus, tip of tongue, thyroids, lungs, heart, thymus, lymph nodes, stomach, pancreas, duodenum, ileum, jejunum, colon, adrenals, kidneys, urinary bladder, liver, ovaries/uterus/testicles, prostate, spleen, muscle, bone marrow, skin, and brain) should be placed in 10% buffered formalin, remembering to section completely through the tissue. For example, the kidney samples should include from the cortex down through the renal pelvis. The intestines should be opened to examine the contents and the mucosal surface. Abnormal areas of any organ should be sampled in addition to the more normal adjacent areas. It is important to have adequate formalin in the containers for the amount of tissue for adequate preservation (one part tissue to ten parts liquid).

After the internal organs have been examined and removed from the body, the head can be disarticulated from the body for further examination. The animal is positioned on its back and the knife or scalpel is used to cut the connective tissue and skin over the left and right side of the atlas (first vertebra) until the atlanto-occipital junction ventral foramen is exposed. The knife is inserted into the atlanto-occipital foramen, incising the spinal cord and cutting from the center, laterally loosening the remaining

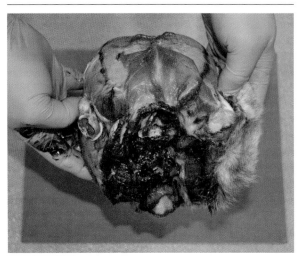

Figure 3.4. Lines (black) demonstrating where to cut the tissue and skull to remove the brain. (Photo courtesy of Dr. Doris Miller.)

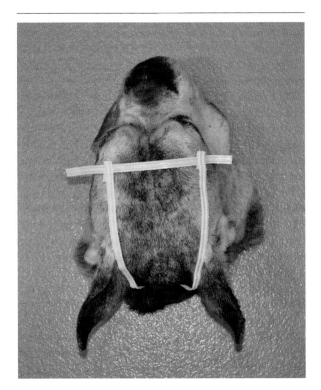

Figure 3.3. Cutting lines for brain removal. (Photo courtesy of Dr. Doris Miller.)

attachments. Slight pressure is applied to the tip of the jaw until a release of the attachments is felt. The head is bent backwards and the remaining tissues of the dorsal neck and skin are severed.

After the head is disarticulated, the skin is removed dorsocranially over the skull. The musculature is removed, exposing the calvarium. The choice of cutting instruments depends on the individual and if a source of electricity is available. For small or young animals and birds the calvarium and caudal wall of the cranial cavity may be broken away piecemeal from the foramen magnum with scissors, bone cutting forceps, or shears. In larger or older animals, once the calvarium is exposed, three cuts with a hand saw, hatchet (large animals), or Stryker saw (small animals) can be used to loosen the calvarium. The first line is parallel and behind the orbits. The other two lines are perpendicular to the first line and connect to the foramen magnum. These last two lines should reach the foramen magnum (Figures 3.3 and 3.4).

The skull is reflected caudally by pushing the front edge of the cut skull caudally, leaving the brain in the head. The dura mater is removed with scissors. If indicated, culture swab samples can be taken at this time of areas between the

cerebellum and brainstem prior to removal of the brain. The skull is held upside down or the rostral part of the head is elevated (large animals) and the cranial nerves cut so the brain is allowed to fall out caudally onto the hands or a clean surface. The pituitary gland also can be removed from the skull at this time. After removal, the brain is sectioned longitudinally along the midline to create symmetrical sections. One half can be saved for microbiology or other testing and one half can be placed into formalin. The brain placed into formalin may need to be further sliced or sectioned depending on its size. If there is a specific lesion in the brain samples of the lesion may need to be taken for both microbiology and histopathology. Special samples also are required in sheep, goats, and cattle in certain states for scrapie and bovine spongiform encephalopathy (BSE) testing. To examine the nasal sinuses, the rostrum may be sectioned along the sagittal midline. It may be preferable for a veterinary diagnostic laboratory to perform the internal cranial exams. The laboratory should be contacted regarding submission of the head and/or brain.

The heart can be examined while still attached to the lungs or it can be removed and then further examined. The surface of the heart, including the epicardial fat, should be examined for any indications of serous atrophy which may appear less white, more gray, and gelatinous. The presence of a small volume of blood-stained fluid in the pericardial sac may be a postmortem artifact related to freezing and thawing. The heart is positioned with the left ventricle on the right, the right ventricle on the left, and the left longitudinal groove vertical. A vertical incision is made in the left ventricle from the ventricle up through the left atrioventricular (AV) valve. The valves should be transparent and not nodular. A second similar vertical incision is made in the right ventricle which extends into the pulmonary valves. This incision is continued in a "U" or "V" shape to the right AV (tricuspid) valve. One should look for any septal defects and vascular shunts. The myocardium should be incised in several areas looking for hemorrhage, mineralization, or fibrosis. If cardiomyopathy is suspected, a horizontal cut should be made across both ventricles midway between the apex and atrium. Samples from the heart for histopathology should include sections from both ventricles, papillary muscles, interventricular septum, atria, and valves.

The joints of the limbs can be opened and examined for signs of inflammation or trauma. The synovial, joint capsule, ligaments, and articular surfaces can be examined and samples collected. The skin is reflected away from the joint to ensure cleanliness. The leg should be moved and manipulated to locate the articulation, and an incision made on the medial joint capsule and ligaments. With additional manipulation and downward pressure on the distal portion of the extremity the joint should pop open. The stifle joint can be opened by cutting along the proximal and medial edges of the patella and reflecting the patella laterally. If samples for toxicology are needed, as in determination of barbiturates or other drugs used in race horses (see next section), fluid can be withdrawn from the joints with a needle and syringe. If bacterial infection is suspected, swabs should be taken of the joint fluid. Sterile technique should be used when opening the joint and the joint immediately swabbed upon opening.

Often the extent and manner in which the spinal cord is removed and examined depends on the history and the size of the animal. To show dorsal or ventral dislocations of vertebrae, fractures, extruded disks, or ventral exostoses the entire vertebral column is cut longitudinally on a band saw. An electric reciprocating saw may be used if the body is suspended by the rear legs or hand saws may be used, although it is much slower than electric saws.

To remove the spinal cord, the remaining limbs and ribs are removed from the spinal column. The remaining muscle and connective tissue are trimmed away from the dorsolateral surface of the spinal column. Bone rongeurs or a Stryker saw are used to cut through the dorsal vertebral wall (dorsal arches) to expose the spinal cord. Once all the dorsal vertebral arches have been removed, the cord is examined *in situ* for any discolorations or abnormalities. The dura surrounding the cord is grasped and the spinal nerves gently

cut. After removing the cord, the floor of the vertebral canal and intervertebral discs are examined. In large animals (see below) an axe, hatchet, or cleaver can be used to firmly but gently remove the lateral processes of the vertebrae in a systematic fashion, slowly shaving off more and more of the processes until the vertebral canal is opened enough to expose the spinal cord. If only a portion of the cord is needed, in large animals the vertebral column can be sectioned into several small pieces and the cord removed from one end of the spinal canal. In small animals, once the cord is removed the entire cord can be placed into formalin. For large animals, the dura should be split and the cord can be sectioned every 30 cm, leaving a small piece of dura connecting the sections together to help with identification. Alternately, the cord can be sectioned and wrapped in paper towels, marked with pencil to identify the cranial and caudal ends, and then placed into formalin.

Additional samples from any wounds, injuries, lungs, trachea, intestines, kidneys, liver, spleen, skin with fur attached, feces, and half the brain should be placed in individual containers to be held for cultures, toxicology, or further testing. Stomach contents and urine should be saved in glass or leakproof containers for toxicology. The femur can be cracked to allow the formalin to penetrate the tissues better during fixation. In starvation cases, a bone may be refrigerated or frozen for bone marrow fat analysis (Chapter 11). If the animal is small (especially with young cats and dogs), right and left femurs, humerus, and ribs may be required to obtain the minimum 5 gm of bone marrow needed for testing.

Based on the nature of the case, investigation information, and exam findings, specific tissue samples may be collected for histopathology examination. For strangulation cases this may include tongue, larynx, neck muscle, and surrounding neck tissues. Histopathology may be needed to distinguish between areas of bruising or imbibition and any vital reaction. Fractures should be preserved and examined to determine antemortem or postmortem injury, evidence of healing, and the degree of healing.

If the eyes are to be removed for histopathologic examination, samples for fluid analysis should be collected first. The third eyelid (membrane nictitans) should be grasped with forceps and while pulling outward, blunt tip scissors or a scalpel should be used to cut through the extraocular soft tissues surrounding the globe in a 360° circle. The tissue is gradually clipped around the eye, loosening the globe until the optic nerve can be clipped and the globe removed intact. The ideal fixative for eyes is Davidson's fixative but formalin fixation is acceptable and routine in most laboratories.

The severely decomposed, skeletonized, or burnt body should be handled very carefully. Depending on the level of decomposition it may still be possible to gather significant information from a postmortem exam, including necropsy and osteology examination (see Animal Forensic Osteology below and Chapter 14). Previously buried bodies should be evaluated for live or deceased burial (Chapter 9). Skin and muscle reflection may show areas of hemorrhage which may vary in discoloration from dark red-brown to black, depending on the breakdown of hemoglobin. Gross exam may reveal evidence of trauma. Depending on the decomposition, samples of organs may be taken for microscopic examination and toxicology testing such as ethylene glycol poisoning. Stomach contents may be collected for toxicology analysis. Examination of bones may reveal evidence of trauma. With decomposition, appropriate samples are needed for DNA testing (Chapter 4).

Once the necropsy examination is complete the organs should be replaced in the body cavity and the skin sutured. This is not only respectful of the cadaver and the owner but it also preserves the body and organs in the event a re-examination is required. The area should be thoroughly washed down with water and disinfected, regardless of the necropsy location (i.e., within a building or at a farm). Depending on any pending tests and the circumstances surrounding the case, the body may be held in refrigeration or frozen. The body is considered evidence and cannot be disposed of without permission from the appropriate legal authorities, either the investigating or prosecuting agency. Disposal is usually contingent upon: there has been full photographic documentation of the exam and any evidence of injury, all testing is complete, all samples have been collected, there are no further tests needed where the body is required, and there is no request from the opposing counsel to have a separate examination performed.

Necropsy examination of food animals and horses

The same initial protocols are followed as previously discussed regarding case information, history, and documentation. Considerations for the external exam include nasal exudates, oral ulcers, eye lesions, skin abrasions, foot lesions, swollen joints, umbilical hernias, evidence of diarrhea, body condition, tattoos, etc. Food animals are placed with their left side down so that the rumen is down in cattle, sheep, and goats, while for pigs the spiral colon of the pig should be visible when the abdominal cavity is opened. Horses are placed on their right sides so the liver, cecum, left dorsal, and left ventral colon with diaphragmatic and pelvic flexures are visible when the abdominal cavity is exposed.

Incisions are made in the right front axillary and right rear coxofemoral joints. If the animal had recently died, blood can be collected from the axillary area. Unless the hide needs to be preserved, a cut is made from the chin to the inguinal area connecting with the previous incisions. The skin is reflected dorsally and ventrally. Mammary glands, umbilicus, lymph nodes, and subcutaneous tissues are examined for edema, trauma, and hemorrhage along with the adjacent musculature. The abdominal musculature is incised through just caudal to the ribs, with care exercised to avoid puncturing the internal organs. The abdominal wall is reflected ventrally. If there is any fluid in the peritoneal cavity, one should stop and collect samples for culture and measure and estimate or measure the volume. The color and consistency of the fluid should be recorded. The abdominal organs are examined carefully, noting any evidence of hemorrhage or trauma. After incising and reflecting the muscle tissue, the ribs are cut with the rib-cutters in a line from the dorsal end near the spinal column of the first rib to the last rib. The entire thoracic wall is removed in one piece by cutting at the costosternal junctions. In a field necropsy this thoracic wall may be used as a place to lay out organs during the exam.

With the thoracic and abdominal organs exposed, the condition of the animal should be assessed and note made of any abnormalities. The presence or lack of body fat and muscle mass, the degree of postmortem autolysis, sex of animal, displacement of organs, hemorrhages, tumors, presence of urine, discolorations, etc. are noted.

The lips, teeth, and oral cavity should be examined. The tongue is removed by making two incisions medial to the right and left mandible. A finger is inserted to pull the tongue ventrally to the exterior while continuing to the connections to the tongue. In horses or animals with narrow jaws, it may be necessary to saw through the mandibular symphysis to remove the tongue. While pulling the tongue toward the thoracic cavity, the articulation of the hyoid bones at the "V" formed by these bones should be cut. One should continue to reflect the larynx, esophagus, and trachea. The guttural pouches in horses are to be examined at this time. The esophagus, trachea, and lungs are removed as previously described for companion animals. The rostral tip of the tongue should be cut and examined for vitamin E-selenium responsive conditions.

After examination, the abdominal organs can be removed and sampled. The omentum should be removed in ruminants. The end of the colon and the end of the proximal duodenum should be tied off and cut, allowing the small and large intestines to be removed as a unit. Next, the rumen, reticulum, omasum, and abomasum can be removed as a single unit. The contents of the stomachs and intestines can be examined and sampled for parasitology, microbiology, and toxicology, including the mucosal surface of the opened sections of intestines. Tied-off sections of intestine can be saved for fresh/frozen tissue examination. The color, consistency, and odor of the contents to the forestomachs should be noted (Thacker 1986; Andrews, Van Alstine, and Schwartz 1986).

In the horse, after opening the abdomen the position and displacement of any organs should be noted. Distention of organs with gas, discolorations, volvulus, and torsions should be noted. The spleen, left kidney, and left adrenal should be removed and set aside. The distal colon is detached at its distal aspect close to the rectum in the pelvic canal and pulled it until the transverse colon is reached; it is then cut close to the right dorsal colon. Next, the ileum is located at the base of the cecum and cut close to the ileocecal valve. The ileum is detached and pulled until the caudal duodenum is reached. Most strangulations occur in the caudal portion of the jejunum and are more easily identified if the small intestine with the ileum is examined first rather than the duodenum. As the small intestine is removed, it can be laid out in a curved or zig-zag pattern for further examination later.

The stomach is removed. The abdominal aorta is located and opened, beginning caudal to the diaphragm and continuing to the iliac bifurcation. It is examined for thrombi or evidence of verminous arteritis. The aorta with the root of the mesentery is cut, and with the help of gravity the remainder of the large intestines is removed. The cranial mesenteric artery should be opened and observed for evidence of verminous arteritis. All the removed organs are examined and the appropriate samples taken. One should look for evidence of gastric ulcers and gastric bots in the stomach. The small and large intestines are opened and the mucosa observed. One should also look for parasites, foreign material, sand, or discolorations. Each region of the gastrointestinal tract is to be sampled for histopathology, culture, toxicology, etc.

Routine necropsy procedure for avian species

As previously mentioned it is important to review the history and case information with any avian submission. Information should include whether this is a single-animal problem or herd problem, clinical signs, species, age, history of trauma or disease, history of any treatment, and time of death if known. Proper routine protective clothing, gloves, and mask are indicated for avian necropsies and if possible conducted using a biosafety hood or downdraft table.

The animal should be weighed and examined for external lesions of the skin, feathers, eyes, nares, comb, wattles, beak, legs, feet, or keel bone. The body should be examined closely for evidence of ectoparasites (and collection), trauma, swollen joints, and tumors. Any leg band numbers should be recorded. Depending on the history, before opening the body swabs should be collected of the choana, trachea, and cloaca.

The feathers are moistened with soapy water to wet all of them and decrease the dander. The animal is placed on its back with the feet facing the veterinarian and the wings are reflected back. The skin is incised between the medial surface of each thigh and abdomen. The legs are reflected laterally and the coxofemoral joints disarticulated. A transverse skin incision is made across the middle of the abdomen and then the skin reflected cranially over the breast and caudally over the abdomen. Samples are taken of the thigh muscle, sciatic nerves, and breast muscle. The shape of the keel bone and amount of breast muscle is noted. Scissors are used to cut through one lateral commissure of the mouth so the oral cavity can be examined.

One should continue with a longitudinal incision through the skin of the neck to the thoracic inlet. The oral cavity, esophagus, trachea, and crop are examined. A longitudinal incision is made through the pectoral muscles on each side of the keel over the costochondral junctions. The abdominal cavity is opened with scissors and the incision continued anteriorly through the costochondral junctions using rongeurs if necessary to cut through the coracoids and clavicle bones at the shoulder. The breast is removed in one piece and the air sacs observed for cloudiness, thickening, and other lesions. All internal viscera should be examined for any abnormalities such as hemorrhage, discolorations, organ enlargements, adhesions, lack of adipose tissue, etc. The spleen can be located and removed for sampling at this time. It is located by lifting the left margin of the gizzard and reflecting it to the right. The spleen is located between the proventriculus and gizzard.

The esophagus is removed at the anterior border of the proventriculus and the entire gastrointestinal tract is removed posteriorly to the cloaca. The contents of crop and gizzard should be noted and can be saved for toxicology. Samples should be collected of the duodenum/pancreas, ceca, bursa of Fabricius, and all other major organs. The kidneys are located close to the dorsal body wall (backbone). The reproductive tract lies on top of the kidneys and varies in size depending on the age of the bird and season. Only the left ovary and oviduct are developed in females. The lungs are located close to the ribs and may be removed by gentle traction on the trachea or reflecting them medially from between the ribs with their color and consistency documented. The femur can be sectioned longitudinally with shears for examination of the bone marrow and growth plates. Removal of the brain is performed as previously described (Schwartz 1986).

General considerations for sample collection and analysis

There are several protocols for collection of fluid specimens from the body. A clean needle and syringe should always be used. Blood, stomach contents, urine, bile, and vitreous should be placed in glass containers. Plastic polymers can be leached out by these fluids, which can cause interference on gas chromatography where their peaks can mask certain compounds.

Collection of blood should be attempted from peripheral vessels for toxicology testing because of redistribution artifacts that are possible when taking blood from near the heart (Di Maio and Di Maio 2001). In descending order of preference, the collection locations are the femoral vessels, subclavian vessel, aortic root, pulmonary artery, superior vena cava, and heart. The blood should be placed in a glass tube (red top tube, lavender top) unless the blood is to be analyzed for volatiles; then the blood should be put in a tube with a Teflon®-lined screw top to avoid volatiles diffusing through a rubber stopper. Other fluid sampling guidelines include: all the vitreous should be collected (see Ocular Analysis); all the urine due to large quantities needed for certain drug testing such as steroid screens; and 10–20 ml of bile (Di Maio and Di Maio 2001). Appropriate DNA samples should be collected based on the level of decomposition (Chapter 4). There should be considerations for viral testing samples such as the bone marrow, which can be tested for certain viruses, and the spleen and small intestine, which can be tested for parvovirus.

Tests may be run on blood samples or blood clots to determine antemortem disease or correlate other necropsy findings. Postmortem blood chemistry may be affected by the decomposition process; therefore, blood should be drawn immediately after death. Alternatively, the vitreous may be of better use for certain tests (see below). Blood clots can be harvested and frozen in cases of suspected poisonings.

There are several documented findings of postmortem chemistry changes in humans that may be associated with antemortem medical conditions or cause of death; they are discussed in more detail in the following chapters. Elevated glucose levels have been found in fatal hypothermia cases. In humans, glycosylated hemoglobin, which is stable, and fructosamine, which slowly declines postmortem, may be used to help diagnose diabetes mellitus. Urea and nitrogen have been shown to be stable postmortem in blood, cerebrospinal fluid (CSF), and vitreous humor, even with moderate decomposition. On the other hand, serum electrolytes begin to decline shortly after death.

Antemortem dehydration may be determined with findings of both electrolyte imbalances (vitreous) and elevated urea nitrogen (Chapter 11). Calcium levels in the serum and vitreous rise slowly postmortem but are relatively stable in CSF the first ten hours after death. Total serum cholesterol remains stable and can correlate with high and low antemortem values. Serum total protein values are similar to antemortem levels except with significant hemolysis. Serum bilirubin may have a minor increase postmortem and may be used to correlate antemortem levels. Postmortem urine urobilinogen is reflective of antemortem concentrations. Serum strontium levels may be helpful in diagnosing saltwater drownings (Chapter 9). Serum enzymes increase rapidly after death for both humans and animals; these include alkaline and acid phosphatase, amylase, creatinine phosphokinase, lactic dehydrogenase, and transaminase. One exception is cholinesterase, which is stable for an extended postmortem interval (PMI), even under room temperature storage, and for ten days when refrigerated. Thyroid-stimulating hormone (TSH) is stable for up to twenty-four hours after death but thyroxin (T_4) decreases after death and triiodothyronine (T_3) is variable. Serum cortisol is stable in the early postmortem period. Urinary catecholamines (adrenaline and noradrenaline) may be increased in fatal hypothermia but hyperthermia cases have shown elevated noradrenaline and low adrenaline (Chapter 11). Serum insulin decreases postmortem. In dogs, blood gas analysis was conducted when fatal cardiac or respiratory arrest was induced. In cardiac deaths the PO_2 was more than 25 mm Hg compared with lower levels found in the respiratory deaths (Sturner 2006).

Aging injuries

To determine whether a wound was antemortem (before death), perimortem (at or near the time of death), or postmortem (after death) requires gross and/or microscopic exam. The aging of certain types of injuries are discussed in the following chapters. The presence of hemorrhage is indicative that the heart was still beating when the injury occurred and indicates antemortem injury. There is the possibility of postmortem hemorrhage associated with postmortem trauma such as when the vitreous is withdrawn from the eye using a syringe and needle. Decomposition can affect microscopic determination of hemorrhage requiring special testing (Chapter 14). The finding of blood ingestion or inhalation signs, such as blood in the alveolar airways, may help with determination of perimortem injuries.

If there is a sufficient survival time after the injury prior to death, there may be evidence of an inflammatory response, i.e., vital reaction, in the injured area seen on histopathology examination. In humans, this may take several hours (Di Maio and Di Maio 2001; Chapter 5). An injury without an inflammatory response is indicative that it occurred in close proximity to death. The nature of any inflammatory response may also determine a time interval, such as in the case of peritonitis resulting from intestinal rupture caused by blunt force trauma which may have evidence of chronic inflammation, including fibroblasts and hemosiderin (Dix and Graham 2000). The inflammatory responses can be affected by the age of the animal, tissues affected, medications, and health of the animal. The precise timing of the repair process is variable depending on the size of the wound and whether or not secondary infection develops. Typically, within twenty-four hours neutrophils appear at the margins of the wound and fibrin clot. Within twenty-four to forty-eight hours there is proliferation and migration of epithelial cells to begin to fuse the incision. By day three the neutrophils generally have disappeared and been replaced by macrophages. Granulation tissue invades the wound and by day five has filled the wound. The surface epithelium is back to its normal thickness with a mature epidermal architecture with surface keratinization. During the second week there is continued proliferation of fibroblasts and collagen (Table 3.2).

The presence of hemosiderin may be an indicator of antemortem hemorrhage. Hemosiderin often forms after a bleeding event. When blood leaves a ruptured blood vessel, the red blood cell dies and the hemoglobin of the cell is released into the extracellular space. The macrophages phagocytize the hemoglobin and degrade it, producing hemosiderin and porphyrin. Hemosiderin may be found as soon as forty-eight hours after injury in macrophages. It also may be found in scar tissue, indicating a longer time line for injury (Munro and Munro 2008).

The analysis of enzyme activity at the wound site using histochemistry, enzymology, and biochemistry can help differentiate antemortem vs. postmortem injury in humans. The use of the proximity ligand assay has been studied in humans. This assay provides reactivity when two marker proteins are in close proximity to each other. This has potential use for markers associated with transient reaction after injury, which are not seen in uninjured tissues. The platelet selectin, which shows rapid dynamics in the early phase of an injury, and platelet endothelial cell adhesion molecule showed a discrete early time window. Different

Table 3.2. Histologic changes with wound healing.

Histologic changes	Age of wound
Serum/clot with congestion, swelling, and leukocyte infiltration	24 hours
New capillaries	36 hours
Spindle-shaped cells at right angles to the vessels	48–72 hours
Fibrils parallel to the vessels	5–6 days
Birefringence developing in newly laid down collagen	21 days

Source: Munro, R. and H. Munro. 2008. Wounds and Injuries. In: *Animal Abuse and Unlawful Killing: Forensic Veterinary Pathology*, pp. 30–47. Edinburgh: Elsevier.

antibody combinations of the coagulation and complement systems consistently produced a negative reaction in uninjured samples and injuries of older age (Cedergren and Jepsen 2012). Enzyme activity can be detected up to five days postmortem and can be used to date the injury. In antemortem wounds, there is a zone of increased enzyme activity at the periphery that occurs over a set time interval for different enzymes.

Other markers, such as DNA, C3 factor, catecholamines, and vasoactive amines, have been used; histamine and serotonin are elevated in antemortem wounds (Di Maio and Di Maio 2001). The detection of tenascin and ubiquitin through immunohistochemistry has been used to estimate wound age in humans, including blunt force, sharp force, and gunshot wounds. Tenascin is an extracellular matrix glycoprotein that plays an important and unique role in the wound healing process.

Ubiquitin, also known as heat shock protein, is a small protein required for ATP-dependent non-lysosomal intracellular protein degradation. It plays a key role in heat shock response, protein breakdown, and regulation of immune responses (see Determination of Perimortem Stress, below). It is rapidly induced with traumatic stress acting as a cytokine-like protein with anti-inflammatory properties. It is expressed in the nuclei of neutrophils, macrophages, and fibroblasts in the wound area. Tenascin was reported positive in 91.8% of cases with wound age greater than twenty-four hours and negative in 98.3% with wound age less than twenty-four hours. Ubiquitin was reported in 26.14% of cases with wound age greater than twenty-four hours and 4.25% with wound age less than twenty-four hours. For wounds over forty days, tenascin was negative and ubiquitin was still expressed in fibroblasts (Guler et al. 2011).

Determination of perimortem stress: measurement of heat shock proteins

Determining survival time and cause of death is a challenge for forensic pathologists. One important task for the veterinarian or forensic pathologist is to document the concomitant physical and mental load of the victim's suffering, especially after a violent or painful death (Chapter 4). The determination of the length and/or intensity of the agonal period following various causes of death have been researched in humans, which has applications in veterinary forensic pathology, especially in situations where suffering is suspected to have occurred. The determination of the adrenaline levels and the amount of glycogen in the liver and adrenal glands as a measurement of stress is well documented in human forensic medicine. Recently, studies have shown that the measurement of heat shock proteins may be used to determine the level of stress during the time before death (Nogami et al. 1999).

Immunohistochemical investigation of these proteins can be of great value for diagnosing not only the cause of death but also the pathophysiological changes and the victim's past history (Nakasono 2001). The heat shock protein, ubiquitin, exerts an essential role in the cellular response to stress. Nogami et al. (1999) reported the usefulness of the ubiquitin expression in the locus coeruleus, located in the brainstem, as a marker for the evaluation of agonal stress. The immunohistochemical expression of ubiquitin was also examined in human locus coeruleus and significant differences in the number of ubiquitin-immunoreactive neurons were noted with respect to the length of the agony with a higher density of positive neurons reported in cases with a pronounced and extended death struggle or in cases of hypothermia (Preuß et al. 2008). The study by Quan et al. also reported that intranuclear ubiquitin immunoreactivity of the pigmented substantia nigra neurons in the midbrain was induced by a fatal severe stress on the central nervous system in asphyxiation and drowning deaths (Quan et al. 2001).

Ocular analysis

The vitreous of the eye may be analyzed for antemortem toxicology, certain disorders, and measurements for time of death estimates. The aqueous is commonly used in large animals for glucose, urea nitrogen, and toxicology testing. The vitreous is acellular, less susceptible to biochemical changes, and more resistant to decomposition than blood. In humans and dogs, the vitreous can be analyzed for electrolytes postmortem. The postmortem blood concentrations change as a result of cellular breakdown but most antemortem electrolyte abnormalities are reflected in the vitreous. The potassium measurement cannot be used to diagnose antemortem hyperkalemia because of the cellular potassium that is released postmortem. The measurement of this potassium release is sometimes helpful in determining time of death (Chapter 14). Hypokalemia may be reflected in the vitreous but this is uncommon because of the postmortem rise of potassium masking antemortem values. In addition, decomposition can lower the sodium and chloride levels (Di Maio and Di Maio 2001).

There are four patterns of abnormal vitreous electrolytes:

- Dehydration (hypertonic): high sodium and chloride with moderate increase in urea nitrogen
- Uremia: normal sodium and chloride with marked elevation of urea nitrogen and creatinine
- Low salt (hypotonic): decreased sodium and chloride with low potassium (less than or equal to 15 mEq/L)
- Decomposition: low sodium and chloride with increased potassium (greater than or equal to 20 mEq/L).

The sodium, chloride, and potassium must be measured at the same time (Sturner 2006).

The vitreous glucose levels of humans have a wide range (0–180 mg/dl) and are significant if elevated. Ketones may be measured in the vitreous and together with elevated glucose can confirm diabetic ketoacidosis (Sturner 2006). Vitreous bilirubin, alkaline phosphatase, serum glutamic oxaloacetic transaminase (SGOT), and calcium are of no value diagnostically (Di Maio and Di Maio 2001).

The vitreous is also useful for toxicological analysis in humans. The vitreous can be tested for a variety of drugs, including cocaine, morphine, propoxyphene, and tricyclic antidepressants (Di Maio and Di Maio 2001).

Mulla et al. showed that in humans there is no significant difference for potassium, sodium, chloride, or calcium levels between the same pair of eyes at the identical postmortem intervals for different subjects (Mulla 2005). This has also been shown in dogs with regard to potassium (Chapter 14). The sample should be aspirated carefully with a syringe and small needle, applying gentle pressure to minimize contamination. To collect the vitreous, a 12-ml syringe and needle should be used and a scleral puncture is performed on the lateral canthus; one should aspirate gently, avoiding tearing loose tissue fragments surrounding the vitreous chamber. It is recommended that a majority of the vitreous be removed, leaving behind a residual amount to avoid this contamination (Jashinani, Kale, and Rupani 2010). In cases where the eyes do not contain fluid, the interior of the globes can be rinsed with saline and the fluid

submitted for toxicological analysis (Perper 2006). Only clear, colorless samples should be analyzed. The sample is centrifuged and then the supernatant is tested. It is recommended to analyze the vitreous, only using clear fluid, as soon as possible because prolonged storage, either refrigerated or frozen, can affect the concentration of electrolytes. For potassium, refrigeration of the sample for lengthy periods does not deteriorate the levels (Jashinani, Kale, and Rupani 2010) and the sample may be frozen and held prior to testing.

SPECIAL CONSIDERATIONS

Animal forensic osteology

The examination of bones may be required to identify an individual animal, determine evidence of trauma, or determine the cause of death. The species of animal may be determined by macroscopic examination or through histological examination, even in cases where only pieces of bones are found. The age of the animal can be estimated based on tooth eruption, bone ossification, and growth plate closures (Table 3.1). There are a variety of circumstances in which bone examination may be indicated such as cannibalism, traumatic injury, animal fighting, fire victims, and buried remains (Chapter 2). There may be times when the species identification and number of individual animals is needed to consider additional animal cruelty charges. The medical history is invaluable to identify previously documented medical conditions that can be recognized on the skeleton including arthritic changes, healed fractures, and dental extractions. Bones may aid in the detection of drugs or toxins. Drug detection has been conducted successfully in human bones. The drugs include morphine, codeine, oxycodone, antidepressants, antihistamines, diazepam, and nordiazepam (McGrath and Jenkins 2009).

Examination of human bones falls under several disciplines, such as forensic anthropology and archeology. There has been a growing documentation of forensic osteology findings in animals with regard to cause of death, trauma, and investigations related to predator-human attacks. All bones, regardless of species, are similar in characteristics and responses to the environment, trauma, or modification of any kind. The study of osteology requires special training and experience. Forensic anthropologists and zooarcheologists may offer invaluable assistance. Because the interpretation of findings requires knowledge of the animal species, behavior, husbandry, and environment, forensic anthropologists need to consult with veterinarians when asked to evaluate animal skeletal remains. In addition, the understanding of soft tissue findings is very important to understand and interpret osteological findings.

Only recently has this collaboration gap and the potential impact on forensic analyses been recognized in the human forensic field. One retrospective study found disparity regarding the mechanism of trauma and number of impacts between autopsy and forensic anthropology findings. Only 76% of the cases were consistent with mechanism of trauma and 12% of the skeletal examinations were unable to determine the mechanism of trauma though it had been determined on autopsy. Only 27% of the skeletal findings were consistent with the number of impacts found on autopsy (Morcillo 2012). The following is a general overview of osteology including documented findings in animals.

Pseudotrauma

Insects and animals can create pseudotrauma and pseudopathology. In addition, roots may displace bones and artifacts. During excavation of buried remains, the presence and location of roots in relation to the bones *in situ* should be noted. Roots can reach great depths, and acid-secreting roots can modify bone and dental enamel, causing abnormalities that can be misinterpreted as trauma. Small roots may travel through the medullary canals, splitting the shaft of bones as they expand. They may also grow, destroying articulations and occasionally penetrating the cortex of the bone. Fine rootlets may cover the surface, creating a lace-like pattern (Saul and Saul 2002). Roots may create openings in bones that may be misinterpreted as wounds caused by projectiles or other penetration trauma. Depending on the projectile and type of bone, entrance wounds into bone may be smaller on entrance surface and larger on the exit surface. Exit wounds through bone may cause the bone to bevel outward. Both entrance and exit wounds may have associated fracture patterns from the site of straight or curved lines, tapering, radiating, beveling, or concentric (Chapter 8). Roots can cause weakening of the bone, causing more jagged and random fractures (Saul and Saul 2002). Erosions on the surface of the bone may be misinterpreted as incised defects. The grooves caused by roots usually are wavy and have rounded floors, whereas incised trauma usually has straight, often parallel grooves that are V-shaped (Saul and Saul 2002).

Blood vessels on the surface of the bone may be misinterpreted as incised wounds. On close inspection blood vessel impressions have smooth channels and pores for branching vessels rather than the striae associated with incisive trauma (Saul and Saul 2002).

General considerations for trauma

As previously discussed for live and deceased animal examinations, information about the case and the animal's history should be obtained prior to examination of skeletal remains. The consideration of documented soft tissue injuries is important to provide context for interpretation of osteology findings. The specific types of skeletal trauma are discussed in the following chapters. The bones should be carefully evaluated to try to determine antemortem, postmortem, and perimortem injuries. Antemortem and perimortem injuries, i.e., injuries that occurred at or around the time of death, can provide evidence regarding the circumstances surrounding the death, contributing cause of death, and the type of weapon used. The vital reaction of bleeding from bone is a perimortem indicator, and evidence of bone remodeling is indicative of antemortem injury. The microscopic analysis of fractured bone, including "dry" bone, can determine vital reaction and survival time post-injury.

Staining and/or immunohistochemistry can detect the presence of clots, red blood cell residues, fibrin clots, and new bone deposition that is not visible macroscopically. These findings can be present even after decomposition and maceration (Cattaneo et al. 2010). It may be difficult to macroscopically determine perimortem vs. postmortem damage to fresh or nearly fresh bone due to the moisture content which tends to respond to modification as if it were fresh (Sorg and Haglund 2002). This time frame for fresh bone characteristics can last several weeks postmortem, making perimortem determination more difficult. As the bone loses moisture, is exposed to the elements, and undergoes changes caused by exposure, it becomes stained in the outer layers. At this stage postmortem vs. perimortem changes are more easily distinguished where postmortem modifications typically disrupt the outer layers, exposing the unstained bone underneath.

Bone fracture patterns have been reported to help differentiate perimortem and postmortem injuries. These patterns include sharp edges, presence of fracture lines, the shape of the broken ends, fracture surface morphology, fracture angle on the Z-axis, and butterfly fractures. The analysis of fracture characteristics in fresh and dry bone is listed in Table 3.3. A study on deer femora found there is some overlap and variability. The study found one characteristic, jagged fracture outline, that was unique to perimortem injury but not found in every case. For postmortem injuries, two characteristics of transverse fractures and right angled edges were found, but not in every case. The findings did show statistically significant differences

between fresh bones fractures less than four days old and dry bones fractured forty-four days or one year postmortem (Wheatley 2008).

Taphonomic processes can affect bone trauma characteristics, making bone trauma very difficult to evaluate. These include freeze-thaw cycle, effects of rain or snow, animal activity, bleaching, grass and soil staining, and soil protection and erosion. These variables can decrease the chance of identifying characteristics of blunt force trauma such as the number of lesions, the direction and force of blows, patterns and timing, and the location of lesions. Typical blunt force trauma indicators such as radiating, concentric, or hinge fractures may be disguised due to the effects of environmental stress (Calce and Rogers 2007).

Sharp force injury

Sharp force injury to bone can be perimortem, resulting from stabbings or cuts, or postmortem, usually resulting from mutilation or dismemberment. Various tools may be used to cause sharp injury, including knives and saws. Saw marks are commonly created postmortem, involving repetitive movements for dismemberment or mutilation. All marks on the bone should be analyzed for evidence of perimortem or postmortem injury. If there are cuts to the cartilaginous ends of the bone, there may be a pattern imprint related to the weapon. Any patterned injury should be preserved using casting material for tool mark comparison to any recovered weapon (see Forensic Necropsy). Vital reaction on bone may be seen as bone remodeling or bone staining from hemorrhage. Hinged, bent areas of bone indicate perimortem trauma such as elevations of slivers of bone (Saul and Saul 2002). Perimortem cuts into bone usually are the same color as the rest of the surface bone, whereas postmortem cuts usually are lighter in color than the rest of the bone. However, if the bone with postmortem cuts has been exposed to the elements for a period of time, both the surface and the cuts will be the same color, such as those caused by scavengers (Symes et al. 2002).

Knives are the most common weapons in sharp-force trauma, although any instrument or tool with a sharp edge or point may be used. Knife wounds may be classed as knife-stab wounds (KSW) or knife-cut wounds (KCW). Knife-cut wounds are incisive wounds resulting from the actions of a slash, flick, tear, chop, or hack. Knives have at least one sharpened edge on a thin blade, sometimes terminating in a point, and a blade bevel (blade tapering). Other tools can be classified as knives, such as box cutters and razor blades. Blades from machines do not have a thin blade with edge beveling and tend to cause lacerations in

Table 3.3. Fracture characteristics of fresh and dry bone.

Morphology	Fresh bone characteristics	Dry bone characteristics
Outline	Radial pattern circling diaphysis	Fracture perpendicular or horizontal fracture surface
Surface	Homogeneous color with external cortical bone	Heterogeneous color with external cortical bone
Surface	Smooth	Rough
Angle	Obtuse and acute angles	Right angles
Other	Loading point present	Loading point absent
Other	Fracture fronts never crosscut epiphyseal ends	Fracture front can crosscut epiphysis

Source: Wieberg, D.A.M. and D.J. Wescott. 2008. Estimating the Timing of Long Bone Fractures: Correlation Between the Postmortem Interval, Bone Moisture Content, and Blunt Force Trauma Fracture Characteristics. *Journal of Forensic Sciences.* 53(5):1028–1034.

soft tissue and possible scraping, incised injury, or fractures to the bone. The blunt side of the blade, or the spine, may cause shaving wounds to the bone. Knife stab wounds also may cause fractures (Symes et al. 2002). If a knife has a serrated edge it may cause a jagged pattern on one side of the cut bone.

Saws have teeth that cut a groove (kerf) into the bone that is defined as the walls and floor of the cut. There are different types of saws but the majority have flat-edged teeth so the cut created is actually chiseling or shaving versus cutting. This creates a square cross-sectioned kerf floor that is larger than the blade width. Cross-cut saws have different teeth that create a W-shaped kerf floor. Saws are further characterized by the number of teeth per inch (TPI). The striae on the walls of the kerf provide information about the sides of the teeth, the shape, and the motion of the blade. The direction of the motion may be determined by examination of the kerf. There may be indicators of false starts and a breakaway spur that help indicate direction (Symes et al. 2002).

When examining bones, it must be considered that scavengers can cause similar marks that may be misinterpreted as sharp force trauma (see below). During the processing of bones for forensic analysis, marks may be created on the bone by the tools used to remove the soft tissue of the bone. Scalpel blades are very thin and should be easily distinguished from true knife cuts or stabs.

Animal fighting

Bone injuries may be seen related to different types of animal fighting based on the species and weapons used. In dog fighting, the dogs exert tremendous bite pressure that can result in bone fractures, punctures, or scoring of the periosteum. These types of bone injuries are not associated with other types of dog aggression with the possible exception of predator attacks. The location of the bite injuries to

the head and legs are characteristic of dog fighting (Chapter 13). Head injuries include punctures or fractures of the maxilla, palatine, incisive, and zygomatic process of the frontal bone. The leg injuries include punctures, fractures, or scoring of the periosteum. The scoring is typically 1–2 mm wide, linear to semi-curved with tapering, and oriented horizontal or diagonal to the diaphysis. Occasionally, circular scoring may be seen created by the tip of a tooth. Injuries similar to those found in the legs may be seen in the bones of the feet. As with soft tissue injuries, there may or may not be opposing bite injuries found with punctures to the bone. Because the dogs may be fought repeatedly, evidence of bone remodeling may be present in some of the injuries. In hog-dog fighting, these same bite injuries may be found on the hog bones. There may be additional bone injuries seen associated with the method of killing the dog such as hanging or gunshot (chapters 8 and 9).

In cockfighting, bone injuries are seen related to the knives or gaffs used (Chapter 13). Evidence of sharp force trauma and fractures may be seen. Injuries may be seen associated with the method of killing the rooster, which is typically cervical dislocation.

Fire victims

In the bone analysis of fire victims, it is important to differentiate perimortem trauma from postmortem damage caused by heat and fire. The extremely high temperatures on the scene can alter non-osseous material such as glass, leather, insulation, and wood in such a way as to resemble bone. It is important to examine the bones *in situ* to determine their relationship to the fire and other evidence at the scene.

Color changes found in human bones can provide evidence of the fire temperature or duration. At temperatures of 200°C (392°F) the bones show a gradual darkening to dark brown; at 300°C (572°F) they turn black; at 300°C (572°F) the color shifts to tan and then to gray, depending on the environmental conditions. Bones burned in open air are gray by 600°C (1112°F) and develop a purple hue at 1,100°C (2012°F). Bones burned surrounded by topsoil turn dark gray at 800°C (1472°F) to 900°C (1652°F). Bones that are calcined in color indicate the bone was exposed to intense high temperatures for an extended period of time (Dirkmaat 2002). A fire temperature determination based on bone color changes should only be an approximation. The availability of oxygen and the insulating effects of muscle mass each play a larger role in the calcination process than the fire temperature (Correia and Beattie 2002). The use of powder X-ray diffraction (XRD) to analyze microscopic changes in bone and teeth may be used to estimate the temperature and duration of a burning event (Piga et al. 2009).

The saw marks striae on bone may be affected by fire exposure but distinguishable features may still be present, including false starts. With handsaws, the bow saw, keyhole saw, and hacksaw were found to be consistently recognizable. With power saws, the chainsaw, jigsaw, and reciprocating saw were identifiable (Marciniak 2009).

Scavengers: bone modification and postmortem interval determination

Scavengers usually are drawn to a decomposing body as a food source. The types of animals may vary and include wolves, coyotes, dogs, foxes, opossum, birds, pigs, and rodents. It is important to avoid misinterpretation of tooth marks on bones as tool marks. It has been observed that the primary feeding target on human remains for wolves, dogs, coyotes, and pigs is the visceral contents of the body (Berryman 2002). Postmortem scavenging of humans by pets within enclosed environments may show a different pattern of feeding. It is not uncommon for the facial area to be the main target. Pets will normally feed on their deceased owner after a considerable time delay, presumably due to hunger, though it may begin immediately after death regardless of food access (Rothschild and Schneider 1997). The bones may have a variety of tooth marks on the surface, including fractures.

When examined under a microscope, rodent teeth create a more hollowed out groove where cut marks have cleaner and sharper margins. Carnivores tend to cause four different types of tooth mark artifacts: punctures, pits, scoring, and furrows. The tooth marks may be conical, which can also occur with knife stabbing. Pigs tend to cause elongated and usually parallel scoring on the bone from their incisor teeth dragging along the surface or when turning the bone. They also may cause punctures to the bone. In addition to the viscera, pigs have been found to focus their

scavenging on the face and throat of human remains (Berryman 2002).

Rodents will feed on the remains at different times based on the species and level of decomposition. This may be used for estimating the postmortem interval. Scavenging modification of bone by rodents is typically paired, broad, shallow, flat-bottomed grooves. The brown rat (*Rattus norvegicus*) modifies fat-laden cancellous bone, targeting bones at loci with minimal cortical thickness for easy access to nutrients. Gray squirrels (*Sciurus carolinensis*) gnaw on bones only after the fats have leached away to acquire minerals, targeting the thicker bone cortices at the edges or protuberances. Studies in eastern Tennessee have documented that gray squirrel modification was found on human and non-human skeletal remains where the postmortem interval was more than thirty months. Exceptions were noted where skeletal elements were more exposed and therefore more dried in time periods less than months. The findings of gray squirrel modification may be used to estimate the postmortem interval of more than thirty months depending on the environmental conditions (Klippel and Synstelien 2007).

Vultures start feeding approximately twenty-four hours postmortem and completely skeletonize a carcass in three to twenty-seven hours. Their scavenging greatly accelerates the rate of decomposition. Vultures leave scat and feathers at the site. They feed on soft tissue through natural openings using their talons as leverage and their beaks to carry elements without leaving marks. The beaks are used to rip flesh from bone, yet they have been observed using them in a delicate and deliberate manner. The body is typically disarticulated in the sequence similar to canids except the mandible is first followed by the cranium, scapulae, front limbs, then the ribs, vertebrae, and lower extremities. The eye orbits do not typically have damage or markings. The bone markings found associated with vulture scavenging are shallow scratches, up to 4 cm in length, which are relatively linear but irregularly shaped and characteristic of vulture modification. These scratches may be found on the mandible, cranium, scapula, ribs, long bones, and vertebrae. As bones weather, exposure and flaking can obscure these markings which appear similar to root etching. Surface scratches may also be seen with vulture feeding. These scratches are without depth and can be washed away by rain or cleaning (Reeves 2009).

Taphonomic effects on bone

Taphonomy refers to the study of the processes that transpire postmortem and how they affect the remains. Bones become discolored over time due to their exposure to different kinds of environments. External and cross-section bone color analysis may be used to interpret the sequence of events surrounding body disposition. Soil staining occurs from prolonged contact with the soil and may be brown, tan, black, or other colors depending on the organic and mineral contact of the soil. Contact with green algae, brass, or copper may stain various shades of green. The bone surface colors reported in a Canadian study are: light yellowish brown denotes soil staining; dark reddish brown denotes hemolysis; white denotes sun bleaching; greenish gray and olive indicate common fungi; and dark reddish gray denotes decompositional staining. Examination of the bone cross-section colors may help determine the sequence of exposure. Bone buried then exposed exhibits a pattern of light to dark color from the outer to inner cortex. Bones exposed then buried exhibit a pattern of dark to light or dark/light/dark from the outer to inner cortex. Buried bones and buried-then-exposed bones have identical staining, making bone surface analysis important. Decomposition of tissue creates minimal color staining and tends to be small and localized without penetration into the interior of the bone (Huculak and Rogers 2009).

Fungal growth, depending on the species, can indicate the exposure sequence of the remains. Fungi found on buried remains may indicate exposure to the surface prior to burial. The fungi are found on the inferior surface of the bones and tissue in a burial environment (Huculak and Rogers 2009).

The positioning of the bones in the grave may provide information about the body movement. Skeletal remains that are not in anatomical position indicate the body must have decomposed for a period of time in an environment that allowed bone movement. This includes a container, which prevents soil infilling that would hold the elements in place during decomposition, or above ground. Missing bones may indicate natural disarticulation due to decomposition above ground prior to burial or dissolution of small bones in acidic soil. It may also indicate dismemberment (Huculak and Rogers 2009).

Bone-modifying effects of water environments

The aquatic environment can have an effect on the bones of bodies that have been placed in the water. Water that has significant current and heavy sediment can cause abrasions and round off any projections normally present on the bone. This may be caused by the sediment or the current causing the bone to abrade against other objects. These abrasions may obscure or obliterate indicators of trauma, including incisive and penetration signs. Fractures may occur if the bones have been subjected to heavy currents

where they have been forcefully pushed against solid objects. These signs of trauma may be difficult to differentiate from perimortem injury. Marine organisms may encrust the bones at and above the waterline. Based on the species and environment, it may be possible to establish a timeline for how long the bones have been in the water. Dissolution, which is the pitting and corrosion of the bone surface, may result from water environmental bioturbation, such as the erosions caused by gastropods (Haglund and Sorg 2002).

THE FORENSIC REPORT

The reports generated for any legal case are of utmost importance. A report is written for the entire community of law enforcement, prosecutor, defense attorney, defendant, judge, and jury. These reports are legal documents and are examined throughout the legal process of the case. For criminal cases, they are submitted to the investigating and prosecuting agency. As the case progresses, the report is examined by the defense counsel, the defendant, their expert witness, and the judge. It is from these reports that decisions are made by both sides, including whether or not to prosecute and how to charge the defendant. The forensic report is used to map out defense and prosecution strategies and may be used to determine plea bargains or sentencing. Based on the contents and how the report is written, it can reveal how the veterinarian will testify. Approximately 95% of criminal cases are resolved without trial.

The purpose of the forensic report is to provide a clear understanding of the veterinary evidence. It should include information provided by investigating authorities and/or anyone else connected to the investigation, exam findings, procedures, samples/evidence collected, test submissions and results (medical and forensic), medical diagnoses, treatments, and outcomes and conclusions. The forensic report collates all the findings including their interpretation and provides a well-balanced professional opinion. It should be clear, methodical, and laid out in a logical manner.

The terminology used in the forensic report is very important, as it is with testimony. Unless there is medical or scientific proof that something occurred, the veterinarian may not be able to make certain statements. The best test to apply to any statement is "how do you know." Even with eye witness statements, the information is still not necessarily considered fact. Certainly, statements may be made by the veterinarian based on a reasonable degree of scientific or medical certainty. Statements also may be made with an explanation for the basis and context.

Absolute statements should be made with caution and only with certainty of the analysis. Peer discussion of findings may be helpful to consider all theories prior to reaching a conclusion (see General Considerations at the beginning of this chapter).

For multiple animal cases, there may be one report with each animal's findings listed (see below) or separate reports. When writing separate reports, each report will be analyzed and compared so it is important to have continuity of descriptions and terminology. Sometimes a report is needed prior to the receipt and analysis of all test results and the final determination of conclusions. In these cases, a verbal report may be given to the investigating officer or a preliminary report issued. If a written preliminary report is required, it should be written with extreme caution and should not contain anything other than known facts, confirmed findings, and pending tests. Conclusions, if any, should be carefully drafted in preliminary reports and based on only confirmed information. If these conclusions are altered in the final report, the basis for the changes must be explained. Both the preliminary and final reports should be kept as separate files. They are both considered evidence and part of discovery to be turned over to the opposing counsel. All electronic communications and documentation made at the scene or during the examination, laboratory results, forensic testing, expert consultations, photographs, radiographs, and any treatment or medical records must be preserved as evidence for the case.

The reports for animal cruelty cases should be titled "Examination Report" or "Necropsy Report" for a live or deceased victim, respectively. For consultations, the report may be titled "Expert Opinion Report." There are templates of report forms that are useful when creating the report, which follows the exam form templates (Appendices 20–21).

Report format

The following is a general description of recommended headings and subheadings to be used in forensic reports. It is appropriate to use medical terminology in the first sections of the report but it is important to switch to lay terminology beginning at the Summary of Findings section.

Heading

The top of the report should have information about the investigating agency, lead investigating officer, and case number. This should be followed by the examining veterinarian information, including the name, address, phone number, fax number, and date of the exam.

Subject of exam

This section should contain a full description of the animal, including the species, breed, sex, whether spayed or neutered, known or estimated age, all coat coloring, any distinguishing marks, microchip number, tattoos, and animal ID. The basis for the age determination should be included such as dentition, growth plate closures, or medical records. For the multiple animal exam report, the number of animals and species are listed here and the animal IDs along with the rest of the information are placed under the Exam Findings section.

Reason for exam

This section should contain a sentence describing the reason for the examination or report. This may be animal cruelty investigation or expert opinion analysis.

Method of arrival and description of packaging

Record the information from the examination form regarding arrival of the animal. This section should contain a list of all material provided, including the source, that is associated with the animal or case. This may be materials provided by the investigating agency, attorney, or the owner.

Crime scene/forensic findings

This section is the context for the analysis of the exam findings and should contain any pertinent crime scene or forensic findings. These may be from personal observations during on-scene investigation work by the veterinarian or information provided by the investigator. If the information is provided verbally by the investigator, it should be clearly noted: "According to Officer (name)…," followed by the date and the information that was conveyed verbally. A summary of the information contained in the materials provided for review should be noted in this section. This includes photographs, videos, reports, and witness statements. Any conclusions from this information may be documented here or under the Conclusions section of the report. All weather data recorded at the scene or from a weather station should be documented here, including the time of the readings.

Medical history

Any known medical history should be documented in this section. This includes medical records and any treatments at another facility prior to exam. It may include a verbal medical history provided by the owner or investigator but should be noted as a verbal source and who provided that information. All medical history related to the victim's injuries should be described in this section, including initial examination findings, response or lack of response to treatment, all medications given, radiographic findings, and if the animal died or was euthanized.

Abbreviations

It is appropriate to use medical abbreviations in the report only if a key is provided. This key may be modified based on the abbreviations used by the veterinarian in the report.

Definitions

To facilitate better understanding by the non-veterinarian reader, a section for definitions should be included for the medical terms used in the report. Some medical terms may be common enough for lay understanding and are not required to be defined. Any terminology unique to animals vs. humans should be defined in this section or within the body of the report. The body condition scoring system used should also be included. A definition for each of the scores may be attached to the report (Appendices 13–14).

Examination findings

This section may have several subsections depending on the type of report, type of exam (live or deceased), nature of the injuries, and medical procedures performed. Any section heading not used may be deleted.

External exam (necropsy) and examination findings (examination report)

For the live animal, this section should include all the documented findings from the live animal exam form. For the deceased animal, this section should include all the documented findings from the external findings section on the necropsy exam form. For multiple animal reports, the findings for each animal may be listed in alpha-numeric order by the animal ID. For each animal, the subject of exam info (breed, age, sex, etc.), exam findings, and test results are documented using abbreviations. This is followed with a line beginning with Summary and a list of the summary of findings for the individual animal, using lay terms (see Summary of Findings section, below). For large scale cases, instead of alpha-numeric order the animals may be grouped based on the crime scene location where the animals were removed from. For example:

Location A
ID A2D5-001: Chihuahua, adult, female, tan, 6#, BCS 2, mm-pink, crt 2s, HLA-UR, long nails, severe dental dz; Labwk: HW-pos, anemia, hookworms
Summary: very thin, long nails, severe dental dz, heartworms, anemia, hookworms

Evidence of medical and/or surgical intervention

This section should contain any findings of medical and/or surgical intervention on the animal such as intravenous catheters or chest tubes.

Radiographic interpretation

Any radiographic procedures should be noted, including views and the interpretation described.

Internal exam

For the necropsy report, all the findings under this section on the necropsy exam form should be placed here.

Evidence of injury

This section is optional and is most helpful with complicated injuries such as multiple stab or gunshot wounds. It is not necessary to repeat the descriptions in the external or internal exam sections. For gunshot cases, the trajectory description may be placed in this section or as a separate heading.

Photographs and diagrams

The use of photographs and/or diagrams in the forensic report is extremely useful to illustrate exam findings. The photo selection should be the most representative of the injury, disease state, or abnormal finding. Diagrams may be inserted into the photo using Word document tools to highlight or explain the areas of interest.

Medical treatment and results

For live animal exams, any treatment or procedures performed should be recorded. A summary of hospitalization, medications, and treatment response including a timeline should be documented. The reasons for the animal's progress, recovery, or failure to respond to treatment should be addressed in this section.

Procedures and results

All evidence collected from the animal, including samples, and tests conducted should be listed in this section. Any samples collected and held for possible future testing should be noted.

Entomology findings

All entomological evidence collected should be described in this section. The location of the collected insect evidence on the body should be noted. The weather data submitted with the insect samples should be kept as evidence in the case file. The results reported by the forensic entomologist should be listed in this section and submitted with the report.

Summary of findings

Beginning at this section of the report, every effort should be made to use lay terms instead of medical terms. All the pertinent findings should be listed numerically in this section. This should include exam findings (normal and abnormal), test results, and a summary of the injuries. Descriptive qualifiers should be used to describe each finding such as mild or severe. For example, in a neglect case: "1. Emaciated (BCS 1) 2. Mild anemia 3. Severe matting and fecal soiling."

This section is also where the exam findings, materials reviewed, and the crime scene/forensic findings can be brought together. For example, in blunt force trauma: "1. Blunt force trauma to the head, a minimum of three blows." A statement may be made regarding a particular weapon based on information provided by the investigator, results of forensic analyses, or exam findings that are indicative of a type of weapon. For example: "Blunt force trauma to the head, a minimum of three blows, consistent with a cylindrical object." Unless there has been forensic evidence or investigation findings proving that a particular weapon was used, the veterinarian does not know for a fact it caused the injuries. Usually, at most, it can be stated as "consistent with" a weapon type or alleged weapon.

For a multiple animal report, the list should include the number of animals associated with the listed findings. For example: "1. Anemia (twelve dogs)" with the total number of animals examined listed in parentheses next to the section title. For large scale cases where animals are listed under different crime scene locations, a location Summary of Findings should be listed followed by a sum total Summary of Findings for all the animals.

Survival period

If any exam or investigation findings, including witness statements, indicate that the animal survived for a period of time prior to death, then the estimated time should be noted in this section. This section also may be used for live animal reports when an estimate may be made for the time of injury or disease. In this case, the estimate refers to the period the animal has survived after the onset of disease or infliction of trauma. The survival period estimate is often based on the exam findings and the veterinarian's experience and knowledge. The basis for the estimate, e.g., medical findings or witness statement, should be documented.

Time of death

The known or estimated time of death should be noted in this section. This may be based on the investigation findings, witness statements, postmortem exam findings, and/or forensic analyses (e.g., forensic entomology). The basis

for this determination should be documented. The term "unknown" is appropriate if the time of death determination is not possible. The next section is known as the Death/ Injury Statement. The final determinations regarding the death or injury are made in this section. For each category, the word "death" may be replaced with "injury" for the live examination report.

Cause of injury (necropsy report)

This section is used when there are injuries present that were not a contributory cause of death or part of the cause of death (see below).

Manner of injury (necropsy report)

This section is required when there is a cause of injury section on the necropsy report.

Mechanism of death

This refers to the biochemical or physiological abnormality or derangement that resulted in death; for example, shock, septicemia, cerebral edema, ventricular fibrillation, or cardiorespiratory arrest.

Cause of death

This refers to the injury or disease that began a sequence of events that ultimately led to the death of the animal; for example, gunshot wounds, stab wounds, and blunt force trauma. If the animal was euthanized due to the nature and extent of the injuries or illness, the injury or illness is listed as the cause of death. For cases where the available information is sparse but not to the extent where using "undetermined" as the cause death is appropriate, the term "probable" may be used before the cause of death opinion. This serves to convey the fact that while there is some degree of certainty, this opinion may change based on any future information provided.

Contributory cause

This refers to any condition the animal had that could have contributed to death or injury. For example, in a case where the cause of death was multiple stab wounds and the mechanism of death is exsanguination and hypovolemic shock, a contributory cause may be a clotting disorder that contributed to the hemorrhage. In a starvation case where an emaciated animal died from hypothermia (cause of death), the contributory cause would be starvation.

Manner of death

This refers to the circumstances surrounding the death. Traditionally, the classifications in humans are homicide, suicide, accident, natural, and undetermined. In animals, the classifications are non-accidental, accident, natural, and undetermined. "Natural" refers to death caused exclusively by disease, "accident" refers to death caused by violent means, not due to an intentional or criminal act by a person, "non-accidental" refers to death caused by a person which may be a criminal offense under the animal cruelty laws, and "undetermined" is used when a reasonable classification cannot be made. However, the term "probable" may be used in certain circumstances (see Cause of Death).

Conclusions

This section is where the veterinarian ties all the exam and crime scene/forensic findings together and provides the medical opinions. Medical opinions are based on facts as they are known at the time the opinion is formulated. Some of these facts may not change such laboratory tests. Some facts may change, such as witness statements or other investigation findings. If any facts change which were the foundation for the original medical opinion, then the opinion may change. Opinions are written with consideration of degrees of probabilities. The highest degree of probability is absolute certainty or certainty beyond a *possible* doubt where every other imaginable contingency is impossible.

The next is a reasonable degree of certainty where the probability of reasonable degree far exceeds 50% and the reasonable certainty is that degree of assurance that a reasonable person relies upon. Next is the preponderance of evidence which means "more likely than not" and permits reasonable doubts. It may also be defined as *probable* with a likelihood exceeding 50%. Because the medical opinions will be used in legal forums, a higher degree of certainty than probable causes is often required. This higher standard may be met by developing a larger factual database or using brevity and broadly defined terms in the medical opinions.

There are two categories of probabilities of less than 50%: reasonable possibilities and speculation. Reasonable possibilities may be discussed in courtroom proceedings and have a probability of less than 50%. Speculation refers to possibilities that are so improbable that they have no basis in reason. Speculation may not be allowed in criminal proceedings (Adams, Flomenbaum, and Hirsch 2006).

The conclusions should address everything listed in the Summary of Findings section. This section should be written with a clear explanation of how the conclusions were reached and the basis for each. It should contain factual findings as well as the veterinary opinion of all the information documented in the report. It is important to know the language of the applicable laws, and if applicable, make appropriate statements using that language within the conclusions. This is also the area to educate the reader on the importance of certain findings, clarifying any interpretations and explaining certain processes such as starvation. The pain and suffering of the animal should be thoroughly discussed (Chapter 4). The use of terminology is important, such as "consistent with."

The terms "unique" and "indicative of" should be used cautiously and only with basis for absolute certainty. It is not appropriate to comment on the rights or wrongs of the actions of the person who allegedly committed the abuse. It is also not appropriate or within the veterinarian's purview to speculate in the report on a potential weapon without having been asked by law enforcement or the attorney to consider if a certain weapon could have been used . The veterinarian can only consider the information provided by the investigating agency or the persons for whom the report is being written. It is the strength of this final section that may determine if charges will be filed or the case proceed, and it may reveal how the veterinarian will testify.

Finalization

The report should be finalized with the veterinarian's name, signature, and the date of the report.

REFERENCES

Adams, V.I., M.A. Flomenbaum, and C.S. Hirsch. 2006. Trauma and Disease. In: *Spitz and Fisher's Medicolegal Investigation of Death: Guidelines for the Application of Pathology to Crime Investigation*, Fourth edition, W.U. Spitz and D.J. Spitz, eds. pp. 436–459. Springfield: Charles C. Thomas Publisher, Ltd.

Andrews, J.J., W.G. Van Alstine, and K.J. Schwartz. 1986. A Basic Approach to Food Animal Necropsy. *Veterinary Clinics of North America: Food Animal Practice.* 2(1):1–29.

Balkin, D. 2012. Animal Legal Defense Fund. Personal communication.

Berryman, H.E. 2002. Disarticulation Pattern and Tooth Mark Artifacts Associated with Pig Scavenging of Human Remains: A Case Study. In: *Advances in Forensic Taphonomy*, W.D. Haglund and M.H. Sorg, eds. pp. 487–495. Boca Raton, FL: CRC Press.

Burkhard, M.J. and D.J. Meyer. 1995. Causes and Effects of Interference with Clinical Laboratory Measurements and Examinations. In: *Kirk's Current Veterinary Therapy XII Small Animal Practice*, J.D. Bonagura and R.W. Kirk, eds. pp. 15–20. Philadelphia: W.B. Saunders.

Calce, S.E. and T.L. Rogers. 2007. Taphonomic Changes to Blunt Force Trauma: A Preliminary Study. *Journal of Forensic Sciences.* 52(3):519–527.

Cattaneo, C., S. Andreola, E. Marinelli, P. Poppa, D. Porta, and M. Grandi. 2010. Detection of Microscopic Markers of Hemorrhaging and Wound Age on Dry Bone. *The American Journal of Forensic Medicine and Pathology.* 31(1):22–26.

Cedergren, L. and M. Jepsen. 2012. Age Estimation of Wounds Using the Proximity Ligand Assay. Presented at the American Academy of Forensic Sciences, 20–25 February, Atlanta, Georgia.

Correia, P.M. and O. Beattie. 2002. A Critical Look at Methods for Recovering, Evaluating, and Interpreting Cremated Human Remains. In: *Advances in Forensic Taphonomy*, W.D. Haglund and M.H. Sorg, eds. pp. 435–450. Boca Raton, FL: CRC Press.

Di Maio, V.J. and D. Di Maio. 2001. *Forensic Pathology*, Second edition. Boca Raton, FL: CRC Press.

Dirkmaat, D.C. 2002. Recovery and Interpretation of the Fatal Fire Victim: The Role of Forensic Anthropology. In: *Advances in Forensic Taphonomy*, W.D. Haglund and M.H. Sorg, eds. pp. 451–472. Boca Raton, FL: CRC Press.

Dix, J. and M. Graham. 2000. *Time of Death, Decomposition and Identification: An Atlas*. Boca Raton, FL: CRC Press.

Gerdin, Jodie. 2011. Necropsy for the Forensic Veterinarian. Presented at 4th Annual Veterinary Forensic Sciences Conference of the International Veterinary Forensic Sciences Association, 2–4 May, Orlando, Florida.

Gilliland, M.G.F. 2011. Infant Death Evaluation: What is the Constellation of Abusive Injuries? Presented at the 63rd Annual Scientific Meeting of the American Academy of Forensic Sciences, 21–26 February, Chicago, Illinois.

Guler, H., E.O. Aktas, H. Karali, and S. Aktas. 2011. The Importance of Tenascin and Ubiquitin in Estimation of Wound Age. *The American Journal of Forensic Medicine and Pathology.* 32(1):83–89.

Haglund, W.D. and M.H. Sorg. 2002. Human Remains in Water Environments. In: *Advances in Forensic Taphonomy*, W.D. Haglund and M.H. Sorg, eds. pp. 201–218. Boca Raton, FL: CRC Press.

Huculak, M.A. and T.L. Rogers. 2009. Reconstructing the Sequence of Events Surrounding Body Disposition Based on Color Staining of Bone. *Journal of Forensic Sciences.* 54(5):979–984.

Jashnani, K.D., S.A. Kale, and A.B. Rupani. 2010. Vitreous Humor: Biochemical Constituents in Estimation of Postmortem Interval. *Journal of Forensic Sciences.* 55(6):1523–1527.

Klippel, W.E. and J.A. Synstelien. 2007. Rodents as Taphonomic Agents: Bone Gnawing by Brown Rats and Gray Squirrels. *Journal of Forensic Sciences.* 52(4):765–773.

Latimer, K.S. and H. Tvedten. 1999. Leukocyte Disorders. In: *Small Animal Clinical Diagnosis by Laboratory Methods*, Third edition. M.D. Willard, H. Tvedten, and G.H. Turnwald, eds. pp. 52–74. Philadelphia: W.B. Saunders.

Lewchanin, S. and E. Zimmerman. 2000. *Clinical Assessment of Juvenile Animal Cruelty*. Huntingdon: Biddle Publishing Company.

Lockwood, R. 2004. Cruelty Toward Cats: Who Does What to Whom and Why? Presented at the International Association of Human Interaction Organizations, 6–9 October, Glasgow, Scotland.

Lockwood, R. 2010. Cruelty Toward Cats: A Different Kind of Abuse. Presented at the North American Veterinary Conference, 16–20 January, Orlando, Florida.

Lockwood, R. 2011. Identifying and Investigating Animal Crimes. Presented at Victim to Verdict: Identification, Investigation and Prosecution of Animal Cruelty, Animal Crimes Summit, Oregon Humane Society, 3 March, Portland, Oregon.

M., Paulo and A. de Siqueira. 2011. Brazil Plenary and Poster Sessions. Presented at the 4th Annual Veterinary Forensic Sciences Conference of the International Veterinary Forensic Sciences Association, 2–4 May, Orlando, Florida.

Marciniak, S.-M. 2009. A Preliminary Assessment of the Identification of Saw Marks on Burned Bone. *Journal of Forensic Sciences.* 54(4):779–785.

McGrath, K.K. and A.J. Jenkins. 2009. Detection of Drugs of Forensic Importance in Postmortem Bone. *The American Journal of Forensic Medicine and Pathology.* 30(1):40–44.

Morcillo, M.D. 2012. Skeletal Trauma Observed in Exhumed Skeletons Compared With Trauma Recorded in the Corresponding Forensic Autopsy Reports. Presented at the American Academy of Forensic Sciences Annual Scientific Meeting, 20–25 February, Atlanta, Georgia.

Mulla, A., K.L. Massey, and J. Kalra. 2005. Vitreous Humor Biochemical Constituents Evaluation of Between–Eye Differences. *The American Journal of Forensic Medicine and Pathology.* 26(2):146–149.

Muller, G.H., R.W. Kirk, D.W. Scott, and C.E. Griffin. 2001. *Muller and Kirk's Small Animal Dermatology*. Philadelphia: Elsevier.

Munro, H.M. and M.V. Thrusfield. 2001a. "Battered Pets": Features That Raise Suspicion of Non-accidental Injury. *Journal of Small Animal Practice.* 42:218–226.

Munro, H.M. and M.V. Thrusfield. 2001b. "Battered Pets": Non-accidental Physical Injuries Found in Dogs and Cats. *Journal of Small Animal Practice.* 42:279–290.

Munro, R. and H. Munro. 2008. Wounds and Injuries. In: *Animal Abuse and Unlawful Killing: Forensic Veterinary Pathology*, pp. 30–47. Edinburgh: Elsevier.

Munro, R. and H. Munro. 2011. Forensic Veterinary Medicine: 2. Postmortem Investigation. *In Practice.* 33:262–270.

Nakasono I. 2001. Application of Immunohistochemistry for Forensic Pathological Diagnosis: Finding of Human Brain in Forensic Autopsy. *Nihon Hoigaku Zasshi.* 55(3):299–309.

Newberry, S. and R. Munro. 2011. Forensic veterinary medicine: 1. Investigation involving live animals. *In Practice.* 33:220–7.

Nogami, M., A. Takatsu, N. Endo, and I. Ishiyama. 1999. Evaluation of the Agonal Stress: Can Immunohistochemical Detection of Ubiquitin in the Locus Coeruleus Be Useful? *Legal Medicine* (Tokyo). 1(4):198–203.

Perper, J.A. 2006. Time of Death and Changes After Death, Part 1: Anatomical Considerations. In: *Spitz and Fisher's Medicolegal Investigation of Death: Guidelines for the Application of Pathology to Crime Investigation*, Fourth edition, W.U. Spitz and D.J. Spitz, eds. pp. 87–127. Springfield: Charles C. Thomas Publisher, Ltd.

Piga, G., T.J.U. Thompson, A. Malgosa, and S. Enzo. 2009. The Potential of X-Ray Diffraction in the Analysis of Burned Remains from Forensic Contexts. *Journal of Forensic Sciences*. 54(3):534–539.

Platt, M.S., D.J. Spitz, and W.U. Spitz. 2006. Investigation of Deaths in Childhood, Part 2: The Abused Child and Adolescent. In: *Spitz and Fisher's Medicolegal Investigation of Death: Guidelines for the Application of Pathology to Crime Investigation*, Fourth edition, W.U. Spitz and D.J. Spitz, eds. pp. 357–416. Springfield: Charles C. Thomas Publisher, Ltd.

Preuß J., R. Dettmeyer, S. Poster, E. Lignitz, and B. Madea. 2008. The Expression of Heat Shock Protein 70 in Kidneys in Cases of Death Due to Hypothermia. *Forensic Science International*. 176(2–3):248–52.

Quan, L., B.-L. Zhu, K. Ishida, S. Oritani, M. Taniguchi, M.Q. Fujita, and H. Maeda. 2001. Intranuclear Ubiquitin Immunoreactivity of the Pigmented Neurons of the Substantia Nigra in Fatal Acute Mechanical Asphyxiation and Drowning. *International Journal of Legal Medicine*. 115(1): 6–11.

Reeves, N.M. 2009. Taphonomic Effects of Vulture Scavenging. *Journal of Forensic Sciences*. 54(3):523–528.

Rothschild, M.A. and V. Schneider. 1997. On the Temporal Onset of Postmortem Animal Scavenging. "Motivation" of the Animal. *Forensic Science International*. 89(1–2):57–64.

Saul, J.M. and F.P. Saul. 2002. Forensics, Archaeology, and Taphonomy: The Symbiotic Relationship. In: *Advances in Forensic Taphonomy*, W.D. Haglund and M.H. Sorg, eds. pp. 71–97. Boca Raton, FL: CRC Press.

Schwartz, L.D. 1986. Necropsy of Chickens, Turkeys, and Other Poultry. *Veterinary Clinics of North America: Food Animal Practice*. 2(1):43–60.

Searcy, G.P. 2001. The Hemopoietic System. In: *Thomson's Special Veterinary Pathology*, Third edition, M.D. McGavin, W.W. Carlton, and J.F. Zachary, eds. pp. 325–379. St. Louis: Mosby.

Sorg, M.H. and W.D. Haglund. 2002. Advancing Forensic Taphonomy: Purpose, Theory, and Process. In: *Advances in Forensic Taphonomy*, W.D. Haglund and M.H. Sorg, eds. pp. 3–29. Boca Raton, FL: CRC Press.

Sturner, W.Q. 2006. Time of Death and Changes After Death, Part 2: Chemical Considerations. In: *Spitz and Fisher's Medicolegal Investigation of Death: Guidelines for the Application of Pathology to Crime Investigation*, Fourth edition, W.U. Spitz and Da.J. Spitz, eds. pp. 128–148. Springfield: Charles C. Thomas Publisher, Ltd.

Symes, S.S., J.A. Williams, E.A. Murray, J.M. Hoffman, T.D. Holland, J.M. Saul, F.P. Saul, and E.J. Pople. 2002. Taphonomic Context of Sharp-Force Trauma in Suspected Cases of Human Mutilation and Dismemberment. In: *Advances in Forensic Taphonomy*, W.D. Haglund and M.H. Sorg, eds. pp. 403–434. Boca Raton, FL: CRC Press.

Takahashi, S., H. Kinoshita, and M. Funayama. 2011. Usefulness of Catheter Guide Wires for Identifying Sites of Vascular Injuries. *American Journal of Forensic Medicine and Pathology*. 32(4):319–320.

Thacker, H.L. 1986. Necropsy of the Feeder Pig and Adult Swine. *Veterinary Clinics of North America: Food Animal Practice*. 2(1):173–186.

Wheatley, B.P. 2008. Perimortem or Postmortem Bone Fractures? An Experimental Study of Fracture Patterns in Deer Femora. *Journal of Forensic Sciences*. 53(1): 69–72.

Wieberg, D.A.M. and D.J. Wescott. 2008. Estimating the Timing of Long Bone Fractures: Correlation Between the Postmortem Interval, Bone Moisture Content, and Blunt Force Trauma Fracture Characteristics. *Journal of Forensic Sciences*. 53(5):1028–1034.

4
Special Considerations in Animal Cruelty Cases

Melinda D. Merck and Richard A. LeCouteur

Truth is incontrovertible
Panic may resent it
Ignorance may deride it
Malice may distort it
But here it is.
        Winston Churchill

LARGE SCALE CRUELTY CASES

Large scale cruelty case responses involve crime scene and animal processing as well as post-seizure care requiring extensive planning and a large number of resources to conduct it properly. These investigations are primarily animal fighting, hoarding, puppy mills, and animal sanctuaries which involve a large number of animals in various stages of neglect or untreated injury. There are several factors that affect the implementation of proper evidentiary procedures. Due to the sheer number of animals and the extensive scene evidence, the processing of the scene and animals needs to be conducted simultaneously. In addition, there are often time constraints imposed by the search warrant and/or limitation of resources. The most important guide for planning is that this is a crime scene with live evidence, not a rescue, and it must be treated as such. With the anticipation and consideration of all factors and potential issues, large scale cruelty cases can be handled successfully for the animals and the criminal investigation.

Incident command system (ICS)

The use of the incident command system (ICS) in these cases, as implemented in disaster responses, is extremely important to maintain a chain of command due to the large number of people conducting simultaneous operations. To better organize and manage the investigation, the ICS structure is implemented with each position filled by function. The structure is set up in modules, with the command module having the positions of incident commander, safety officer, information officer, and liaison. Depending on the size of the incident and organizational needs, each position may or may not be filled.

- Incident commander: This person must have the responsibility, authority, and ability to make and implement decisions.
- Safety officer: This person must have the knowledge, common sense, and ability to prepare and implement a safety plan to cover all aspects of the incident.
- Information officer: This person has the authority to control all public information concerning the investigation, and should be the single "clearing house" for all media and official statements concerning the case.
- Liaison officer: This person is the contact for all other agencies and organizations that are assisting in the investigation.

Veterinary Forensics: Animal Cruelty Investigations, Second Edition. Edited by Melinda D. Merck.
© 2013 John Wiley & Sons, Inc. Published 2013 by John Wiley & Sons, Inc.

The incident management module has the positions of finance, logistics, operations, and planning.

- Finance: This person has the responsibility to account for monies used in the incident.
- Logistics: This person manages all supplies and support for the event including travel and housing for staff.
- Operations: This person has the authority and responsibility to carry out all operational aspects of this incident.
- Planning: This person should have the knowledge and capability to organize and draw up action plans to be approved by the incident commander.

Under operations, the assignment of positions depends on the individual's function in the investigation. This may be divided into enforcement and animal, with the link to both in the evidence position. This would be a law enforcement branch and an animal branch with the position of animal evidence chief as that link. Another option is to have a physical evidence team lead (PEL) and a medical evidence team lead (MEL), which is always a veterinarian, reporting to the animal evidence chief.

- Law enforcement branch: This lead person is in charge of all investigation and enforcement.
- Animal branch: This person must have the knowledge, experience, and ability to organize and manage the entire animal branch.
- Animal evidence chief (AEC): This person manages and is responsible for all aspects of the animal evidence. This may be a veterinarian with forensic training and experience.

Depending on the size of the investigation, additional team assignments would fall under the AEC for assessment, evaluation, and identification of each animal. They may include medical triage, animal identification, and forensic exam teams.

Under the animal branch there are other needs such as handlers to carry the crated and identified animals to the transport unit, a response team for loose and escaped animals, a medic for both humans and animals, and the ability to transport any animal emergency that arises. If the crime scene search reveals a burial site a team(s) will be assigned to handle the excavation. If there is a need for a temporary shelter for the animals, there will be staffing requirements, which also falls under the animal branch.

General considerations

The logistical planning for these cases often requires outside agencies to assist with personnel, equipment, and general and medical supplies. These supplies for the investigation and the operation of the shelter need to be planned for very early in the investigation. All team leaders should be involved in this planning including from the medical, forensic evidence, and shelter units. A supply list should be compiled for each team, unit, and shelter (Appendices 5 and 23). Arrangements should be made to obtain both general and medical supplies during the case response for items that were not anticipated or depleted due to use. Provisions should be made for supplying food to the workers on-scene and at the shelter location. Often, there are local agencies that specialize in this for disaster situations that may be able to assist.

The animal evidence chief, and, if the AEC is not a veterinarian, the medial evidence lead, should be part of the planning stage including all conference calls and meetings. All intelligence related to the case should be shared with the AEC and MEL so that there is proper planning in anticipation of processing the evidence at the scene, identifying the resources needed, and determining what impact it will have on processing the animals. The AEC and the MEL eventually will testify in court and must be part of the early investigation, which can help determine investigation strategy, possible charges, and trial strategy. Usually a prosecutor will be assigned to the case in the early planning process to guide the planning and facilitate warrants, bonds, and forfeiture procedures. It is helpful to have the prosecutor or a representative from the prosecutor's office on site when the search warrant is executed to observe the scene directly and assist with any legal issues that may arise.

Security is another consideration, both on site and at the shelter location. This may be provided by local law enforcement or a private security agency and may be required twenty-four hours a day. The security risk surrounding these cases may come from the defendant, his or her acquaintances, the community, or those interested in stealing the animals for other purposes, such as with animal fighting cases. Depending on the case issues, it may be determined not to disclose the location of the shelter and/or the animals for safety reasons.

Crime scene processing

The crime scene processing involves two stages: initial walk-through followed by full documentation and processing of physical evidence. Although the animals are evidence, they are processed simultaneously under separate teams and protocols. The walk-through team should be a small group of people comprised of, at a minimum, the lead investigator(s), lead veterinarian (AEC or MEL), AEC, removal team lead, videographer, photographer, scribe, and safety officer. The purpose of the initial walk-through of the scene is to assess the size of the scene, number of animals, general conditions, safety hazards, and key evidence areas. These areas must be secured and pathways for all personnel traffic identified within the scene. The walk-through team (scribe, AEC, or MEL) will create a general map of the scene to be used by the animal identification teams (see Mapping section, below). Video and photography of the general scene will be taken during this initial walk-through. Any evidence that may be altered by the walk-through, such as ammonia levels, should be obtained during this process. After the walk-through is completed, the team will meet with all team leads to share the information gathered and make any necessary adjustments to the operation and logistics plan.

The next step is the full crime scene processing (Chapter 2). This may be a single evidence team or multiple teams based on the size of the scene and amount of evidence. This team is responsible for the identification, collection, packaging, labeling, and documentation of the evidence. In addition, the team is responsible for detailed mapping of the scene. The number of team members may vary based on the case and evidence present. A minimum of two people are needed for mapping and measurements (Chapter 2). Each team is comprised of an evidence technician and a photographer/videographer. A lead evidence tech should be designated to be responsible for logging all evidence, including medical forensic evidence, for the entire scene and animal examination site(s). It is advantageous to create a specific area for evidence to be processed and securely held.

Animal mapping and identification system

The purpose of animal mapping is to create an identification system that provides a unique animal ID number that corresponds to the exact location where the animal was found at the scene. By using the map as a key, the animal ID is an "address" for the animal. This is extremely useful for several reasons: It provides the prosecutor the needed information for drafting indictments (animal location), it shows the relationship of animals in each area based on the identification alone, and it provides rapid information needed for treatment plans based on diagnostic test results and in the event of disease outbreak. Most importantly, it follows proper evidence identification and chain of custody

protocols, which are required for the admissibility of evidence in court.

The animal identification is a four-digit series of alternating letters and numbers that provide the location, followed by a hyphen and the assigned number for that individual animal. The first letter designates the building or area. It is the responsibility of the initial walk-through team to provide a general map of the scene, both buildings and areas, assigning a letter for each building or area that contains animals. If there is only one building or area that contains animals then the letter is "A". Each animal identification team is responsible for assigning the rest of the numbers and letters for their designated building or area and sketching a map that shows each number and letter assigned to serve as a key for the entire case (see the animal ID team section below).

Following the first letter is a number. This numbering system is assigned to each room within the building. This number assigned to an animal corresponds to the room where the animal was located. If there is only one room within the building, the number is 1. Following this number is a letter which is assigned to each row or section of cages or runs within that room. This letter assigned to an animal corresponds to the row or section where the animal was located. If there is only one row or section, the letter is A. Following this letter is a number. This numbering system is assigned to individual cages or runs, even if they are empty. This is to maintain continuity and show empty cages/runs that may have previously been occupied. The number assigned to an animal corresponds to the cage or run where the animal was located. If there is only one cage or run, the number is 1. This number is followed by a hyphen and an animal number which is based on the number of animals within that cage or run, i.e. 1, 2, 3, etc. The animal ID of B2C3-1 indicates the animal was in building/area B, room 2, row/section C, cage/run 3, and was the first animal removed from that cage/run.

For situations where the animals are free roaming in a single-room building, as discussed above, the defaults of A or 1 apply: e.g., A1A1-1, A1A1-2, etc. For animals that are free-roaming outside, the area may be given a letter designation and the following number-letter-number assigned will be defaults of A or 1. For example: the first free-roaming animal found around the house, designated area D on the map, will have an ID of D1A1-1. For situations where juveniles are located in the same cage as their mother, the juveniles' ID will include their mother's ID followed by a letter corresponding to the juvenile species (P for puppies, K for kittens), followed by the juvenile's animal number. For example: B2C3-1P1 indicates a puppy belonging to female B2C3-1 and that both were located in the same cage. After the animal ID is assigned, it is written on a label (duct tape) that is placed on the transport carrier (see Animal Removal section).

This unique animal ID is permanently assigned to the animal to be used throughout the case: on all paperwork, exam forms, laboratory forms, and reports. This system works for any species of animal in large scale seizures. From an evidentiary standpoint, it is extremely important to use this system when dealing with multiple animals of the same breed and coloring to differentiate them from each other.

The use of a color-coded system for triage and animal removal

The use of color codes is important for large scale cases to implement a visual system of communication at the scene, from scene to the shelter, within the shelter, and for forensic examinations. The colors are used to designate triage categories, initial on-scene temperament issues, and conditions that determine placement and housing within the shelter. The assignment of color categories may vary with each case based on the availability of the color devices used. Colored duct tape is easily used and readily purchased at home improvement, hardware, office supply, and general merchandise stores. The use of colored flagging tape is sometimes used but poses several problems and risks: animal ingestion, difficult removal from the transport cage/carrier after tied for transfer with the animal to the shelter cage, and difficult removal from the cage within the shelter when the color no longer applies or needs to be changed.

The color-coded system often used is:

Red: bite case (has bitten a human)

Yellow: handle with caution (this is for animals that have exhibited shyness, fear, or aggression and is intended for handlers to be cautious, especially at shelter intake)

Pink: pregnant (suspected at the scene or confirmed on exam)

Green: infectious (suspected at the scene or confirmed on exam)

Blue: priority exam (in determining which animals are to be examined first by the forensic exam teams, the blue animals are the priority exams)

Orange: first general exam (these animals are examined next after the blue priority exams are completed)

Black: emergency (to be transported to off-site veterinary facility)

A piece of the appropriate colored duct tape is placed on the animal ID label located on the transport carrier. Note that some animals may have more than one color assigned.

The primary use of the color system is at the scene but some colors may continue to be used within the sheltering system. The color system and their assigned categories should be posted at the scene, within each forensic examination area, and at multiple areas within the shelter. It is helpful for each team lead, especially the animal identification and removal teams, to have a notebook with the color system written on the inside cover for easy reference.

Animal ID, animal removal, and transport teams

The Animal identification team is comprised of two scribes: one to sketch the maps and assign the letter-number designations, and one to create the animal ID label for the carrier and the animal ID collar, and maintain an animal inventory log of the animal IDs assigned. Copies of these final maps must be made and distributed to the appropriate team leads including the lead veterinarian, lead investigator, and shelter manager. The scene animal inventory logs are a backup system for the transport manifest and shelter intake log and should be given to the overall animal ID team lead. The best way to create the animal ID label is by using silver duct tape (the most common color and easiest to obtain) and writing the animal ID on the tape, leaving an area for color code tape assignments. This duct tape label may be placed on the clothing of the person removing the animal and then transferred to the transport carrier.

The animals may be removed after the animal ID team has assigned the animal ID. The animal removal team is comprised of several skilled animal handlers who are responsible for removing the animal from the cage, transferring into the transport carrier, and placing the animal ID label on the carrier. The appropriate animal handling is critical at the scene (see Sheltering and Animal Handling section). In addition, couriers are needed to take the carrier to the transport vehicle.

Each animal must be photographed with a frontal face view and the case board (which contains the case number, date, and animal ID) in the picture. This may be done as the animal is removed or prior to placement in the transport carrier. The photographer may be part of the animal ID team, the animal removal team, or a separate photography team. Absorbent material, such as newspaper, should be placed in the bottom of each carrier prior to placing an animal inside. After the animals are removed, it is the physical evidence and/or medical evidence team's responsibility to document, through photography/videography and mapping, the conditions within the housing environment that the animals were removed from, including the collection of any evidence.

The transport team is comprised of the load master, assistants, and transport driver. This team is responsible for the transport manifest, carrier placement, and safe transportation of the animals to the designated shelter site. The transport of animals from the scene to the shelter site should be done in such a manner to minimize stress on the animals and that is compliant with any applicable state or federal laws.

Considerations should be given to the environmental conditions, the time required to fully load the vehicle, and the effect on the animals first loaded. The spacing of the animal transport carriers within the transport unit should be planned to provide adequate ventilation around the animals. The individual transport carriers should be of sturdy construction, put together properly to prevent animal escape or injury, have adequate ventilation, and consist of a design that allows stacking of carriers. Special areas may need to be designated toward the off-loading area for animals requiring immediate veterinary care upon arrival to the shelter. Planning for animal carrier placement based on infectious disease is difficult and usually unnecessary with most cases when there has already been ongoing exposure between animals based on their living conditions.

The driving time for transport is important and should be kept to a minimum. For extended drive times, the driver or an additional designated person riding with the driver may be needed to periodically stop and check on the animals. Any transport unit should have solid walls and adequate ventilation to reduce the buildup of carbon dioxide during transport. The unit should have adequate temperature control for the health and safety of the animals. Additional external lighting may be needed if the loading or unloading process begins or extends beyond daylight hours. After unloading at the shelter, if additional transport is needed from the scene, the carriers may be re-used after cleaning and placing fresh newspaper inside.

The transport manifest is an important legal document comprised of a log of each animal ID and physical description as they are placed in the vehicle. In addition, this manifest should include the date and time of departure from the scene and arrival at the shelter. It is to be filled out by the driver and serves as part of the chain of custody. A copy of the truck manifest is sent with the driver and the other copy is given to the lead investigator to be used as part of the evidence receipt, which is required to be given to the person who is the subject of the search warrant. Upon arrival at the shelter, a separate intake log will be maintained for each transport arrival. This, together with the transport manifest, documents the chain of custody of each animal. The transport manifest and shelter intake logs are extremely important legal documents and it is imperative that the responsible persons are meticulous in their documentation.

For animals that have received on-scene medical examinations, a copy of the exam paperwork should accompany the animal in transport. This paperwork for each animal may be placed inside a plastic sheet protector and secured with duct tape to the top of the carrier or given separately to the driver to provide to the lead shelter veterinarian. If attached to the carrier, the transport load master should place the animal on the vehicle where the paperwork is protected and will be the first to be unloaded at the shelter site. Ideally, the blue-colored priority exam animals should be loaded in a manner to facilitate first removal at shelter intake for the shelter forensic exam teams to assess.

Medical teams

Critical triage team

The purpose of the critical triage team (CT) is to identify any animals in need of urgent care. The triage team is comprised of veterinarians with or without veterinary technicians. The CT team assesses animals after the initial walk-through as the physical evidence (PE), animal ID (AI), and animal removal (AR) teams begin their work. Any critical animals are priority for ID assignment and removal. After identifying any critical animals, the CT team works with the AI and AR teams to assign the animal ID, photograph the animals, and place them in carriers. At the veterinarian's discretion, the normal animal ID protocol may be delayed and assigned after removal to facilitate urgent medical care.

Provisions for an on-site critical exam area should be made. This may be in a vehicle, such as a mobile veterinary clinic, a mobile operations vehicle or trailer, a mobile temporary building, a tent, or one of the buildings located within the scene. Any animal that is examined on site and subsequently transported to the shelter should receive a blue color code. Local veterinary and emergency hospitals should have been identified to receive critical cases. Due to the confidentiality of the case, these hospitals should not be contacted until the day the search warrant is executed unless the local veterinarian is part of the medical teams. There should be a designated person and an available vehicle for emergency transports. Euthanasia decisions are made per the established medical protocol (see below). Part of the planning should include provisions for holding of any euthanized or deceased animals for possible necropsy.

Forensic exam team

The forensic exam teams (FE) are responsible for examinations of all the animals. The teams are comprised of a veterinarian skilled in the animal species involved in the investigation, a scribe, and animal handler. Depending on the species, a courier may be needed for transport of carriers to and from the exam areas. It is important that all animals are examined in a timely fashion, no longer than seventy-two hours, to ensure the examination evidence is representative of the animal's condition at the original scene and any health issues are addressed as quickly as possible. This is the purpose of the color-coded system, to establish the examination sequence. Each FE team can usually process four to six animals/hour depending on the severity of injury or illness, the ease of handling the animals (temperament or socialization issues), and the size of the animals. The exam and treatment process should be complete and efficient. These teams work best when the scribe, who must be familiar with medical terminology, fills out the examination form and the veterinarian dictates exam findings. The creation of additional types of teams can improve this efficiency and free up the veterinarian to focus on examination and documentation.

These additional teams include a laboratory team comprised of one person (usually a veterinary technician) to perform in-house testing, such as viral and heartworm snap-tests and fill out laboratory submission forms, a treatment team comprised of two people who provide vaccinations and treatment per the established medical protocol and specific instructions for an animal from the examining veterinarian, an exam photographer who may float between several exam stations taking the requisite animal photos (see Chapter 3), and any areas of interest noted on exam.

It is important that each veterinarian use the same exam form (Appendices 24–25). It is the responsibility of the scribe to ensure that the entire form is complete and the veterinarian's responsibility to review it for accuracy. In addition, the veterinary teams should use consistent terminology and abbreviations, which may be posted in the exam areas. A series of conference calls and briefings for all FE team members (at minimum the veterinarians) should be conducted prior to the day of seizure to facilitate communication and understanding of all forms, protocols, assessments, and descriptions.

The breed descriptions should be done carefully. Unless the breed is known, it is often best to use "breed-type" or predominant "breed-mix." The body condition scale to be used should be posted in each exam area so that the veterinarians can refer to it. Often, it is very difficult to age adult

animals. For this reason, it is best to designate the animal as adult unless the age is known. For juvenile animals, in which the age estimate is possible due to dentition, the age estimate may be documented along with the basis for the determination. After the examination is completed, a check mark should be placed on the animal ID duct tape to create a visual indication that the animal has been examined. Any color-coded markers should be assessed and removed or changed based on the exam. Any change that affects the shelter operation should be communicated to the shelter manager by the animal courier.

The medical protocol for the animals should be established during the planning stages (Appendix 22). This includes vaccinations, testing, deworming, and flea treatment. It should cover the protocol for euthanasia and handling of deceased animals. Because the animals are evidence, and out of sensitivity to the case responders and public sentiment, the criteria and parameters of euthanasia decisions should be discussed with the lead investigator and prosecutor prior to the day of seizure. The decision for euthanasia should first be agreed upon by the examining veterinarian and the case lead veterinarian, either the animal evidence chief or the medical evidence lead. The lead veterinarian should obtain permission from the lead investigator to euthanize. Another factor to address in the planning phase is the use and storage of controlled drugs including, euthanasia solution and sedatives. A controlled drug log must be maintained per the state and federal laws.

The exam forms should be in triplicate: the original goes to the lead veterinarian, the other two copies go to the shelter manager. One copy stays with the shelter paperwork and one copy will go with the animal as part of its medical record when transferred for placement or adoption. Diagram forms may be used to document injuries or scars (Appendices 15–18, 33–34). The diagram forms may be single or in duplicate, in which case both copies go to the lead veterinarian. As the supervisor of all the FE teams, the lead veterinarian is responsible for writing the final examination report of all the animals based on the exam forms, laboratory tests, any hospital records, scene notes, and photographs/video taken of the scene and animals. It is important to have a person designated to collect all exam forms daily and organize them in alpha-numeric order.

It is important to plan for an FE team to be at the shelter for the arrival of the first animal transport. This team may be comprised of one veterinarian and assistant, preferably a veterinary technician. The shelter FE team is responsible for visually assessing the animals as they are placed in the shelter and addressing any issues that may have emerged during transport. In addition, any animals that were identified during critical triage and examined at the scene but deemed safe for transport should be re-assessed by the shelter FE team (blue coded and with medical paperwork). Examination areas should already be set up in preparation for the full FE teams. Depending on situation, the shelter FE team may elect to begin forensic examinations of the blue priority animals. For a two-person team, this may require additional assistance from shelter staff to handle or courier animals.

Sheltering and animal handling

The full planning and design of a temporary shelter is beyond the scope of this textbook. Organizations such as the American Humane Association offer training in disaster sheltering which are the same principles used for large scale cruelty sheltering (Appendix 37). The primary difference is that the animals are evidence in a criminal case. Protocols must be in place for monitoring, treatment, daily assessment, and progress documentation. There should be a shelter mapping system to identify and track the location of every animal, including when moved. It is important to have the veterinarian's input on the initial design and any adjustments needed based on the animal findings during the seizure or forensic examinations. The shelter should be designed to be flexible based on changing conditions with the animals, either medical or behavioral.

Planning of the shelter design should consider the species of animal (see Appendix 28 for small bird sheltering guidelines), infectious disease, temperature control, airflow, foot traffic, noise issues, animal stress, and environmental enrichment. Continued assessment and reassessment of animal behavior and temperament should be conducted with changes made to improve any issues.

The proper handling of animals at the scene, during examination, and in the sheltering environment is extremely important. Many of these cases involve animals that lack proper socialization and/or have been under severe stress. They may exhibit fear or aggression, or they may be completely shut down (Figure 4.1). Some animals may exhibit subtle behavioral clues of extreme distress. It is the initial handling at the scene that can set the animal up for success or failure for future adoption, though a negative setback can occur during the examination or shelter handling process. The key to successful handling of animals involves the accurate appraisal of behavior, having an adequate number of properly trained staff, and using the appropriate equipment in the appropriate area, with proper training being the most important aspect.

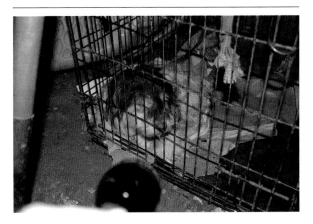

Figure 4.1 Dog that is completely shut down during a hoarding seizure.

The Animal removal teams should exercise extreme patience and discretion in their animal handling. Resistance to animal handling and restraint is almost always the result of fear or anxiety, which is compounded when force is used. It is better to take several hours if necessary to remove an animal than to force the issue and reinforce the animal's fear and negative associations. It is important to recognize that these animals may have reactions to novel stimuli that animals raised in normal homes would not. The simple act of petting may cause extreme distress. The animal may avoid foreign substrates, such as walking on grass for dogs. Sounds such as music may cause distress. It is not uncommon for dogs to react negatively to leashes. All of these potential issues are important for the animal handlers and shelter staff to recognize and handle appropriately. The assistance of an animal behaviorist can be highly beneficial for the animals' well being.

Organization of large scale grave excavation and on-site necropsy analysis

Team composition

Several types of experts should be considered to assist in these types of cases: veterinarians, veterinary pathologists, anthropologists, entomologists, archeologists, crime scene investigators, and mapping experts (by hand and/or use of total station; Chapter 2). Additional expertise may be needed such as IT and crime scene photography/videography. There may be several teams based on the number and size of the burial sites and the number of animals buried. Additional team members may include: scribes, assistants for the experts, sifters, and experienced grave excavators. Local universities are a great resource for the needed experts and often have experienced students who can assist with the case. As described above, other personnel are needed for certain roles and responsibilities including evidence technicians, security, and a medic.

Excavation and animal examinations

The process may be divided into excavation, radiology, examination of the remains, and storage of the remains. There are section heads for each section, who are assisted by specialists, and they should be involved with the set-up. A zone system should be established for the site, separating different work areas to limit foot traffic and protect the grave site. This provides a secure and efficient workflow as well as respectful treatment of the remains. Tents, RVs, and portable trailers may be used for working space in the different areas. Portable toilets and wash areas are needed for all the teams. Security badges that are numbered and color coded can be assigned to the different team members. The color codes designate the zone areas the team members may enter and the numbers are recorded by security at the site entrance with each arrival and exit. The excavation site may be secured with fencing, establishing the inner zone, and twenty-four-hour security personnel. Tool storage, an office, and facilities may be set up for the excavation team within the inner zone that can only be entered when team members change into work clothing and appropriate full personal protective equipment.

Once a set of remains is uncovered, it is identified with an evidence marker and animal ID, photographed, recorded on the evidence log, and mapped (Chapter 2). The remains are then moved to the processing area where they are recorded on the intake evidence log. At the processing area the remains are radiographed and examined. Every effort should be made to keep the body in the original position in which it was found for the examination. Digital radiology may be set up inside a dark tent with a controlled light source to facilitate reading of the radiographs. Light-colored tents are preferred for necropsy examinations due to the natural lighting. If the examination will be delayed, the bodies should be placed in body bags in their original grave positions. There should be a refrigerated storage area, which can be a refrigerated trailer, to hold bodies before and after examination. All movement of bodies in and out of the storage area should be recorded on an evidence log. A system of tagging the bags to identify completed and pending examination should be implemented. All evidence collected from the excavation site and necropsy exams, including any special instructions for evidence handling or further testing such as pathology, toxicology, or DNA, should be turned over to the designated evidence technician. After all examinations are completed, the remains are transferred to the appropriate authority for final storage or disposal (Figure 4.2).

Several additional considerations can enhance the excavation and necropsy process. Plastic sheeting may be placed on the ground in all work areas to facilitate clean-up and create clean areas for equipment and supplies. It is helpful to have a person(s) who has experience with tools and craftsmanship to create needed items at the scene using wood, plastic, etc. Exam tables may be built on-site by covering plywood with plastic sheeting and placing it on sawhorses. Writing and supply tables may be created the

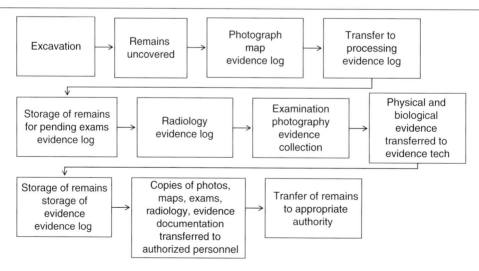

Figure 4.2 Operation structure of large scale grave excavation and on-site necropsy analysis.

same way. A stretcher may be made from plywood covered with plastic sheeting with rope handles on each end for transporting the bodies from the burial to the examination site.

Additional considerations for large scale cases

There are several additional considerations for planning and implementing large scale responses. Planning for the handling of the media is extremely important and should be part of the briefings for all personnel associated with the case (Chapter 1). This should include no pictures or videos, including from cell phones, of any animals, the scene, or investigators. The case documentation is most important and copies (paperwork, photographs, videos) should be given to the appropriate and authorized personnel. A secure area should be identified for daily briefings, debriefs, and team lead meetings. A secure, private area at the staff lodging location, which may be used for the serving of breakfast and dinners, creates the ideal confidential place for discussions. Having these meals catered with set times greatly reduces the staff stress and decreases the need for multiple vehicles to transport people to restaurants. One can consider creating a place for staff to have down time at the shelter site that is free from animals and noise. Inclement weather should be planned for, with a protected area for staff gear and supplies and a temperature controlled area for staff breaks provided. Stainless steel rolling tool carts may be used as exam stations. For slippery exam surfaces, bath mats are ideal to create traction, are easily cleaned, and may be disposed of at the end of examinations. Lastly, when the time for animal removal will be extensive, provisions for the feeding and watering of the animals at the scene must be made.

TRACE EVIDENCE

Overview

When examining an animal or the crime scene, the veterinarian and investigators are searching for evidence that provides links between the suspect, victim, weapon, and scene, including evidence that can assist with re-creation of the incident. Edmond Locard (1877–1966), considered the founder of forensic science, developed the rule that "every contact leaves a trace," known as the Locard Exchange Principle. This principle is based on the transfer theory that any time two or more surfaces come in contact with each other, there is a mutual exchange of trace matter between the surfaces. Trace evidence is by definition very small pieces of evidence found on objects or surfaces and is found in a variety of forms that can be virtually limitless

Table 4.1 Types of trace evidence.

Hair	Skin
Fur	Tape
Fiber	Tape residue
Paint	Fire debris
Chemicals	Fire accelerants
Gunshot residue	Glass
Soil	Feathers
Pollen	Plastic
Metal	Sand
Brick dust	Sawdust
Plant material	Bodily fluids

(Table 4.1). Trace evidence can provide the linkages answering what, where, how, and when through microscopic examination and forensic analysis.

The basis for trace evidence analysis is that humans and/or animals could not interact or have been present at a crime scene without leaving behind associated evidence or taking evidence with them. Evidence may be transferred by direct deposit or secondary transfer. Direct deposit is from direct contact with the source. Secondary transfer refers to a transfer of evidence through an intermediary person, animal, or object to a surface such as an animal, person, object, or location. With secondary transfer, there is no direct contact between the source of the evidence and the surface from which the evidence is recovered.

Trace evidence on the animal

There are some positive and negative attributes of an animal's body and behavior for retention and retrieval of trace evidence, also called trace. Animals' fur can hold embedded trace in the same manner as human hair, with entire body coverage in which trace evidence can be found. However, depending on the density and length of the fur, it may be more easily dislodged and lost and precautions should be taken to preserve any potential trace evidence starting at the scene (Chapter 2). The persistence of trace is affected by the size and texture of the material being transferred, the surface on which it is retained, and how easily it may be removed. The ability to retrieve trace evidence is also affected by the length of time since the incident and the activity of the suspect or victim.

In humans, trace evidence can be found on the body after a prolonged period of time, surviving environmental elements including heavy rains and submersion in water. There are different considerations when looking for trace evidence on animals. The human nail has a pocket under which trace evidence may become trapped. In animals, trace may be found embedded in frayed nails, the fur between the claws, or around the foot pads, especially if there are skin injuries. Evidence on the feet can be easily lost, especially if the animal was mobile or groomed the feet.

It is important to consider the possible behavior of the animal during and after the incident. In response to injury, the victim may hide, roll around, rub on surfaces, and lick or bite at painful injured areas. During the assault, the animal may have responded defensively by biting or scratching the assailant. Alternatively, the suspect may have taken precautions to prevent this by using restraints to control the mouth, body, and/or feet of the animal.

Collection and analysis of trace evidence

As discussed in Chapter 3, it is important to have all information from the case investigation prior to the examination of the animal. This includes what the suspect was wearing, any wounds on the suspect, crime scene photos, and the different environments in which the animal may have been kept prior to examination. The elements of the crime and the alleged events help direct where to search for trace evidence. As examples, bindings may leave distinct fibers behind on the victim and at the scene; weapons and toenails may contain important hair, fiber, or microscopic DNA evidence (skin, blood). There are several other considerations when assessing the significance of trace evidence. These include possible contamination, the transfer and retentive properties of the material, the degree of specificity and certainty attached to the identification of the material, commonness of the material, level of discrimination in material comparison, and one-way vs. two-way transfer (Houck 2001). The significance of any recovered trace evidence is based on all the information gathered from the investigation. It is important to have all this information for the laboratory to be able to decide which evidence to test and what tests to perform. It also can determine the order in which the evidence is analyzed to prevent contamination. Any assessments made usually are subjective, with a high level of confidence supported by the overall data.

Because animals and humans often occupy the same environments it is not uncommon to find animal hair associated with criminal investigations as a secondary transfer from either the victim or suspect or where the animal was involved in the crime. Microscopic hair or fur examination may be conducted to determine the species and for comparison to samples of interest. Human hair is easily distinguished from non-human hair by examining the core

that runs through the center of the shaft (medulla). Humans have a thin medulla and animals have a thick medulla. There are large databases of animal hair including an online resource for the forensic analysis of animal hair called HAIRbase™ (Appendix 37). This is a digital database containing mammalian primary and secondary guard hairs from three different body regions: dorsal, ventral, and tip of the tail. For microscopic hair analysis, the examination cannot conclusively determine if a questioned hair came from a particular source. If the questioned and reference sample demonstrate a similar range of features it may be stated that the hairs are consistent with one another and could have originated from the source of the reference sample. If the sample is determined to be consistent, then mtDNA or nuclear DNA testing may be considered (SWG-MAT 2009).

Soil has many chemical and physical properties that may be analyzed and provide valuable information for the investigation. Another area of research is the biochemistry of soil. This involves the extraction of microbial DNA and fatty acids to develop of soil "fingerprint." The soil microbial community can change rapidly, which presents difficulty in comparison analysis after several weeks have elapsed since the event and/or sample collection. Fresh samples or stored samples at -20°C or -80°C are best for this analysis (Larson and Patel 2012).

Appropriate steps should be taken to avoid evidence transfer or contamination of evidence on the victim and at the crime scene, including avoiding contact with the suspect and wearing clean, protective equipment when examining the animal or collecting trace evidence (Chapter 2). The examining table should be thoroughly cleaned and a clean sheet or white roll or butcher paper placed underneath the animal (see below).

The face, lips, teeth, torso, legs, and feet should be carefully examined for any obvious trace evidence. The use of a UV light source can assist with identification of foreign evidence (Chapter 2). An indirect light source, such as a flashlight held at an angle, can help identify especially small pieces of trace evidence. A magnifying device is useful to detect and collect evidence. The physical context of the trace evidence is paramount to the value of the analysis. It is important to first photograph the evidence prior to collection and document the description and location. Once evidence is removed from its original location it can never be put back exactly where it was.

Certain tools are needed to collect trace evidence (Appendix 5). Evidence collection tweezers are best to retrieve hair and fibers. These plastic tweezers have ridges on the tips that have increased contact with applied pressure providing a more secure grip on fine objects. Clean tissue, such as Kimwipes®, may be used to retrieve hair or fibers. Evidence collection lifters with protective backers can be used to pick up hair, fur, fibers, dust, pollen, and other trace evidence. The lifter is similar to clear tape with an adhesive side that is pressed onto the evidence and then placed down on a vinyl cover or siliconated paper, which is the backer. A Belgian study of different products for forensic fiber sampling evaluated fiber uptake and saturation, fiber recovery, and the ease of analysis. It was concluded that the product that performed best in all of these categories was High Tack Etilux (De Wael, Gason, and Baes 2008). If lifters are not available, regular clear tape may be used with wax paper or a similar slick surface used as backing. It is not recommended to fold the tape onto itself, which can cause damage to the evidence when the tape is pulled apart. Any trace evidence lifting tape should be stored in a separate container or protective packaging to prevent contamination prior to use.

Precautions, such as blocking moving air, should be taken to prevent loss of trace evidence during the collection process, especially in outdoor situations. The evidence should be packaged separately using an appropriate sized paper envelope or pharmaceutical fold and labeled properly (Chapter 2). Any loose fur at the scene should be collected for potential mtDNA or species analysis (see DNA section). Control samples of the victim's fur should be taken, one of each color and with the root intact, for potential comparison to other evidence found. This includes samples of primary and guard hairs from each color pattern and length, with the root intact, taken from the dorsal and ventral body regions and the tail.

Trace evidence may not be grossly visible and may be embedded in the fur. After examination for obvious evidence, the animal, live or deceased, should be placed on top of white roll or butcher paper that is taped down to the table. The animal should be combed in sections with a clean fine tooth comb, collecting any obvious trace evidence separately and then any remaining debris for laboratory analysis. Another option is to use a special evidence vacuum on the body. There are several kinds of vacuums that capture all the debris into a special filter assembly that is then sent for analysis. The nails on the animal's feet can be scraped with a scalpel or special evidence scraper over a tissue or pharmaceutical fold to collect any potential trace evidence. In deceased animals it is best to remove the entire claw by disarticulation or cutting the nail off at the base.

In addition to fur, trace may be found on items related to the victim, suspect, or scene including collars, leashes, bowls, toys, dog houses, and pet carriers. Any collars, leashes, or tie-outs should be inspected for obvious trace evidence and the items collected as evidence.

FORENSIC BOTANY

Overview

Forensic botany refers to the forensic analysis of botanical evidence including plant anatomy, plant growth and behavior, plant reproductive cycles and population dynamics, and plant classification schemes to species identification. It can help confirm or refute an alibi, place a suspect/object/victim at a scene, and determine time of death or burial. Because plant material is ubiquitous, it is often found on bodies or at crime scenes as trace evidence. Types of botanical evidence include seeds, grass stains, plant leaves, plant stems, fruit, petioles, roots, and pollen (see Forensic Palynology). Plant matter may be found in stomach contents or feces, and on fur or clothing. Forensic botany can also involve analyzing plant growth around a body or area and wood from a weapon. Plant material also can be associated with poisoning. This botanical evidence may be from direct contact with the plant or as secondary transfer. Plant-derived evidence can be linked to specific locations and certain seasons, which can be used to verify an alibi, track movements of the suspect or victim, aid in determination of time of death, or determine the primary crime scene in cases in which there is a secondary body dump site.

Plant DNA may be linked to a specific tree or plant. The same DNA testing performed on animal tissue may be performed on plant tissue, including mitochondrial DNA. In addition, DNA tests may be performed on specialized organelles called chloroplasts, which are more resistant to environmental insult (Budowle 2005).

Because plant matter is ubiquitous, it is important to recognize botanical evidence. The location of the evidence and the types of samples collected depend on the nature of the crime. It may be easier to recognize significant botanical evidence in indoor crime scenes. In both outdoor and indoor scenes, botanical evidence should be compared to the surrounding plants to identify displaced leaves, seeds, or pollen that are foreign to the scene. There may be broken branches or leaves removed from a plant that may or may not be associated with the crime scene. Botanical evidence may be found surrounding the body, on a suspect, on the victim, or inside the body. The evidence found may help with crime scene reconstruction based on the point of entry, travel path of the perpetrator, area in which the crime occurred, site of the body dump, and point of exit (Ladd and Lee 2005).

Collection of evidence

The evidence location and condition must be documented prior to collection (Appendix 26). Documentation should include weather conditions, photographs, sketches, diagrams, and written notes. The approach to the scene and the crime scene area should be photographed 360° including close-ups of the plants and leaves. The location of surrounding vegetation and its condition should be documented including items such as broken branches, trampled areas, and fruit or flowering plants. A sketch should be made of the crime scene including all vegetation and a scale reference (Chapter 2).

Collection of botanical evidence should be performed by hand and in a manner to minimize contamination. It should include whole plants (with entire root structure if possible), any fragments that may be used for a physical match, and any pieces on the body. To provide a reference of what plants should be associated with that environment, collection should include ten to twelve samples of the largest or most common plants at the scene, and for trees, a 6- to 10-inch piece with obvious leaf arrangement for identification. For burial sites, the soil on the surface of the grave should be examined for plant fragments from the fill (original plants disturbed during the creation of the grave) and any new growth of plants collected (growth after burial).

After collection, the plants need to dry to stop metabolism and prevent mold and mildew. The plants should be packaged flat to dry using a field press; this can be done by wrapping the plants in newspaper and securing them between cardboard. Large plants may be folded accordion style and packaged. For fruits, a slice can be taken and placed on wax paper or slick paper (e.g., magazine) so it does not stick to the surface. Each sample should be packaged separately in a paper bag or cardboard box.

In addition to normal evidence packaging information, the sample should be include the type of plant, flower color, shape of fruit, and where it was found at the scene. The plant evidence should be stored in a cool environment for three to five days for drying. Mothballs may be placed in the box and sealed tightly to prevent insects from eating the plant. Plant material that has additional biological evidence (e.g., blood or feces) should be kept cool, not frozen, and analyzed within three days, after which the plant begins to deteriorate. Plant matter from stomach contents should be collected separately. Any plant matter for microscopic analysis may be placed in 10% formalin. For plant DNA testing, the size of the plant fragment can be a factor in the ability to obtain a DNA profile. A large quantity of the plant material should be collected, avoiding cross-contamination. The sample can be placed in a paper bag and should be stored frozen.

Forensic palynology
Overview

Forensic palynology is the study of pollen, spores, and other acid-resistant microscopic plant bodies (known as palynomorphs) as it relates to matters of law. Pollen and spores are valuable forensically because of their microscopic size, they are produced in vast numbers, they can be identified to a plant taxon, and they are highly resistant to decay (Milne et al. 2005). Pollen and spores are so morphologically complex that they can be linked to a specific plant type, site, region, or country. They are often called "the fingerprints of plants" (Milne et al. 2005). The value and significance of pollen and spore evidence depend on the case, types of pollen present, amount of pollen produced, prevalence of the particular pattern, and dispersal pattern. The same questions and linkages may be answered with pollen or spores as with all botanical evidence.

Because of their vast numbers and ubiquitous nature, pollen is often microscopically present on a body or object. Pollen may be found on shoes, clothing, fur, rope, or carpet, and inside the nasal cavity or upper airways when inhaled. Submerged water plants also rely on pollination to reproduce. Pollen may be valuable evidence when a victim is associated with a body of water in which the submerged plants may be pollinating.

Collection of evidence

It is important to take appropriate samples with consideration that pollen and other botanical evidence may become significant later. Because pollen can be recovered from almost any surface that has been exposed to air, it is critical to prevent contamination during the collection and storage of samples. Sterile gloves should be used. All instruments should have been cleaned and stored in sealed, airtight containers prior to use. All samples should be placed in sterile, airtight containers and sealed immediately.

Control samples are needed from the scene as well as the places where the victim and suspect live or work. This provides a baseline pollen record for later comparison to any recovered pollen of forensic interest (Milne et al. 2005). The control samples may be surface soil, mud, or water, including plant reference material associated with these areas. A minimum of 15 to 20 grams of soil or mud samples should be collected in a glass or plastic container or sterile plastic bags. The soil is collected by ten to twenty regularly spaced "pinch samples" (1/2 to 1 teaspoon) from the top 1 cm layer of soil by walking back and forth in a particular sampling area, placing the samples together in a container and shaken to mix. Several soil samples should be collected starting at 1 to 2 m2 from the target area of the crime scene, then 50 to 100 m2 for the locality sample; then 50 to 100 m away from the scene for a regional sample. Sample areas should include any entrance and exit points to the crime scene. For water, a minimum of 0.5 to 1 L is sufficient for analysis (Milne et al. 2005).

Storage should be done to prevent contamination and prevent bacterial and fungal growth, which can feed on pollen and hinder analysis. Dry pollen samples can be stored at room temperature and moist or damp samples should be refrigerated or frozen. With water and sludge samples, a small amount of alcohol or phenol should be added prior to refrigeration. Any water or soil samples may be frozen, which will not damage pollen or spores (Milne et al. 2005).

Surrounding plants and vegetation should be photographed and reference samples collected and packaged for identification as discussed above and should include any flowering plants. Smaller plants (less than 30 cm in height) may be collected intact, and for larger plants a 30-cm section should be collected, preserving attached leaves, flowers, or fruits (Milne et al. 2005).

DNA: DEOXYRIBONUCLEIC ACID

Overview

Animal DNA has been proven to be unique to the individual animal and the results have been used successfully in court. Animals live in close contact with humans and animal-derived trace and DNA evidence is often found at a crime scene or on a suspect. The uniqueness of animal DNA has profound implications in all criminal cases. The U.S pet ownership statistics from the American Pet Products Association 2011–2012 National Pet Owners Survey found that 39% of households own at least one dog and 33% own at least one cat, with a majority owning more than one dog or cat (60% and 52%, respectively). There are several types of information that can be obtained from DNA testing including species, sex, and maternal or paternal linkages. Breed determination is possible depending on identifiable unique DNA markers for the particular breed. Research has shown that inbreeding in dogs does not affect the ability to match DNA to a particular animal (Halverson and Basten 2005). Similar results have been shown in cats. In response to a criminal case in Canada, DNA testing was conducted on an island population of cats that were by

definition isolated with significant inbreeding. The test results reported by Dr. Stephen O'Brien from the National Cancer Institute found that there was a 1:70,000,000 chance of another cat having the same genetic profile.

There are three categories of animal DNA evidence: the animal as victim, perpetrator, or witness. The animal as victim can occur in cases of animal abuse, theft of an animal, or identifying a lost pet. DNA from an animal may be matched to a weapon, toys, bedding, brushes, bowls, and other items related to the crime or animal. Situations in which the animal is a perpetrator include animal attacks, property damage caused by an animal, or an unrestrained animal causing an accident. DNA from the animal may be found on wounds, clothing, or property. In animal attacks, this testing is important to identify the animals involved and prevent innocent animals from being euthanized for aggressive behavior (see below). The animal as a witness involves the animal's presence during the commission of a crime. The use of animal DNA has been used successfully in several criminal cases to link a suspect with a crime. During the commission of the crime, there can be transfer of hair, saliva, blood, urine, or feces from the victim's animal to the suspect and/or crime scene and from the suspect's animal to the victim and/or crime scene.

Mitochondrial DNA (mtDNA) is often used when the sample of nuclear DNA is too small or degraded. The mtDNA is unique in that it is maternally inherited and shared by the offspring along the maternal line. The mitochondria are more plentiful than nuclear DNA, making this test very important when there is a lack of usable nuclear DNA, especially in older remains. It is also a valuable analysis for dog hairs. Studies of canine mtDNA show substantial variation within and among dog breeds, making it a discriminating piece of forensic evidence (Gundry et al. 2007; Webb and Allard 2009).

Examination of the animal

When examining a case of animal cruelty, consideration should be given to the type and location of DNA evidence transfer that could have occurred between the animal and the suspect. This includes events during the abuse and any defensive actions by the animal such as biting or scratching. The body of the animal should be examined for DNA evidence, including blood, hair, saliva, urine, and semen (Chapter 3). A UV light can help detect evidence not grossly visible (Chapter 2). Special attention should be given to the mouth, feet, wounds, and any blood evidence present, especially if there are no obvious wounds on the animal. In sharp force trauma, it is possible that the perpetrator slipped and cut his or her hand, leaving blood evidence behind. A control sample of the victim's DNA always should be collected for comparison testing.

Collection of DNA evidence

General considerations

Samples of DNA should be collected by veterinarians, law enforcement, or other authorities who can testify to the collection procedures. Evidence should be collected and packaged as discussed in Chapter 2. Clean gloves should be worn during collection of DNA samples to avoid contamination. Gloves should be changed between handling different pieces of evidence.

The DNA laboratory should be contacted prior to shipment of any samples to determine what tests will be needed, the priority of testing, and to ensure that their preferred and submission procedures are followed. It is preferable to submit the entire item of evidence for testing. Care should be taken to prevent the object from having contact with other surfaces which may cause a stain to flake off. Alternatively, cuttings or swabs of the item may be taken when that is not possible, using sterile swabs (Chapter 2). Care should be taken to avoid dirt or leaf material contamination, which can inhibit DNA analysis. It is recommended to collect a control sample prior to collecting the sample of interest unless submitting the entire item to the lab. This reduces the chance of contamination from other materials. For this reason, the same solution should be used for both control and evidence samples when moistening the swabs. Moist samples should be stored in a cool, dry environment away from direct sunlight. Some samples may be stored frozen. DNA laboratories usually have preferred procedures for sample preservation so it is recommended to contact them for directions. It is also recommended to create a readily available manual for DNA collection and packing, including information provided by the laboratory.

The use of adhesive tape for recovery of DNA, especially shed epithelial cells, from crime scene items may be more advantageous than swabbing for selected areas on items. It is important to use a tape that is suitable for biological trace evidence collection as well as DNA extraction. The use of three-layer adhesive tape has been used successfully (see Trace Evidence) (Barash, Reshef, and Brauner 2010). Another adhesive, Gel-Pak® "O", was found to be ideal. It is a thin adhesive that only removed the newest or loosest particulate that is usually the most relevant forensic evidence; it also picks up mostly epithelial cells and little extraneous material. It is colorless, which allows staining and transmitted illumination, and can be mounted on different collection surfaces such as glass slides. The gel film allows easy removal of the cells and does not interfere with polymerase chain reaction (PCR) analysis (Vigil and Kelley-Primozic 2011).

There are four factors that affect the ability to obtain and interpret a DNA profile: sample quantity, sample degradation, sample purity, and ratio of major and minor contributors from DNA mixtures. Heat, cold, sunlight, bacteria, and mold can adversely affect DNA. It should be noted that usable DNA evidence has even been recovered from human fire victims and from the teeth of animals that have been buried for two years. Each source of DNA requires special collection and submission procedures. Sources of DNA include fresh collected blood, dried blood stains, wet blood stains, buccal (cheek) swabs, bones, teeth, hair/fur, feces, muscle, organs, hide, saliva, semen, sweat, and urine. Animals sweat through their nose and footpads, which can be another source of DNA. Touch DNA refers to the DNA left behind when a person touches an item. Because human skin is constantly shedding cells, when a person touches something he or she leaves skin behind. A sample as small as six to eight skin cells is enough to develop a DNA profile (Warrington 2010). In animal investigations, areas where the suspect may have touched items related to the animal, such as the collar, should be collected for possible DNA testing.

Blood evidence

Fresh blood collected by venipuncture should be placed into an EDTA or ACD tube, refrigerated, and shipped overnight to the laboratory. For dried blood stains, the entire object should be submitted if possible. It should be placed in a paper envelope and shipped at room temperature. Alternatively, swabs or cuttings may be submitted (Chapter 2). Blood that is found frozen in snow or ice should be placed in a tightly sealed tube and kept frozen.

Buccal swabs

Buccal (cheek) swabs are a non-invasive method for collecting animal DNA samples. Sterile swabs may be used or special brush swabs may be provided free by the DNA laboratory. Food and water should be withheld for twenty minutes prior to sampling. The swab is placed inside the cheek and swirled ten times, collecting two swabs from each animal. The swab should be air dried briefly and returned to the provided wrapper and/or paper envelope, leaving the end of the wrapper open.

Teeth and bone

Teeth are useful sources of DNA when the soft tissue is too degraded. The pulp of the teeth is well protected from decomposition. Viable DNA has been found in teeth up to two years postmortem. It is preferable to submit at least two molars in good condition without any cracks or chips. If there are no available teeth, then a 3- to 4-inch piece of long bone may be submitted. The teeth or bones should not be cleaned or bleached. If the samples are wet they should be tightly wrapped to prevent fluid leakage during shipping.

Hair (fur)

Hair may be submitted for DNA testing. Approximately ten to twenty hairs should be pulled from the animal (mane for horses, tail force horses or cattle, and neck guard hairs for elk and deer), taking care to obtain the roots (do not cut the hairs) and the sample placed in a paper envelope. If the postmortem interval is greater than twenty-four hours, then hair samples should not be collected. Shed hair may also be a source of DNA testing in animals, including mtDNA. Because animals groom themselves there is a chance that DNA may be obtained from the deposited saliva; this usually requires a larger number of hairs for testing. In multi-animal households there may be a chance of mixed DNA from mutual grooming, in which case a sample of each animal's DNA should be obtained. It may be possible to perform mitochondrial DNA testing on hair without roots. Loose hairs found on the body, objects, or other surfaces may be collected individually or with trace lifting tape and placed in paper envelopes (see Trace Evidence). Hair samples on non-porous surfaces can be lifted with conventional fingerprint tape. The lift should be placed sticky side down onto a piece of paper or microscope slide. Mounted hairs may be shipped in slide mailers.

Muscle, organs, and hide

Muscle, organs, and hide samples may be used for DNA unless it has been more than seventy-two hours postmortem and/or there has been significant decomposition. Spleen and muscle are good sources for DNA. The fresh tissue should be frozen in an airtight container and shipped overnight with a cold pack. Paraffin-embedded tissue is usually an adequate source of DNA. A 1-cm square piece of tissue should be submitted in a sealed container. Formalin fixation can inhibit DNA analysis, but tissues fixed for up to ten days in formalin may be acceptable.

Saliva, semen, feces, and urine

Swabs from dried saliva, semen, and urine evidence may be collected, but it is preferred that the entire item be submitted. Saliva samples may be air-dried or frozen. Fresh semen or urine should be placed in a leak-proof container and frozen. At least 50 ml of urine are needed for DNA testing. Feces also can be used for DNA testing. Dried feces should be placed in a paper container. Wet feces should be collected in a leak-proof container, immediately frozen, and shipped overnight. Moldy feces should not be submitted.

Predator attacks

There are special considerations when collecting DNA from a victim of a predator attack. The goal is to get the samples as soon as possible. The body should be kept cool and dry; ideally it will not have been exposed to rain. The target areas for collection should be where there is the best chance for isolated DNA from the predator. If the victim was wearing a collar it may contain DNA from the attacking animal. Any wounds where there was little to no bleeding should be swabbed because hemorrhage can wash away the predator's DNA. Any areas of fur where there is evidence of saliva deposition from the predator's mouth should be swabbed or the fur carefully clipped with sterile scissors and removed (Chapter 6). If there is evidence of frayed nails with or without fur embedded in them, the nails or claw should be removed using a sterile instrument, as discussed in Trace Evidence. Depending on the amount of DNA recovered and any degradation, the lab may be able to do a species identification or have an individual profile to compare to the suspected predator's DNA. Quantitative real-time PCR assays have been used successfully on mixed-species samples to quantify canine DNA and have facilitated successful profiling of individual dogs while minimizing the consumption of the sample (Evans et al. 2007).

If the suspected predator is available, several things may be of value for DNA testing comparison. For cases where there is evidence of feeding on the victim, radiographs may reveal bone fragments in the gastrointestinal tract. DNA analysis of the bones can be performed to compare to the victim's DNA. The feces of the suspected predator may be of DNA value for comparison depending on the time elapsed since the alleged attack. Any areas of injury on the suspected predator may have been caused by the victim and steps taken to collect potential transferred DNA evidence.

ANIMAL DEATH/INJURY IN HUMAN SUSPICIOUS DEATH/INJURY CASES

In human suspicious death or injury cases, the victim's animal(s) may be found dead or injured. The investigation tends to focus on the human side and often overlooks the value of animal evidence. The animal may have been killed or injured in a manner similar to that of the human victim;

thus, the animal examination could provide vital information for investigators.

One key question to answer is why the animal was killed or injured. The animal may have been defending the property or the owner, or otherwise became a target during the incident. The injuries may have been inflicted accidentally by either the victim or perpetrator. The animal may have been an unknown victim of the crime such as in arson cases, where the perpetrator did not know the animal was in the house.

The presence of an animal at the scene of a crime offers an opportunity to look for animal evidence on a suspect. There is a high likelihood that there was a transfer of animal fur to the suspect's body, clothes, or shoes. The suspect may have the animal's urine or feces on the bottom of his or her shoes from walking through an area where the animal normally urinated or defecated (usually outdoors) or from fear release of urine and feces during the incident (indoors or outdoors). During the assault of the animal, or in the process of defending the property or the owner, the animal may have attempted to or successfully scratched or bitten the suspect. This could result in transfer of animal saliva or blood to the suspect, transfer of human blood or hair to the animal, transfer of human DNA to the animal's nails or teeth, or findings of scratches or bite marks on the suspect. The animal's body, including the mouth and feet, should be closely examined for biological fluids and trace evidence. The teeth should be swabbed for possible human DNA and bacterial profiles (Chapter 6). The tail should be inspected for injury because it is often used to grab or throw an animal. The fur should be collected as discussed under Trace Evidence.

OTHER UNIQUE IDENTIFIERS OF ANIMALS

Some other unique characteristics of animals can be used to identify an individual animal. The most obvious identifiers are microchips and tattoos. All victims of animal cruelty should be scanned for a microchip, making sure to use a scanner that can read international chips and following the proper scanning method. The body should be inspected for tattoos, which usually are located on the ears or caudal ventral abdomen. There may be tattoo ink at spay incisions from a local trap-neuter-release (TNR) program. The nose print of the dog has been found to be unique to the individual dog, just as a fingerprint is to humans. The surface of footpads in cats is similar to a human palm in that they are covered with patterned creases that could be uniquely identifying; this is an area for future research. The dentition of animals may be useful for bite mark comparison provided there are unique characteristics such as size and shape of the teeth, occlusion, and dental arcade. One study was unable to distinguish members of the same family of animals by using the shape of the jaws or bite mark patterns (Murmann et al. 2006).

Paw prints may be useable depending on the purpose of analysis. Intraspecies paw prints of the same breed and size may not be distinguishable unless there are unique characteristics of the foot such as a deformity or missing toes. In cases of skinning or mutilation of the Canidae Family, where the species of the animal cannot be easily determined grossly, the paw prints may be analyzed in lieu of genetic testing of hair samples.

The wolf, coyote, and domestic dog have different characteristics based on the side, claws, and rear margin of the heel pad. The Western coyote paw print measures 2.25–3.25 inches, including the claws, with the front claws usually close together, not attached to the toe marks, and the claws from digits two and five usually not seen in the paw print. The forelimb heel pad has a pronounced three-lobed rear margin. The hindlimb heel pad rear margin is circular in shape with two slightly forward pointing lateral crescents. When compared to the coyote, wolf print differences include the size range of 3.75–5.75 inches, the toe marks are more rounded, and the four claws often register. The forelimb heel pad is arrowhead shaped and the two lateral lobes point rearward, which is unique to the wolf. The hindlimb heel pad rear margin has a pronounced three-lobed rear margin. The domestic dog has similarities with both the coyote and wolf. The four claw marks often register and the hindlimb heel pads have a pronounced three-lobed margin. The size overlaps with both the coyote and wolf due to the variety of dog sizes. The difference in claw marks for the domestic dog is that the inner claws often spread outward (Stern and Lamm 2011).

The animal tracks are different in the domestic dog when compared to the coyote and wolf. Dogs tend to have a sloppy pattern and tend not to walk in a straight line. This is referred to as a double register, where the animal's hind paw does not fall directly on the front track. Wolves and coyotes tend to walk in a straight line and have direct register where the hind paw overprints the forepaw (Stern and Lamm 2011).

MÜNCHAUSEN SYNDROME BY PROXY

Overview

Münchausen syndrome by proxy (MSBP) is a specific type of abusive syndrome perpetrated on children. The name Münchausen comes from Baron von Münchausen, who was a reputed teller of exaggerated lies and who later became addicted to the attention from his tales. This syndrome is characterized by an adult providing falsification of illness in a proxy, the child, to deceive the medical professionals so they will believe the child is ill. In the veterinary setting the proxy is the animal. Based on fictitious symptoms, doctors may hospitalize a patient, run a myriad of tests to investigate the symptoms, and render treatment. The motive of the perpetrator is to gain sympathy and attention. In child abuse cases, a high proportion of these perpetrators have been abused as children (Munro and Thrusfield 2001).

One of the warning signs of MSBP in children is the sudden death or unusual illness of the family pet. The index of suspicion of MSBP in animals may be raised when the symptoms or signs are deliberately produced or invented by the owner, the owner initially denies falsifying or causing the symptoms or signs, the symptoms are reduced or resolved when the pet is separated from the owner (Munro and Thrusfield 2001), and the pet is repetitively taken to a doctor for medical assessment and treatment, being subjected to multiple unnecessary procedures (Platt, Spitz, and Spitz 2006). There are three different stages of falsifying the illness. The first stage is false illness story alone, which does not cause any direct harm but may cause unnecessary tests and treatments. The second stage is false illness story plus fabrication of signs, which involves manipulating records or tampering with samples. The last stage is induced illness, which involves causing physical harm to the animal, producing a myriad of clinical signs (Munro and Thrusfield 2001).

It is the very bizarre nature of the symptoms and the complexity of the problem that makes detecting MSBP difficult. There are several things to consider in these cases: the animal victim who is being abused, the owner, whose mental state may be unstable, and the relationship between the owner and the veterinarian, which may hinder the doctor's ability to recognize the symptoms. These owners may present themselves as very caring, nurturing, and believable while actually injuring or facilitating the injury of the pet. They seem to find great emotional satisfaction when their pet is hospitalized, whereas most owners have anxiety related to this event. These owners believe that by hospitalizing their pet the doctors and hospital staff think that they are good owners. The perpetrators are often very calm when informed of the unusual medical symptoms and tests. They want diagnostic tests done and tend to be very involved with the care and treatment. They may excessively praise the staff. They may seem to have a medical background and seem knowledgeable about the pet's illness (Hanon 1991). It is important that the veterinarian

maintain objectivity and avoid manipulation by the owner. It also is important to remember the perpetrator's entire motive is to receive attention and sympathy.

Symptoms

The symptoms of MSBP victims can be anything, depending on what was used to induce the illness. Because any number of things may be used to make the animal sick, the range and degree of symptoms are limited only by the imagination of the owner. One hallmark sign of MSBP is when the test results are bizarre (failing to fit with any clinical picture), contradictory, or previously never reported in the veterinary literature. A study by Munro and Thrusfield (2001) found nine suspected cases of MSBP out of 448 reported cases of non-accidental injury. The features of these cases included attention-seeking behavior by the owner characterized by repeated requests for treatment, abnormal laboratory findings (electrolytes), recovery of the animal upon hospitalization (separation from the owner), interference with and breaking of an orthopedic intramedullary (IM) pin, unexplained and suspicious circumstances of serial pet deaths in one home, serial incidents, fear of owner by the animal, frequent veterinarian changes, and admission of the deliberate injury by the owner.

Deliberate poisoning and suffocation then revival may be one of the forms of abuse used to induce the desired symptoms. The most common clinical signs in children include hematuria, hematemesis, seizures, central nervous system depression, apnea, failure to thrive, diarrhea, vomiting, fever, rashes, and hypertension (Munro and Thrusfield 2001). The perpetrator may add his or her personal blood or blood from uncooked meat to the urine, vomit, or even feces and present the samples to the veterinarian. Over-the-counter medications, veterinary prescriptions, the owner's personal prescriptions, salt, or chemicals may be administered to the animal, producing gastrointestinal signs, neurological signs, biochemical changes, or even death. The owner may interfere with equipment used for treatment in the hospital or sent home with the animal. If the perpetrator has access to a syringe, he or she may inject foreign substances under the skin, including bodily fluids or feces. A feature in children MSBP cases is that the parent will shop around for physicians (Munro and Thrusfield 2001). One of the biggest clues that MSBP is the problem is the resolution of clinical signs once the pet has been removed from the owner for a period of time. The veterinarian should consider that the environment or another individual in the home might be the source of the problem and not the presenting caregiver.

Outcomes

Abuse by MSBP has high morbidity, high mortality, and high re-abuse in children. The long-term outcome is considered poor when the proxy remains with the caregiver inflicting the abuse. Of the nine cases reported in the Munro and Thrusfield study, three resulted in death and two required euthanasia. In addition, two of the cases had serial animal involvement over an extended period of time. When MSBP is suspected, the animal should be kept under constant watch and the owner should not be allowed alone with the patient. The primary goal is the safety of the victim. When discussing the medical situation for the animal, it is important to consider the perpetrator of MSBP may view the pet as a surrogate child. Emphasis should be placed on the welfare of the animal and the possibility of a fatal outcome unless the doctor knows what was done to the animal (Hanon 1991). The perpetrator may confess to his or her actions after initial denial.

Evidence

Evidence must be obtained to determine what the animal was being subjected to, administer correct treatment, and pursue criminal action. Because the perpetrators of MSBP may take advantage of any opportunity to continue the abuse and induce symptoms while the animal is examined or hospitalized, any place the owner had access to in the veterinary hospital needs to be searched for evidence. The offender may have taken certain items to use in the future, such as syringes, needles, and medications. Certain items should be collected as possible evidence and testing, including the sharps containers, trash can contents, which may contain syringes and needles or poisons, all IV lines and catheters, and all medication the owner had access to for the pet. All food and water in the cage should be inspected for evidence of foreign material, such as powders or tablet fragments, and collected for toxicology testing. Any vomitus, urine, or feces collected from a hospitalized animal should be examined for foreign material and/or tested.

SUFFERING

Overview

Many animal cruelty laws incorporate animal suffering as an element of the crime, sometimes defined as "unjustifiable" or "unnecessary" in the statute. It is the degree of this suffering that can determine the level of charges filed and impact the sentencing. Five freedoms were recognized for animals by the Farm Animal Welfare Council in 2009 that provide the basis for animal suffering: freedom from hunger and thirst, discomfort, pain, injury or disease, and fear of distress, and to express normal behavior (Table 4.2). Veterinarians are considered the experts on the animal's condition, including pain and suffering (see Pain section below), and are often asked to provide time estimates for the length of any negative or adverse conditions, physical or environmental, which are a component of the length of suffering. In addition to pain, it is important to recognize there are other forms of suffering that have can have mental and physical effects including stress, boredom, distress, and emotional maltreatment.

In daily practice, veterinarians are often asked about animal suffering by the caregiver. This is typically within the context of making medical decisions for the patient such as treatment options, euthanasia, anesthesia, analgesics, after care, and long-term prognosis. There is usually some level of animal suffering that occurs in routine veterinary practice and with certain medical conditions that is considered acceptable and manageable for various lengths of time. This is commonly based on a more positive outcome and acceptable quality of life for the animal. This is also based on an ongoing patient-client relationship with the opportunity to mitigate suffering with appropriate medical treatments. This assessment of suffering is in a completely different context than in an animal cruelty case or similar legal forum. It is important the veterinarian be mindful of these differences and objectively assess suffering within the proper context.

Suffering has been defined as different unpleasant states that one would avoid or remove themselves from if they could (Dawkins 2005). Suffering also has been defined as an unpleasant state of mind that disrupts the quality of life. This mental state is associated with unpleasant experiences, including pain, malaise, distress, injury, and emotional numbness (Gregory 2004), and must be either severe or prolonged. Causes of suffering include hot or cold environments, lack of food or water, confinement, space restriction, lack of social companions, lack of stimulation, injury, and disease (Dawkins 2005). There are physiological and behavioral manifestations of suffering as well such as increased corticosteroid levels (stress), respiratory rate, heart rate, or blood pressure; vocalizing; and the sudden release of urine or bowels (fear reaction). These manifestations must be contextually evaluated, because some of these same responses can result from pleasurable experiences.

Animals may have severe or prolonged experiences of fear, pain, hunger, boredom, thirst, and so on. Suffering can be further defined by looking for evidence that the animal attempted to or would have taken steps to change the

Table 4.2 The five freedoms for animal welfare.

Freedom from hunger or thirst	by ready access to fresh water and a diet to maintain full health and vigor
Freedom from discomfort	by providing an appropriate environment including shelter and a comfortable resting area
Freedom from pain, injury, or disease	by prevention or rapid diagnosis and treatment
Freedom to express normal behavior	by providing sufficient space, proper facilities, and company of the animal's own kind
Freedom from fear and distress	by ensuring conditions and treatment which avoids mental suffering

Newberry, S., M.K. Blinn, P.A. Busby, C. Barker Cox, J.D. Dinnage, K.F. Hurley, N. Isaza, W. Jones, L. Miller, J. O'Quin, G.J. Patronek, M. Smith-Blackmore, and M. Spindel. 2010. Guidelines for Standard of Care in Shelter Animals, p.10. Association of Shelter Veterinarians.

situation, either by escaping or to gain access to something wanted or needed (Dawkins 2005). Comparison of the animal's behavior after removal from the situation can reveal the extent of the suffering. It should be considered that the animal may be too weak to exhibit the behavior of escape, avoidance, or to otherwise seek change.

Learned helplessness may occur in animals that have been subjected to prolonged abuse. Learned helplessness refers to a condition in which the animal will not escape from a negative situation, even when able to do so. This occurs in animals that have been subjected to prolonged abuse without any opportunity to escape or effect change. They "learn" that they are "helpless" to change their situation. Eventually, when presented with an opportunity to escape or effect change, the animal will not attempt to do so.

Stress

Overview

Stress may be defined as an abnormal or extreme adjustment in physiology and/or behavior in response to prolonged or intense aversive stimuli (Griffin and Hume 2006). To recognize stress, the veterinarian must have an understanding and appreciation of the physical, psychological, and behavioral needs of the animal. These needs are affected and determined by species, gender, reproductive status, age, and environment. They include appropriate space, ability to locate to a safe area, light, suitable bedding, environmental enrichment, sanitary environment, appropriate food, and clean water.

An animal's response to stress is usually to develop coping behaviors such as hiding or escaping. The ability to cope varies with the individual animal and type of stressor. The unpredictability of the stressor may induce chronic fear and anxiety. Depending on the severity of the stressor

and the animal's coping ability, the animal may adapt over time and the stress response may no longer be activated (Griffin and Hume 2006).

The psychological impact of stress on housed cats is primarily caused by the lack of opportunity for active behavioral coping responses. The impact of the stressor is directly related to the degree the cat can exert a behavioral response to the stimulus. The most severe stress response is when the stressor is perceived as uncontrollable or inescapable (Griffin and Hume 2006). This is especially important in hoarding situations and whenever cats are housed with unfamiliar dogs.

Several factors affect the stress response, including novelty, severity, predictability, chronicity, and duration. The animal's prior experiences, socialization, personality, and genetics affect the individual stress response. Multiple stressors can have a cumulative effect. The physiological effects of stress are compounded by poor nutrition (Griffin and Hume 2006).

Physical manifestations

Acute stress causes the release of epinephrine and norepinephrine through the activation of the sympathetic branch of the autonomic nervous system. This catecholamine release can be triggered by several different stimuli in dogs and cats. However, in cats, apprehension is the most potent stimulus for its release (Griffin and Hume 2006). Triggers for apprehension can be anything unfamiliar to a cat presented in any form, including visual, auditory, and olfactory stimuli.

Persistent stress causes the activation of the hypothalamic-pituitary-adrenal (HPA) response pathway causing glucocorticoid secretion. Under chronic stress, the glucocorticoid secretion reduces over time and the animal actually becomes more sensitized to new stressors. When a chronically stressed animal is stimulated by a new stressor, the HPA system responds. Chronic activation of these pathways can have deleterious effects on the body, including insulin resistance, mental depression, increased susceptibility to infection, peptic ulcers, decreased reproductive capacity, promotion of dehydration, and sudden death. The pathology of disease of the urinary bladder, gingiva, lung, gastrointestinal tract, and skin may be affected by the increased endothelial and epithelial permeability caused by the stress response pathways. The metabolism may be altered because of chronic stress, resulting in weight loss, lack of normal growth, and abnormal behavior that may be harmful to the animal (Griffin and Hume 2006).

Acute or chronic stress can have potentially irreversible effects on the animal's health. Stress has behavioral, endocrine, and immune effects. Higher levels of prolactin are seen in dogs with chronic stress and high anxiety, whereas lower levels are seen with acute fearful and phobic events. Hyperglycemia and increased lactate are seen in stressed cats. Acute stress, including fear and anxiety, can result in decreased appetite, anorexia, vomiting, diarrhea, and/or colitis along with anxiety and displacement behavior. Recurrent or chronic stress results in alteration of the immune system, inflammation, increased sensitivity to pathogens, cellular aging, neurologic disease, and respiratory disease (especially in cats). Acute or chronic stress can cause urinary tract disease due to altered bladder permeability and is linked to feline interstitial cystitis. It can also cause dermatologic conditions as a result of increased immune cells in the skin, increased opioid levels which potentiate pruritis, and increased epidermal permeability.

Chronic stress can alter the bacterial flora, decrease gastric emptying time, increase colonic activity, and increase intestinal permeability to antigens. This can result in inflammatory bowel disease, gastrointestinal reflux, heartburn, and stress-induced hypersensitivity. Anorexia, pica, polyphagia, and polydipsia may also be seen. Behavioral manifestations of chronic stress include anxiety disorders, panic disorders, phobias, and compulsive disorders (Landsberg 2010).

Stress can produce primary physical injury or secondary-to-stress-induced behaviors. Escape behaviors can result in worn teeth from chewing on tethers or barriers due separation anxiety, phobias, and territory or barrier frustration. Stress can produce aggression and trauma such as maternal cannibalism (Figure 4.3). Frustration or conflict may lead to displacement behaviors that are out of context, which may progress to compulsive disorders, such as self-mutilation, if the animal cannot achieve homeostasis.

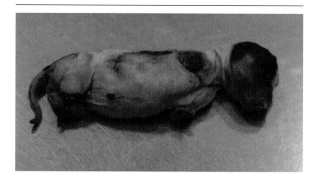

Figure 4.3 Maternal cannibalism in response to stress in a hoarding environment. (Photo courtesy of Dr. Doris Miller.)

Anxiety can decrease the left brain perfusion that improves with behavior therapy combined with anxiety drug therapy (Landsberg 2010).

Boredom

Animals have an innate need to interact with their environment, explore, and play. Juvenile animals are prone to develop arousing behavior that is part of the cognitive and neurological maturation. Confinement and lack of stimulation lead to another form of suffering, i.e., boredom, which has physical and psychological impacts on the animal. Prolonged confinement can lead to behaviors of self-mutilation; aggression toward other animals; tension; restlessness; agitation; coprophagy; over-grooming or fur pulling; and licking, sucking, or chewing at cage surfaces (Wemelsfelder 2005). A study was conducted on the effect of feeding enrichment using the Kong™ feeding toy with kenneled military working dogs in the U.K. It was found that there was no negative effect on the overall working ability, health, or behavior. The study did find there was a significant increase in the dog's ability to learn from being rewarded. Furthermore, the dogs showed an increase in cortisol levels when the feeding toy was removed and a decrease when it was re-introduced (Gaines, Rooney, and Bradshaw 2008). To recognize boredom, one must understand that the criteria are fluid and changing for the animal. The degree of boredom for an animal is most evident when one observes the behavior after the environment is changed to enriched conditions.

Distress

Consideration should be given to the distress of animals as a form of suffering. The definition of distress is as follows:Distress may be conceived as the unpleasant affective state, akin to or the same as anguish, resulting from an inability to control or otherwise cope with or adapt to the unpleasant affect generated by altered or threatened homeostasis (McMillan 2005a).

Examples of distress are boredom, pain, thirst, hunger, loneliness, fear, and any function of how an animal copes with the unpleasant affect. The term "affect" refers to any feeling, emotional or physical, in origin. Evidence of unpleasant emotions in animals are fear, phobias, anxiety, separation anxiety, loneliness, boredom, frustration, anger, grief, helplessness, hopelessness, and depression (McMillan 2005a).

Emotional maltreatment

Emotional maltreatment refers to the link between emotional states and physical health. Emotions can cause distress, anguish, and suffering. Long-term problems associated with emotional maltreatment may be separation anxiety, decreased learning, depression, difficulty with social interactions, or even physical manifestations of illness (McMillan 2005b). Because the idea of maltreatment in animals is analogous to children, the terminology associated with child maltreatment may be used. The U.S. Department of Health, Education, and Welfare defines maltreatment as actions or inactions that are neglectful, abusive, or otherwise threatening to an individual's welfare (McMillan 2005b). Note that the term maltreatment includes both neglect and physical abuse. Maltreatment should be considered from the perspective of the victim, i.e., the animal, in which the animal is harmed or at risk of harm.

Emotional suffering is generated along the same or similar pathways as physical pain, and the same drugs alleviate emotional and physical pain (see Pain, below). Studies have been conducted to determine which hurts more: physical and emotional pain. When the animals are presented with a choice to endure or relieve physical pain in response to separation anxiety, i.e., emotional suffering, they chose to endure the physical pain to alleviate the emotional suffering. A study of capuchin monkeys found they chose social companionship over food. There are reports of cats that have shown they will continue to enter a burning fire to retrieve their kittens despite enduring repetitive physical harm (McMillan 2012).

Traditionally, neglect is considered to be a passive act or act of omission by the caregiver to provide basic physical and emotional needs of a dependent being (McMillan 2005b). Most animal cruelty laws include neglect as a form of animal cruelty. It is estimated that greater than 80% of cruelty cases are classified as neglect. Commonly, neglect

has been characterized by a lack of intent considered a result of ignorance or poor judgment. However, a reasonable-person standard should be applied: What would a reasonable person think and do in a given situation? For example, when someone does not provide food or fresh water for an animal, a reasonable person would expect the result of death, or at minimum physical harm, due to imposed starvation and/or dehydration.

Sometimes proving intent by the abuser is required to meet the animal cruelty statute in certain states. Physical and emotional abuse is considered an active maltreatment characterized by intent to harm. These overt acts or acts of omission also are characterized by the caregiver's knowledge that the action or inaction will result in harm to the animal (McMillan 2005b).

There are four categories of maltreatment: emotional neglect, physical neglect, emotional abuse, and physical abuse. There can be crossover of neglect to abuse depending on the caregiver's intent and the animal cruelty laws.

Emotional neglect

An emotional need may be defined as any need that is signaled by an emotional affect (McMillan 2005b). The emotional needs of animals have similar properties as physical needs and are shared regardless of species, gender, etc. The physical needs of animals include food, water, shelter, temperature regulation, oxygen, health care, and exercise. Failure to meet both emotional and physical needs of an animal results in harm to the animal. The emotional needs of most animals include the following (McMillan 2005b):

- Sense of control and the ability to exert meaningful change to situations, especially those of an unpleasant nature
- Ability and resources to cope with aversive events
- Sufficient living space
- Mental stimulation
- Safety, security, and protection from danger
- Social companionship for social animals
- Adequate predictability and stability to life events

It is an accepted fact that dogs are pack animals and need social companionship. Studies on cats confirm that they are social animals as well, forming close social bonds between siblings and their mother. It also was found that given an option, cats prefer to live in colonies with other cats rather than living alone. The mental stimulation required depends on the age, sex, species, and specific traits of the animal (McMillan 2005b).

Emotional abuse

Emotional abuse may be defined as the deliberate inflic-tion of emotional distress on another individual. It includes acts of commission or omission that have caused or may cause serious behavioral, cognitive, emotional, or mental disorders (McMillan 2005b). A study was conducted in dogs on the physiological reactions to fear provocation, specifically assessing fear of floors and fear of gunshots. The dogs with fear of floors demonstrated higher heart rates than the fearless group. In the gunshot fear group, the study found elevations in heart rate, hematocrit and plasma cortisol, progesterone, vasopressin, and beta-endorphins compared to the fearless group, with cortisol and progesterone the most drastically increased (Hydbring-Sandberg et al. 2004). The following catego-ries of emotional abuse used for children may be applied to animals (McMillan 2005b):

- Rejection: Emotional deprivation, active refusal to provide emotional support and nurturing with the knowl-edge that the individual is harmed
- Terrorism: Deprivation of safety and security, hostility, or creation of a "climate of fear"
- Taunting: Teasing, provocation, or harassment causing frustration, anger, or mental anguish
- Isolation: Deprivation of social interaction and companionship
- Abandonment: Termination of care or desertion
- Overpressuring: Excessive demand or pressure to perform or achieve

Physical abuse

Physical abuse can cause emotional maltreatment if it causes emotional distress. There is evidence that emotional maltreatment produces harm that is often worse than physical abuse. This is seen in children with long-term effects resulting from emotional maltreatment, with simi-lar findings in dogs (McMillan 2005b). The harm depends on the animal's coping ability to the event. In animals, the long-term consequences may be seen as behavioral prob-lems under otherwise normal conditions, similar to post-traumatic stress syndrome in humans.

PAIN

The vital role of veterinarians trained in forensic sciences in interpreting biological, trace, and other evidence in criminal investigations is clear, and cannot be disputed. However, the role of forensic veterinarians in interpreting such evidence in the context of animal abuse and cruelty

investigations may be less well defined. The overriding issues in animal abuse and cruelty investigations hitherto have been somewhat inaccessible, namely, (1) do animals feel pain, and (2) what is the conscious experience of pain in animals?

For many years the subject of pain in non-human animals has been approached as mysterious and enigmatic by the judicial system. It has been difficult for prosecutors to convince judges and juries that *conscious experience* is a feature of animal life. Consequently, consideration of pain in non-human animals as an aspect of animal abuse often has been difficult to quantitate and communicate.

Prosecution of animal cruelty cases generally may be considered the exclusive purview of law enforcement offi-cials and veterinary forensic scientists. However, veterinar-ians who routinely examine and treat sick and injured animals have a unique role in the legal process of identifying cruelty and bringing its perpetrators to justice.

Determining the cause, severity, and duration of an animal's injuries (or the cause of death), as well as the extent to which the animal suffered or experienced pain, are vital legal elements of an animal cruelty case. Yet these elements cannot be established without the expertise of the veterinar-ian who has examined or treated the animal in question. For the veterinarian, this unanticipated status as a critical resource (and often witness) in animal cruelty investigations and prosecutions brings both rewards and frustrations.

The goal of this section is to summarize for veterinari-ans, veterinary forensic scientists, and prosecutors of animal cruelty cases the essential aspects of pain percep-tion in non-human animals. In turn, this will provide all parties involved in the prosecution of animal cruelty cases with a framework for the presentation and discussion of pain in non-human animals. Most importantly, the infor-mation that follows will assist a judge and jury to accept that animals do "feel" pain, and that there is a conscious experience (e.g., fear, suffering, stress) associated with feeling that pain.

The responsibilities of veterinarians in assessing animal pain

Beyond understanding local statutes and laws relating to animal abuse, veterinarians involved in animal cruelty investigations must understand the current views and scientific evidence regarding pain in animals. Pain is a sensory and emotional experience often caused by intense or damaging stimuli. Pain is a conscious experience involv-ing "unpleasantness" (i.e., suffering). For a non-human animal to experience pain, by that definition, the animal must be *capable of* consciousness and suffering.

The standard measure of pain in a human is that person's testimony, because only he or she can know the quality and intensity of the pain, and therefore, the degree of suffering. Non-human animals, without human language, cannot report their feelings in this way. Therefore, knowledge of aspects of animal behavior and physiology must be used to make the case that an animal is experiencing, or has experienced, pain and suffering.

A veterinarian is the person in the community best qualified to offer evidence with regard to pain in non-human animals. Pain assessment is part of a routine physical examination for most veterinarians, who recognize the importance of pain assessment as part of daily patient evaluation and often obtain a pain score as a fourth vital sign (temperature, pulse, respiratory rate, and pain). In addition to the owner's assessment, a veterinarian uses a behavioral assessment and the assessment of physiologic measures (heart rate, respiratory rate, etc.) as indications of pain. A veterinarian also may attempt to quantify pain in non-human animals by using one of the several pain scoring systems that are available. To illustrate the method involved in determining a pain score, some of the observations that may contribute to pain scoring are included in Table 4.3. A visual analog scale (VAS) to evaluate pain, similar to that used to assess the efficacy of pain management strategies, may be used. A VAS is a scale that goes from "no pain" to "worst pain ever," based on a numeric scale from zero to 100.

Questions that should be asked and answered by a veterinarian conducting a forensic investigation in which animal pain and suffering are being considered include (Table 4.4):

- Is there situational evidence that pain exists (e.g., a recent injury)?
- Are there altered behavioral responses that suggest the animal may have been subjected to abuse (e.g., increased aggressiveness, avoidance behavior, reluctance to be touched, decreased appetite, decreased activity, lethargy, vocalization, crying/yelping, lameness)?
- Are there physiological changes consistent with animal suffering (e.g., altered autonomic functions such as increased heart rate, increased blood pressure, increased respiratory rate, increased sweating, salivation)?
- Are there biochemical changes supportive of an animal having been subjected to painful stimuli (e.g., increases in cortisol or adrenaline in the blood)?

Objective data gained in this way permits a veterinarian to support or refute any claim of animal cruelty or abuse. This data also provides a platform for discussion of the

Table 4.3 Behavioral categories used to assess visual analog scale pain score in dogs.

Demeanor	Response to people	Response to food
Anxious	Aggressive	Disinterested
Depressed	Fearful	Eating hungrily
Distressed	Indifferent	Picking
Quiet	Sullen	Rejecting food
Posture	Mobility	Activity
Curled	Lame	Restless
Hunched	Slow/reluctant	Sit/lie still

emotional aspects of animal abuse, which are more difficult to assess in many cases.

Do animals "feel" pain?

All vertebrates (and some invertebrates) are capable of nociception, a neural response to intense or damaging stimuli. Nociception may be observed using modern imaging techniques, and a physiological and behavioral response to nociception may be detected, but presently there is no objective measure of the emotional aspects of animal nociception (i.e., suffering). An understanding of pain and the manifestations of pain (including suffering) in animals is an essential consideration in the processing of forensic cases in which animal cruelty is suspected. Yet pain, by definition, is a *subjective* phenomenon known to humans only by experience and described by illustration. Therefore, this apparently straightforward subject in humans becomes complex when applied to animals, particularly when accurate and subjective details must be included in a forensic record or report. Pain is something a judge and jury can appreciate based on their personal experience, and because of this, documentation of apparent pain is vital for the successful prosecution of animal abuse cases.

Whether animals are capable of feeling pain has been a matter of controversy for many years. Animals and humans share similar mechanisms of pain detection, have similar areas of the brain involved in processing pain, and manifest similar pain behaviors; however, it is notoriously difficult to assess *how* animals actually experience pain. We know *about* pain in an animal but we do not necessarily know *of* pain in an animal. The ascription of pain perception to animals is feasible only by *inference* and *reasoning from analogy*.

One of the principal objectives of veterinarians is to prevent unnecessary pain from occurring in animals, or to relieve suffering from chronic pain in animals. This is part

Table 4.4 Signs of pain.

Cat/dog	Cats	Dogs
Increased RR	Purr, groom	Whine, whimper
Increased BP	Growl, hide	Timid, aggressive
Increased HR	Squint eyes	Fixed stare
Blanched mucous membranes (vasoconstriction)	No change of body position	Arched posture
Muscle splinting (thoracic pain)	Laying sternal, balled up	Restless
Stress leukogram	Decreased human interaction	
Catabolism		
Change in vocalization		
Attention seeking		
Guarding of painful areas		
Lick, chew, paw at painful area		
Change in voiding behavior		
Change in grooming behavior		

Tranquilli W.J., K.A. Grimm, L.A. Lamont. 2004. Pain Management for the Small Animal Practitioner. Jackson: Teton NewMedia.

of the oath taken by veterinarians entering the profession. In fact, if all aspects of pain are considered, it may not be possible to have either an animal or a human in a "pain-free environment." It is therefore absolutely essential that a veterinarian be knowledgeable regarding the neural mechanisms involved in the perception of pain.

What is pain?

The biomedical definition of pain is an "unpleasant sensory and emotional experience associated with actual or potential tissue damage." The word "unpleasant" suggests an intangible quality. Pain, however, is experiential and subjective. It may be considered to have two components:

1. Physical hurt or discomfort caused by injury or disease
2. Emotional suffering

Each of these aspects of pain is relevant for a veterinarian completing a report in a case of suspected animal abuse: the former is *tangible* while the latter is somewhat *intangible*.

Physical hurt or discomfort caused by injury or disease

Should an event or situation cause pain to a human, it is reasonable to conclude that a similar event is likely to cause pain to an animal. Stimuli that elicit the subjective response of pain in humans, and by inference in animals, are referred to as *noxious stimuli*, meaning that the stimuli either produce damage to tissue or are potentially damaging to tissue.

Noxious stimuli may be divided arbitrarily into four categories:

- Physical injury from strong mechanical or thermal injury. Examples include strong pressure from tight ligatures or a burn from a branding iron.
- Inflammation of the tissues that may follow physical injury, but may also arise from local tissue reaction to chemicals. Examples include exposure to strong chemicals or caustic agents.
- Ischemia, which arises from impairment of normal blood supply.
- Strong electrical stimuli.

In all of the above circumstances pain arises because the receptors of neurons conducting nociceptive impulses are stimulated. This aspect of pain is the most straightforward for humans to understand. Most people agree that animals are capable of feeling pain that results from a physical injury or from the discomfort caused by disease; however, they also express the notion that they do not know anything about the "content or experience" of that pain (e.g., is it the same as that experienced by humans faced with a similar injury?).

There are three aspects that must be considered when testing hypotheses for the perception of pain in non-human animals:

- Animals possess neurotransmitters, biochemical pathways, and neural systems homologous to nociceptive pathways in humans. Arguments for pain perception in animals have been based on genome searches for genes that code for products such as substance P or prokinectins, or for receptors that may be involved in pain modulation such as opioid receptors. While this argument may be compelling for some, others have argued that DNA sequences are deeply rooted in evolution, and that the products from similar DNA may differ substantially from humans to non-animals. Simply stated, the presence of matching DNA sequences does not guarantee matching function, and the presence of identical neurotransmitters in animals and humans does not prove identical signaling function. Opioid receptors occur in many diverse animals; however, their presence does not necessarily argue for perception of pain as a general phenomenon among animals.

- The fact that analgesics used in humans are known to reduce the pain response in animals supports the hypothesis that the biochemical basis for pain perception and response is similar between humans and animals.
- Behavioral avoidance by animals of situations known to be painful to humans supports the notion of nociception in animals.

Animals meet all three of the above criteria supporting pain perception, and the evidence for pain as a physiological response to help an animal avoid injury is widespread and accepted.

Emotional suffering

This aspect of pain perception in animals is less clear to most humans, and is the subject of discussion and controversy. The basic question is: Does pain "feel" the same to non-human animals as it does to humans? The truth is, we will probably never know the answer to this question, just as we will never know whether "sadness" feels exactly the same to every human. However, attempting to answer this question, and to develop objective methods of assessing pain in animals, is an essential consideration in the world of forensics. The well-intentioned avoidance of anthropomorphism in this discussion may overstep reasonable scientific boundaries, because anthropomorphism may be an essential aspect of understanding the emotional suffering associated with pain in non-human animals.

Anthropomorphism refers to attributing human qualities to animals. In the scientific community, using language that suggests animals have intentions, desires, and emotions has been severely criticized as lacking objectivity. One of the worst sins a biologist could commit was to assume that animals shared the same mental, social, and emotional capacities as humans. Scientists would go out of their way to overlook evidence of mindedness, selfhood, and personality in non-human animals. The irony, of course, is that the more non-human animals have been studied, the more we have learned about their complex cognitive and emotional capabilities. We have learned that many animals have preferences and intentions, can solve problems, display emotions, are self-aware, and can create shared meanings with humans. Of course, anyone with affection for companion animals knows this intuitively. The discovery of these qualities has serious moral implications for how we treat our fellow creatures, including issues related, but not limited to, animal experimentation. If non-human animals are a "somebody," and not simply a "something," then what are the ethical obligations of humans to them?

Of course, we have to be careful not to go too far with this argument. Non-human animals are not little people in fur. They are what they are, with their own unique needs and desires. Attributing human qualities too freely or inappropriately to non-human animals could lead to misunderstanding them, and worse, to mistreating them. So anthropomorphism, if used wisely, does not have to be one of science's most serious transgressions. In fact, it may be the key to understanding emotional suffering in animals. If we can employ anthropomorphism critically to reach reasonable conclusions, without misrepresenting the animal's nature or needs, then it could help us not only understand non-human animals better, it might influence how to approach the documentation of animal abuse and cruelty.

What can forensic scientists and veterinarians learn about pain from the biomedical research community?

It is interesting to compare and contrast some of the issues experienced by forensic scientists involved in animal cruelty cases and the issues faced by scientists involved in biomedical research. Both forensic scientists and biomedical researchers have embraced the fact that the ability to experience pain in an animal cannot be determined directly. However, both forensic scientists and biomedical researchers agree that pain may be inferred through physiological and behavioral reactions (Tables 4.5–4.8). While this approach has been widely accepted by the research community, and by veterinary forensic scientists, it has yet to be widely accepted by those prosecuting (or defending) cases of animal cruelty.

Despite the inexact and subjective nature of pain, scientists have undertaken voluminous research concerning nociceptive stimuli, pain thresholds, nociceptors, nociceptive pathways, biochemistry, and avoidance behavior, all of which assume that animals do indeed feel pain. It is uncommon, however, to read discussions regarding the behaviors or the experiences associated with pain in animals (other

Table 4.5 Areas of psychological and biological deprivation associated with pain, stress, and suffering in animals used for research.

Denial of:

Social relations
Contact comfort
Privacy
Sensory stimulation
Food
Water
Space
Executable environmental challenge
Aggressive outlet

Table 4.6 Types of environmental variables whose range and quality may cause pain, stress, and suffering in animals.

Noise (quality and level)
Quiet
Temperature
Luminosity
Humidity

Table 4.7 Situational variables that may cause pain, stress, and suffering in animals.

Unpredictability
Forced exercise
Invasive procedure
Manipulatory procedure
Change
Electric shock
Burning or heat
Freezing or cold
Radiation
Inhalation or ingestion of foreign, toxic, irritative, or pathogenic agents
Externally and internally applied toxic, irritative, or pathogenic agents
Physical and psychological trauma
Abuses from co-animals under stress

than in the pages of animal use and care protocols), yet this is an essential consideration for the forensic scientist. For animal cruelty cases, this lack of objective information regarding the emotional aspects of nociception has impeded the ability of forensic scientists and veterinarians, because there is little scientific information regarding emotional suffering of animals. Unless it is the object of the scientific study, pain inherent in animal research is rarely addressed in journal articles.

The reasons for this reluctance by biomedical researchers to address the emotional aspects of pain in animals stems from a number of underlying issues, including:

- The pragmatic denial by biomedical researchers of subjective animal reality in an attempt to objectify animal life to reduce it to measurable data
- Frequent intensive, circumscribed, relatively exclusionary experimental focus on questions of critical experimental interest and manipulation, for which the latter can entail varying degrees of unpreventable animal suffering
- The human tendency to dissociate from pain-provoking circumstances. It is emotionally uncomfortable to keep animal suffering in the forefront of one's concerns
- The extension of traditional ideas that humans may use animals in the service of human interest and design
- Human conditioning to the incongruous position that considers animals dissimilar to humans with respect to drive, need, or sensation, yet similar enough to be used as models for the study of humans themselves. The doctrine of biological materialism dictates accepting verifiable pain based on the great similarities between animals' and humans' pain receptors, pathways, and centers. Pain neuro-structural similarities, in fact, are more striking than those of morphology, chemistry, or behavior specificity and breadth, all of which are used by researchers to draw conclusions from animals to humans.

Significantly, variations of these same issues are faced frequently by forensic scientists and veterinarians and by those prosecuting animal cruelty cases. Non-human animal pain is sentience, sensation, and feeling that humans can understand through observing either behavior or the lack of behavior. To know how and what an animal is doing affectively, cognitively, psychologically, and behaviorally, and to know whether it is in pain, humans (especially veterinarians) must carefully observe it and know about it in the way we know or think about other humans and ourselves; that is, with feeling and interest (i.e., anthropomorphically).

For veterinarians, forensic scientists, biomedical researchers, prosecutors, and others involved in the judicial system, recognizing animals in pain requires empathic observation, which in turn engenders identification with, sympathy for, and positive regard for non-human animals.

Table 4.8 Some behaviors that may be associated with suffering, pain, stress, distress, anxiety, and fear in animals.

Aphagia	Hyperphagia
Adipsia	Polydipsia
Lack of motivation/ability to reproduce	Self-imposed isolation
Continuous sleep or sleep-like state	Little or fitful sleep
Lack or care of coat or body surface	Staring, lack of blinking reflex
Ears flattened maximally	Body drawn in or continuously extended
Unusual positioning	Agitation, lethargy, listlessness
Head shaking	Grunting in expiration
Rapid, shallow breathing	Deep and staggered breathing
Facing away from surroundings	Muscle rigidity, lack of muscle tone
Convulsions	Unsteady gait
Self-mutilation, gnawing at limbs	Twitching, trembling, tremor
Panting, shivering	Hissing, spitting, biting, baring teeth
Growling	Scratching, kicking, struggling
Whimpering	Struggling
Baring teeth	Howling
Reduced awareness and response to environmental stimuli	Hypervigilance
Exaggerated startle response	Immobility, crouching
Apathy	Grimacing

SUGGESTED READING ON PAIN IN ANIMALS

Kitchell, R.L. 1983. Animal Pain: Perception and Alleviation, American Physiological Society Animal Welfare Series. Erickson, H.H., E. Carstens, and Lloyd E. Davis, eds. Baltimore: Wilkins & Wilkins.

Kitchen, H., A. Aronson, J.L. Bittle, C.W. McPherson, D.B. Morton, S.P. Pakes, B. Rollin, A.N. Rowan, J.A. Sechzer, J.E. Vanderlip, J.A. Will, A.S. Clark, and J.S. Gloyd. 1987. Panel Report on the Colloquium on Recognition and Alleviation of Animal Pain and Distress. *Journal of the American Veterinary Medicine Association.* 191:1186–1191.

Morton, D.B. and P.H.M Griffiths. 1985. Guidelines on the Recognition of Pain, Distress, and Discomfort in Experimental Animals and an Hypothesis for Assessment. *Veterinary Record.* 116:431–436.

Mroczek, NS. 1992. Point of View: Recognizing Animal Suffering and Pain. *Lab Animal* 21(9):27–30.

Rollin, B.E. 1989. *The Unheeded Cry; Animal Consciousness, Animal Pain, and Science.* Oxford: The Oxford University Press.

REFERENCES

Barash, M., A. Reshef, and P. Brauner. 2010. The Use of Adhesive Tape for Recovery of DNA from Crime Scene Items. *Journal of Forensic Sciences.* 55(4):1058–1064.

Budowle, B. 2005. Foreword. In: *Forensic Botany: Principles and Applications to Criminal Casework.* H.M. Coyle, ed. pp. vii–ix. Boca Raton, FL: CRC Press.

Dawkins, M.S. 2005. The Science of Suffering. In *Mental Health and Well–Being of Animals*, F.D. McMillan, ed. pp. 47–56. Ames, IA: Blackwell Publishing.

De Wael, K., F.G.C.S.J. Gason, and C.A.V. Baes. 2008. Selection of an Adhesive Tape Suitable for Forensic Fiber Sampling. *Journal of Forensic Sciences.* 53(1):168–171.

Evans, J.J., E.J. Wictum, M. Cecilia, T. Penedo, and Sreetharan K. 2007. Real–Time Polymerase Chain Reaction Quantification of Canine DNA. *Journal of Forensic Sciences.* 52(1):93–96.

Gaines, S.A., N.J. Rooney, and J.W.S. Bradshaw. 2008. The Effect of Feeding Enrichment upon Reported Working Ability and Behavior of Kenneled Working Dogs. *Journal of Forensic Sciences.* 53(6):1400–1404.

Gregory, N.G. 2004. *Physiology and Behaviour of Animal Suffering.* Oxford, UK: Blackwell Science.

Griffin, B. and K.R. Hume. 2006. Recognition and Management of Stress in Housed Cats. In: *Consultations in Feline Internal Medicine.* J.R. August, ed. pp. 717–734. St. Louis: Elsevier Saunders.

Gundry, R.L., M.W. Allard, T.R. Moretti, R.L. Honeycutt, M.R. Wilson, K.L. Monson, and D.R. Foran. 2007. Mitochondrial DNA Analysis of the Domestic Dog: Control Region Variation Within and Among Breeds. *Journal of Forensic Sciences.* 52(3):562–571.

Halverson, J. and C. Basten. 2005. A PCR Multiplex and Database for Forensic DNA Identification of Dogs. *Journal of Forensic Sciences* 50(2):352–363.

Hanon, K.A. 1991. Child Abuse: Münchausen's Syndrome by Proxy. *FBI Law Enforcement Bulletin*.

Houck, M.M. 2001. *Mute Witnesses: Trace Evidence Analysis*. San Diego: Academic Press.

Hydbring–Sandberg, E., L.W. von Walter, K. Hoglund, K. Svartberg, L. Swenson, and B. Forkman. 2004. Physiological Reactions to Fear Provocation in Dogs. *Journal of Endocrinology*. 180(3):439–448.

Ladd, C. and H.C. Lee. 2005. The Use of Biological and Botanical Evidence in Criminal Investigations. In: *Forensic Botany: Principles and Applications to Criminal Casework*. H.M. Coyle, ed. pp. 97–115. Boca Raton, FL: CRC Press.

Landsberg, G. 2010. Behavior, Health, and Welfare: How Stress and Behavior Can Affect Disease. Presented at the North American Veterinary Conference, 16–20 January, Orlando, Florida.

Larson, S. and N. Patel. 2012. Storage and Handling for Using Soil Molecular Biology as Trace Evidence. Presented at the American Academy of Forensic Sciences, 20–25 February, Atlanta, Georgia.

McMillan, F.D. 2005a. Stress, Distress, and Emotion: Distinctions and Implications for Mental Well–Being. In: *Mental Health and Well–Being of Animals*. F.D. McMillan, ed. pp. 93–112. Ames, IA: Blackwell Publishing.

McMillan, F.D. 2005b. Emotional Maltreatment of Animals. In: *Mental Health and Well–Being of Animals*. F.D. McMillan, ed. pp. 167–180. Ames, IA: Blackwell Publishing.

McMillan, F.D. 2012. The Psychological Aspects of Abuse and Neglect in Animals. Presented at the North American Veterinary Conference, 14–18 January, Orlando, Florida.

Milne, L.A., V.M. Bryant Jr., and D.C. Mildenhall, 2005. Forensic Palynology. In: *Forensic Botany: Principles and Applications to Criminal Casework*. H.M. Coyle, ed. pp. 217–252. Boca Raton, FL: CRC Press.

Munro, H.M. and M.V. Thrusfield. 2001. Battered Pets: Münchausen Syndrome by Proxy (Factitious Illness by Proxy). *Journal of Small Animal Practice* 42:385–389.

Murmann, D.C., P.C. Brumit, B.A. Schrader, and D.R. Senn. 2006. A Comparison of Animal Jaws and Bite Mark Patterns. *Journal of Forensic Sciences* 51(4):846–860.

Newberry, S., M.K. Blinn, P.A. Busby, C. Barker Cox, J.D. Dinnage, K.F. Hurley, N. Isaza, W. Jones, L. Miller, J. O'Quin, G. J. Patronek, M. Smith–Blackmore, and M. Spindel. 2010. Guidelines for Standard of Care in Shelter Animals, p. 10. Association of Shelter Veterinarians.

Platt, M.S., D.J. Spitz, and W.U. Spitz. 2006. Investigation of Deaths in Childhood, Part 2: The Abused Child and Adolescent. In *Spitz and Fisher's Medicolegal Investigation of Death: Guidelines for the Application of Pathology to Crime Investigation*, Fourth edition. Werner U. Spitz and Daniel J. Spitz, eds. pp. 357–416. Springfield: Charles C Thomas Publisher, Ltd.

Scientific Working Group on Materials Analysis Position (SWG-MAT) on Hair Evidence. 2009. Letter to the Editor. *Journal of Forensic Sciences*. 54(5):1198–1202.

Stern, A.W. and C.G. Lamm. 2011. Utilization of Paw Prints for Species Identification in the Canidae Family. *Journal of Forensic Sciences*. 56(4):1041–1043.

Tranquilli, W.J., K.A. Grimm, and L.A. Lamont. 2004. *Pain Management for the Small Animal Practitioner*. Jackson, MS: Teton NewMedia.

Vigil, B.N. and K.T. Kelley-Primozic. 2011. Evaluation of Three Different Adhesive Tapes for the Collection of Epithelial Cells and the Subsequent Micro-Isolation for PCR Analysis. Presented at the 63rd Annual Scientific Meeting of American Academy of Forensic Sciences, 21–26 February, Chicago, Illinois.

Warrington, D. 2010. Touch DNA. *Forensic Magazine*, December edition, pp. 1–2.

Webb, K.M. and M.W. Allard. 2009. Mitochondrial Genome DNA Analysis of the Domestic Dog: Identifying Informative SNPs Outside of the Control Region. *Journal of Forensic Sciences*. 54(2):275–288.

Wemelsfelder, F. 2005. Animal Boredom: Understanding the Tedium of Confined Lives. In: *Mental Health and Well–Being of Animals*. F.D. McMillan, ed. pp. 79–92. Ames, IA: Blackwell Publishing.

Willard, M.D. 2003. Disorders of the Stomach. In: *Small Animal Internal Medicine*, R.W. Nelson and C.G. Couto, eds. pp. 418–430. St. Louis: Mosby.

5
Blunt Force Trauma

Melinda D. Merck, Doris M. Miller, Robert W. Reisman,
and Paulo C. Maiorka

In forensic medicine, eye the most, hand the next and tongue the least.

From the forensic medicine practical notebook prescribed for undergraduate students at the Department of Forensic Medicine, Al-Ameen Medical College, Bijapur, India

OVERVIEW

Blunt force trauma occurs as a result of the impact of an animal's body against a blunt surface, or the impact of an object with a blunt surface against an animal's body. In order for a blunt force impact to occur there must be motion of the blunt object, or motion of the animal, or motion of the blunt object and the animal. Kinetic energy is the type of energy of motion (Whiting 1998).

Mechanics is the branch of physics that describes the effect of the application of force to an object. Force applied to an object causes change in an object's form (deformation) and direction of motion (acceleration). Force causes a free body to accelerate. The acceleration of a body is directly proportional to the force acting on the body (Newton's second law: $F = M * A$).

Biomechanics is the branch of physical science that describes the effects of intrinsic and extrinsic physiological and non-physiological forces on living tissue (with specific material and structural properties). Load is another term for an external force applied to a body. Body tissues continuously experience loads during normal activity with no obvious injury. These loads are within a physiologic range. The probability of injury increases when loads exceed the physiological range (overload).

Blunt force applied to biological tissue can cause blunt force trauma injuries. The mechanisms causing injury are:

- Excessive energy transfer (kinetic energy) to body tissues
- Acceleration/deceleration of the body and its constituent tissues
- Direct physical disruption of tissue (crushing injuries)

The composition and the mass of individual organs influence how they are affected by a blunt force impact. Different tissues/organs are affected differently by the application of force.

Energy cannot be created or destroyed; it can only change form (conservation of energy, the first law of thermodynamics). At the time of blunt force impact there is a transfer of kinetic energy from the blunt object to living tissue where all of the energy delivered to tissue is absorbed and changed. The injuries caused by blunt force trauma depend on the amount of energy delivered and transferred to the body, how it is delivered, and the body's reaction to the forces. Factors involved are the amount of force delivered, the time over which the force is delivered, the region struck, the size of the impact area, the specific tissues involved, and the nature of the weapon (Di Maio and Di Maio 2001).

When a weapon breaks or is deformed on impact, the energy delivered to the body is reduced because part of the energy was used in the break or deformation of the weapon. The severity of the injury may be reduced if the body moves with the blow, which increases the time over which the energy is delivered. Regardless of the amount of force,

Veterinary Forensics: Animal Cruelty Investigations, Second Edition. Edited by Melinda D. Merck.
© 2013 John Wiley & Sons, Inc. Published 2013 by John Wiley & Sons, Inc.

the larger the area over which the energy is delivered, the less severe the injury. A weapon with a broader surface will inflict less injury than a narrower weapon. If there is an object at the end of the weapon, all the energy will be concentrated at the end, creating a more severe injury. A blow to a flat portion of the body dissipates energy over a larger area than a blow to a rounder portion of the body, such as the head, which even with apparent superficial injuries can result in coup and contrecoup lesions that can affect the brain stem and lead to the death of the animal.

Veterinarians are familiar with variable tissue interaction with energy. The images created by ultrasound (sound energy) and X-rays (X-ray energy) are created because there is a variable interaction of body tissues with these types of energy. There is a variable interaction of tissue when there is a transfer of kinetic energy from a blunt force impact.

With the application of force all tissues/organs of the body experience acceleration. Different organs have different masses and accelerate at different rates. They do not move en masse in an organized fashion. Deceleration of body organs and tissues occurs when the body comes to rest. With rapid change from acceleration to deceleration, organs can be avulsed from fixed attachment points and blood vessels can be torn. As a result, organ disruption such as liver lacerations, pulmonary contusions and lacerations, and brain injury can occur.

Blunt force injuries can be characterized as mild, moderate, and severe. With mild injuries there is negligible structural involvement, no visible injury, mild local inflammation, and minimal tissue dysfunction. These injuries generally resolve within days. When there is a moderate degree of injury there is partial structural involvement, visible swelling, and inflammation with variable tissue dysfunction. These injuries may take weeks to resolve. With severe injury, there is complete structural involvement, gross swelling and inflammation, and clear tissue dysfunction. Severe injuries may take weeks to resolve or they may not resolve, resulting in permanent injury and loss of function.

Blunt force trauma can be the result of accidental or non-accidental causes. It is important to examine the entire animal for clues as to the incident and sequence of events. There may be evidence of repetitive abuse such as older bruises, scars, or healing fractures. External signs of bruising in animals may not be present, even when a blunt force impact has caused significant internal injuries. The causes of blunt force trauma are motor vehicle accidents (MVA), high-rise falls (i.e., falls greater than two stories for cats and one story for dogs), injuries of activity (e.g., running, jumping, falling), and physical assault injuries (non-accidental injuries).

The types of injuries caused by blunt force impacts are contusions, abrasions, lacerations, and fractures. The type and distribution of injuries should be determined when examining a victim of blunt force trauma. Each separate injury represents a separate impact. The number of visible blunt force lesions (abrasions, contusions, and lacerations) should be interpreted as the *minimum* number of impacts. Secondary impacts occur, such as when a dog's body contacts the pavement after being hit by a car. Secondary impacts may cause additional blunt force trauma lesions. It is during this second impact that deceleration occurs.

The type of event that caused the observed injuries should be considered and determined. This determination can be made by comparing both the type and distribution of the injuries with what is typically seen in other accidental or non-accidental cases. For example, if the injuries are severe, they can be compared to injuries sustained in known MVA victims or high-rise syndrome cases. It is important to use analogies in court to explain the amount of force required to cause observed injuries.

BRUISING/CONTUSIONS

Overview

A contusion or bruise is an area of tissue hemorrhage caused by a blunt force impact that ruptures the blood vessels. The size and severity of the contusion depends on the blunt force applied and the vascularity of the tissue. Gravity may affect the spread of the underlying hemorrhage away from the original site of injury (Munro and Munro 2011). Similar to the protection clothes provide the skin of people, an animal's hair coat protects the skin and may minimize surface injury. Additionally, because animals have a reduced blood supply to their skin compared with humans, external bruising is not as commonly seen on the skin surface. When it is seen in animals, it is usually caused by severe force that may not only cause bleeding in the skin but also in the underlying tissue structures. It is frequently necessary to shave the hair coat to identify the full extent of skin contusions. Other causes for apparent bruising include clotting disorders. In addition, the apparent surface bruise may be a result of hemorrhage where the blood source is from a deeper or adjacent area of injury, such as a fracture, which has followed a path of least resistance through tissue planes.

Contusions also may be present in the internal organs and internal body walls. The appearance of bruising may be delayed for several hours, especially if it is located in an anatomical site in which there is reduced blood supply. Bruising may take minutes to several hours to form in animals and may fade quickly depending on the extent of damage. The appearance may appear much later than the time of impact depending on blood pressure, position of the body, and blood loss. In general, the shorter the survival time after injury the less prominent the contusion.

A special case is that of pulmonary contusions in which lung hemorrhage may progress for forty-eight hours post-impact. Continued monitoring of the live animal is essential to detect bruising. Photographs should be taken of the bruising pattern periodically as it forms to capture the full representation. It is possible that early on the bruise may be more reflective of what caused the contusion and as bleeding continues, especially from the deeper tissue, the pattern may become obscured.

The absence of a bruise does not indicate the absence of blunt force trauma. A live animal may have suffered severe blunt force trauma but not have any external signs except for the possibility of tenderness in the injured areas, which may be difficult to discern. In suspected blunt force trauma cases, as with all suspected cases of abuse, radiographs and blood work may reveal evidence of acute and chronic injuries. In all cases in which blunt force injuries are present, radiographs should be a standard part of the forensic evaluation with special attention to areas with significant soft tissue injury. Rib fractures, both recent and old, and zygomatic bone fractures are relatively common findings in blunt force trauma cases and these areas should be included in the radiography studies. Special photographic and imaging equipment may enhance visualization of deeper injuries (see Chapter 3 and next section).

Thermal imaging: detecting hidden trauma

Thermography, or thermal imaging, has been used extensively in veterinary medicine. Similar to how a regular camera uses visible light to form an image, a thermographic camera, or infrared camera, forms an image using infrared radiation technology measuring the surface temperatures of an object. The cooler areas appear blue, black, green, or purple, and warmer areas appear orange, red, yellow, or white. Thermal imaging cameras are used by a variety of agencies where heat detection is needed such as the military, law enforcement, firefighting, and building inspection. Thermography is most commonly used in veterinary medicine for lameness exams in working animals such as horses or dogs to detect areas of inflammation. It is also used for wildlife and exotic animals in situations where physical exam is difficult and remote sensing is useful. The United States Department of Agriculture Animal and Plant Inspection Service (APHIS) began using thermography in 2009 during horse inspections as a diagnostic tool for the detection of soring.

Thermal imaging may be used in live animals with suspected blunt force trauma. Thermography can detect areas of inflammation in cases in which there is no visible bruising or the physical exam and diagnostic imaging does not reveal areas of trauma. The thermal scan should be performed as soon as possible on animals with suspected trauma because the inflammatory response may have a short duration. Detection of inflammation does not necessarily indicate acute trauma but may be due to chronic inflammation. The area should be rescanned to rule out chronic inflammation and detect resolving acute inflammation. Thermal imaging may confirm accidental injuries. An animal with a broken leg due to allegedly falling down the stairs should have other areas of inflammation due to impacting the stairs.

Several cameras are available and the costs vary widely. Most companies offer training on the use of their camera. It is advantageous to perform scans on animals that are not part of legal cases to establish a baseline for the camera images. For legal cases the images should be captured for documentation. Some cameras come with the ability to capture the image on a digital card which can be downloaded to a computer.

Postmortem finding of contusions

Postmortem exam can reveal the true extent of the bruising, which is usually larger than what was apparent on the skin surface. As with live animal evaluations of skin injuries, the hair may be shaved to look for bruising. It is possible to see bruising even in dark-pigmented skin. The skin should be reflected over the entire body to look for subcutaneous or deeper tissue bruising. Reflection of muscle layers may be needed to detect deeper injuries. Hemorrhage from the area of injury may gravitate along fascial planes and provide the false impression that the injury occurred at the apparent bruised area.

Microscopic exam of a bruise will have findings due to crushing of the tissue and homogeneous infiltration of blood into all layers of the skin vs. just the fascial planes (Spitz 2006). There may be significant underlying tissue damage caused by the weapon. Bruising is larger than normal with certain types of death: electrocution, drowning, and all forms of asphyxia deaths. This is due to the intense congestion associated with these conditions (Spitz 2006).

Contused areas should be photographed as soon as possible because the bruising tends to become less defined and fade with time and there is risk of contamination with blood leakage from other tissue or body cavities during the exam (Munro and Munro 2011). In contrast, undetected contusions may become more visible in humans twelve to twenty-four hours after the initial autopsy and after drying for wet bodies (Chapter 9).

At first appearance, contusions may be grossly difficult to differentiate from postmortem lividity (Chapter 14). A contusion involves hemorrhage into the soft tissue and the blood cannot be wiped or squeezed out when incised. This is not the case in areas of lividity (Di Maio and Di Maio 2001). Over time, decomposition can make it extremely difficult to differentiate antemortem bruising and lividity. Hemolysis of the red blood cells creates diffuse discoloration of the soft tissue. The blood within the vessels and the erythrocyte leakage caused by the breakdown of the blood vessels from decomposition hemolyze. The erythrocytes in the soft tissue from antemortem bruising also hemolyze, making it impossible to distinguish from an area of livor mortis. The lack of other areas of lividity in expected associated regions of the body can help with determination of bruising (Chapter 14).

Patterned bruising

A patterned contusion may be seen that reflects the shape and sometimes details of the object that was used to cause the bruise. Asymmetry to the bruise may be an important indicator due to the fact that bleeding follows the path of least resistance. Depending on the area of skin and gravity, it tends to flow from the center outward, forming irregular or blurred lines. Bruising may extend beyond the site of impact, obscuring the pattern created by the object. If the contusion was caused by a weapon, it may be possible to find evidence of the weapon within a bruising pattern or indentation of the skin, underlying tissue, or even bone (Figure 5.1). A linear object, depending on the width, may cause two parallel, train track lines, or tramlines, of bruising with the skin between uninjured (Figure 5.2). This is due to the hemorrhage under the skin being displaced laterally by the pressure of the blow. The same findings can be seen associated with blows from other type of objects such as a baseball, which results in a circular bruise and a pale center. If the weapon has a rough texture there may be parallel abrasions present with or without bruising (Spitz 2006). Blows from a weapon also can cause skin lacerations if used with enough force or if the skin is more susceptible to tearing, such as with young or geriatric animals and certain species. The imprint of a shoe or fingertips may be seen from stomping, grabbing, or holding the animal.

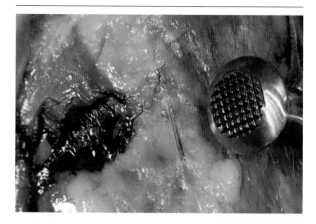

Figure 5.1. Patterned injury in the deeper tissue reflecting weapon pattern without skin penetration.

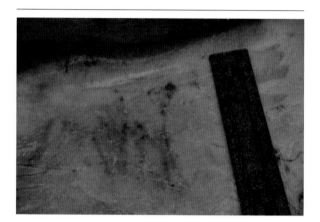

Figure 5.2. Patterned bruising of tramlines seen on skin reflection due to blunt force trauma from a belt.

It is important to find out if investigators have a suspected weapon that was used in the incident, either seized as evidence or through interview statements. A weapon may be identified or discovered later in the investigation, so it is important to preserve any evidence that may be linked to the weapon for later comparison or confirmation. The patterns and indentation of the skin may fade or resolve very quickly, so it is important to take photographs as soon as possible, with and without a photographic scale, for a forensic specialist to analyze for weapon comparison. For any indentations, a cast may be taken. Mikrosil™ is a rubber casting material that is inexpensive and easily used for this purpose. It may be ordered from any forensic supply company with brown the preferred color for tool mark examiners.

Aging bruising

Microscopic examination may be used whenever the aging of a bruise is required. The healing of a bruise depends on the number of bruises in the area, vasculature of the injured area, amount of subcutaneous tissue and fat, type and severity of the force that caused the bruise, and any underlying disease that may impair local tissue reactions. In humans, perivascular neutrophils appear within three to four hours and peak in one to three days, macrophages peak in sixteen to twenty-four hours, and hemosiderin within macrophages may be seen as soon as twenty-four hours after injury. In animals it is reported in macrophages forty-eight hours after injury (Munro and Munro 2008b). Intracellular hematoidin may be seen after several days or one week and appears as amorphous yellow granules or sheaves of crystals. It does not react with Prussian blue stain like hemosiderin (Spitz 2006).

Contusions undergo color changes over time because of the breakdown of hemoglobin, but the color change and time for change are variable and may at best offer estimates of acute, recent, or older. In animals, bruising initially may appear red, purple, or dark blue. As time progresses the bruise may fade and turn brown. Research has been conducted on farm livestock (lambs and calves) and poultry (chapters 16 and 17) to age bruises but this does not necessarily apply to other species (Munro and Munro 2011). At best, one can usually say the bruise appears recent or is older (Di Maio and Di Maio 2001).

It is possible to cause postmortem contusions if a severe enough blunt force is directed at the body within a few hours after death. This causes rupture of capillaries and forces blood into the surrounding tissue. Antemortem contusions that occur immediately prior to death may or may not have had enough time to show a vital reaction detectable by histology. If the contusion occurred antemortem with enough time for the body to mount a response, evidence of a vital reaction may be seen with microscopic examination of the injury.

A recent study on rats found that the use of electric impedance spectroscopy can differentiate between vital and postmortem bruising and determine the survival time after injury. Electrical impedance spectroscopy has been used in the medical setting to diagnose disease and determine the state of organs. When tissue is injured tissue fluid increases and progresses over time due to inflammation. The electrical impedance decreases in impaired muscle tissue as the liquid content increases. The study limited the impedance values measured using a frequency range of 100–1,000 Hz with twenty-one frequency points (Mao et al. 2011).

ABRASIONS

Overview

An abrasion is due to blunt force injury when the superficial (epithelial) layer of skin is removed by contact with another object. The severity and size of an abrasion does not always correlate with the severity of an underlying injury. An animal's hair coat protects the skin and may minimize surface injury. Abrasions are caused by blunt force trauma, dragging, or anything that causes crushing and tearing of the skin. Abrasions result from compression and destruction of the epidermal layers or friction of the skin against a rough surface. They usually leak tissue fluid but do not bleed unless the injury extends deep enough to expose and damage the dermal papillae (Munro and Munro 2011). Abrasions in animals are initially wet in appearance, then darken and become drier with time (Munro and Munro 2011). Ante-mortem abrasions are pink, red, or reddish-brown in animals. In humans, postmortem abrasions are yellow, translucent, and have a parchment-like appearance (Di Maio and Di Maio 2001). Drying of the area may change the coloring from pink or red to pale yellow-brown, dark brown, and even black. Abrasions may not be initially detected in bodies recovered from water until drying occurs (Spitz 2006).

Types of abrasions

The types of abrasions are grazes, scratches, scrapes or brush abrasions, grating or sliding abrasions, impact abrasions, and patterned abrasions. Graze abrasions may be seen when an object, such as a bullet, sideswipes the body. Scratch abrasions are caused by a sharp edge or finger nails. These may be mistaken for burns and require microscopic examination for accurate determination (Spitz 2006). Scrape or brush abrasions are created when a blunt object scrapes off the superficial layers of the skin, sometimes exposing the deeper dermal layers and causing fluid leakage from the vessels. This causes a serosanguineous fluid covering on the abrasion. When the area is incised, there usually is no hemorrhage in the underlying soft tissue, indicating the injury is confined to the epidermis. Grating or sliding abrasions are caused when the body slides across a rough surface such as pavement. Ligatures, nooses, and dragging a body may cause sliding abrasions. Abrasions may have gross or microscopic debris embedded in the wound related to the object or surface that caused the injury or the area in which the injury occurred. Evidence of bunching of the epidermis at one end of the injury may be seen, indicating the direction of movement of the body or object.

Impact abrasions are crushing injuries caused when the blunt force impacts perpendicular to the skin. This may

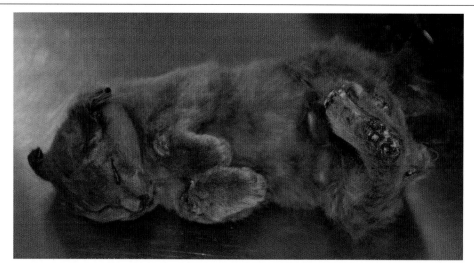

Figure 5.3. Cat that died in a clothes dryer. Note the impact abrasions from the expected points of contact (bony prominences) and ear crumpling due to thermal injury.

occur from a weapon or a fall. Impact abrasions usually affect the skin over bony prominences in which there is less underlying protective tissue (Figure 5.3).

A patterned abrasion shows the imprint of the weapon or surface that caused the abrasion. This may be seen with ligature injuries that leave a patterned imprint, revealing the type of ligature used. In humans, intermediary material on the body such as clothing may leave an imprint from the crushing force of the weapon used. The impact surface, such as gravel, can exhibit characteristic patterned abrasions. If the weapon has a rough texture there may be parallel abrasions present with or without bruising (Spitz 2006).

Artifacts that mimic abrasions

Postmortem artifacts may be misinterpreted as abrasions. Insect feeding postmortem from ants and roaches may be mistaken for abrasions or burns. The hair shaft remains intact with ant feeding and is snipped off with roach feeding. The drying of areas of skin may resemble abrasions. Careful examination should determine between true abrasions and artifacts.

Aging abrasions

The aging of abrasions may be limited to a determination of ante- or postmortem injury. There may be skin or subcutaneous hemorrhage associated with ligature abrasions, indicating the victim was alive when the ligatures were present, though the lack of hemorrhage does not indicate the ligatures were applied postmortem. The best place to find this hemorrhage is over bony prominences.

Hard ligatures, such as electrical cord, are more likely to cause hemorrhage than smooth, soft, or wider materials. Hemorrhage may not be seen with superficial abrasions, though hemorrhage into the surrounding tissue usually indicates antemortem injury. Gravitational bleeding from injuries located in areas of livor mortis may be difficult to differentiate from antemortem hemorrhage (Spitz 2006).

In humans, the aging of abrasions is possible with histological examination by documenting the stages of healing. The length for healing is affected by the extent of the injury, secondary infection, and any repeated trauma to the area. A fresh abrasion is moist and leaks serum for one to two days before scab formation, which may trap some red blood cells (Spitz 2006). The deposit of serum, red cells, and fibrin indicate survival after the injury. The appearance of red blood cells, serum, and fibrin occurs in less than two hours. Infiltration of neutrophils in a perivascular formation may start in two hours but is clearly visible in four to six hours, indicating the injury is four to six hours old. Under the area of epithelial injury, a zone of infiltrating neutrophils in the bed of the scab is present by eight hours. A surface zone of fibrin and red cells, followed by a zone of infiltrating neutrophils and then a layer of damaged abnormally staining collagen appear by twelve to eighteen hours. In impact abrasions, the surface zone is comprised of crushed epithelium (Di Maio and Di Maio 2001).

Epithelial regeneration marks the second stage of healing. The regeneration comes from the margins of the abrasion and the surviving hair follicles. In scrape abrasions, this growth of epithelium may appear in as little as thirty hours. In most other abrasions, it is visible by seventy-two hours (Di Maio and Di Maio 2001).

The third stage of healing is subepidermal granulation, which occurs only after epithelial covering of the abrasion is complete. Perivascular infiltration and chronic inflammatory cells are present. It becomes prominent during days five to eight. During days nine to twelve, changes in the overlying epithelium are most prominent as it forms keratin and becomes progressively hyperplastic. Collagen fibers may begin to appear (Di Maio and Di Maio 2001).

The fourth and final stage of healing is regression, which starts around the twelfth day. The epithelium is remodeled, becoming thinner and atrophic. The collagen fibers become more prominent. The vascularity of the dermis decreases, and a definitive basement membrane develops (Di Maio and Di Maio 2001).

LACERATIONS

A laceration is due to blunt force trauma that results in a tear in soft tissue caused by a crushing or shearing force. This can occur on the skin, mucous membranes (such as the gingiva, especially over a maxillary canine), or internal organs (e.g., a disruption of the liver parenchyma is a laceration, and not a fracture). Skin lacerations may be caused by blunt force directed by an object, the terminal end of body movement such as a fall impact, or an impact from a vehicle. The margins of skin lacerations tend to be bruised, abraded, and irregular. This is in contrast to an incised wound in which the wound edges are well defined and there is minimal bruising of the surrounding skin (Table 5.1). Incised wounds, in which blood vessels are cut, bleed more than lacerations, in which blood vessels are crushed.

Most veterinarians easily recognize incised wounds because of their experience performing surgery. The laceration may have a pattern that mirrors the offending object. Long, thin objects tend to produce linear lacerations but may produce a Y-shaped laceration. The wound should be examined for deeply embedded material related to the weapon or impact surface.

Lacerations usually are present in areas where the skin is fixed and more easily stretched and torn. The underlying blood vessels and nerves are stronger than the skin, forming a visible "bridge" of the underlying tissue. This tissue bridging is a distinguishing feature that differentiates a laceration from an incisive wound (Di Maio and Di Maio 2001). Tissue bridging also may be seen in the internal organs and indicates crushing injuries. This may not be seen in organs with little to no interstitial tissues such as the liver, kidney, pancreas, or spleen (Spitz 2006). The

Table 5.1. Comparison of characteristics in laceration and incised wounds.

Characteristics	Laceration	Incised
Margin	Irregular	Defined
Abrasion	Usually present	None to minimal
Bruising	Usually present	None to minimal
Tissue division	Bridging	Cleanly divided
Debris	Frequent	Usually absent
Hemorrhage	Slight	Notable

Source: Nelson, S.J. 2008. Blunt Force Trauma. Presented at the Veterinary Forensics Conference, 9–11 April. Orlando, Florida.

edges of the laceration may be undermined due to the crushing and shearing force, especially against bone. A laceration resulting from an angled impact may have undermining of one edge of the laceration, indicating the direction of the impact, whereas the finding of equally distributed undermining wound edges indicates a perpendicular force. The opposite side of the angled impact laceration may be beveled and abraded (Di Maio and Di Maio 2001). The shape of a laceration depends on the shape of the striking object or impact surface and the body characteristics at the impact area such as the curvature of the skull or bony protuberances (Spitz 2006).

If the object was heavy and had a sharp edge, a wound laceration may appear to be an incisive wound. Careful examination will reveal some margin contusion or abrasion and deeper tissue bridging. The use of a dull knife may cause injuries that appear grossly similar to lacerations. The use of a dissecting microscopic can help differentiate it from a laceration. Decomposition can make differentiation from lacerations and incisive wounds extremely difficult (Di Maio and Di Maio 2001).

Lacerations can occur in deeper tissues such as muscle lacerations with or without skin penetration. This is commonly seen in predator attacks and may be located in the deeper neck muscles, the torso, or limbs. The internal organs may have laceration injuries, which indicates that considerable forces were applied (Munro and Munro 2011). These may be seen in accidental cases such as motor vehicle impacts or falls from significant heights, or non-accidental cases from deliberate, directed force such as a kick or punch.

LIGATURE INJURIES

It is not uncommon for ligatures to be used as a form of abuse or to control the victim, especially in blunt force

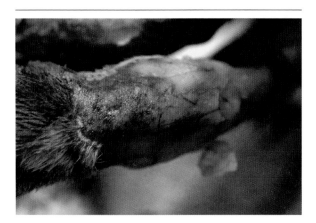

Figure 5.4. Hemorrhage present underneath area where the legs had been bound with duct tape.

trauma. The types of injuries depend on the type of ligature, location on the body, amount of compression and constriction, animal movement, and length of time the ligature was on the animal (Chapter 9). Ligatures may be placed around the mouth, ears, neck, legs, feet, torso, genitalia, or tail. If left in place for a period of time, ligatures cause compression and constriction of the skin and vessels, creating tissue swelling and edema with eventual necrosis. Injuries associated with ligatures depend on the type of ligature and movement or struggle of the victim including areas of hair loss, subcutaneous hemorrhage, contusions, abrasions, lacerations, and tissue necrosis (Figure 5.4). When examining the animal, the ligature should be carefully removed by cutting the ligature on the opposite side to preserve all potential trace or DNA evidence on the surface of the ligature or within any knots, twists, or fasteners. Often the joined areas of the ligature have trace evidence or skin cells related to the perpetrator.

If the ligature is no longer present, the area of injury should be carefully examined for embedded trace evidence related to the ligature, such as tape adhesive. There may be patterned injuries such as abrasions or contusions which may retain the ligature pattern. Evidence of ligature or patterned injury may be more evident after skin reflection during the postmortem examination. The pattern should be thoroughly photographed with a photographic scale in each photo.

Geographic information systems (GIS) are used as a forensic tool to evaluate marine mammal entanglement wound patterns and may have application in other species and criminal cases. Developing maps of unique characteristics of fishing gear and entanglement wounds can help in the identi-

fication of the fishing source for animals that strand without fishing gear attached. A database of information regarding season, gear, and location of commercial fisheries along the U.S. Atlantic coast is available to stranding networks. Photographs must be properly taken at a 90° angle to the wound and close-up views must be clear enough to identify wound characteristics (Burdett, Adams, and McFee 2007).

The depth and width of the ligature wound should be measured. Cultures should be taken of any infection. A time estimate for the ligature to have been on the animal should be given based on healing and infection. This is possible by evaluating the granulation tissue (see Embedded Collars, Chapter 11).

AVULSION INJURIES

Avulsion injuries to the external body involve a blunt force impacting the body at a tangential or oblique angle, ripping skin and/or soft tissue off the underlying fascia or bone (Di Maio and Di Maio 2001). Avulsion also can occur with internal organs that are partially or completely torn from their attachments. Shearing forces also can cause the underlying soft tissue, connective tissue, and fascia to be avulsed from the overlying skin and subcutaneous tissue. The skin can appear normal except for a pocket of blood or blood-tinged fluid underneath. This can occur when an animal is picked up by the scruff of the neck and shaken. Forcible stretching of the neck may result in tracheal avulsion near the bifurcation of the mainstem bronchi with associated hemorrhage. This may be caused by attempted wringing/breaking of the neck or due to blunt force trauma to the neck or thorax resulting in hyperextension of the neck (Munro and Munro 2008b).

Shearing and degloving injuries of the limbs or other areas of the body are commonly seen resulting from motor vehicle accidents or dragging injuries. They also may be caused by ligatures or any other means that can compress, twist, or otherwise strip the overlying tissue. These injuries may be simple lacerations or more extensive with severe loss of skin and the underlying soft tissue damaging the associated bones and joints. These wounds, by the very nature of their cause, are contaminated and typically contain a significant amount of foreign, forensically important material embedded in the tissue.

This wealth of trace evidence may link the victim to a crime scene, weapon, or a suspect. The potential evidence includes soil, vegetation, debris, glass, and fibers. The non-vital tissue with avulsions becomes necrotic within forty-eight hours after the trauma (Beardsley 2000). In animals with these injuries it is critical to do a complete physical exam for additional forensic evidence and injuries. It is has been reported that 70%

of dogs with shearing and degloving injuries had concurrent injuries, including fractures, skin lacerations, and cardiopulmonary problems (Beardsley 2000).

FRACTURES

Forces and determining directionality

The term fracture should be reserved for catastrophic disruption of bones and teeth. Bone fractures can be classified based on the amount of energy that causes the structural failure: low-energy, high-energy, and very-high-energy impact fractures (Radasch 1999). The associated soft tissue injuries are informative as to the impact energy. The greater the energy of blunt force impact, the greater the degree of bone and associated soft tissue injury that result. The soft tissue injury and fracture displacement help with determination of the direction of force (see below).

Fractures may be caused directly or indirectly by blunt force trauma. There are five basic forces that act on bone: tension, compression, bending, shear, and torsion. When a long bone is struck, it tends to bend, causing a fracture in the opposite side of the bone where there is greatest tension on the convex aspect of the bend. With significant force, crushing of the concave side of the bone can occur. Focal or crushing fractures can occur as a result of blunt force trauma depending on the amount of force and size of the area to which it is directed. A focal fracture results from a small force applied to a small area, usually causing a transverse fracture when applied perpendicularly. The overlying tissue often has associated injuries such as contusions, abrasions, or lacerations. In the lower leg areas, where two bones are present, usually only one bone is fractured (Di Maio and Di Maio 2001).

With larger forces, a crush fracture may be produced and the overlying tissue injury is usually extensive. A variety of fractures can result from a severe impact depending on the type of force applied, including oblique, transverse, comminuted, spiral, longitudinal split, segmental, tension wedge, and compression wedge. A tension wedge fracture occurs when the fracture begins at the opposite side and then radiates back at a 90° angle, creating the wedge. The point of the wedge indicates the direction of the force, and the base indicates the points of impact. On radiographs, tension wedge fractures may appear to be oblique fractures (Di Maio and Di Maio 2001). Radiographic reports should describe fractures exactly.

Additional information about the nature of the fracture may become apparent at surgery and should be described in the surgery report. During an open surgical repair of a bone fracture, scar tissue may be removed from the fracture site. This tissue should be submitted for histopathology. In cases in which a leg is amputated because of a blunt force trauma injury, the section of the leg that was injured should be submitted for histopathology.

The pelvic ring creates great stability of the pelvis. It requires immense force to disrupt this ring and cause fractures. Disruption of one part of the ring usually causes disruption in another part because of their strong connections. Pelvic fractures should be described as high-energy impact fractures.

Indirect fractures are caused by the application of force distant from the fracture site. Bone is weaker to tension forces than compression forces. The classifications of indirect fractures are traction; angulation; rotational; vertical compression; angulation and compression; and angulation, rotation, and compression. In traction fractures the bone is pulled apart by traction. In angulation fractures the bone is bent, creating compression on the concave surface and tension on the convex surface, which causes it to break. The resulting fracture usually is transverse. Rotational fractures are spiral fractures produced when bone is twisted. The direction of the spiral indicates the direction of the torque that caused the fracture. Vertical compression fractures are produced when the shaft of the long bone is driven into the cancellous end. This causes an oblique fracture of the long bone and may cause a T- or Y-shaped fracture of the end of the bone. Angulation and compression fractures have a transverse and oblique component caused by the two forces. In angulation, rotation, and compression fractures the angulation and rotation forces together produce an oblique fracture, while the compression increases the tendency toward fracture (Di Maio and Di Maio 2001).

A study was conducted on human long bones to determine fracture patterns and directionality by evaluation of complete and incomplete fractures that were created by the application of controlled perpendicular force. The patterns of complete fractures were 60% oblique, 27% transverse, and 13% comminuted. No determination of the force direction was possible without soft tissue displacement evaluation. The patterns of incomplete fractures were butterfly (tension wedges) 80%, transverse initiated on tension side 80%, failing angle shifts (shallowing at 45° and running parallel) 87%, and breakaway spurs on compression side 73%. The direction of force was able to be determined with the incomplete fractures. It should be noted that bone fractures may contain a combination of complete and incomplete fracture patterns (Fenton 2012).

Evidence of repetitive abuse

The presence of multiple injuries (soft tissue and bone) in different stages of healing is highly indicative of repetitive abuse (i.e., battered animal syndrome) (Munro 1997). There may or may not be skin injuries in cases in which there is an underlying bone fracture. If the bone fracture is acute, there will be hemorrhage from the marrow and adjacent tissue injury in the immediate vicinity of the fracture site and into the surrounding tissue. The rate of healing callus formation depends on several factors: the age of the animal, amount of displacement of the fracture site, and stability or amount of movement at the fracture site. Production of a callus begins with the external callus produced by the periosteum and the internal callus produced by the endosteum. Periosteal proliferation may be underway within twenty-four hours of injury. Mineralization can begin in three days, but this early fibrocartilaginous callus may not be visible in radiographs for two weeks. It may be palpated as a hard thickening but should be differentiated from a resolving hematoma.

Disuse atrophy of the muscle of an injured leg results in muscle mass that is clearly smaller than that of the opposite leg. Muscle atrophy can be determined by palpation and radiography. The value of using radiography to identify muscle atrophy is that it serves as a permanent record of the animal's compromised state. It is best if both legs (i.e., the injured and the healthy leg) are included in the radiograph, where the comparison can be dramatic. Once the fracture is repaired and the animal regains function, lost muscle mass is regained and visualization and/or palpation of muscle atrophy are no longer possible.

Bone remodeling seen radiographically can help differentiate between a recent fracture and a fracture that is weeks old or older. On postmortem exam a gross and microscopic exam of the fracture area should be conducted to determine the stage of callus formation. At best, a time estimate for the fracture may be given as acute, recent, or older.

MOTOR VEHICLE ACCIDENT (MVA) INJURIES

MVA victims have characteristic injuries related to the dynamic incident. A motor vehicle accident causes injury not just by the direct crushing effect of the part of the body that sustains the impact, but also by the other mechanisms that cause injury: excessive energy transfer and acceleration/deceleration injuries. These mechanisms can cause injury to body areas that are remote from the impact site. The impact of the vehicle to the body can cause several injuries depending on the speed of the vehicle, where the animal was hit, if the animal rolled under the car or inside the wheel well, how far it was projected away, and where it

landed. At higher vehicle speeds, the impact can cause severe, devastating injuries. In the U.S., 80% of animals are hit be a vehicle on the left side of the body, which is thought to be due to the animal getting hit when crossing the first lane of the road and decreased driver reaction time. A coup-contrecoup effect may be seen in the thorax where the heart impacts the left thorax and bounces into the right middle lung lobe, resulting in lung contusions and middle lung lobe collapse.

In addition to the blunt force injuries, characteristic findings associated with MVAs include frayed nails, dirt or debris embedded in the fur or mouth, and abrasions. The abrasion injuries are usually drag or sliding abrasions located on more than one area of the body. They almost always present as lateral on one side of the body and medial on the opposite side. They are reported in the extremities in 79% of cases and to the head in 35% of the cases (Kolata and Johnson 1975).

Primary impact injuries are caused by the first impact of the vehicle to the victim. After this, the victim may be thrown under the vehicle or projected away or up onto the car, causing secondary impact injuries. These injuries are due to impact with the vehicle undercarriage or wheels, surface impact(s) or landing, and/or sliding or dragging and include head trauma, additional fractures, abrasions, debris, or glass from the site of injury embedded into the fur or wounds. After a secondary impact with the vehicle the terminal ground surface contact causes tertiary injuries. If the animal is lying on the ground and run over by a vehicle, there may or may not be impact injuries, depending on the point of body contact, and are more typically crushing, avulsion, or laceration injuries.

Studies have been conducted on MVA injuries in dogs. A study of the records of 600 dogs presenting for MVA trauma found that young males were more frequently injured. In 31% (190) of the dogs, superficial injuries were the only injury found. For the remaining 410 dogs, 87% had skeletal injuries (pelvis most frequently affected) and 27% had soft tissue injuries (liver most frequently affected). Multiple areas of injury were found in 36% of all 600 dogs (Kolata and Johnston 1975).

Another study of 267 dogs looked at thoracic trauma and association with other injuries. The study found 38.9% had thoracic wall and pulmonary trauma with pulmonary contusions, pneumothorax, and fractured ribs the most common injuries. In 57.7% there was more than one type of thoracic wall or pulmonary injury. Of the dogs with thoracic injury, 24% had extrathoracic injuries while 16.5% of dogs without thoracic injury had extrathoracic injuries, not including fractures. Thoracic injuries were seen in 36.3% of the dogs with fractures of one bone and 42.3% of the dogs with fractures of more than one bone. The prevalence of thoracic wall and pulmonary trauma was significantly associated with the site of the fracture, i.e., cranial vs. caudal and ipsilateral vs. contralateral (Spackman et al. 1984).

A study of MVA injuries in 100 dogs that were examined within twenty-four hours found pelvic fractures (twenty), limb fractures (fifteen), hip joint luxation (seven), spinal injury (five), pulmonary contusions (thirty-one), pneumothorax (twenty-one), hemothorax (five), head trauma (ten), and retroperitoneal injury (one). In addition, fourteen dogs had skin lacerations requiring surgical repair, of which four were degloving injuries in the distal limbs (Boysen et al. 2004).

FALL INJURIES

When evaluating victims of falls, it is important to consider how the animal fell, the distance, the mass of the animal, the species, and age. In addition, it is important to know how the animal landed and if the animal could have landed on any objects or surface protrusions. All information regarding the fall incident is crucial to supply context for the analysis and interpretation as to the cause of the injuries.

Cats develop air-righting reaction while falling as kittens beginning at four weeks of age continuing for the following two weeks. By six to seven weeks of age they are able to right themselves and land on their feet. As a result, head injuries in cats over six to seven weeks with a "fall" explanation are less likely to be accurate, especially if they occurred inside a home (Munro and Munro 2008a).

With injuries related to falls, it is important to consider that it was non-accidental and may be due to the animal being thrown or dropped. Blunt force injuries due to falls to the ground or similar circumstances should be distributed over bony prominences and have a pattern of injuries along one plane of body impact. Injuries found to recessed or protected parts of the body are suspicious indicators for non-accidental causes.

To know what injuries to expect, it is important to know how the fall occurred and the surface on which the animal landed. Frayed nails may be seen as a result of frantic clawing at the surrounding surface edges before or during the fall. Depending on the circumstances surrounding the fall and investigation findings, frayed nails may or may not be present in accidental or non-accidental falls. The animal should be examined for other injuries that may be inconsistent with the fall and possibly more indicative that they occurred prior to the fall. For example, a fractured lower spine is not expected in a cat that accidentally fell from a first-story balcony to smooth asphalt; it is more consistent with blunt force trauma to the spine prior to the fall. As

with all suspected animal cruelty cases the animal always should be examined for evidence of repetitive abuse.

High rise syndrome is a term given to a complex of injuries as a result of severe deceleration trauma due to falls from a significant height (cats that have fallen two to thirty-two floors and dogs that have fallen one to six floors). The triad of injuries associated with this syndrome is facial, thoracic, and extremities. In cats, the presenting facial trauma is epistaxis and fracture (or split) of the hard palate. The hard palate injury is caused by the force of the lower canines being thrust upward between the upper dental arcade. The thoracic trauma most commonly found is pneumothorax. Examination findings also may include skin abrasions, pulmonary contusions, limb fractures, and possible bladder rupture resulting from the acute increase of intra-abdominal pressure on impact. Rib fractures are an uncommon finding.

A study conducted on known high rise injuries in dogs found that fall injuries differ from cats in degree and nature, with height of the fall being the most significant factor (Table 5.2). The position of the dog, i.e., jump vs. fall, influenced the distribution of injuries including extremities. Dogs that jumped sustained more head, thoracic, spinal, forelimb, and extremity soft tissue injuries than those that fell. Dogs that jumped were more likely to

Table 5.2. Comparison of injuries in dogs and cats with high rise syndrome.

Injury	% of 132 cats (falls 2–32 stories)	% of 104 cats (falls 1–6 stories)	% of 80 dogs (falls 1–6 stories)
Thorax	90	80	83
Pulmonary contusions	88	52	37
Pneumothorax	83	43	25
Facial	57	NA	45
Hard palate fx	17	NA	0
Dental fx	17	19	14
Mandibular fx	9	NA	3
Extremity fxs	81	83	80
Forelimb	54	41	80
Hindlimb	46	28	41

NA = not available

Source: Gordon, L.E., C. Thacher, and A. Kapatkin. 1993. High-Rise Syndrome in Dogs: 81 Cases (1985–1991). *Journal of American Veterinary Medical Association*, 202 (1):118–122.

have forelimb injuries and those that fell were more likely to have hindlimb injuries. Dogs are more likely to have extremity injuries than cats. Facial trauma in dogs is less severe than in cats and usually only skin abrasions are found. This may be attributed to their larger and stronger legs which can absorb most of the impact and lessen the head injury. Dogs are less likely to survive falls from heights greater than six floors.

SWINGING/DRAGGING INJURIES

It is not uncommon for animal abuse to involve swinging or dragging the animal, either by the tail or a limb(s), which often results in multiple injuries. Features may include contusions, abrasions, lacerations, avulsion injuries, fractures, dislocations, ligament injuries, and muscle tearing. Bruising and fractures may occur from surface impact or when the animal is struck with an object. Dislocations of the limb joints or tearing of the limb attachments may be seen. If the scapula is completely avulsed from the thoracic wall, the scapula will protrude dorsally, higher than the opposite scapula, when the animal bears weight on that limb. Dislocation of the elbow joint, without fracture to the anconeal process, is caused by traction and torque forces created by pulling and twisting the lower arm, which may be seen if the animal was swung or was suspended by the leg. Normal dislocation of the femur from the coxofemoral joint results in cranio-dorsal displacement of the femoral head, whereas caudal displacement is indicative of tearing the muscle attachments as a result of force applied caudally to the hindlimb. This may be seen if the animal was swung or suspended by the hind leg.

The tail is a common location for abusers to grab the animal. This can result in separation of the coccygeal vertebrae, usually in the proximal tail vs. distal. Vertebral fractures may be seen if the tail was forced dorsally or laterally. Distal tail fractures are more commonly associated with accidental causes such as tails caught in a door closing or stepping on the tail, though these actions can be intentional and non-accidental. Contusions may be seen around the site of tail injury or with fractures; especially near the caudal pelvis, hemorrhage may dissect through fascial planes away from the area of injury.

Abrasions from dragging an animal usually are more circular or elongated in shape, typically located over the points of the body that had ground surface contact. These abrasions usually contain embedded debris from the surface over which the body was dragged, which should be collected for forensic analysis. It is important to try to determine if the animal was alive when the injuries occurred through gross evidence of healing or infection and microscopic examination for vital reaction.

GROOMING-ASSOCIATED INJURIES

Injuries associated with professional grooming need to be investigated to determine accidental or non-accidental cause. Grooming services may be performed at veterinary hospitals, grooming shops, or mobile facilities. The grooming service may encompass a variety of procedures that the animal may resist including nail trimming, ear hair plucking, bathing, shaving, and drying. Restraint procedures may be implemented to protect the animal and the groomer. Resistance by the animal may lead to frustration by the groomer, which may be heightened when the groomer works alone without available assistance.

The injuries most commonly associated with grooming are due to blunt force trauma. They may be related to hitting (with a hand, fist, or object), kicking, and/or throwing the animal, and can result in mild to severe injury or death. The animal may also be strangled (manual, ligature, or hanging) to the point of losing consciousness or death. A study in Brazil of 111 animals that died during grooming reported that 28% died of trauma of mechanical origin and 72% died of respiratory failure. Of the trauma group, 87.1% died of brain injury, 67.7% from hematoma in the cephalic region, 38.7% from skull fractures, and 12.9% from dislocation of the atlanto-occipital joint. Of the respiratory failure group, 96.3% had pulmonary edema, 90% had pulmonary hemorrhage, 80% had pulmonary congestion, 52.5% had splenomegaly, 53.1% had renal congestion, and 52.5% had hepatic congestion. It is thought that the cause of these respiratory deaths may be due to neurogenic shock where stress may have played a role either as the cause or contributing factor. Young animals, males, and small breeds are all more prone to stress (Maiorka, Maria, and Rego 2011).

The detection of trauma may be delayed due to the time required for visible bruising depending on the amount of force used and the location of the injury. It often goes undetected by the owner after grooming for several possible reasons: the lack of visible signs hidden by the haircoat, behavior of hiding by the animal after returning home, or lack of handling by the owner which may have elicited symptoms of pain. The common explanations offered for grooming injuries include falls from a table or bathtub, accidental drop while holding the animal, and extreme agitation by the animal during bathing on a slick tub surface. However, these scenarios are known to occur in the veterinary practice setting without resulting in injury or severe injury to the animal.

BLUNT FORCE INJURIES TO SPECIFIC BODY REGIONS

All areas of the body are susceptible to injury from blunt force impact. The next sections will look at injuries to the head, neck, spine, and body cavities. It is important that when there is any indication of blunt force trauma to one part of the body that the entire body is evaluated for injuries. The initial impact force can create additional force mechanisms resulting in remote injuries. With intentional blows, there are often multiple impacts which may vary in force, location, and degree of injury and may be the result of one or more causes such as kicking, punching, and/or the use of a weapon (Figures 5.5 and 5.6). In addition to

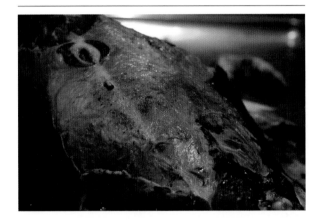

Figure 5.5. Bruising on the abdomen of a dog as a result of blunt force trauma due to kicking. The dog suffered severe internal organ damage. (Photo courtesy of Dr. Doris Miller.)

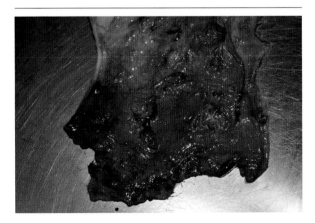

Figure 5.6. Bruising on reflected abdominal skin due to blunt force trauma from punching with a fist. (Photo courtesy of Dr. Doris Miller.)

blunt force trauma, consideration should be given to the possibility of evidence of other actions by the assailant such as the use of ligatures.

Head trauma

Overview

Both live and deceased animals can present with blunt force trauma head injuries. Traumatic injury to the head causes direct and immediate damage that is primarily mechanical in nature. These injuries may vary due to the force of the blow and the cause of the injury. Head injuries may include soft tissue injuries such as skin contusions, abrasions, and lacerations; eye injuries (sclera/conjunctival hemorrhage, hyphema, lens luxation, retinal detachment, and glaucoma); pulpal hemorrhage, tooth fractures; gingival contusions; ear injuries; tongue and gingival lacerations; frenulum tears; skull fractures; and brain injury (see Examination of Head Trauma Victims section). Brain injury may be very obvious if there is the presence of anisocoria and the animal has an abnormal mentation. A kitten with a brain injury may present with a sedate attitude and sit on an exam table without any restraint. As with any blunt force trauma case, an animal with obvious head injuries should have a full body evaluation to identify other traumatic injuries which may include radiographs and abdominal ultrasound.

Animals with a history of sudden death should be inspected during necropsy for lesions in the head and cervical area because minimal lesions can lead to neurogenic shock and present as sudden death. Other injuries may be found such as spinal cord injury. The key assessment in the postmortem examination of head injuries is the animal's time of consciousness and suffering: the determination if the blow caused immediate unconsciousness or death or if there was any level of suffering prior to death (Munro and Munro 2011).

Traumatic brain injury (TBI) is the term used to indicate a blunt force injury to the brain. The degree of brain injury depends on the acceleration, deceleration, and rotational impact forces that may cause shearing injury of the nerve fibers or diffuse axonal injury (Braund 2003). It also depends on the characteristics of the impacting object or surface, amount of force applied, and age of the animal. Another consideration is the area of the injury because occipital lesions, even those that seem to be superficial with minimal alterations in cerebella, can lead to a contrecoup brain lesion that can cause death.

Often, the animal lacks evidence of external trauma to the head yet has severe brain injury. In deceased animals subcutaneous bruising may be found on skin reflection during necropsy examination. A lack of bruising may be an indicator of postmortem injury or acute death without enough time elapsed for hemorrhage to occur subcutaneously. The presence of bilateral symmetrical skull bruising may be a postmortem artifact or normal anatomical feature. Marked or extensive intramuscular hemorrhage in the temporalis muscles of dogs and cats suggest high-energy trauma (Munro and Munro 2008b). There may be significant brain trauma with little to no associated subcutaneous hemorrhage if the force was dissipated over a larger area such as broad surface impact or soft weapon or if the force was not sufficient to cause subcutaneous hemorrhage but the transfer of energy was sufficient to cause brain injury.

A study of the activation of dural mast cells was conducted in rats. In response to trauma the mast cells will degranulate and induce the histamine receptor H3 expression in the cerebrum. The study found a significant decrease in toluidine blue-stained dural mast cells at the site of impact and a significant increase in the immunoreactivity and mRNA expression of histamine receptor H3 at days one and four. This finding on histological examinations of the dura can provide evidence of head trauma (Kibayashi 2011).

Skull and brain injuries include fractures, bone fragments embedded within the brain tissue, edema, ischemic laminar necrosis of the cerebral cortex, brain lacerations, contusions, and hemorrhage within the brain parenchyma with focal or multifocal malacia, and intracranial hemorrhage (Figure 5.7). Skull fractures usually result in extradural hemorrhage due to rupture of the meningeal artery (Munro and Munro 2011). There may be separation of the suture lines (diastasis) which may be difficult to detect on radiographs. Fractures or diastasis of the cranium floor can result in significant hemorrhage flowing through the nasal cavities and out the nose (Munro and Munro 2008b). There may be epidural, subdural, subarachnoid, and intraparenchymal hemorrhages (Fenner 1995). This hemorrhage can lead to large clot formation that will compress brain parenchyma and result in the death of the animal. Antemortem fractures of the zygomatic arch are associated with local soft tissue injury and hemorrhage. The junction of the zygomatic processes may remain open in adult dogs and be misinterpreted as fractures.

There are also species differences related to the type of head injuries sustained from blunt trauma. Head trauma injuries in cats more commonly involve mandibular symphyseal fractures, hard palate separation, and other maxillary injuries. In cats, there can be a different presentation than dogs with blunt force trauma to the rostral muzzle. The lip conformation in cats is typically tighter with less flexibility than dogs, which results in skin abrasions from

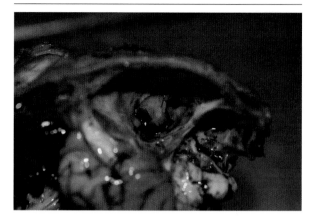

Figure 5.7. Bone hemorrhage associated with skull fractures.

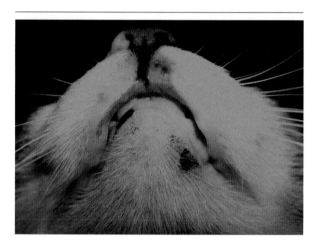

Figure 5.8. Characteristic abrasion and puncture injuries associated with blunt force trauma to the rostral muzzle of cats

their canine teeth, with or without punctures, due to blunt impact. In addition, distal fractures of one or more canine teeth may be seen (Figure 5.8). Fractures of the parietal crest indicate a direct and heavy blow due to the prominence and strength of the crest in certain species such as dogs and pigs (Munro and Munro 2008b).

Blunt force trauma to the head may cause damage to the central nervous system (CNS) or peripheral nervous system (PNS) or both. Animals that sustain CNS damage are defined as having craniocerebral trauma (CCT) and may have reversible or irreversible injuries. Patients with PNS injury usually have a better prognosis of survival and less chance of serious sequelae than those with CNS injury

(Fenner 1995). Victims of head trauma should be evaluated carefully to document injuries, determine cause of injuries, determine prognosis in live victims, and institute appropriate treatment. Continued monitoring of vital signs is crucial to detect worsening symptoms when lesions of minimal hemorrhage progress to a space-occupying hematoma or clot compressing brain parenchyma.

Examination of head trauma victims

Overview

Animals with head injuries may have no outward signs of trauma or neurological dysfunction. The only indicators of head trauma may be found in the eyes, ears, nose, or mouth. The skull should be palpated for swelling and possible fractures. Skull radiographs may reveal injuries and full body radiographs should be taken to detect additional injuries. Computed tomography (CT) scans and MRI are becoming more available in veterinary practice, providing the opportunity for greater evidence documentation. This imaging allows a better understanding of head trauma lesions in animals, especially because they have less rotational movements than is seen in humans. The outcome of head trauma injuries is affected by location, severity, and progression of injury resulting from edema and ischemia.

Ocular injuries

Ocular injuries are primarily the result of blunt force trauma to the head causing closed trauma to the eye. Sometimes the only injury in head trauma is to the eye. It is important to do a complete eye exam, including the cornea with possible fluorescein stain, anterior chamber, fundis, and possible measurement of the intraocular pressure. Eye trauma may present as hemorrhage in the conjunctiva, nictitating membrane, sclera, or periorbital tissues (Figure 5.9). There may be anterior uveitis present with hyphema, hypopyon, or fibrin clots. Evidence of anterior uveitis may not be as obvious after the acute event and fibrin and blood clots may be found in the ventral anterior chamber. Other findings may include traumatic lens luxation, retinal hemorrhage, and retinal detachment. Retinal scarring may be seen from previous retinal injury. It is important to consider causes for exam findings such as clotting disorders, hypertension, and other causes of anterior uveitis.

In child abuse, postmortem orbit pathology can be an indicator of abuse vs. accidental injury. The combination of optic nerve sheath and orbital hemorrhage was significantly more common in abuse head trauma than accidental head injury. Retinal hemorrhage is the most common form of ocular damage in child abuse with head injury and is predominantly found in the superficial retinal layers and sub-

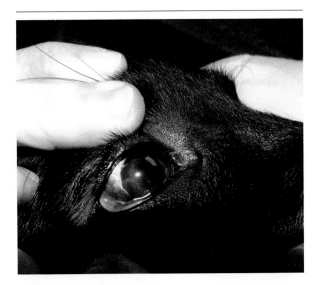

Figure 5.9. Scleral hemorrhage due to blunt force trauma.

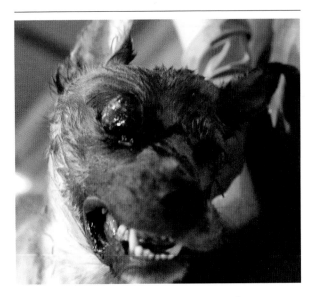

Figure 5.10. Proptosed eye due to blunt force trauma from a blow to the head. (Photo courtesy of Dr. Doris Miller.)

retinal space. The intraretinal and periretinal hemorrhages are most prevalent at the posterior pole. Retinal hemorrhages are more commonly found with inflicted head injury than accidental injury or natural disease (Gilliland et al. 2007).

Traumatic proptosis occurs when the globe of the eye is displaced rostral from the orbit because of blunt force trauma (Figure 5.10). It requires substantial force to induce

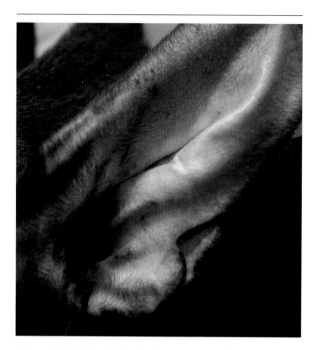

Figure 5.11. Petechiae in the pinna due to blunt force trauma. (Photo courtesy of Dr. Doris Miller.)

proptosis in cats and non-brachycephalic dogs (Ramsey 2000). Usually concurrent injuries are found, including severe craniofacial, CNS, and intraocular trauma.

In dogs, the most common problems with traumatic proptosis include strabismus, chemosis, exposure keratitis, corneal ulceration, and hyphema. In cats, they include corneal perforation, hyphema, and facial fractures (Ramsey 2000). Important forensic evidence such as debris may be embedded in the globe or surrounding tissues. A traumatic proptosis in a cat or non-brachycephalic dog has a poor prognosis for vision and it is uncommon for cats to regain vision after replacement of the proptosed eye. Other poor prognostic indicators include optic nerve transection, no visible pupil, extensive hyphema, facial fractures, and avulsion of three or more extraocular muscles (Ramsey 2000).

Ear injuries

Injury to the ear may be the only evidence found in blunt force trauma to the head. Petechiae may be found on the surface of the pinna or the base of the ear (Figure 5.11). The tympanic membrane may be ruptured with evidence of bleeding, though this finding is less common in dogs and cats with head trauma. Due to the conformation of the vertical and horizontal ear canal, the concussive force from a blow to the head can create stretching of the horizontal

canal instead of tympanic membrane rupture. This stretching of the canal ruptures the capillaries within the lining, creating petechial hemorrhages. This finding is unique to animal victims of head trauma. Frank hemorrhage may be found in the ear canal. Bleeding from the inner ear may be associated with intracranial hemorrhages in dogs and cats (Braund 2003). Clotting disorders should be considered with findings of petechial hemorrhages. Unilateral presentation of hemorrhages or injuries can support trauma vs. systemic causes.

Nasal and oral injuries

Blunt force trauma to the nasal area may or may not result in epistaxis. There may be a delay before epistaxis is seen or the blood may only flow caudally and be swallowed or aspirated. Evidence of blood may be found in the trachea, lower airways, deeper airways on microscopic exam, esophagus, and stomach with possible signs of blood digestion (blackened) depending on the elapsed time period. Obstruction of the nasal cavity may develop due to the presence of blood clots and subsequent edema, forcing open-mouthed breathing which may last for several days until the swelling subsides. Fractures of the nasal bone and maxillary bone may be found, which reduces the patency of the nasal cavity. Subsequent secondary infection and necrosis of the conchae may develop over time. Due to the extensive nasal cavity in some species of animals, especially dogs, blunt force trauma to the nasal area can result in severe, life-threatening hemorrhage that usually flows caudally to the pharyngeal area and may or may not include signs of epistaxis. Fracture of the hard palate and the palatine symphyses can be seen as a result of blunt force trauma or a fall and cause nasal hemorrhage (see Fall Injuries section). Edema and hemorrhage of the palatine mucosa may obscure the cleft until tissue necrosis develops several days later (Bedford 1995).

Examination of the oral cavity may reveal injuries related to head trauma. These include lacerations to the gingiva, buccal mucosa, tongue, lips; palate injuries; teeth fractures; and contusions of the surrounding skin, lips, or mucosa. Blood may be found secondary to oral injuries or from nasal injury draining into the pharyngeal area.

Neurological assessment

It is important to classify the CNS injury based on the location of the affected area in the brain. This can help determine the prognosis, such as with brainstem injury patients, who have a poor prognosis even with treatment. The animal's level of consciousness and whether it is abnormal or normal should be noted. A coma lasting forty-eight hours or longer is considered a grave prognostic sign (Braund 2003). It is very important to note if there is a change in the level of consciousness over a period of time. Deteriorating clinical signs indicate progressive brain swelling or possible brain herniation (Braund 2003). Even a minimal continuous hemorrhage that progresses to a large hematoma/clot can create a space-occupying lesion and compress brain parenchyma. The animal may appear awake but does not respond properly to the environment, indicating an abnormal level of consciousness as a result of cerebral injury. An animal that is in a stupor or coma has an abnormal level of consciousness, which is indicative of either cerebral or brainstem injury. Cardiovascular and respiratory function should be monitored because they can be affected by minimal lesions from the brainstem injuries and lead to the death of the animal by neurogenic shock.

The eyes should be examined for pupillary light responses (PLRs), pupil size and symmetry, physiological nystagmus (doll's eye maneuver), and ocular injury (see Ocular Injuries). When interpreting eye test results it is important to rule out injury to the optic nerve. With optic nerve injury, normal physiological nystagmus should be present. There may be abnormal pupil size in either cerebral or brainstem damage. In cerebral injuries, the animal has small pupils with normal PLRs and normal physiological nystagmus. In brainstem injuries, the animal can have small or large pupils, abnormal or absent physiological nystagmus, and usually abnormal PLRs. In cerebellar injuries, there may be abnormal pupil size but there is usually normal consciousness and normal physiological nystagmus (Fenner 1986). Animals that are stuporous or comatose with dilated pupils have a poor prognosis (Braund 2003).

Peripheral nerve injury must be ruled out in suspected cerebellar injuries. The posture of the animal and response to stimuli may help determine the location of the injuries. In rostral brainstem injuries, the animal may have episodes of decerebrate posturing that can appear similar to the opisthotonic posturing caused by cerebellar injury. The level of consciousness helps differentiate the site of injury where stupor or coma is associated with brainstem injury in animals (Fenner 1986). Lastly, the cranial nerves and spinal reflexes should be examined to determine sites of injury and whether there are multiple locations.

The primary brain injury actually sets off a cascade of secondary biochemical events that can exacerbate the neurological problems known as secondary injuries. These changes can occur within hours to days after the primary event. These injuries are believed to be caused by progressive ischemic brain injury and are affected by several factors including decreased blood flow autoregulation, altered cerebral metabolism, inadequate cerebral perfusion pressure, hemorrhage, increased cytokine and free radical production, increased excitotoxins, depletion of neuronal adenosine triphosphatase (ATP) levels, decreased intracellular magnesium levels, intracellular accumulation of calcium and sodium leading to astrocytic swelling, and cytotoxic edema (Braund 2003). The result of these events is increased intracranial pressure (ICP) and progressive damage to the brain parenchyma. In addition, some secondary events are thought to be related to the activation of the sympathetic nervous system, causing a further increase of intracranial pressure (ICP), systemic hypertension, myocardial necrosis, cardiac arrhythmias, increased nutritional requirements, and non-cardiogenic pulmonary edema (Fenner 1995).

Respiratory distress associated with head trauma may be caused by indirect injury to the soft tissues of the neck. The blow to the head may cause rapid acceleration of the skull, resulting in tearing of the soft tissues of the neck, the hyoid apparatus or larynx, and cervical spine fracture or subluxation (Braund 2003). Systemic hypotension or hypovolemia exacerbates the autolytic processes in the brain, resulting in further parenchymal damage and edema with a resultant rise in ICP (Dewey 2005). In human patients with severe head trauma, mortality is doubled with concurrent secondary injuries of hypoxia and hypotension (Braund 2003).

The increased ICP is caused by intracranial hemorrhage and brain edema. The high ICP is further compounded by the decreased cerebral blood flow because of the compressed dural veins. If not ameliorated, increased ICP may cause brain herniation and also may result in secondary spinal cord myelomalacia (Dewey 2005). Brain edema may be caused by cytotoxic edema, which accumulates primarily in neurons and astrocytes because of cellular hypoxia. Vasogenic edema, which primarily affects the white matter, may be another component of brain edema. This type of edema is extracellular and is caused by leakage across the injured blood-brain barrier. The increased ICP also causes CNS hypoxia. The hypoxic animal then may develop hypercarbia, which in turn increases the ICP even more. Seizures are common in craniocerebral trauma patients and may be seen early on or develop later because of the brain injury (Fenner 1995).

Impact injuries

Head injuries may be categorized as impact injuries or acceleration/deceleration injuries. Impact injuries are caused when the head strikes an object or surface, or the head is struck by an object. The surface or weapon that is relatively soft and yielding will absorb a large proportion of the impacting energy by way of deformation as compared with a hard unyielding surface or weapon. Impact injuries can cause soft-tissue injuries, fractures, brain contusions, epidural hematomas, and intracerebral hemorrhage. Impact soft-tissue injuries include abrasions, contusions, and lacerations. These injuries may reflect the weapon or surface that struck the head (see Patterned Abrasions and Bruising). Unlike humans, lacerations to the cephalic area of a dog or cat do not tend to bleed profusely.

Fractures

Impact injuries can cause skull fractures, which may or may not have concurrent brain injury. Skull fractures and fragments may cause lacerations and penetrating wounds of the brain without lacerations of the overlying skin. The fracture produced depends on several factors including the fur covering, thickness of the skin, thickness and configuration of the skull, and elasticity of the bone at the point of impact. It also depends on the object's shape, weight, and consistency that impacts the head along with the velocity with which the blow was delivered or the head struck the object (Di Maio and Di Maio 2001).

When a broad, flat object impacts the head, the skull flattens at the point of impact to conform to the surface. The flattened area bends inward, and the adjacent and more distant areas bend outward. This can cause fractures distant from the point of impact. In the area of sharp curves, linear fractures occur at the site of the outbending. Then the inbended area tries to rebound back, causing the fracture line to extend toward the area of impact as well as in the opposite direction. This fracture line may not completely extend to the area of impact or may extend through it. A low-velocity impact with a large area of contact between the head and the object may cause simple linear fractures (Di Maio and Di Maio 2001).

Circular fractures, either complete or incomplete, may be seen with higher velocity and force. Stellate fractures are caused by an even higher velocity and force, causing a depression in the bone at the site of impact. This area of severe inbending causes fractures on the inner surface that radiate outward from the impact site. The outbending areas fracture and radiate back toward the area of impact joining the inbending fractures. There may be circular fractures at the outbended area. They may be incomplete, stopping at a linear fracture, and indicate that the linear fracture preceded the circular. If the linear fracture stops at the circular, it indicates the linear fracture occurred after the circular fracture (Di Maio and Di Maio 2001).

Blows to different parts of the head can produce different effects. If the head is struck with a large amount of force by an object that has a small surface area it can cause a depressed skull fracture, sometimes with fragmentation. This also can be caused when the skull is impacted in a small area by a large amount of force. There are no large deformations of the skull distant from the impact associated with this type of fracture, such as linear fractures. Basilar fractures are caused by blows to the base of the skull. Hinge fractures are transverse fractures that completely bisect the base of the skull, creating a "hinge." These are usually caused by impacts on the side of the head and occasionally from the front of the mandible (Di Maio and Di Maio 2001). Ring fractures are circular fractures that surround the foramen magnum at the base of the skull. They are caused by the head being driven down onto the vertebral column or the column being driven into the base of the skull. If the suture lines are not completely fused in the skull, then fracture lines can follow along these lines. These are called diastatic fractures.

A contrecoup injury occurs in the area opposite the site of impact. A coup injury occurs at the site of impact. Contrecoup fractures are located at the opposite point of impact and are associated with contrecoup brain injury, primarily seen in human deaths caused by falls (Di Maio and Di Maio 2001).

Brain contusions

Brain contusions may be produced by impact injuries to the head. They are typically more severe when associated with skull fractures. Brains with diffuse axonal injury usually have less severe contusions. It is possible to have severe open skull fractures with massive brain lacerations or evisceration without any contusions. Contusions are composed of hemorrhage and usually are associated with necrosis of the brain tissue. It is possible to have necrosis with minimal to no associated hemorrhage. The amount of hemorrhage depends on the type and size of vessel involved. Brain contusions usually are multiple, densely arranged, and streak-like in appearance. Overlying subarachnoid hemorrhage may be present (Di Maio and Di Maio 2001).

There are six types of contusions: coup, contrecoup, fracture, intermediary coup, gliding, and herniation. Coup contusions are located at the site of impact. They are caused by the inbending of the bone rebounding back, causing tensile force injury to the brain. Contrecoup contusions are located opposite the point of impact and are caused by the brain rebounding back from the skull after impact. It is possible to see both coup (from the direct impact) and contrecoup contusions, but contrecoup injury is more extensive than the coup. This may be seen in head injuries caused by a fall. A blow to the head usually produces coup contusions, although it is possible to see associated but less extensive contrecoup contusions (Di Maio and Di Maio 2001).

Fracture contusions are caused by skull fractures. They may or may not be at the site of impact because fractures can occur remotely. Intermediary coup contusions are located in the deeper structures of the brain and follow the line of impact. Gliding contusions are areas of focal hemorrhages in the dorsal surface of the cerebral hemispheres, specifically involving the cortex and underlying white matter. They are usually associated with diffuse axonal injury and are not associated with the direction and site of impact. Herniation contusions are caused by brain herniation and are also independent of the direction and site of impact (Di Maio and Di Maio 2001).

The aging of brain contusions may be possible based on microscopic patterns of neuronal and glial injuries, granulocytic response, vascular changes, and the presence of fat and hemosiderin within macrophages. In humans, within minutes of injury neuronal change may be seen as dark neurons with wavy apical dendrites which develop into eosinophilic shrunken cells within two to three days. Diffuse cytoplasmic eosinophilia and decreased nuclear basophilia may be detected as soon as one hour after injury and may be present for weeks. Axonal swelling may be seen after two to five days. Oligodendroglia may be detected within a few minutes to four to five days after injury. Necrotic glial cells with eosinophilic nuclei are seen at six to twelve hours. Reactive changes in astrocytes may be seen at five days with gemistocyte transformation at ten to fifteen days. Extravascular karyorrhectic granulocytes may be observed at forty-eight hours and longer. Hemosiderin and fat within the macrophages may be detected at the injury margins at three to four days. Endothelial swelling may be seen after twelve to twenty-four hours with development of new capillaries after three to four days (Perper 2006).

Epidural hematomas

Epidermal hematomas are caused by the primary impact and are usually associated with skull fractures. The skull is bent inward on impact, causing stripping of the dura and laceration of the meningeal vessels. They are usually unilateral and have a thick, disk-shaped appearance. Death from an epidermal hematoma is caused by brain displacement and compression of the brainstem (Di Maio and Di Maio 2001).

Subarachnoid hemorrhage

Subarachnoid hemorrhage is the common injury of head trauma in humans. It occurs in all penetrating injuries of the brain and may be present along with extradural and subdural hemorrhage (Munro and Munro 2008b). It can range from minor to severe and be focal or diffuse. Hemorrhage is of mostly venous origin and is usually diffuse over the cerebral hemispheres. There may be some pooling of blood on the ventral surface of the brain. Massive brain injury, including lacerations, may be present with little to no subarachnoid hemorrhage because of vessel spasm.

Some artifactual hemorrhage may be caused on necropsy when removing the skull cap, diffusing blood into the dependent portion of the subarachnoid space. Subarachnoid hemorrhage also can be produced by decomposition because of lysis of blood cells, breakdown of the vessels, and leakage into the subarachnoid space (Di Maio and Di Maio 2001).

Lacerations of the internal carotid, vertebral, or carotid arteries can produce subarachnoid hemorrhage over the base of the brain. The carotid artery may be damaged within the cranium in conjunction with skull fractures. It also may be damaged in the neck with cervical fractures or hyperextension injury. The vertebral arteries can be injured because of blunt force trauma to the neck (see below). This can cause subarachnoid hemorrhage to the base of the brain or thrombosis within the artery, resulting in brain infarction (Di Maio and Di Maio 2001).

Brain swelling

Swelling of the brain can occur because of severe head trauma. The swelling may be focal or diffuse and results from vasodilation causing an increase in intravascular cerebral blood volume, cerebral edema, or both. This swelling causes a space-occupying mass effect. If the swelling becomes severe, herniation of the brain, brainstem hemorrhage, infarction, and necrosis can result.

Subdural hygromas

A subdural hygroma may be seen when brain trauma causes the effusion of spinal fluid to the subdural space. This fluid may be blood tinged. The accumulation of spinal fluid can cause the same space-occupying effects of a subdural hematoma (see below) (Di Maio and Di Maio 2001).

Acceleration/deceleration injuries

Acceleration or deceleration injuries result from the sudden movement of the head, immediately after the impact, imparting shearing and tensile forces to the brain and creating intracranial pressure gradients. One type of injury produced is subdural hematomas, which are caused by the tearing of the subdural bridging veins. The second type of injury is diffuse axonal injury, which is secondary to injury of the axons (see below) (Di Maio and Di Maio 2001).

An impact to the head can produce linear or rotational (angular) acceleration or a combination of both. Linear acceleration is caused by the force passing through the center of the head, which causes the head to accelerate in a straight line. When the impact force does not pass through the center of the head it causes rotational or angular acceleration. This causes the head to rotate about its center (Di Maio and Di Maio 2001). In theory, acceleration or deceleration injuries do not require an impact but virtually all are associated with an initiating impact force (Di Maio and Di Maio 2001).

Blunt force trauma to the head can cause intracerebral hemorrhage. This hemorrhage is located within the cerebral parenchyma and does not involve the surface of the brain. These areas present as a collection of blood and usually are well demarcated. Intracerebral hemorrhage is caused by acceleration/deceleration forces that are usually associated with gliding contusions and diffuse axonal injury (Di Maio and Di Maio 2001).

Diffuse axonal injury (DAI)

Diffuse axonal injury is caused by sudden acceleration or deceleration of the head, usually started by an impact to the head. The severity of injury depends on the force, the time over which the acceleration or deceleration occurs, and the direction of the movement. In humans it has been shown that lateral motion of the head causes severe injuries vs. those due to forward or backward motion, which tend to cause milder injuries (Di Maio and Di Maio 2001).

The longer the time period over which acceleration or deceleration occurs, the more likely it is to see diffuse axonal injury vs. subdural hematomas. Injuries can range from mild to severe and may result in death. There may only be physiological dysfunction without disruption of the axons at low acceleration or deceleration. When there is reversible physiological disruption it is known as a concussion (Fenner 1995). With increasing force, there is increasing physiological and structural disruption of axons. The cell membranes are damaged, which may be reversible in some cells (Di Maio and Di Maio 2001).

Histologically, diffuse axonal injury (DAI) may be seen as axonal swelling, initially dilated, then club shaped, then finally round balls called "retraction balls" (Di Maio and Di Maio 2001); it is often surrounded by a clear halo (Perper 2006). If the victim survives for weeks or months, clusters of microglia and demyelination may be seen in the white matter (Perper 2006). In humans, a minimum post-injury survival time of fifteen hours is required to detect DAI using hematoxylin and eosin stain. Using the immunostain β-amyloid precursor protein decreases this time to two hours (Spitz 2006).

Subdural hematomas

Subdural hematomas are always due to trauma and often are not associated with skull fractures (Munro and Munro 2008b). There may or may not be cerebral contusions or grossly obvious brain injury. They are caused by a head impact to a hard surface, which causes the brain to accelerate. This produces stretching and tearing of the bridging veins that drain the surface of the cerebral hemispheres into the sinus. The more rapid the acceleration or deceleration and the shorter the time for the acceleration or deceleration, the more likely subdural hematomas will occur vs. diffuse axonal injury. There is no association of skull fracture location with the location or presence of a subdural hematoma. Typically these hematomas are more lethal because the same acceleration and deceleration forces produce diffuse axonal injury to the cerebral parenchyma. They also may cause brain displacement, possible cerebral edema, and compression of the brainstem (Di Maio and Di Maio 2001).

Shaken baby syndrome (SBS)

The violent shaking of infants can cause major damage of the brain. This shaking causes the head to flop back and forth, producing extensive intracranial (often subdural) and retinal hemorrhages. The injuries result from the indirect acceleration and deceleration traction stresses from the whiplash action. The violent forces can produce stretching of axons in the cerebral white matter strong enough to shear off the axons. These ends then retract into globoid shapes, known as retraction balls. The cause of the retinal hemorrhages is not known but is believed to result from increased retinal venous pressure, extravasation of subarachnoid blood, and traction caused by angular deceleration of the retinal vessels at the vitreoretinal interface (Di Maio and Di Maio 2001). Intrascleral hemorrhage at the optic nerve-globe junction and optic nerve sheath hemorrhage are also reported. The most common site for optic nerve sheath hemorrhage is the immediate retrobulbar portion of the optic nerve with most hemorrhage located in the subdural space. There appears to be a positive correlation between the findings of retinal hemorrhage, retrobulbar optic nerve sheath hemorrhage, and intrascleral hemorrhage at the optic nerve-globe junction and SBS (Gilliland et al. 2007).

In several reported cases of shaken baby syndrome, evidence has been found of head impact trauma. This has caused some pathologists to switch to the use of shaken impact syndrome. In these cases, the retinal and intracranial hemorrhage is caused by the shaking; then the head is impacted against a hard surface, causing further intracranial bleeding, contusions, and possible fractures. Although these same forces would be expected to cause cervical fractures and/or spinal cord damage it has not been found in human cases (Di Maio and Di Maio 2001).

Neck and spinal injuries

Neck injuries

The pharyngeal area, larynx, and trachea may be an area of trauma resulting from bite wounds from a predator attack, strangulation, blunt or sharp force trauma, or grabbing and wrenching of the neck or head. The pharyngeal injuries may include edema of the pharynx and surrounding tissue, hematoma, laceration, or fracture of the hyoid bone. A fractured hyoid bone in a surviving animal may present with symptoms of painful swallowing (Venker-van Haagen 1995). Laryngeal injuries may lead to life-threatening edema, causing upper airway obstruction. The laryngeal cartilage can be damaged, causing further narrowing of the airway. Lacerations of the larynx can result in tissue emphysema (Venker-van Haagen 1995). Tracheal injuries include tears in the tracheal wall or fractures of the tracheal rings that typically cause subcutaneous emphysema. Depending on the location of the tracheal lesions, other findings may include pneumomediastinum and peritracheal or intermuscular emphysema (Brayley and Ettinger 1995). There may be evidence of swelling in the dorsal neck due to cellulitis or tissue hemorrhage which may be caused by blunt force trauma. It also may be the result of compression, stretching and/or tearing injuries associated with grabbing, squeezing, and/or shaking the animal by the neck, either by another animal or person. On necropsy exam there may be evidence of injury to the muscles and surrounding tissue, the vertebrae and associated ligaments, and possible avulsion injuries.

Spinal injuries

Blunt force trauma to the head can cause cervical vertebrae injuries. Atlanto-occipital dislocation is caused by the separation of the craniocervical ligament attachments. There may or may not be osseous injury to the vertebra and there may be associated ventral brain lacerations. On the axis, C2, a fracture of the neural arch between the superior and inferior articular processes is called the hangman's fracture in humans. It is caused by axial loading forces with flexion or extension. Atlantoaxial dislocations may be difficult to detect (Di Maio and Di Maio 2001).

Hyperextension of the head of an animal may be due to accidental or non-accidental causes. Non-accidental scenarios include swinging or throwing the animal by the head or throwing or kicking the animal with enough force to cause hyperextension movement at the beginning or upon surface impact. Severe hyperextension may result in injury to the brainstem which can vary from tears and hemorrhage to complete avulsion. Subarachnoid hemorrhage is a common finding with severe hyperextension. In humans, these injuries usually are associated with fractures of the upper cervical vertebrae and the base of the skull. Lacerations of the brainstem can occur without cervical or cranial fractures and usually are associated with subarachnoid hemorrhage around the brainstem (Di Maio and Di Maio 2001).

Hyperextension of the head of an animal can result in traumatic atlantoaxial luxations. This can occur in all breeds of dogs and cats and is a result of the rupture of the atlantoaxial ligaments or fracture of the dens at its junction with the axis (LeCouteur and Child 1995). Clinical signs usually are acute and are associated with the incident or may be delayed in onset. In three reported cases of injuries to dogs, two presented with mild neurological deficits and cervical pain, and one had vestibular abnormalities and tetraparesis (LeCouteur and Child 1995). The clinical signs can vary and include sensitivity to the head, cervical pain, tetraparesis, and tetraplegia. This type of injury can cause spinal cord trauma leading to hemorrhage and edema to the brain which may cause dysphagia, facial paralysis, vestibular deficits, opisthotonos, or respiratory paralysis and death (LeCouteur and Child 1995).

Spinal injuries may be a result of blunt force trauma which may be associated with motor vehicle accidents, direct blows, animal fighting, predator attacks, or falls. The types of injuries found may include vertebral fractures, luxations, subluxations, dural tearing, or disk extrusion resulting in spinal cord concussion, compression, laceration, or distraction (Braund 2003). Reports of subluxation injuries at C5–C6 associated with dog fighting injuries indicate a possible anatomical predisposition for subluxation at this level (Braund 2003).

Fractures of the axis appear to be more common than fractures of other cervical vertebrae (Braund 2003). There is direct primary injury to the spinal cord resulting from mechanical disruption of the nerve pathways, followed by secondary injury caused by ischemia, edema, hypoxia, and multiple biochemical deleterious events, including reduced spinal blood flow. The end result is membrane destruction, ischemia, edema, cell death, and possibly permanent neurological dysfunction (Braund 2003).

Table 5.3 The four classes of hemorrhage.

Class 1	Loss of up to 15% (approximately 10–12 ml/kg)* of the circulating blood volume. Clinical symptoms are minimal as suggested by mild tachycardia; no changes in arterial blood pressure, pulse pressure, or respiratory rate
Class 2	Loss of 15%–30% (approximately 12–25 ml/kg)* of the circulating blood volume. Clinical signs include tachycardia, tachypnea, and a decrease in pulse pressure
Class 3	Loss of 30%–40% (approximately 25–32 ml/kg)* of the circulating blood volume. Clinical signs include pale mucous membranes, prolonged capillary refill time, tachycardia, tachypnea, depression, and a decrease in arterial blood pressure
Class 4	Loss of more than 40% of circulating blood volume. A potentially life threatening event. Clinical signs include very pale or white mucous membranes, prolonged capillary refill time, cold extremities, tachycardia, tachypnea, rapid thread pulse, markedly decreased arterial blood pressure, delirium, and depression

*Assumes a total blood volume of 80 ml/kg (i.e., 8% of BW)

Source: Muir, W. 2006. Trauma: Physiology, Pathophysiology, and Clinical Implications. *Journal of Veterinary Emergency and Critical Care Society.* 16(4):253–263.

A complete neurological exam should be performed to determine the level of spinal injury. This exam should be repeated periodically to detect progression of damage and deteriorating neurological function. Radiographs, CT, and MRI can document the presence of fractures, luxations, or subluxations. Evaluation of spinal abnormalities should include consideration of congenital deformities, underlying nutritional factors, or metabolic disorders.

Body cavity trauma

Blunt force trauma to both body cavities is common. Diagnostic imaging is necessary to understand the extent of the injuries in live animals. Chest and abdominal radiographs should be routinely performed. Abdominal ultrasound may be a better choice than radiography for abdominal evaluation (Boysen 2004).

One of the primary concerns with body cavity injury is intra-cavity hemorrhage. Assessment for abdominal hemorrhage in live animals is best done using ultrasound. Blood loss can affect the degree of hemorrhage from subsequent injuries which can help determine the sequence of injuries (Chapter 6). Blood loss should be estimated in the live animal (Chapter 3). Free blood identified in body cavities at necropsy should be quantified. The percentage blood loss should be estimated by using estimated total blood volumes of 5% to 6% of body weight (kg) in cats and 8% to 9% of body weight (kg) in dogs (Muir 2006). Blood loss can be divided into four classes representing increasing blood loss and progressively deteriorating health (Table 5.3). Significant clinical signs are first seen with Class 2, which represents a 15% to 30% loss (approxi-

mately 12 to 25 ml/kg) of total estimated blood volume. Clinical signs include tachycardia, tachypnea, and a decrease in pulse pressure. Blood loss greater than 40% is fatal without treatment.

Chest injuries

Blunt force or sharp force trauma to the thorax can result in bone fractures, hemothorax, myocardial trauma, lung injury, tracheobronchial fractures or avulsions, damage to the major vessels, pneumomediastinum, pneumothorax, or diaphragmatic rupture. Injuries to the lungs include contusions, hematomas, lacerations, lung torsions, or lung collapse. If the surface of the lung at the site of impact does not absorb the full force of the blow, the energy can be transferred to the opposite side, usually fixed, causing contrecoup contusions (Di Maio and Di Maio 2001). The coup or coutrecoup lung lesions may have an indentation or bruising pattern from rib impact. Pulmonary contusions may take as long as twenty-four hours to develop radiographically.

The thorax may have rib fractures, flail chest, sternal fractures, or thoracic vertebral fractures. The pliability in the chests of animals, depending on age and/or conformation, allows transmission of kinetic energy which can result in significant damage to the intrathoracic structures without fractures of the ribs or sternum. Rib fractures may damage the internal chest structures during the compressive phase of the blunt force impact, and then rebound back into position. Rib fractures may lacerate or puncture the lungs, vessels, or heart. Myocardial injuries include contusions, lacerations, hemorrhage, pericardial effusions, cardiac tamponade, or myocardial necrosis. The primary clinical signs of injury, which may not develop for twelve to twenty-four hours, are ST-T abnormalities on the electrocardiogram and cardiac arrhythmias (Sisson and Thomas 1995). Severe grinding force (compression and rotation) to the chest can cause multiple fractures and maceration of the lungs.

Ribs are designed to protect vital organs in the chest and abdomen, and rib fractures are a marker of severe trauma (Kraje 2000). Ribs are good at absorbing energy and are difficult to break. Puppy and kitten ribs are less bony and more elastic than those of adult or older animals and are very difficult, but not impossible, to break. Rib fractures are a common abuse finding in cats and dogs. They can be found in both neglect (e.g., starvation) and physical assault cases. In motor vehicle accidents, it is more common to have intrathoracic injuries (e.g., pneumothorax, pulmonary contusions) than rib fractures (Boysen 2004, Sigrist 2004, Lisciandro 2011). In animal abuse cases, rib fractures may occur due to focal application of force, which includes the animal being struck, kicked, stomped, or thrown against a blunt object. With physical assault, the blunt force impact is delivered to a smaller area compared to blunt force from a motor vehicle accident, which typically is delivered to a larger area.

Rib fractures frequently occur in groups of two or three adjacent ribs. The presentation of more than one grouping of rib fractures indicates more than one blunt force impact and any explanation offered for the cause of injuries must account for these findings. The finding of bilateral rib fractures is a strong suspicious indicator of abuse. With severe compressive blunt force, such as stomping, rib fractures are most commonly found at the neck of the rib at or near the vertebral attachment.

Commotio cordis is the term for cases of sudden cardiac death due to non-penetrating chest trauma without evidence of underlying myocardial disease or injury. It is been demonstrated to occur in studies of anesthetized dogs, cats, and rabbits. Commotio cordis means "disturbance of the heart" and refers to cardiac concussion in the absence of injury. The blunt trauma causes disruption of the heart rhythm including ventricular tachycardia, bradyarrhythmias, idioventricular rhythms, complete heart block, and asystole (Marshall, Gilbert, and Byard 2008).

Animal studies have shown that the heart is vulnerable to electrical instability when struck early during ventricular repolarization and involves adenosine triphosphate (ATP)-dependent potassium channels. A study in pigs reported the electrophysiologic consequences of chest wall impacts were critically dependent on the precise timing of the impact during the cardiac cycle. When the impact occurred in a narrow 15-msec window during cardiac repolarization, just before the peak of the T wave, ventricular fibrillation was consistently produced. Ventricular fibrillation was induced instantaneously and was not preceded by premature ventricular contractions, ischemic ST-segment changes, or heart block. In contrast, chest-wall impact during ventricular depolarization (the QRS complex) did not produce ventricular fibrillation and instead produced transient complete heart block followed by ST-segment elevation and, in some pigs, left bundle-branch block (Link et al. 1998).

Abdominal injuries

Abdominal injuries may be caused by blunt force trauma due to blows to the abdomen, crushing injury, dog bites, or falls. In child abuse, abdominal injuries are the second most common cause of death, which may be caused by the delay in recognition of the injury and initiation of treatment. The same may be true in animals due to lack of the presence or detection of external bruising and their tendency to hide symptoms of pain and injury. The abdominal walls are lax and compressible, which readily transmit the force from a blow to the internal viscera while showing little to no evidence of bruising (Munro and Munro 2011). The injuries associated with blunt force to the abdomen depend on the organ affected. The liver and spleen are highly affected viscera and ruptures can lead to hypovolemic shock that can result in death.

Microscopic analysis of liver lacerations may show histologic response to the injury. A human study of traumatic liver lacerations associated with fatal motor vehicle accidents found that these changes of neutrophilic infiltrate, pyknotic nucleus, and necrosis appeared approximately fifty-one minutes after injury. Cases with shorter survival time did not have evidence of histologic response (Kohlmeier et al. 2008).

The absence of external injury does not exclude the possibility of injury, which is sometimes massive, to the abdominal organs. Blunt force trauma to the abdomen may cause rupture of hollow organs (gastrointestinal tract, bladder, and uterus); lacerations or complete avulsion of solid organs, blood vessels, diaphragm, and abdominal wall; hemorrhage within organs; free hemorrhage; and leakage of organ contents into the peritoneal cavity (Figure 5.12). Pancreatitis may be seen secondary to blunt force trauma to the abdomen. Hemorrhagic pleural effusions may be caused by abdominal trauma. Urinary tract trauma (bladder, urethra, ureter, and kidneys) may be seen because of compressive forces to the abdomen or due to impact or penetration from fractures of the pelvis or os penis. Major vessels may be injured and organs may be

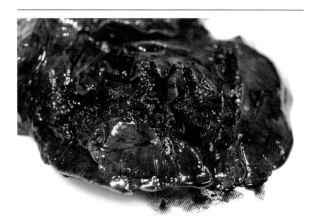

Figure 5.12 Liver lacerations due to abdominal blunt force trauma. (Photo courtesy of Dr. Doris Miller.)

avulsed from their attachments. The omentum may be bruised or torn, or major vessels damaged. Subcapsular hematomas may be present on the liver or spleen. The rupture of hollow organs usually occurs when the organs are distended with food or fluid (e.g., urine) at the time of the impact (Di Maio and Di Maio 2001).

Results of physical examination alone are insensitive and unreliable in the detection of intra-abdominal injury. Radiographically, intra-abdominal hemorrhage may take several hours to become apparent. Fluid volumes of as much as 8.8 ml/kg (4 ml/lb) of body weight are required before a consistent diagnosis of hemoperitoneum can be made on radiographs in dogs. Abdominal ultrasound is a much more sensitive diagnostic tool to identify intra-abdominal hemorrhage (Boysen 2004). The FAST (Focused Assesment with Sonography for Trauma) exam which was first used in human medicine to rapidly identify intra-abdominal hemorrhage in emergency rooms is now a diagnostic procedure in veterinary medicine (Boysen 2004, Lisciandro 2011).

REFERENCES

Bedford, P.G.C. 1995. Diseases of the Nose. In: *Textbook of Veterinary Internal Medicine: Diseases of the Dog and Cat*, Vol. 1, Fourth edition. S.J. Ettinger, and E.C. Feldman, eds. pp. 551–567. Philadelphia: W.B. Saunders.

Boysen, Søren R., E.A. Rozanski, A.S. Tidwell, J.L. Holm, S.P. Shaw, and J.E. Rush. 2004. Evaluation of a Focused Assessment With Sonography for Trauma Protocol to Detect Free Abdominal Fluid in Dogs Involved in Notor Vehicle Accidents. *Journal of American Veterinary Medical Association.* 225(8):1198–1204.

Braund, K.G. 2003. Traumatic Disorders. In: *Clinical Neurology in Small Animals: Localization, Diagnosis and Treatment*, K.G. Braund, ed. Ithaca, NY: International Veterinary Information Service (www.ivis.org).

Brayley, K.A., and S.J. Ettinger. 1995. Diseases of the Trachea. In: *Textbook of Veterinary Internal Medicine: Diseases of the Dog and Cat*, Vol. 1, Fourth edition, S.J. Ettinger and E.C. Feldman, eds. pp. 754–766. Philadelphia: W.B. Saunders.

Burdett, L.G., J.D. Adams, and W.E. McFee. 2007. The Use of Geographic Information Systems as a Forensic Tool to Investigate Sources of Marine Mammal Entanglement in Fisheries. *Journal of Forensic Sciences.* 52(4):904–908.

Dewey, C.W. 2005. Emergency Treatment of Head/Spinal Trauma. In: Proceedings of the Eleventh International Veterinary Emergency and Critical Care Symposium. Atlanta, GA, September 7–11, 2005. pp. 493–497.

Di Maio, V.J. and D. Di Maio. 2001. *Forensic Pathology*, Second edition. Boca Raton, FL: CRC Press.

Fenner, W.R. 1986. Head Trauma and Nervous System Injury. In: *Current Veterinary Therapy IX Small Animal Practice*, R.W. Kirk, ed. pp. 830–836. Philadelphia: W.B. Saunders.

Fenner, W.R. 1995. Diseases of the Brain. In: *Textbook of Veterinary Internal Medicine: Diseases of the Dog and Cat*, Vol. 1, Fourth edition, S.J. Ettinger, and E.C. Feldman, eds. pp. 578–629. Philadelphia: W.B. Saunders.

Fenton, TW. 2012. Determination of Impact Direction Based on Fracture Patterns in Human and Long Bones. Presented at the American Academy of Forensic Sciences Annual Scientific Meeting, 20–25 February, Atlanta, Georgia.

Gilliland, M.G.F., A.V. Levin, R.W. Enzenauer, C. Smith, M.A. Parsons, L.B. Rorke-Adams, J.R. Lauridson, G.R. La Roche, L.M. Christmann, M. Mian, J. Jentzen, K.B. Simons, Y. Morad, R. Alexander, C. Jenny, and T. Wygnanski-Jaffe. 2007. Guidelines for Postmortem Protocol for Ocular Investigation of Sudden Unexplained Infant Death and Suspected Physical Child Abuse. *The American Journal of Forensic Medicine and Pathology.* 28(4):323–329.

Gordon, L.E., C. Thacher, and A. Kapatkin. 1993. High-rise syndrome in dogs: 81 cases (1985–1991). *Journal of American Veterinary Medical Association*, 202(1):118–122.

Kibayashi, K. 2011. Responses of Mast Cells in the Dura to Traumatic Brain Injury in an Animal Model. Presented at the 63rd Annual Scientific Meeting of the American Academy of Forensic Sciences, 21–26 February, Chicago, Illinois.

Kohlmeier, R.E., V.J.M. Di Maio, F. Sharkey, E.A. Rouse, and K.E. Reeves. 2008. The Timing of Histologic Changes in Liver Lacerations. *The American Journal of Forensic Medicine and Pathology.* 29(3):206–207.

Kolata, R.J. and D.E. Johnston. 1976. Motor Vehicle Accidents in Urban Dogs: A Study of 600 Cases. *Journal of American Veterinary Medical Association*, 167(10):938–41.

Kraje, B.J., A.C. Kraje, B.W. Rohrbach, K.A. Anderson, S.L. Marks, and D.K. Macintire. 2000. Intrathoracic and

Concurrent Orthopedic Injury Associated with Traumatic Rib Fracture in Cats: 75 cases (1980–1998). *Journal of American Veterinary Medicine Association.* 216(1):51–54.

LeCouteur, R.A. and G. Child. 1995. Diseases of the Spinal Cord. In: *Textbook of Veterinary Internal Medicine: Diseases of the Dog and Cat*, Vol. 1, Fourth edition, S.J. Ettinger, and E.C. Feldman, eds. pp. 629–696. Philadelphia: W.B. Saunders.

Link, M.S., P.J. Wang, N.G. Pandian, S. Bharati, J.E. Udelson, M.-Y. Lee, M.A. Vecchiotti, B.A. VanderBrink, G. Mirra, B.J. Maron, and N.A. Mark Estes. 1998. An Experimental Model of Sudden Death Due to Low-Energy Chest-Wall Impact (Commotio Cordis). *New England Journal of Medicine.* 338:1805–1811.

Lisciandro, G.R. 2011. Abdominal and thoracic focused assessment with sonography for trauma, triage, and monitoring in small animals. *Journal of Veterinary Emergency and Critical Care Society.* 21(2):104–122.

Maiorka, P., A. Maria, and A. Rego. 2011. Brazil Plenary and Poster Sessions. Presented at 4th Annual Veterinary Forensic Sciences Conference of the International Veterinary Forensic Sciences Association, 2–4 May, Orlando, Florida.

Mao, S., F. Fu, X. Dong, and Z. Wang. 2011. Supplementary Pathway for Vitality of Wounds and Wound Age Estimation in Bruises Using the Electric Impedance Spectroscopy Technique. *Journal of Forensic Sciences.* 56(4):925–929.

Marshall, D.T., J.D. Gilbert, and R.W. Byard. 2008. The Spectrum of Findings in Cases of Sudden Death Due to Blunt Cardiac Trauma—"Commotio Cordis." *The American Journal of Forensic Medicine and Pathology.* 29(1):1–4.

Muir, W. 2006. Trauma: physiology, Pathophysiology, and Clinical Implications. *Journal of Veterinary Emergency and Critical Care Society.* 16(4):253–263.

Munro, H.M.C. 1997. The Battered Pet Syndrome: Signs and Symptoms. In: *Recognizing and Reporting Animal Abuse: A Veterinarian's Guide*, pp. 76–81. Englewood: American Humane Association.

Munro, R. and H. Munro. 2008a. Non-Accidental Injury. In: *Animal Abuse and Unlawful Killing: Forensic Veterinary Pathology*, pp. 6–10. Edinburgh: Elsevier.

Munro, R. and H. Munro. 2008b. Wounds and Injuries. In: *Animal Abuse and Unlawful Killing: Forensic Veterinary Pathology*, pp. 30–47. Edinburgh: Elsevier.

Munro, R. and H. Munro. 2011. Forensic Veterinary Medicine: 2. *Postmortem Investigation. In Practice.* 33:262–270.

Nelson, S.J. 2008. Blunt Force Trauma. Presented at the *Veterinary Forensics Conference*, 9–11 April. Orlando, Florida.

Perper, J.A. 2006. Microscopic Forensic Pathology. In: *Medicolegal Investigation of Death*, Fourth edition, W.U. Spitz and D.J. Spitz, eds. pp. 1092–1134. Springfield: Charles C. Thomas Publisher.

Radasch, R.M. 1999. Biomechanics of Bones and Fractures, Fracture Management and Bone Healing. *The Veterinary Clinics of North America.* 29(5):1045–1082.

Ramsey, D.T. 2000. Exophthalmos. In: *Kirk's Current Veterinary Therapy XIII Small Animal Practice*, J.D. Bonagura, ed. pp. 1086–1089. Philadelphia: W.B. Saunders.

Sigrist, N.E., M.G. Doherr, and D.E. Spreng. 2004. Clinical Findings and Diagnostic Value of Posttraumatic Thoracic Radiographs in Dogs and Cats with Blunt Trauma. *Journal of Veterinary Emergency and Critical Care Society.* 14(4):259–268.

Sisson, D.D. and W.P. Thomas. 1995. Myocardial Diseases. In: *Textbook of Veterinary Internal Medicine: Diseases of the Dog and Cat*, Vol. 1, Fourth edition. S.J. Ettinger and E.C. Feldman, eds. pp. 995–1032. Philadelphia: W.B. Saunders.

Spackman, C.J., D.D. Caywood, D.A. Feeney, and G.R. Johnston. 1984. Thoracic Wall and Pulmonary Trauma in Dogs Sustaining Fractures as a Result of Motor Vehicle Accidents. *Journal of American Veterinary Medical Association*, 185(9):975–7.

Spitz, W.U. 2006. Blunt Force Injury. In: *Medicolegal Investigation of Death*, Fourth edition, W.U. Spitz and D.J. Spitz, eds, pp. 461–531. Springfield: Charles C. Thomas Publisher.

Taylor, S.M. 2003. Abnormalities of Mentation, Loss of Vision, and Pupillary Abnormalities. In: *Small Animal Internal Medicine*, R.W. Nelson and C.G. Couto, eds. pp. 983–990. St. Louis: Mosby.

Venker-van Haagen, A.J. 1995. Diseases of the Throat. In: *Textbook of Veterinary Internal Medicine Diseases of the Dog and Cat*, Vol. 1, Fourth edition, S.J. Ettinger and E.C. Feldman, eds. pp. 567–575. Philadelphia: W.B. Saunders.

Whiting, W. and R.F. Zernicke. 1998. *Biomechanics of Musculoskeletal Injury*, First edition. Champaign: Human Kinetics.

6

Sharp Force Injuries

Melinda D. Merck, Doris M. Miller, and Paulo C. Maiorka

There is nothing more deceptive than an obvious fact.

Sherlock Holmes

GENERAL CONSIDERATIONS

Sharp force injuries (SFI) are a result of penetration of the skin and underlying tissues by pointed objects or objects with sharp edges. They are characterized by a relatively well-defined traumatic separation of tissues. The subtypes of sharp force injuries include stab wounds, incisive (incised) wounds (cuts), and chop wounds. There are specific types of cruelty associated with SFI including predator attacks, mutilations, and ritualistic crimes.

By the very nature of sharp force injury cases, close contact is usually required between the perpetrator and the victim with the highly likely exchange of trace evidence and DNA. The body should be carefully inspected for trace evidence before it is disturbed at the scene and prior to examination. All potential weapons recovered from a crime scene should be tested for blood and tissue, both human and animal. Initially, the suspected weapon may not be found at the scene but discovered later in the investigation. It should be anticipated that a weapon and/or suspect will be found and DNA samples should be taken from the animal to use for comparison testing. Also, it should be noted that the assailant may slip and cut him- or herself during the assault, potentially leaving his or her blood on the animal's body or at the scene. All blood found on the animal and at the scene should be sampled separately and saved for testing.

In addition to the protocols for examining animal cruelty victims in Chapter 3, there are additional techniques and considerations for SFI victims. Shaving of the hair should be considered to detect hidden injures, especially partially penetrating wounds or important superficial cuts. The elasticity or laxity of the skin can change the wound appearance, either increasing or decreasing the size. The wound margins should be re-approximated to identify weapon characteristics and accurate measurements. Photographs should be taken before and after re-approximating the wounds using photo scales. This can be performed by holding the margins together, using clear tape over the wound, or using superglue to bind the subcutaneous tissues together. Radiographs should be taken of all areas of SFI to identify the presence of retained weapons or portions of weapons. A thorax view can be evaluated for the presence of air embolism. Advanced decomposition may result in skin defects that may be mistaken for stab wounds. Examination of the underlying tissues and bone can help distinguish true sharp force injuries from decomposition related events.

The location of each sharp force injury and pathway should be identified, documented, and described in the same manner as discussed for gunshot wounds in Chapter 8, including flap dissection for wound track identification. Probing is rarely necessary and can create false tracks. It is helpful to use a diagram to record the injuries (see Appendices 15–16). The overall wound length, width, depth, and directionality should be described, including the wound's margins and angles.

In some cases of multiple stab wounds, it may be appropriate to group the wounds in the Evidence of Injury section in the forensic report (Chapter 3). The directionality of the long axis of a sharp force wound can be described as

Veterinary Forensics: Animal Cruelty Investigations, Second Edition. Edited by Melinda D. Merck.
© 2013 John Wiley & Sons, Inc. Published 2013 by John Wiley & Sons, Inc.

vertical, horizontal, or angled, with a general or specific measurement of the angulation. This directionality refers to the orientation of the long axis and does not refer to the direction of the cutting. One method is to describe the directionality based on a clock-face configuration as used in gunshot wounds. The long axis is described as running between two clock positions, such as between the 1:00 and 7:00 positions. The pathway into or through the body should be described using reference planes (Chapter 8). A perforated wound goes completely through a specific body part and a penetrating wound only goes partly into a body part.

It is important to know if the investigation has determined the weapon used or if there is a suspected weapon. When evaluating SFI, the veterinarian must consider that the investigators will eventually have the weapon and properly collect and document evidence than can be used for weapon comparison and identification. In addition to the skin surface and soft tissue wound track, the bone or cartilage may contain tool-mark impressions which can be initially casted (Chapter 3) and then should be removed and preserved in formalin for analysis.

The amount of blood loss should be measured as discussed in Chapters 3 and 5. The blood loss due to SFI can affect where to search for evidence at a crime scene and bloodstain pattern analysis, and can help determine the sequence of injuries, especially with multiple sharp force injuries. A victim of SFI may be able to move for a substantial distance, depending on the injuries sustained. A blood trail may be found at the scene that leads to the site of the assault. If the animal suffers multiple assaults, the wounds may have progressively less associated soft tissue hemorrhage with significant blood loss. The last perimortem wound may appear bloodless, which can be impossible to differentiate from postmortem wounds.

With a deceased animal there may be minimum drainage of blood from the wounds depending on the nature of the injuries. When the body is moved blood may escape through the wounds, which can alter pre-existing bloodstains on the body or wash away surface evidence. Consideration should be given to preventing this by wrapping wounds with clean towels, sheets, or a separate plastic bag. There may be substantial internal blood found if a large vessel located in the dependent part of the body was severed, allowing drainage from other vessels postmortem (Di Maio and Di Maio 2001). If the body has been immersed in water for a prolonged period of time, the blood from the wounds can be leached out by the water. This can give the wound the appearance that it was postmortem vs. antemortem.

Therapeutic or diagnostic wounds can be misinterpreted as SFI. It is important to obtain the medical history information including procedures that were performed and any resuscitative measures. The original wounds may have been obscured or obliterated by surgical procedures, they may have been used for chest tubes, or resuscitation may have caused additional injuries or hemorrhage. All tubes, intravenous lines, and drains should be left in place upon death of the animal until a necropsy is performed. Healing wounds and scars may dehisce during the bloating phase of decomposition and mimic stab, incised, or gunshot wounds (Chapter 14).

STAB WOUNDS

Stab wounds are characterized by the depth of the wound exceeding the length of the wound. They may be caused by a variety of sharp or pointed objects, including knives, scissors, screwdrivers, pens, forks, broken glass, and ice picks. The most common weapon used is a knife, primarily a single-edged blade, which also can produce incisive wounds. The use of more than one weapon should be considered in cases of multiple stab wounds.

The force needed to cause the entrance wound depends on the sharpness of the instrument and the thickness of the skin. Some knives, including single-edged knives, have a sharp edge on both sides of the point, making entrance into the skin easier. Once the tip of the knife penetrates the skin, the amount of force needed to penetrate or perforate underlying structures is greatly reduced. Depending on the weapon characteristics and length, the depth of the stab wound can indicate the level of force used (see below).

Interpretation of stab wound appearances
Knife wounds

The appearance of the stab wound depends on the skin properties, nature of the blade and knife, movement of the victim, and movement of the blade in the wound. With sharp knives, the wound is sharp and regular. If the weapon or part of the weapon is blunt or dull, the wound appears abraded and contused or jagged and contused. If the knife blade enters at an oblique angle, the wound can have a beveled margin on one side with tissue undermining on the opposite margin, indicating the direction the knife entered the body. Superficial stab wounds have a shallow wound track that runs parallel to the body surface. The wound cavity profile may reflect the weapon profile (Ohshima 2005).

To understand knife wound appearances it is important to know the different parts of the knife. First there is the handle, which is comprised of the grip, followed by a guard end and is squared-off or rounded at the other end from the back of the blade (Figure 6.1). This end also may look forked because of tears by the back of the blade. If the ricasso penetrates the wound, then both ends may be squared off and may or may not have tears resembling a forked area (Figure 6.2). These tears can be differentiated from the cutting edge because they are not as clean and sharp and usually are only found in the superficial skin layers (Di Maio and Di Maio 2001).

With a double-edged knife, there are points at both ends of the stab wound. The use of these knives is more rare. It is possible for a single-edged blade to have points at both ends. This can occur after the knife point penetrates the skin and the knife is pulled in such a manner that keeps the squared-off back of the knife from contacting the skin. It also may occur if the point has a cutting edge on the back and the knife is pulled down even slightly, in which case the back of the blade will not contact the skin. The ricasso can cause both ends of the wound to be square because of the blunt edges (Di Maio and Di Maio 2001).

The characteristics of the blade edge, smooth or serrated, may be determined from marks or imprints on the wound margins, within the stab canal, or on the skin surface. Superficial cuts or shallow wounds with these characteristics may be made if the assailant was repetitively attempting to stab the animal and was unable to initially fully penetrate with the knife or was unable to control the animal. A serrated blade is characterized by wavy patterns or striations. These striations are best preserved by staining with 5% neutral red followed by fixation in formaldehyde. Casting, such as with vinyl polysiloxane dental impression material, can be useful for photo documentation (Pounder et al. 2011). Striations may be produced in the wound track on the soft tissues of internal organs. These may vary in consistency and quality and are most easily seen in the liver, heart, and aorta (Pounder and Cormack 2011). Because there are knives with partially serrated blades it is best to describe the stab wound as "impact with a serrated portion of the blade."

The shape of the wound is also affected by the properties of the skin. If the skin is stretched when the stab wound is made, it may appear broader and shorter when the skin relaxes. The Langer's lines also have an effect on the appearance of stab wounds. These are skin tension lines that have different orientations depending on the region of the body. If a stab wound is made perpendicular to the Langer's lines, it will tend to pull apart the edges of the wound. If it is made parallel to these lines, it will create narrow and more slit-like wounds. If a stab wound is made oblique to the Langer's lines it will appear asymmetrical or semicircular (Di Maio and Di Maio 2001).

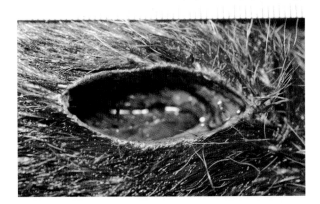

Figure 6.1 Stab wound from a single-edged blade knife.

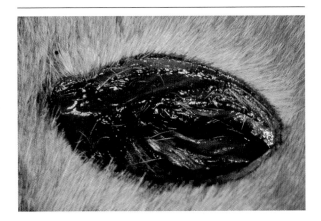

Figure 6.2 Stab wound with squared ends.

or cross guard. The guard is to protect the person's hand from slipping onto the blade and cutting him- or herself. The bottom portion of the blade is called the ricasso and is blunt on both sides. On a single-edged blade the sharp side is called the edge and the opposite blunt side is called the back of the blade. Where the sharp edge ends along the length of the blade is called the spine. The end of the knife blade is called the point; there may be a sharp edge on both sides of the point (Di Maio and Di Maio 2001).

The appearance of a stab wound depends on what part of the knife penetrates or contacts the skin and how deeply it is thrust into the body. It is not always possible to determine if the weapon was single- or double-edged from examination of a single wound. There is more likelihood of making that determination with multiple stab wounds. With a single-edged knife, a stab wound has a point at one

The edges of gaping wounds should be re-approximated as discussed above. When the knife is withdrawn from the body, it may be twisted by the perpetrator or the victim may move, creating a secondary exit path. This can create a Y- or L-shaped wound if there is substantial movement. If there is only slight movement it can create a V-shaped notch or "fork" at the cutting end of the wound instead of a point (Di Maio and Di Maio 2001). The restoration or reconstruction of oddly shaped wounds, often due to simultaneous cutting and twisting forces caused by the assailant or movement of the victim, is important to properly interpret the pattern. Pliability of dried wounds can be restored by placing a wet paper towel on the wound for twenty to thirty minutes or longer and then working a moisturizing cream into the wound edges (Spitz 2006).

The force needed to cause the entrance wound depends on the sharpness of the instrument and the thickness of the skin. Some knives have a sharp edge on both sides of the point, making entrance into the skin easier. Once the tip of the knife penetrates the skin, the rest of the blade penetrates more easily into the body. The depth of the wound depends on the force applied, level of penetration, and whether the blade met increased tissue resistance such as contact with bone. The depth may be equal, less, or greater than the length of the knife. If the knife is plunged into the body with great force, it may penetrate deeper than the length of the blade, creating associated surface evidence from the knife guard. If the knife is plunged straight and perpendicular to the skin, the mark from the guard is symmetrical. If the knife enters at an angle from the right, the mark is to the right of the wound. If the knife enters at a downward angle, the mark is above the stab wound. If the knife enters at an upward angle, the mark is below the wound (Di Maio and Di Maio 2001). The guard pattern imprinted on the skin may be matched to a particular type of knife.

The surface length of a knife stab wound does not necessarily correlate with the width of the knife. It can be greater than the blade width if the blade is drawn against the skin as it penetrates the skin or as it is withdrawn, creating a larger wound. This often occurs due to the movement between the assailant and the victim. The blade may be larger than the wound length if there was not full penetration of the knife. The width of the stab wound and characteristics at the wound margins and within the deeper wounds can provide information about the thickness of the blade. The width of the back or spine of the blade is retained within the wound and the stab canal as a squared off end that is more visible in dry wounds than wet. This weapon pattern may be less apparent for very thin blades and require magnification.

Making a determination of the type of weapon used in stabbings should be done with extreme caution. The most information that can be given is usually an approximation of the blade width and length and whether it was a single- or double-edged blade. A weapon only can be matched to the wounds if a piece of the blade or weapon broke off in the body. This may be the tip of the knife when it penetrates bone. The recovered tip may be matched conclusively to a weapon by a forensic tool examiner.

Stab wounds from other weapons

The overall shape of a stab wound tends to mimic the object that caused the wound. Stab wounds made with weapons other than knives usually contain unique characteristics and configuration of the weapon. Identification requires careful examination of the penetrating wound margins, track, and pattern along with any superficial or deep tissue wound patterns. Consideration of the possible types of weapons used may be based on information from the investigation and crime scene findings, such as weapons of opportunity.

The size and shape of the wound and associated injuries are affected by a number of factors including the shape and the blunt/sharp edges of the weapon, location on the body (skin tension, thickness, bony protuberances), age and neuter status of the animal (skin fragility, increased skin thickness in some areas), dynamic movement during the stabbing by the victim and/or assailant, and the amount of force applied by the assailant. Some attempted stabbing may not penetrate the skin or only partially penetrate, creating more blunt force type injuries to the underlying tissues which may retain weapon characteristics. The edges and/or terminal end of the wound track may display the weapon features. Penetration of the weapon may extend through the body, creating a perforating wound with weapon characteristics observed at the entrance and exit wounds. Experiments with the alleged weapon on comparable tissue or surfaces may be needed, taking into consideration the above factors to determine if the injuries are consistent.

There are obviously a variety of weapons that may be used in animal cruelty cases and are usually based on the ease of access, such as household items or tools. Wounds made with ice picks are less common because they are no longer commonly used in households. Ice pick wounds or similar weapon wounds can be easily missed and are sometimes mistaken for gunshot wounds caused by shotgun pellets or .22 caliber bullets. A fork may be used for stabbing, although it is very hard for the prongs of a kitchen fork to penetrate the skin. The perforations seen with fork stabbings correspond to the number of tines or prongs on the weapon and are evenly spaced. The wounds made by scissors depend on if the blades are open or closed with consideration that the scissors may have been open to varying degrees during the stabbing. If the scissor blades are open, then two stab wounds may be produced. If the blades are closed, the wound produced is caused by splitting the skin versus cutting. The stab wound created is linear and has abraded edges. The screwlock connecting the scissor blades protrudes out and may create an angular laceration or abraded margins along one edge of the wound. Broken bottles may be used as weapons and tend to create sharp and ragged wounds. They tend to be in clusters with a variety sizes, shapes, and depths (Di Maio and Di Maio 2001).

When screwdrivers are used in stabbing, the wound can show the characteristics of the type of screwdriver. A Phillips®, or cross-tipped, screwdriver produces a circular wound with abraded margins and four equally spaced cuts. A slit-like wound is produced by a flat-blade screwdriver with angular or squared ends, sometimes rounded, and often with abraded margins. This wound can be difficult to differentiate from one caused by a dull knife blade that is plunged up to the guard. There may be non-penetrating lesions from screwdriver stabbing, causing intra- or subcutaneous hemorrhages.

Injuries to the underlying or adjacent bones may be seen with screwdriver penetrating wounds, which can help identify the type of screwdriver used, especially in bodies with advanced decomposition. A study was conducted on the thorax of pig cadavers creating stab wounds at different angles using flat-tipped and Phillips® screwdrivers. The underlying fat layer was partially removed to create a uniform depth of 15 mm to simulate human fat layers, which may correlate to other species of animals. Fabric covering of cotton and denim were added to some of the samples. The skin of pigs has similar properties to that of humans, while other species of animals have tougher skin, which can simulate certain types of clothing in humans.

The main categories of trauma to the skeletal material were punctures wounds and fractures. Grazing or minor surface splintering was also seen in adjacent bones when stabbing was at an angle. Embedding of electroplating from the screwdriver surface may be seen without associated trauma. The study found the primary characteristic of screwdriver trauma was fractures. The primary fractures of the flat-tipped screwdriver were transverse, complete or incomplete, and direct and indirect, with 69% being direct. The cross-tipped screwdriver more consistently caused trauma than the flat-tipped. The most frequent fracture type

for both was transverse, concluding it is a characteristic of screwdriver trauma. Longitudinal fractures were attributed almost exclusively to cross-tipped screwdrivers. Indirect fractures were seen with flat-tipped screwdrivers and are suggestive of a higher level of force used. As the fabric thickness increased, the number of fractures declined using the flat-tipped screwdriver and increased for the cross-tipped (Croft and Ferllini 2007). This may simulate expected findings in animals with thicker skin than pigs and humans.

The cross-tipped screwdriver tended to inflict more puncture wounds than the flat-tipped one except when greater force was applied in the study. The punctures exhibited cruciform impressions visible macroscopically and many had further associated trauma. The cruciform impression could be seen on both external and internal bone surfaces, though if the shaft passed into the bone the impression was still visible on the internal rib surface and within the wound structure.

Puncture wounds from flat-tipped screwdrivers were typically rectangular in shape and visible on both internal and external rib surfaces. Both wastage (fragments of bones detached from the body of the bone) and protrusions (bone fragments that maintain their attachment with the bone) were primarily seen with puncture wounds on the edge of the rib. Protrusions indicate that the periosteum and other soft tissue were present at the time of injury. Wastage was more associated with oblique angle penetrations (Croft and Ferllinni 2007).

In some animal cruelty cases, multiple types of weapons may be used on the animal, including power tools. The injuries seen may be due to a combination of assaults such as stabbing, shooting, strangulation, or blunt force. In addition, these actions may have taken place over a period of time. Injuries from different mechanisms may appear similar and be difficult to differentiate, requiring careful examination. Power tools can create injuries with characteristics of the cutting or penetrating blade. The animal's fur can provide important clues to the type of weapon used. For power drills, the fur can get caught in the drill bit and be found as detached circular swirls that are embedded at the wound margins or subcutaneous tissue and possibly deeper in the wound track (Figure 6.3). This differs from gunshot wounds, where the fur is usually attached to the skin and spirals into the wound track. Some gunshot projectiles may cause the fur to detach and have a swirl pattern but this is usually a small amount of fur compared to the larger amount typically caught in the drill bit.

Arrows or crossbow bolts often cause severe internal injuries and bone fractures. The arrowhead configuration

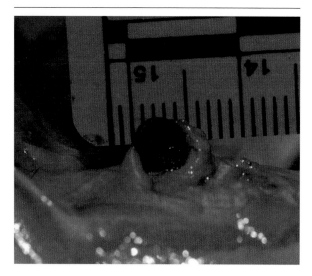

Figure 6.3 Coiled hair embedded in tissue from use of a drill weapon.

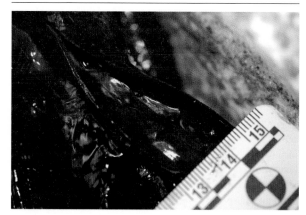

Figure 6.4 Chest stab wound that penetrated the aorta.

determines the appearance of the wounds. In target arrows, the end is pointed and conical. These produce circular entrance wounds similar to gunshot wounds. In hunting arrows, the ends have two to five knife-like edges. In four-edged arrows, the wounds are X-shaped or cross-like and the edges appear incised without evidence of abrasions (Di Maio and Di Maio 2001). Impaling injuries may be purposefully inflicted or due to accidental or non-accidental falls. A determination should be made if the injuries are perimortem or postmortem. It is important to have all the case information to interpret the findings, including when the animal was last seen alive.

Considerations in removal of the object

As with all penetrating injuries, care should be taken not to remove the foreign object in a live animal without proper preparation for treatment. The object often causes compression and prevents hemorrhage. Withdrawal of the object may not only allow life-threatening hemorrhage, it may also cause more tissue damage. The object should be removed carefully, protecting the integrity of potential associated evidence including fingerprints, biological fluids, and trace. The item should be held in areas where it was least likely to be handled by the suspect.

Evaluation of injuries

Stab wounds may inflict severe damage to the internal structures of the body. The cause of death depends on the injuries but often results from exsanguination. In the chest, there may be lacerations of the major blood vessels, lungs,

heart, diaphragm, trachea, or esophagus (Figure 6.4). Rib fractures, hemothorax, and pneumothorax may be found. In the heart, the ventricular muscle can contract, slowing or terminating bleeding (Di Maio and Di Maio 2001). Stab wounds to the abdomen can cause lacerations of the organs or major blood vessels. If the intestinal tract is lacerated, death may be secondary to peritonitis.

Stab wounds to the neck can produce exsanguination, air embolism, trachea laceration, or asphyxia caused by soft tissue hemorrhage compressing the trachea and vessels of the neck. Arterial thrombosis is possible. Stab wounds to the head penetrating to the brain are uncommon and usually are through the eye or temporal region in humans (Di Maio and Di Maio 2001). These stab wounds can produce intracerebral, subarachnoid, and/or subdural hemorrhage. Stab wounds to the spine may occur and either cause fractures or spinal cord injury. The extremities may be stabbed, causing muscle, ligament, joint, or major vessel damage. Fractures are possible in the extremities, especially with arrows.

INCISED-STAB WOUNDS

An incised-stab wound is found when a stab wound changes to an incised wound. The stab is made first, but instead of withdrawing the blade, it is pulled along the body, cutting through tissue and creating a wound that is longer than it is deep. The only way to determine the direction is if there are markings at one end indicating where the blade was withdrawn (Di Maio and Di Maio 2001).

INCISED WOUNDS

Incised wounds, also called cuts, are created by sharp-edged instruments or weapons, including knives, glass, or metal implements. The wound produced has a length greater than

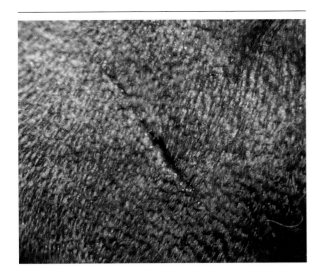

Figure 6.5 Superficial incisive wound created by a serrated blade. Note the wavy pattern on left lower side.

its depth. In contrast to stabbings, the length and depth of the wound do not correlate to the type of weapon used. Incised wounds should not be confused with lacerations. In contrast to lacerations, the edges are typically sharp and clean with no abrasions, contusions, or tissue bridging in the base of the wound. Instruments that have dull, irregular, or nicked cutting edge can produce incisive wounds that are abraded, irregular, or contused because of the pressure required to cut with that particular weapon. However, no tissue bridging is found in the depth of the wound.

Incised wounds typically are superficial at the beginning, become deeper and then ending superficially. When a blade is held at an oblique angle, the wound has a beveled or undermined edge. When the blade is held at an extreme angle a skin flap is created. If the blade cuts along wrinkles of skin instead of a flat area, a straight line of interrupted cuts is seen when the skin is flattened due to the blade cutting just the tops of the wrinkle folds. If the blade draws the skin up into irregular folds as it cuts, the wounds may appear irregular or zigzag when the skin is flattened (Di Maio and Di Maio 2001). Edges of incised wounds tend to gap open and should be re-approximated as discussed above. The amount of the gap is determined on the orientation of the wound to the Langer's lines (see Stab Wounds). The knife characteristics (serration) may be seen along the wound margins and are more visible when the edges are re-approximated. These may be seen especially if the serrated edge is dragged along the skin surface or with multiple, small, superficial, or parallel incised wounds

(Figure 6.5). Serrations also may be detected on underlying bony structures.

Superficial incisive wounds may be found adjacent to deeper incisive wounds. In the past, classification of these incised marks in human cases has been termed hesitation marks. These marks do not necessarily denote a hesitation or lack of intent by the perpetrator, but may instead show a repetitive attempt to perform the cutting. Assigning the term of hesitation gives a misleading description of the events that took place (Symes et al. 2002). In torture cases, the marks may be called "tease marks." These superficial marks also could be caused by the victim struggling during the attack.

Incised wounds of the neck may be produced from behind or in front of the body. Based on the position of the attacker and the victim, wound characteristics may indicate if the individual was right- or left-handed. However, for any scenario offered as an explanation for a particular wound pattern, there are typically several other scenarios that are equally possible.

In human homicides, the wound starts shallow and higher on the left side of the victim, extends deeper, then shallow again, terminating lower on the right side for a right-handed perpetrator. It is equally possible that the attacker was facing the victim, holding the knife in the left hand, and slashing the victim with a backhand motion, from the victim's left to right. If done from the front, a right-handed assailant creates incisive marks on the left side of the victim's neck, and the opposite for a left-handed assailant. Horizontal incisive wounds to the neck may be made from the front if the assailant makes swipes or slashes to the neck. Deep incisive wounds penetrating to the vertebral column are possible and are inflicted from behind the victim (Di Maio and Di Maio 2001). Case and crime scene information is required to more conclusively interpret the wounds and make these determinations. Death from incisive wounds often results from exsanguination. Death from neck incisive wounds may result from exsanguination or massive air embolus (Di Maio and Di Maio 2001).

CHOP WOUNDS

Chop wounds are caused by heavy objects with a cutting edge, such as machetes, axes, and meat cleavers, or by a sharp object wielded with a tremendous amount of force. A chop wound represents a combination of sharp and blunt force injuries. The edge of the object creates a sharp force injury, characterized by cutting of the skin and underlying tissues, whereas the intensity of the force, or the relative bluntness of the object, produces associated abrasions, lacerations, and/or contusions (Figure 6.6). These wounds appear incisive and often have underlying damage to the bone, either fractures or

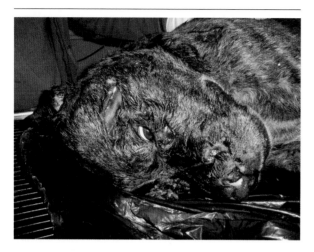

Figure 6.6 Chop wounds from a meat cleaver.

a deep groove from the cutting edge. When the weapon is pulled out of the bone, it may be necessary to give it a sharp twist, which breaks off the adjacent bone or creates fractures. If the instrument strikes at an angle it may chop off disks of bone. Flaking or chattering on the bone can indicate direction of impact. Fractures in long, larger bones may be spiral or curved transverse and with smaller bones fractures may be longitudinal (Lynn and Fairgrieve 2009).

A chop wound's appearance also may aid in determining the type of weapon used. The weapon can leave unique tool mark striations on the bone. Evaluations of the hacking trauma caused by machetes, axes, and meat cleavers have been conducted. Hacking blows to bone have at least one smooth, flat side. If the blow was directed at an angle, there is fracturing of the opposite side. Meat cleavers create clean, narrow wounds without fractures. Microscopically they create sharp, distinct, fine striations in the bone. Machetes produce wider, less-clean wounds with fractures in the bed of the cut and small fragmented bone at the entrance site. Microscopically they produce more pronounced striations than cleavers but they are coarse and less distinct. Axes produce crushing, fragmented wounds with fractures. Microscopically, they create no striations in the wounds of bone (Di Maio and Di Maio 2001).

MUTILATIONS, PREDATOR ATTACKS, AND DOG ATTACKS

Community considerations

Mutilation of a live or deceased animal may be seen. These cases are often caused by predators, such as foxes and coyotes, which prey on pets that are allowed outside. They

also may be pranks using already deceased animals or the result of animal cruelty. DNA testing in predator or dog attacks is important to identify species and the specific individual animals involved (Chapter 4). Analysis of foreign hair/fur found on the victim or scene from the attacking animal may identify the species, providing the community with the information needed to determine if wildlife authorities or animal control may assist with the removal of the predator.

Veterinarians and forensic odontologists are often called to assist with the investigation of dog and predator attacks on humans. These cases require a thorough investigation by the investigating officers which can benefit from the assistance of dog bite and aggression experts or animal behaviorists (Appendix 28). The assessment and examination of a suspected dog involved in a fatal dog attack should include information about the circumstances, the scene, and a complete internal and external exam (Table 6.1). Underlying factors or disease that may have precipitated the attack should be noted such as recent pregnancy, blindness, or central nervous system (CNS) disorders. Necropsy examination of the suspected attacking animal may reveal human biological evidence or non-biological evidence ingested by the animal. The gastric contents also may provide clues to whether the dog is a pet, stray, or feral animal (Tsokos, Byard, and Püschel 2007). Bite mark analysis has been shown to be useful in distinguishing between wolf, dog, and large cat attacks (Pomara et al. 2011). It is important to conduct a forensic odontological exam to include, identify, or exclude certain dogs accused of the crime, especially when multiple dogs are implicated. This analysis should be conducted for both witnessed and unwitnessed attacks.

The injuries found on humans from fatal dog attacks often include multiple blunt and sharp force injuries to various body locations with extensive craniofacial trauma (Tsokos, Byard, and Püschel 2007). The distinctive feature of cutaneous dog bites is a puncture and a tear. The hole is from the canine teeth that allows for anchorage as the other teeth produce a tear while biting, shaking, or pulling. These are often associated with superficial, parallel, and linear abrasions. The injuries include lacerations, crushing injuries, and avulsions of skin and soft tissue (Shields et al. 2009). The analysis of bite mark patterns should be interpreted in the context of the animal behavior.

An average of nineteen fatal dog attacks per year were reported from 1979–2005 in the U.S. and that number appears to be increasing (Pomara et al. 2011). The victims were predominantly children less than twelve years old and elderly more than seventy years old, with the elder majority

Table 6.1 Steps in the necropsy evaluation of a fatal dog attack.

Circumstances

Description of the events leading up to the attack
Description of the attack
Dog characteristics: age, sex, neutered or not, breed, tethered, free ranging
History of the dog's behavior, previous aggressive actions
History of the dog and victim's interaction

The scene

Evaluation/examination of the scene, with photographic documentation of the position of the victim and likely site of the attack

Exam of the dog

External exam for identifying features: collar, tag, tattoos, microchip
External exam for evidence of maltreatment
Weight
Collection of external trace evidence (on body, feet, teeth): victim's blood, clothing, fibers
Exam of oral cavity: dental impressions
Collection of fur reference samples
Collection of DNA reference sample
Radiographs: detection of human biological and non-biological material
Internal exam: stomach/intestinal contents, underlying diseases/conditions, brain histopathology
Samples for toxicology

Source: Tsokos, M., R.W. Byard, and K.Püschel. 2007. Extensive and Mutilating Craniofacial Trauma Involving Defleshing and Decapitation: Unusual Features of Fatal Dog Attacks in the Young. *The American Journal of Forensic Medicine and Pathology.* 28(2):131–136.

being females. In a Kentucky study, the majority of fatal dog attacks involved unleashed dogs on their owner's property and dogs who killed their owner (Shields et al. 2009). Victim behavior can precipitate dog attacks. Running away, kicking, and screaming may provoke dog attacks, especially pack attacks (Tsokos, Byard, and Püschel 2007). The dog breeds implicated in dog bite-related fatalities in the U.S. have been reported as pit bull 21%–28%, mixed breed 13%, Rottweiler 13%–16%, German shepherd 9%, wolf hybrid 6%, great Dane 3%, Rottweiler/chow 3%, and Akita 2% (Shields et al. 2009).

The fatal attack is characterized by repetitive, uninhibited biting with the dog being relatively unresponsive to efforts to terminate the attack. Fatal attacks most often occur when only the victim is present (Pomara et al. 2011). Several factors may interplay in dog bite instigation: defense of territory, heredity, maltreatment, physical health, socialization, and training (Shields et al. 2009). Other factors may include predatory experience; pack-dog experience; assertion of social dominance; and the age, size, and behavior of victims (Pomara et al. 2011).

Canine aggression has been grouped into seven categories: territorial guarding of house and yard, possessive (guarding of toys, bones and food), fearful (overreaction to a fearful circumstance), predatory (enjoyment of chasing moving objects), intrasexual (male to male and female to female), parental (protecting the young), and dominance (attempt to impose one's will on another or resistance to dominance imposed by others) (Shield et al. 2009). Male dogs are 6.2 times more likely to bite than female dogs, sexually intact dogs 2.6 times more than neutered, and chained dogs 2.8 times more than unchained (Tsokos, Byard, and Püschel 2007).

Pack attacks are more likely to result in severe injury than a single-dog attack due to the greater number of wounds inflicted and the role of social interaction between the dogs that may escalate the attack (Shields et al. 2009). Dog pack attacks are rare, accounting for 6.9% of all fatal attacks (Pomara et al. 2011). There are several reported causes of dog attacks: the dog senses its position in the family is threatened, usually with children or new babies, making them more susceptible to attack, the dog is fearful, with warning growls or postures often unrecognized by children, the dog senses that its territory of food is being threatened, making unaware children more susceptible, vocalization or physical activity may stimulate aggressiveness, especially in packs, and medical illness may cause aggressive behavior such as CNS or metabolic disorders (Pomara et al. 2011).

A study was conducted on college students regarding the antisocial behaviors and psychological characteristics of vicious dog owners. The sample study was divided into four groups: vicious dog owners, large dog owners, small dog owners, and controls. Owners of vicious dogs differ from the other groups in terms of antisocial behaviors and psychopathic traits. The study revealed that vicious dog owners reported significantly higher criminal behavior, especially violent criminal behavior. They were higher in sensation seeking and primary psychopathic traits such as carelessness, selfishness, and manipulative tendencies. No differences were found between the groups regarding attitudes toward animal maltreatment or secondary psychopathy such as impulsiveness or self-defeating behaviors. The study concluded that these findings suggest that vicious dog ownership may be a simple marker of broader social deviance (Ragatz et al. 2009).

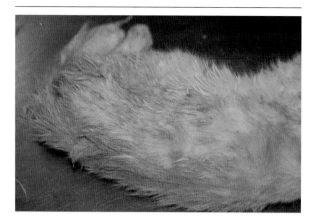

Figure 6.7 Clumping of fur as a result of predator saliva deposited during the attack.

Examination of the Animal Victim

Cases involving animal mutilation, predator, or dog attacks may be criminal investigations or potentially involve eventual civil litigation. The exam of the victim should begin with consideration of DNA collection, animal predator or human, and predator species identification. The external body should be examined for foreign hair/fur and evidence of saliva, where the use of UV light or alternate light source (ALS) may be of value (Chapter 3). In predator attacks, it is common to find wet or dry clumping of the body fur on the victim, which is from the predator's saliva (Figure 6.7). This important finding, which provides valuable DNA evidence, may be overlooked or misinterpreted as evidence the body was "washed" by a suspected human perpetrator. The teeth and any wounds or indentations from non-penetrating teeth due to grab holds should be swabbed for DNA. The nails should be inspected for evidence of fur and the entire nail may be removed for DNA testing (Figure 6.8).

It is important to determine and document antemortem, perimortem, and postmortem injuries. The types of injuries and evidence associated with predator attacks depend on the species and/or breed of predator, whether claws and/or teeth were used, the dentition of the predator, the victim's skin, and the struggle or action between the attacking animal and victim. Typical findings include abrasions on the head or muzzle from dragging and impact injuries, dirt or debris in the mouth, and other findings typical of head trauma such as fractured teeth and ocular injuries (Chapter 5) (Figure 6.9).

Bite marks may be found on the skin surface. The bite mark may be used for comparison with the suspected attacking animal. Photographs of any bite marks should be

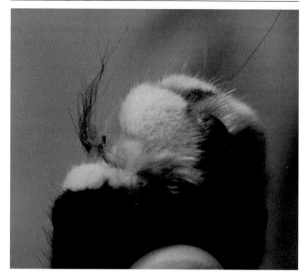

Figure 6.8 Hair caught in a frayed cat nail from a predator attack.

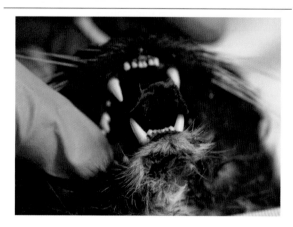

Figure 6.9 Chin abrasions sustained from dragging during a predator attack.

carefully taken at 90° angles with and without the ABFO (American Board of Forensic Odontology) no. 2 photo scale (Chapter 2). The use of UV/IR (infrared) photography may be considered to enhance any impression information. Skin penetration by the canine teeth typically is characterized by elliptical puncture wounds. The skin should be reflected to identify underlying injuries such as punctures, evidence of hemorrhage, or contusions. Depending on the incisive properties of the teeth, the canines may not penetrate the skin but through compressive force still create elliptical wounds in the underlying tissue (Figure 6.10).

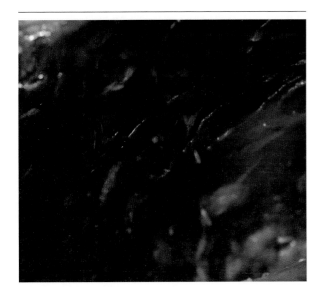

Figure 6.10 Elliptical punctures in the deeper tissue from predator attack.

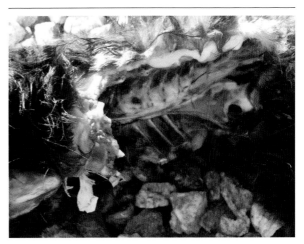

Figure 6.11 Predator attack with characteristic triangular-type defects along tissue margins.

There may be deep punctures or tears in the muscle and/or internal organs due to the struggle during the attack and/or shaking of the victim by the predator. Skin reflection must be performed to reveal these characteristic injuries. Bone fractures or punctures, often characterized by crushing and splintering, may be seen due to a direct bite force. Distant fractures may be present, such as rib neck fractures, due to compression. Frayed or avulsed nails are a distinct characteristic associated with rapid leg movement or as resistance to slow down forceful body movement; this is most commonly seen in cats (Chapter 5). In predator attacks, the finding of frayed nails may be due to several reasons including an attempt by the victim of a violent struggle to escape and defend itself or the tossing or dragging of the victim, or the victim's rapid, frantic foot movements during any preceding chase in which the nails are splintered.

The discovery of partial animal body remains may be a result of predator or human mutilation. The finding of a decapitated body, with the head missing, may be evidence of a ritualistic crime (see below), animal cruelty, predator, or human opportunistic action for a trophy. Some species of predators, such as foxes, may decapitate the victim and carry the head away. There may be significant tearing of the skin and small to large sections removed along with organs damaged, pulled out, or missing. Some predators are capable of biting the body of an animal in half, leaving behind one-half of the body and carrying off the other. These cases are usually first believed to be mutilations caused by a human

perpetrator. This type of predator attack typically produces very little blood at the scene, which is thought to be due to a combination of factors which include compression of the bite, the tearing and retraction of blood vessels, reduced skin blood supply of animals, the physiological stress response of vasoconstriction during the chase and/or attack, and the rapid or instant cardiac arrest which ceases active hemorrhage.

Predation as the cause of death is usually easily determined by close examination of the body. In addition to the findings already discussed in predation injuries, the primary evidence of predator causation is found along the wound margins. The edges may initially appear linear without defect, often mistakenly described as appearing to be cut with a sharp knife or scalpel. Careful inspection of every margin reveals one or more areas of irregularity, typically with triangular or V-shaped defects created by the teeth (Figure 6.11). There may be evidence of blunt-triangular defects where the skin was gathered or bunched-up at the site of the bite or due to molar teeth action. These patterns may be seen along the skin or deeper tissues. There may be separate injuries that appear incisive but closer inspection of the wound track often reveals a puncture at the terminal end. There may also be evidence of crushing bone injuries.

Mutilation injuries caused by humans have the same characteristics as discussed in stab, incisive, and chop wounds without predation injuries. They may involve severe injuries to the body or specific areas, or complete or partial dismemberment. The wound characteristics can help identify the instrument used. The presence of hemorrhage or microscopic examination of the tissue can help differentiate antemortem, perimortem, and postmortem injuries. The portion of the body still connected to the torso is needed to determine vital tissue reaction at the time of dismemberment. This is very important to remember in the investigation of ritualistic crimes (see below).

Skinning may be part of the mutilation. The skinning or mutilation may preclude species or breed determination of the victim by gross exam. The skull may be analyzed by a veterinary anatomist or mammologist to determine species and possibly breed. The paw prints may be evaluated to determine species (Chapter 4). Hair or tissue may be analyzed for species identification through microscopy (fur) or DNA analysis. It is important to consider whether the animal was alive for any part of the injuries and what type of restraint, physical or chemical, could have been used. It may be possible the animal was unconscious due to inflicted head injuries (Chapter 5). The skin reflection exam may include searching for injection sites and ligature marks (Chapter 9). Appropriate blood or tissue toxicological analysis may be performed.

Examination of the animal perpetrator

The examination of the suspected animal perpetrator should include collection of DNA and fur. In addition, teeth swabs should be collected for potential bacteria DNA sequence testing for comparison of victim bite wound infections (Kennedy 2012). If there was feeding on the victim, there may be evidence of bone material on radiographs. There may be bone and fur/hair evidence in the feces or found on postmortem examination in the gastrointestinal tract. Depending on the facts of the case, paw print and dental impressions should be taken and consideration given to behavior evaluation by the appropriate expert.

RITUALISTIC CRIMES

Ritualistic crimes involve ceremonial acts that are often related to behavior patterns based on a belief in some occult ideology. These crimes can be not only disturbing, but also frustrating because of the general unfamiliarity with these practices. Several groups perform rituals that involve animal sacrifice and sometimes mutilation that may present issues of animal cruelty. These include Satanism, Vampirism, Voodoo, Santeria, Brujeria, and Palo Mayombe. The common factor of all these groups is the use of blood in their rituals, which they believe contains the life force energy and power. The animals chosen for sacrifice may be based on species and/or coloring. Black or white coloring are commonly preferred and the animals associated with each group discussed below are not limited to those species. The use of domestic animals, such as cats

or dogs, is typically associated with the malevolent side of any group. The determination of animal cruelty charges is usually based on the species killed and the method of killing under the applicable laws.

The evidence found at the crime scene is the key to determining what group is involved. There are several textbooks about the investigation of ritualistic abuse that cover in detail the different paraphernalia and symbols used in ceremonies by the different groups. The scene should be evaluated for symbols, symbolic objects, candles, calendars, the type of animal mutilation, and the species of animal used, which can determine the belief system.

Satanism

Several Satanism categories are linked with animal crimes and additional criminal activity. The traditional/intergenerational Satanist engages in blood rituals, animal and human sacrifice, sexual abuse, kidnapping, child pornography, arson, and ritual murder involving mutilation and cannibalism. The self-styled Satanist is linked with child molestation, animal mutilation, and homicide. The youth subculture Satanists engage in animal mutilation, vandalism, arson, school violence, grave desecration, and sometimes homicide. Their crimes tend to escalate over time. The modern Satanists believe that violence is part of human nature and that ritualistic sacrifice is necessary to defer violence. They perform animal sacrifice and have been linked to human sacrifice (Perlmutter 2004).

Vampirism

The vampirism culture engages in blood rituals, role-playing games, and sadomasochism that can escalate to murder. The purpose of their ritual of bloodletting and drinking is to acquire energy from the blood source. Some use animal blood if it is fresh. They also attribute magical qualities to the blood, believing they will acquire the strength and qualities of their victim. Vampirism has been linked with child molestation, vandalism, animal mutilation, and murder.

Voodoo

Voodoo religion originated from West Africa and evolved on the island of Hispaniola (Haiti and the Dominican Republic). The voodoo belief system is based on a creator deity known as Gran Met Bondye. The focus is primarily on the reverence of deities, known as Loas, which were created by Bondye. The purpose of the ceremonies, called services, is to summon the Loa through the offerings of food, animals, and song. The Loa are believed to eat as humans do. There is a ritual feeding of the animals that are to be sacrificed. If the animal eats the food it is believed the

Table 6.2 Preferred animal sacrifices for Loas.

Loa	Animals preferred
Legba	Molted roosters
Gede family	Black goats, black roosters
Dambala	White hens
Ayida Wedo	White hens
Ezil	Chickens
Ogou Feray	Red roosters, bulls
Agwe	White sheep, hens
Simbi	Black animals, turkeys, hens

Source: Kail, T.M. 2008. *Magico-Religious Groups and Ritualistic Activities: A Guide for First Responders.* Boca Raton: CRC Press.

animal has accepted the sacrifice. The animal is rubbed with sacred herbs and killed. A portion of the blood from the animal is drunk by the person who killed it and then carried to four points of the ritual area. Other participants may rub the blood in the shape of a cross on their foreheads. Then the animal is taken outside to be cooked. There are certain animals for sacrifice preferred by each Loa (Table 6.2) (Kail 2008).

Santeria and Palo Mayombe

Santeria and Palo Mayombe are syncretic religions composed of two or more belief systems. Brujeria refers to the malevolent use of traditional tools of Santeria. Their rituals center around the spirits of the dead and their purpose is to manipulate or threaten a person. Santeria and Palo Mayombe are Afro-Caribbean faiths formed from the Catholicism that was imposed on African slaves. The Africans tried to hide their beliefs by assigning a Catholic saint image to each of their gods. All syncretic religions incorporate the practice of magic and belief in the supernatural. Santeria is known as La Regal de Lukumi (Lukimi's Rule) and is based on Western African religious beliefs originating in the Yoruba region of Nigeria. The word "Santeria" means "the Way of the Saints" and was meant to be a derisive Spanish term to mock followers. Palo Mayombe, known as Las Reglas de Congo, is a branch of Palo. It is from the Congo basin in Central Africa of Bantu origin. Palo is Spanish for "stick" and refers to the use of sticks in their ceremonies. In 2001, more than 20,000 practitioners were estimated to be in the United States (Gill, Rainwater, and Adams 2009).

Santeria rituals include animal and artifact offerings, dance, and sung invocations. The deities, known as Orishas, are characterized by necklaces, symbols, and objects that

Table 6.3 Specific animals sacrificed for Orishas.

Orisha	Animals
Elegua	Turtles, goats, roosters, opossum
Chango	Goats, turtles, quail, roosters, rams
Babalu-Aye	Goats, roosters, pigeons
Oshun	Yellow hens, female goats
Ogun	Opossum, roosters, goats, pigeons, sometimes dogs
Yemaya	Ducks, turtles, rams, roosters
Oya	Female goats, pigeons, hens, any black animals
Aggayu	Castrated goats, guinea hens, pigeons
Obatala	Female goats, hens, doves, guinea fowl

Source: Kail, T.M. 2008. *Magico-Religious Groups and Ritualistic Activities: A Guide for First Responders.* Boca Raton: CRC Press.

correspond to their various functions and powers. Ogun is a worshipped Orisha that is syncretized with Saint Peter and whose patron animal is the dog. The shrines may contain stuffed animals and dog statues. The cauldron of Ogun usually contains the knife used to commit animal sacrifices (Kail 2008). Ebbo is the practice of animal sacrifice which gives the Orisha energy through the blood, called Eje, in exchange for the energy of the Orisha known as Ache. A particular animal is to be sacrificed for each Orisha (Table 6.3). Interestingly, the ceremonial sacrifice is blamed on Ogun. The animal's blood is usually dripped onto stones or tools that represent the Orisha. Traditionally the meat is cleaned, cooked, and eaten by ritual participants. This is not performed with animals that are used to remove sickness or curses (Kail 2008).

The Palo rituals focus on religious receptacles or altars (Nganga or Prenda) that contain earth, sticks, and human or animal remains. The human bones may be from illegal avenues such as looting graves and not necessarily indicate a homicide. The Palo Mayombe incorporates much of the symbolism of Santeria. Alternating colored beads, sea shells, cigars, metals, pennies, bottles of alcohol, and feathers are commonly used in both Santeria and Palo Mayombe rituals. They both use elemental mercury, which is an important crime scene consideration as well as a public health issue for practitioners. The mercury may be contained in vials or poured in an open cauldron (Gill, Rainwater, and Adams 2009). Symbols of "+" and "O" may be found as drawings or on items in Palo Mayombe scenes. Tattoos with these symbols are said to signify allegiance to Palo Mayombe. These drawings, called firmas (signatures), are complex emblems that may contain arrows, circles, crosses, the moon, and other symbols. Their purpose is to give the practitioners powers for various ritual purposes including calling and directing spirits (mpungos). They may be found on the floor, walls, flags, scarves, or other ritual objects such as skulls or knives (Gill, Rainwater, and Adams 2009).

The animal sacrifice ritual is performed to feed the spirits that live in the Nganga with the blood of the animal, called Menga, which is poured onto the objects inside the Nganga. The animal carcass is placed inside the cauldron until the practitioner feels it is necessary to remove it. The animals sacrificed in Palo Mayombe include chickens, goats, rams, sheep, dogs, snakes, and horses, as well as spiders (Kail 2008).

The animal sacrifice ritual for both Santeria and Palo Mayombe is usually associated with a larger problem or event. The animal is normally killed by slicing the throat or breaking the neck. Evidence of animal torture or mutilation is indicative of Brujeria, Palo Mayombe, another occult religion, or a non-religious act of cruelty. Animal sacrifice involving cats, dogs, or large animals such as cows are more commonly associated with Palo Mayombe, Satanism, other occult groups, or disturbed individuals. The animal sacrifice usually involves removing the head from the body. The body may then be stuffed with food and other items. The head, and sometimes the body, are then disposed of in public areas such as beaches, railroad tracks, cemeteries, road intersections, or other locations that may have magical significance. With Brujeria or Palo Mayombe, the animal's body may be left at the entrance to a person's home or business.

Crime scene investigation for ritualistic crimes

Evidence that is crucial to the investigation is anything that can establish time lines or ownership of the animals, or demonstrate that the animal was alive at the time of sacrifice. There may be skeletal remains or heads of previously sacrificed animals in the ritual site or in the refrigerator or freezer. Any animal body or body parts should be collected for examination and DNA. The animal should be examined for any evidence of antemortem injury and appropriate tissue samples taken. Any antemortem reaction only occurs in the parts of the body that were still attached to the cardiovascular system at the time of injury, which makes the collection of decapitated carcasses important. Unfortunately these carcasses are commonly retrieved by animal control or waste management and discarded without recognizing their significance. There may have been severe blood loss, which can make interpretation of injuries difficult.

In addition to written documentation, photographs taken of the scene should include all the names on the candles and any calendars. The scene should be examined for containers used to hold the live animals during the ritual, such as carriers or bags. In addition, ropes or chains may have been used to suspend the animal over the ritual site for blood drainage. Blood spatter is always present, requiring careful documentation for analysis (Chapter 2). Samples of all blood should be collected for DNA testing. Any knives found should be collected for wound comparisons and DNA.

REFERENCES

Beardsley, S.L. 2000. Shearing and Degloving Wounds on the Extremities of Dogs and Cats. In *Kirk's Current Veterinary Therapy XIII Small Animal Practice*, J.D. Bonagura, ed. pp. 1032–1035. Philadelphia: W.B. Saunders.

Croft, A.M. and R. Ferllini. 2007. Macroscopic Characteristics of Screwdriver Trauma. *Journal of Forensic Sciences.* 52(6):1243–1251.

Di Maio, V.J. and D. Di Maio. 2001. *Forensic Pathology*, Second edition. Boca Raton, FL: CRC Press.

Gill, J.R., C.W. Rainwater, and B.J. Adams. 2009. Santeria and Palo Mayombe: Skulls, Mercury, and Artifacts. *Journal of Forensic Sciences.* 54(6):1458–1462.

Kail, T.M. 2008. *Magico-Religious Groups and Ritualistic Activities: A Guide for First Responders.* Boca Raton: CRC Press.

Kennedy, D.M. 2012. Microbial Analysis of Bitemarks by Sequence Comparison of Streptococcal DNA. Presented at the American Academy of Forensic Sciences, 20–25 February, Atlanta, Georgia.

Lynn, K.S. and S.I. Fairgrieve. 2009. Macroscopic Analysis of Axe and Hatchet Trauma in Fleshed and Defleshed Mammalian Long Bones. *Journal of Forensic Sciences.* 54(4):786–792.

Munro, R. and H. Munro. 2011. Forensic veterinary medicine: 2. Postmortem Investigation. *In Practice.* 33:262–270.

Ohshima, T. 2005. Diagnostic value of "superficial" stab wounds in forensic practice. *Journal of Clinical Forensic Medicine.* 12:32–35.

Perlmutter, D. 2004. *Investigating Religious Terrorism and Ritualistic Crimes.* Boca Raton, FL: CRC Press.

Pomara, C., S. D'Errico, V. Jarussi, E. Turillazzi, and V. Finschi. 2011. Cave Canem: Bite Mark Analysis in a Fatal Dog Pack Attack. *The American Journal of Forensic Medicine and Pathology.* 32(1):50–54.

Pounder, D.J. and L. Cormack. 2011. An Experimental Model of Tool Mark Striations in Soft Tissues Produced by Serrated Blades. *The American Journal of Forensic Medicine and Pathology.* 32(1):90–92.

Pounder, D.J., S. Bhatt, L. Cormack, and B.A.C. Hunt. 2011. Tool Mark Striations in Pig Skin Produced by Stabs from a

Serrated Blade. *The American Journal of Forensic Medicine and Pathology.* 32(1):93–95.

Ragatz, L., W. Fremouw, T. Thomas, and K. McCoy. 2009. Vicious Dogs: The Antisocial Behaviors and Psychological Characteristics of Owners. *Journal of Forensic Sciences.* 54(3):699–703.

Shields, L.B.E., M.L. Bernstein, J.C. Hunsaker, and D.M. Stewart. 2009. Dog Bite-Related Fatalities: A 15-Year Review of Kentucky Medical Examiner Cases. *The American Journal of Forensic Medicine and Pathology.* 30(3):223–230.

Spitz, W.U. 2006. Sharp Force Injury. In: *Spitz and Fisher's Medicolegal Investigation of Death: Guidelines for the Application of Pathology to Crime Investigation*, Fourth edition. W.U. Spitz and D.J. Spitz, eds. pp. 532–606. Springfield: Charles C. Thomas Publisher, Ltd.

Symes, S.A., J.A. Williams, E.A. Murray, J.M. Hoffman, T.D. Holland, J.M. Saul, F.P. Saul, and E.J. Pople. 2002. Taphonomic Context of Sharp-Force Trauma in Suspected Cases of Human Mutilation and Dismemberment. In: *Advances in Forensic Taphonomy*, W.D. Haglund and M.H. Sorg, eds. pp. 403–434. Boca Raton, FL: CRC Press.

Tsokos, M., R.W. Byard, and K. Püschel. 2007. Extensive and Mutilating Craniofacial Trauma Involving Defleshing and Decapitation: Unusual Features of Fatal Dog Attacks in the Young. *The American Journal of Forensic Medicine and Pathology.* 28(2):131–136.

7

Burn-, Electrical-, and Fire-Related Injuries

Melinda D. Merck and Doris M. Miller

Take nothing for granted because things are not always what they seem.

LeMoyne Snyder

INTERPRETING BURN PATTERNS

The suspicion of deliberate infliction of burns on an animal is raised when the history offered by the owner does not match the presentation of the burn, the environment, or the expected animal behavior that can result in accidental burns. Some owners may blame the animal laying too close to a hot object as the cause of the burn. Although it is possible for an animal to sustain a thermal burn injury before registering the associated pain, the burn pattern may be inconsistent. Burns should be considered with the presence of any unexplained eschar.

Burns are usually a patterned injury with characteristics that reflect the cause of the injury. They are typically localized or distributed asymmetrically. Biologically abnormal patterns include unusual symmetry, drip configurations, and straight or angular borders. They typically do not progress after five days without repetitive injury, unlike other dermatologic conditions (Munro and Munro 2008).

Proper interpretation of the burn patterns can reveal the exact nature of the incident that may support or refute the history and help direct the investigation. The multiple levels of injury present can provide valuable information. The most severe level may be indicative of where the area had initial, longer, or more intense contact with the burn-causing agent. A determination of where the burn started on the body may be made when there are more severe burns confluent with more superficial burns. Burns from a liquid, such as splashes or spills, typically have flow lines from the liquid impact or gravity, which are usually more superficial than the initial contact area. A burn pattern that is evenly distributed with the same degree of injury is indicative of an even rate of burn, such as with a flash fire or chemical agent. The location of the burn can indicate whether the burn could have been accidental vs. intentional such as protected body areas (Figure 7.1). When an animal is set on fire and the fur burns for a short period of time there may not be large areas of injury to the underlying skin. Instead, there may be a wide distribution of isolated circular burns on the skin where the fur acted as a wick for the fire to reach the skin. There may be a larger burn area on the skin where the fire was initially ignited on the body.

It is common for burn victims to have additional injuries in cruelty cases. The animal should be examined for evidence of trauma, especially blunt force, and the use of ligatures or bindings. The feet should be examined for trace evidence. Because the animal may try to remove the offensive agent through grooming, the oral cavity, alimentary canal, and stomach should be examined for evidence and burn lesions.

RECOGNITION AND COLLECTION OF EVIDENCE

In addition to the crime scene, there may be evidence on the animal or surrounding the burn that can provide information as to the cause of the incident or injury, including the substance or object. Devices used to ignite fires may be

Veterinary Forensics: Animal Cruelty Investigations, Second Edition. Edited by Melinda D. Merck.
© 2013 John Wiley & Sons, Inc. Published 2013 by John Wiley & Sons, Inc.

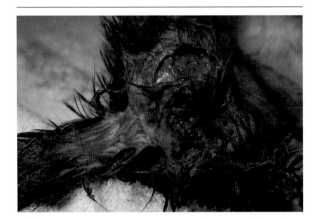

Figure 7.1 Burn injuries on cat due to firecrackers tied to the tail.

cigarette lighters, matches, or blow torches, and they may contain residue of the accelerant on the surface. The soil beneath where the animal was found may contain residue of the burn agent. Soil samples should be taken from under and immediately around where the animal was found and in the area of the suspected incident, along with control soil samples from the nearby area for comparison. Evidence of an accelerant, chemical, or liquid may be found on the animal, body bag or wrappings, or objects at the scene. There may be an odor present on the animal that may indicate the cause of the burn.

The fur and skin may contain residue of the offending agent. Swab samples should be taken of the skin immediately adjacent to the burn area. Swabs and fur samples should be collected in areas of suspicious odors and matted or wet fur. All samples should be collected prior to cleaning and treatment of the injuries. The evidence should be appropriately packaged, especially with possible accelerants, as discussed in Chapter 2.

BURN CLASSIFICATION

The severity of each burn should be determined and classified using systems based on the degree (depth) of the burn and total body surface area affected. The severity of the burn also is assessed based on the location. Burns affecting the face, eyes, ears, perineum, and feet are considered more severe because of the potential for serious disfigurement, loss of function, and severity of the pain associated with burns in these areas. The evaluation of the burn may be hindered by the haircoat, requiring shaving. Evaluation based on the initial burn presentation may be complicated by the fact that skin is slow to heat and slow to cool. Thermal damage continues after the animal is removed

from the source of the heat (Saxon and Kirby 1992). Therefore, it is prudent to overestimate the burn severity rather than underestimate it.

Percentage of total body surface area

Burns are classified by the percentage of total body surface area (TBSA) involved. The TBSA may be quickly determined using the rule of nines. This rule assigns a specific body surface area percentage to each area of the body: forelimb 9%; hindlimb 18%; head and neck together 9%; dorsal and ventral thorax together 18%; dorsal and ventral abdomen together 18%; and perineum 1% (Saxon and Kirby 1992). The burn areas can be documented using a diagram (Appendices 15–16). Another method is to measure the burned area in centimeters and divide it by the body surface area in meters. The body weight can be converted to body surface area using the standard conversion tables available.

Burn degrees

Burns can be classified based on the depth and tissue affected (Table 7.1). First-degree burns are superficial burns that affect only the epidermis. They are characterized by pain, erythema, and desquamation, and are thickened. Erythema is less in animals than in humans with first-degree burns because of the lack of superficial vascular plexus. Healing occurs within five days and most often without scarring. Usually first-degree burns are not included in burn surface calculation unless they exceed 25% of the body surface area (Jutkowitz 2005).

Second-degree burns include superficial and deep partial-thickness burns that involve the epidermis and one-half of the dermis. Superficial partial-thickness burns are painful, blistered, and blanch when pressure is applied (Hedlund 2002). The upper layers of the subcutaneous fat are still present. There is subcutaneous edema present, notable inflammation, and the hair is intact. The burn may appear moist, red, or mottled (Jutkowitz 2005). These burns usually heal in two to three weeks with mild scarring. Deep partial-thickness burns may appear moist, blistered, or dried. The wounds may have a red-mottled appearance, they do not blanch, and hair is easily epilated. They are slow to heal and are associated with serious scarring and loss of function (Jutkowitz 2005). Second-degree burns may vary in areas to third-degree burns, changing in appearance. In the first twenty-four hours there is progressive damage resulting from heat injury and the release of vasoactive substances, prostaglandins, and proteolytic enzymes, causing further edema and tissue destruction. If appropriate therapy is not started or secondary bacterial

Table 7.1 Burn classification.

Classification	Skin layer/tissue	Pain[*]	Signs
First-degree (superficial)	Epidermis	+++	Erythema, desquamation
Second-degree (partial-superficial)	Partial epidermis, mid-dermis	++	Erythema, subcutaneous edema
Second-degree (partial-deep)	Total epidermis, partial dermis	++	Severe inflammation, dry surface, does not blanch
Third-degree (full)	Epidermis, dermis	−	Leathery (eschar), dry surface, blanched
Fourth-degree	Epidermis, dermis, and underlying tissue/bone	−	Blackened, charred with eschar

[*]+ mild, ++ moderate, +++ severe, − none

Source: Saxon, W.D. and R. Kirby. 1992. Treatment of Acute Burn Injury and Smoke Inhalation. In: *Current Veterinary Therapy XI Small Animal Practice*, R.W. Kirk and J.D. Bonagura, eds. pp. 146–154. Philadelphia: W.B. Saunders Company.

infection occurs this burn may progress to a third-degree burn (Hedlund 2002).

Third-degree burns are full-thickness burns characterized by a dark brown, leathery eschar and are dry with white or charred coloration. In these burns there is full destruction of all the skin structures, sometimes extending to the subcutaneous tissue, and the hair easily epilates. There is much less pain than with the other burns because the nerves have been destroyed. Healing occurs by contraction, epithelialization, and granulation, or by surgical intervention. There is subcutaneous edema and necrosis resulting from superficial vascular thrombosis and deep vascular permeability (Hedlund 2002).

A fourth-degree burn extends through the skin to the underlying tissue and/or bone. This tissue may appear blackened or charred with eschar. These burns are associated with severe tissue necrosis and subsequent systemic illness, and are often fatal (Jutkowitz 2005).

SYSTEMIC EFFECTS OF BURNS

Burns may cause severe systemic problems, especially with involvement of large surface areas. Severe burns are characterized by burns involving greater than 20% of the total body surface area (Jutkowitz 2005). Victims of burns often are in shock and develop multiple organ failure due to the loss of fluid and resulting hypovolemia, fluid shifts, electrolyte imbalances, protein loss, myocardial depression, raised peripheral vascular resistance, and increased blood viscosity.

Some animals develop further complications, including sepsis, immunosuppression, renal failure, liver failure, anemia, cardiac abnormalities, and disseminated intravascular coagulation (Hedlund 2002). Sepsis is a major

contributor to death in burn patients. The source of infection comes from the wounds, respiratory infection, and catheter sites. In addition, the gastrointestinal mucosal barrier is compromised, allowing endotoxins and bacteria to penetrate the blood stream, contributing to multi-organ failure (Jutkowitz 2005).

GENERAL MICROSCOPIC EXAMINATION FINDINGS IN BURNS

There are some general findings associated with burns and each section below discusses in detail the associated findings. Areas of erythema without ulceration are the best sites for skin biopsy. Microscopically there is coagulation necrosis of the epidermis, which often extends through the epidermis to the hair follicles. Second-degree burns involve the adnexal glands as well. The dermal collagen is usually less necrotic than the epithelial structures. Third-degree chemical and thermal burns are characterized by full-thickness obliterative acellular necrosis of all dermal structures extending to the panniculus or deeper subcutaneous tissue. Thermal burns often cause deeper injury than chemical burns. Some thermal and chemical burns may be clinically indistinguishable unless residue of the chemical is present on the haircoat or skin. Electrical and microwave radiation can cause lesions that are indistinguishable on histopathology examination.

THERMAL BURNS

General findings

Thermal burns may be caused by situations or objects that radiate heat including fires, heating pads, ovens, hair dryers, hot liquid, steam, microwave ovens, heat lamps, space heaters, or radiators. Thermal damage produced by clothes dryers or hot gases are similar to injuries seen in fire victims (see below). Thermal burns may be produced by contact or near contact to the heat source. Several factors affect the extent of the injury, including the temperature of the heat source, length of contact, and conductance of the tissue. The appearance of contact thermal burns may be delayed. The initial findings may be limited, including matted or moist fur with the eventual loss of hair and skin (Hedlund 2002).

The skin of the animal does not disseminate heat as the human skin does because of the lack of a plentiful superficial vascular plexus. In a direct contact burn injury there is coagulation, cellular protein denaturation, and blood vessel coagulation (Hedlund 2002) with plasma loss and tissue edema. Local tissue ischemia is apparent within three to five days (Smith 1995). A transition area divides the devitalized tissue from healthy tissue, which has potentially reversible tissue damage, reduced blood flow, and intravascular sludging. Due to the release of vasoactive substances there may be continued dermal ischemia, tissue edema, dessication, and secondary bacterial invasion. This transition zone is surrounded by hyperemic tissue. Eschar is the residue of coagulated skin elements comprised of tough, denatured collagen fibers that form a strong protective covering of the wound. Comparatively, scabs are not as protective and are comprised of dead skin cells, blood cells, and fibrin.

Initially, it may be difficult to assess the depth of a burn. Repeated evaluation during the first twenty-four hours may be required, and eschar covering can make this difficult to assess. When raised and bent to reveal the underlying tissue, the eschar will split in first- and second-degree burns. In third-degree burns the eschar may or may not split and the split may extend down to the subcutaneous tissue. Bacterial invasion under the eschar occurs within four to five days (Hedlund 2002).

Radiant heat burns

Radiant heat burns are near-contact burns caused by the heat waves produced from a hot surface such as a flame, heat lamp, fire, oven, or radiator. Depending on the temperature, burns can occur in seconds. Conventional ovens that operate through radiant heat cook from the outside of the body in. Radiant heat causes maximum injury to the outside of the body. Initially, the hair may be intact and the skin may appear erythematous and blistered with possible skin slippage. With prolonged exposure the skin can become leathery with eventual charring (Di Maio and Di Maio 2001).

Solar thermal necrosis

Solar injury associated with UV rays has been well documented in animals, occurring in areas of light pigmentation and sparse fur. Thermal injury due to solar radiation also can be seen in dark pigmented areas. Black skin absorbs approximately 45% more solar radiation than white skin, making dark skin areas more susceptible to thermal radiation damage. Visible radiation penetrates the skin several millimeters and degrades into thermal energy, increasing the thermal burden. The epidermis absorbs almost all of the UV light and therefore does not contribute to the thermal burden (Hargis and Lewis 1999). The application of any topical oil-based product, such as topical flea drops, can exacerbate the thermal injury. Heat stroke, dark-colored fur, and short haircoats can also predispose the animal to these burns. Histologic findings are consistent with a full-thickness burn: epidermal, adnexal, and vascular necrosis and subepidermal vesiculation (Hargis and Lewis 1999).

These cases present with burn lesions along the dorsum, which may contain plaques and eschars (Figures 7.2a and 7.2b). Multi-colored animals may have focal lesions located in the dark pigmented areas. These burns are often mistaken for signs of animal cruelty by the intentional application of a caustic agent to the dorsum, but when examined closely the burn does not have a typical liquid or pour pattern with flow lines. The location is the other indicator of the cause. This solar thermal necrosis is due to prolonged exposure to direct sunlight. Animals normally change positions and seek shade as the radiation heat increases in their skin. Solar thermal necrosis occurs when the animal is unable to escape from the direct sunlight, either through environmental circumstances or physical limitations. Depending on the circumstances, this may result in animal cruelty charges. It should be noted that the burn lesions may not appear for several days to two weeks after the sun exposure.

Microwave ovens

Microwave ovens pass microwave radiation at a frequency of 2,450 MHx, producing heat through molecular agitation primarily through water. The higher the tissue water content, the greater the heat and tissue damage that is produced. Because muscle tissue contains more water than fat, it sustains more thermal injury (Di Maio and Di Maio 2001). The amount of tissue damage also depends on the length of time the body is in the microwave oven and the strength of the microwaves produced. Microwaves produce heat directly to the internal tissue. The external body may sustain partial- to full-thickness burns that tend to be well

(a) (b)

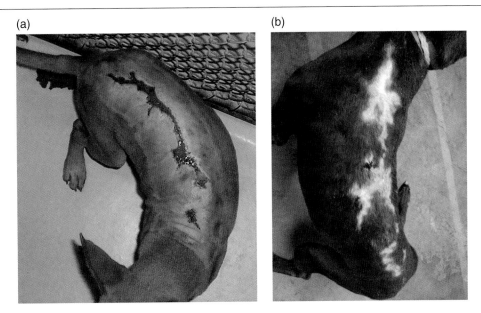

Figure 7.2 (a and b). Solar thermal necrosis.

demarcated without charring (Di Maio and Di Maio 2001), with the thinner, peripheral tissues more commonly affected, such as the ears. Injuries are based on the water distribution in the tissues, with the greatest injury to the internal body. Microscopic examination may show sparing of different tissues, giving a sandwich-type appearance. For example, skin burns may show sparing of the subcutaneous fat and burns of the underlying muscle (Di Maio and Di Maio 2001).

Postmortem findings that are suspicious of microwave damage include: skin fragility that can lead to extensive splitting with well-defined edges and loosening of the hair, flexure of the forelimb at the carpus with or without ex-sheathing of the claws, crumpling and reddening of the tips of the pinnae, absence of burning or singeing of hair, congestion of all lung lobes with or without microscopic alveolar flooding and perivascular hemorrhage, cooked appearance of internal organs depending on length of microwave exposure, tissues that readily disintegrate, and a cooked chicken odor (Munro and Munro 2008).

Cigarette burns

Cigarette burn patterns and injuries have been well documented in abused children. In acute burns the area is red, circular, 0.5–1.0 cm in diameter, and possibly wedge shaped if the cigarette was applied at an oblique angle. Deliberate burns are often full thickness, creating a crater. Older burns may be circular and sunken with thin scar tissue

on the surface; accidental cigarette burns tend to be superficial and usually more eccentric due to the brief contact with the hot ash (Munro and Thrusfield 2001). It is important to consider histopathology to determine other possible causes of the skin lesions.

Scalding burns

Scalding burns are caused by contact with a hot liquid and do not result in singeing of hair. They may be produced by immersion, spills, splashing, or exposure to superheated steam. Water heaters in houses and apartments are commonly set at 140°F (60°C), and full-thickness burns can occur in just a few seconds at this temperature. In animals, scalding can occur when the fluid temperature is 120°F (48.8°C) (Sinclair and Lockwood 2006). In humans, the time and temperature of water required to cause epidermal damage and full-thickness burns has been documented (Table 7.2).

In splash or spill burns, the fluid cools as it flows down the body. The burn is more severe where the fluid had initial contact with the skin, becoming more superficial where the fluid flowed away. Superheated steam causes severe scald-like burns. If inhaled, this steam causes airway injury, including upper, lower, and deeper airways. There may be massive edema in the larynx causing occlusion of the airway and asphyxia (Di Maio and Di Maio 2001). Deliberate immersion burns are typically characterized by a straight burn line caused by the water level (Platt, Spitz, and Spitz 2006), depending on the body part lowered into the liquid

Table 7.2 Water temperature and scalding burn time in humans.

Temp (°F)	Threshold for epidermal injury	Full-thickness burns
120	290 seconds	600 seconds
125	50 seconds	120 seconds
130	15 seconds	30 seconds
140	2.6 seconds	Approximately 7 seconds
150	Less than 1 second	2.3 seconds

Source: Di Maio V.J. and D. Di Maio. 2001. *Forensic Pathology*, Second edition. P. 349. Boca Raton: CRC Press.

and the struggle or resistance of the victim. In legs, this can result in a stocking or glove distribution with the upper margin clearly defined. The scald may be limited to the feet and pads depending on the depth. In cats, the toes retract on contact protecting the areas between the pads. The findings in feet scald include loss of epithelium from the ventral pad surfaces with eventual weeping or darkening, normal non-erythematous areas between the pads and toes, erythematous skin with loss of hair and epidermis on the lateral and dorsal aspects of the toes or foot (Munro and Munro 2008).

CHEMICAL BURNS

Overview

Burns resulting from chemicals that are strong acids or alkalis cause severe tissue damage by interfering with cell metabolism or denaturing proteins. These burns may be external, internal, or a combination of both. Because thermal and chemical burns produce the same injury, the burn must be examined carefully to determine the cause.

Tissue damage occurs through different mechanisms of action with chemical burns. Chemicals that are oxidizing cause injury by coagulation of protein (chromic acid, hypochlorite, and potassium permanganate), dehydrating chemicals desiccate the tissues (sulfuric and hydrochloric acids), denaturing chemicals fix or stabilize tissue through the formation of salts (picric acid, tannic acid, acetic acid, formic acid, and hydrofluoric acid), corrosive agents denature proteins causing erosion and ulceration (sodium-containing drain and oven cleaners, and phenol disinfectants), and vesicants cause the release of tissue histamine and serotonin resulting in blisters (dimethylsulfoxide, cantharides, halogenated hydrocarbons, and gasoline) (Hedlund 2002).

General findings

The degree of injury depends on several factors, including the type of chemical and its action, volume of chemical in contact with the body, strength of the chemical, length of contact time, penetration of the chemical, and whether or not the animal ingested the chemical. Injuries can range from superficial to third-degree burns.

Chemicals that have contact with the eye can cause severe corneal damage, including full-thickness perforation and corneal necrosis. With chemical burns heat is often generated because of the chemical reactions, causing thermal injury (Hedlund 2002). The ingestion of chemicals by an animal may be a result of environmental exposure (intentional or accidental), intentional feeding, or intentional application to the body and subsequent grooming, i.e., licking. Chemical burns caused by ingestion may be found on the muzzle, tongue, palate, gums, oropharynx, esophagus, stomach, and small intestine, depending on the amount and properties of the chemical agent.

Some chemical agents can cause systemic poisoning in addition to chemical burns. These include phenol, yellow phosphorus, and ammonium sulfide. Phenol can cause acute tubular necrosis and phosphorus can cause kidney and liver necrosis (Di Maio and Di Maio 2001). Common compounds can produce chemical burns with prolonged contact. Cement is a very strong alkaline compound with a pH of 12.5–14. Hydrocarbons, such as gasoline, can produce partial-thickness burns with prolonged contact. They have an irritating effect and high lipid solubility, which permits dissolution of fatty tissue (Di Maio and Di Maio 2001).

A wide variety of chemicals have been associated with animal abuse, including battery acid. Lye (sodium hydroxide) has been used intentionally on animals to cause burns. It is found in drain clog treatments and is used in methamphetamine manufacturing. The perpetrator may mix lye with flour or pancake mix to allow it to adhere more effectively to the body of the animal (Sinclair and Lockwood 2006). If ingested, it can produce transmural necrosis of the esophagus with one second of contact. Gastric necrosis is common with the use of liquid lye and may be accompanied by perforation of the small intestine (Di Maio and Di Maio 2001).

ELECTRICAL BURNS

Overview

Electrical burns occur when the body has contact with an electrical current with or without an exit point. The damage caused is from the current, voltage, heat generated, and amount of time the victim is in contact with electricity. Current refers to the quantity of electricity passing through the wire and is measured in milliamperes (mA). The current is actually electrons flowing through the wire and the number of electrons increases with a corresponding increase in current. Amperage is the most important factor in electrocution injuries; it is directly related to the voltage and indirectly related to the resistance. The longer current passes through the body, the greater the damage produced. Exposure to a lower current for a long period of time causes more damage than exposure to a higher current for a shorter period. Heat is also generated by the electrical current, producing thermal injury. Voltage of electricity is another factor in electrocution. This is what causes more electricity to flow through the wire, analogous to water pressure. The higher the voltage, the higher the amount of electricity that passes through.

Upon entering the body, electrical current tends to travel the shortest route from the point of contact to the point of grounding or exit. The pathway depends on the relative resistance the potential exit points and is less dependent on the internal tissues conductivity (Knight 2004). The tissue resistance to electrical current in order of greatest to least is bone, fat, tendon, skin, muscle, blood, and nerves. Current flows along the path of least resistance such as blood vessels, nerves, and wet tissue. The current concentrates in tissues with greater resistance, such as bone, causing greater thermal injury. Oral exposure to electrical current is particularly damaging because the wet oral tissues are in direct contact with the bone (Hedlund 2002).

General findings

Victims of electrocution are often found still in contact with the item that caused the injury. In animals, this is most commonly an electrical cord into which the animal has bitten. In animal cruelty cases, electricity may be used to torture or attempt to kill an animal. The injured animal is often found in a tonic state because of the contraction of striated muscles. In humans, these contractions can be severe enough to cause bone fractures (Di Maio and Di Maio 2001). Vomiting and defecation can occur with generalized tonoclonic activity. This state resolves in the surviving animal once the source of the electricity is removed from the body. The animal may be weak and ataxic afterward. Pulmonary edema may develop secondary to electrocution.

Oral burns can be found on the lips, palate, tongue, and gums, and oronasal fistulas may be present or develop later. Electrical burns cause the release of vasoactive substances and vascular thrombosis, resulting in tissue necrosis. The tissue may appear charred, tan, or pale gray. Tissue edema develops one to two days after the injury, although the extent of injuries may take two to three weeks to fully develop (Hedlund 2002). Local tissue ischemia may be apparent in three to five days (Smith 1995).

In victims of low-voltage electrocution, burns, also called electrical marks, may be found around the area where there was electrical contact (the entry point) and/or the point of grounding (the exit point). These burns also may be completely absent if the point of contact was over a large, broad area that had minimal resistance such as electrocution when the body is immersed in water. The burn size generally is small and may be characterized by a chalky white lesion with a central crater and raised borders, or an area of erythematous blistering. In humans, the pathognomonic indicator of electrical damage is an areola of blanched skin at the periphery of the lesion due to arteriolar spasm which remains after death. Some lesions may have a hyperemic border around the pale area or reddening within the zone (Knight 2004). The burn sites may have yellowish or black discoloration produced by heat. Histologically the changes are generally due to thermal effects and may have a Swiss cheese appearance to the epidermis. There may be minute particles of metal deposited in the burn from the conducting surface. The appearances of antemortem and postmortem electrocution burns are similar, making differentiation difficult except for the presence of vital reaction (Knight 2004).

With high-voltage electrocution, the burns may be extremely severe with charring of the body. Third-degree burns may develop at the contact site. There may be numerous individual and confluent third-degree burns. Multiple small burns may be produced by the arcing of the current, causing a crocodile-skin effect in humans (Knight 2004). If the current is transmitted indirectly through another object the burns may be large and irregular. They are chalky white with a central crater and raised borders. The heat produces yellowish or black discoloration around the burn sites. There may be massive tissue destruction with very high voltage, including loss of extremities and organ rupture (Di Maio and Di Maio 2001).

Death owing to electrocution is usually caused by cardiac arrest. In lower amperage, electrocution causes muscle tremors to painful muscle contractions. As the amperage increases, loss of consciousness, ventricular fibrillation, and death can occur. Electrocution also can produce contracture of all the muscles, causing respiratory paralysis and death. There may be little thermal damage to the largely aqueous internal tissue, creating a diffuse pathway. Evidence of pulmonary edema may be found. The heat that is generated by electrocution may cause profound and massive tissue damage (Hedlund 2002). With high-voltage electrocution, there may be thermal damage to the respiratory center of the brainstem, causing respiratory arrest (Di Maio and Di Maio 2001).

Lightning electrocution

Lightning electrocution may result from a direct strike or a side-flash strike. There are usually entrance and exit burns from the current. There may be cutaneous burns that microscopically show the epidermis separated from the papillary dermis. There may be singed fur and the tympanic membrane may be ruptured. Linear singe marks may be present and are more commonly found on the medial legs in animals (Fraser 1986). If the animal survives, pulmonary edema may be present. Survivors have a pathognomonic skin injury called Lichtenberg figures. These lesions appear fern-like and comprise an area of transient erythema that appears within one hour of the incident and gradually fades in twenty-four hours. These arboreal patterns may be found in animals on the dermal side of the skin as extravasation of blood (Fraser 1986). Death resulting from lighting strike is caused by cardiopulmonary arrest or electrothermal injury caused by the high-voltage current. Depending on the animal's location at the time of the lightning strike, additional injuries may be found related to the body falling.

Taser® and stun gun electrocution

The Taser® is part of a class of electronic control devices or conducted energy weapons designed to incapacitate people by delivering high voltage to the body, causing neuromuscular incapacitation. This is achieved by firing two darts that penetrate the skin. They are attached by wires to the firing device which delivers the electricity in the form of pulsed current output. The effective firing distance is reportedly up to thirty-five feet. Canine studies using the most common Advanced Taser®, Taser® X26, did not induce cardiac arrhythmias (Bleetman, Steyn, and Lee 2004). A device for wildlife, Taser® Wildlife ECD, has been developed that delivers 20,000 volts. Injuries associated with the use of a Taser® are limited to the skin penetration of the darts, which may be located at variable distances apart. A stun gun can deliver 50,000 volts of electricity to the body through two contact points. The distance between the contact points is unique to the individual stun gun. These guns can cause burns on the skin from the two contact points. The distance between the two burns should be measured for comparison to a recovered gun.

Microscopic findings

Electrical burns may be differentiated from thermal burns by several features. Electrical burns have sharp borders with abrupt transition from normal to injured tissue, honeycomb vacuolization of the stratum corneum; subepidermal bullae as a result of detachment of the epidermis from the dermis, denaturation of the dermal collagen, and deposition of vaporized metal on the surface of the skin (metallization) usually associated with lightning and high voltage injuries (Perper 2006).

The use of computerized image analysis in addition to light microscopic exam can be useful to differentiate electrocution, flame burn, and abrasion-type skin lesions. A study of these skin lesions evaluated the epidermal cell nuclei in respect to nuclear area, nuclear perimeter, nuclear form factor, minimum axes of nucleus, maximum axes of nucleus, and minimum axes/maximum axes ratio. The nuclear area was higher in flame burns and abrasion-type lesions than electrocution. The nuclear perimeter for electrocution was considerably higher than flame burns and abrasions. The electrocution nuclear form factor was significantly higher than the others with a mean of 4.0273 for electrocution, 2.2648 for flame burns, and 2.0941 for abrasions.

There was no difference in the nuclear minimum axes between electrocution and flame burn groups, but the abrasion group was higher. The electrocution nuclear maximum axes were the highest over the flame burn or abrasion groups. The nuclear minimum axes/nuclear maximum axes ratio was higher in the abrasion group with no difference between electrocution and flame burn. The long axes/short axes ratio has been used to compare electrocution skin lesions with normal skin in humans. It was found that the normal skin epidermal cell nuclear ratio was 5.9325 and electrocution injuries had 1.4344 (Akyldiz et al. 2009).

FIRE-RELATED INJURIES

Overview

Fires can cause injuries related to burns and smoke inhalation. Burns resulting from fires occur when there is contact with the body and the flame. The severity of the injury depends on the amount of contact time and area of the body that is burned. The damage may range from first- to fourth-degree burns.

Flame burns may produce scorching of the skin and can progress to charring. Flash burns are caused by ignition from flash fires. These flash fires are caused by the sudden ignition or explosion of fuels, fine particulate matter, or gases. The initial flash ignition is usually short, burning the contacting surfaces uniformly. The hair is singed and there are partial-thickness burns. The burn may be superficial if the flash is very short (Di Maio and Di Maio 2001). Additional burns may be seen due to radiant heat injury from the flame, as discussed above. Depending on the circumstances, most fire victims suffer smoke inhalation in addition to burn injuries.

Examination of fire victims

General

When examining fire victims it is important to consider the circumstances found at the crime scene. In fire-related deaths, it is important for the body to be photographed and examined *in situ* to establish the context of the body in relation to the fire scene. Evidence of the cause of the fire may be found on the body of fire victims, including odors from the accelerant used. All potential evidence should be collected from the body (see above and Chapter 2). Full-body radiographs should be taken of all fire victims to look for any evidence of antemortem trauma, such as projectiles or fractures. It should be noted that extreme heat from fires may cause characteristic fracturing of the bone (see below).

Live victims

Surviving victims of fire usually have the smell of smoke on their fur. In addition to external burns, there may be thermal burns to the oral cavity and along the upper and lower airways. Laryngospasm may be present. Findings in the airways may include mucosal erythema, ulceration, hemorrhage, edema, and carbonaceous particle accumulation, even in the terminal airways. In one reported case, a burned hair was found in the lungs on histopathology examination (Gerdin 2011). The animal may have carbonaceous sputum. Findings of carbon monoxide poisoning may be seen, such as cherry red skin and mucous membranes, which also may be due to thermal burns or congestion. Conjunctivitis or corneal abrasions may be found. In moderate to severe cases cytological exam of transtracheal aspirates may reveal burned ciliated cells, strands of mucus, and soot particles (Carson 1986).

Deceased victims

It is important when examining a deceased victim to determine if the animal was alive or deceased prior to the fire and if there is evidence of antemortem injuries. Some bodies may not be charred or disfigured. Some may be seared and some may show little to no external evidence of injury except for the odor of smoke. Bodies that have minimal external injury have usually died from smoke inhalation (see findings below). With searing damage, the skin may be light brown in color and have a stiff, leathery consistency. There may be blisters on the skin with an erythematous rim but they are not indicative of antemortem injury. Blisters with this rim can be produced postmortem by heat causing contraction of the dermal capillaries forcing blood to the periphery of the blister or burn (Di Maio and Di Maio 2001).

The body may be partially charred and swollen from the heat. Heat build-up within the thorax may cause blood to be pressed into the alveoli, airway, mouth, and nostrils, simulating antemortem injury. Blood encrusted to the chest inner linings is usually indicative of antemortem trauma (Spitz 2006). The lung tissue may contain accelerant residue if the animal inhaled the vapors prior to death (Pahor 2012). If the body is severely burned, there may be splitting of the skin due to shrinkage. The skin may be completely burned away, exposing the underlying muscle, which may be ruptured by the heat. Muscle splits due to heat run parallel to the muscle fibers; therefore, any splits across muscle are due to antemortem trauma (Spitz 2006). The skin that is not burned may have a seared, leathery texture. There may be areas of undamaged skin where the body was laying on a flat surface. The internal body walls may be burned away, exposing the viscera, which may be seared or charred (Di Maio and Di Maio 2001).

It is usually impossible to determine antemortem burns from postmortem burns on gross examination. There may be microscopic evidence if the victim survived long enough to develop an inflammatory response, although the lack of this response does not indicate that the burns were postmortem. Heat thrombosis of the dermal vessels can delay inflammatory cells from reaching the area of the burn (Di Maio and Di Maio 2001).

During a fire, blood and marrow often are expressed from the skull and accumulate between the bone and the dura mater, mimicking a traumatic epidural hematoma which is usually large and thick overlying the frontal, parietal, and temporal areas with possible extension to the occipital area. This clot-like mass is chocolate brown in color with a crumbly or honeycomb appearance and can be distinguished from antemortem epidural hematomas (Di Maio and Di Maio 2001). One indicator is the presence of fractures, often due to heat changes, which is usually absent in antemortem epidural hematomas. The finding of subdural hemorrhage is always an indicator of antemortem injury (Spitz 2006).

Burning of the body causes heat coagulation of the muscle tissue and contraction of the muscle fibers. This causes flexion of the limbs, producing a pugilistic posture (pugilistic attitude). This pugilistic posture does not indicate whether the victim was alive or deceased before the fire (Di Maio and Di Maio 2001). This muscle shrinking can also cause bone fractures. The use of multi-detector computed tomography can be very useful to differentiate traumatic or lethal fracture patterns from thermal changes (Levy et al. 2009).

Burning of bones causes color changes and possible heat fractures. Burned bone may have a gray-white color. There may be a fine network of superficial fractures caused by the heat that can crumble with handling. The outer table of the skull can fragment and be completely absent. The feet may not be attached to the body and unrecognized at the scene, especially with severe burning and fragmentation (Di Maio and Di Maio 2001).

Entomology

There may be entomology evidence in the form of live or deceased insects or larvae found on burn victims either externally or internally. After the fire insects may feed on the body postmortem, with the same first waves of insect colonization as fresh remains (Catteneo 2012), which can help determine the postmortem interval. This corresponds to a time estimate of when the fire occurred (Chapter 15). Deceased entomology evidence (blow fly larvae and possibly other types of insects) may be found internally, especially inside the skull or body cavities, which protects them from being consumed in the fire. This indicates the animal was dead for a period of time prior to the fire, with enough time for colonization and egg hatching. The time estimate for the postmortem interval can be determined through entomology analysis (Chapter 15).

Smoke inhalation and thermal injury

Overview

The cause of death in fire victims is most commonly caused by carbon monoxide poisoning, smoke toxicity, thermal damage to the airways or the body, or any combination of these. Immediate deaths may result from smoke inhalation or direct thermal injury to the body. The mouth, nostrils, and upper and lower airways usually contain soot in smoke inhalation victims. Soot may be swallowed and small flakes recovered from the esophagus or stomach lining (Spitz 2006). To avoid contamination from soot particles dropping down from the mouth or laryngeal area, a ball of absorbent cotton may be used to plug the upper airway and the trachea excised and examined *in situ*. When a small amount of soot is trapped in mucus it may be removed by using a scalpel and spread in a thin layer onto a clean, white paper towel for documentation (Spitz 2006). It should be noted that the absence of soot is not indicative of death prior to the fire.

The leading cause of death in human victims of smoke inhalation is respiratory failure (Saxon and Kirby 1992). Damage to the respiratory tract usually results from both thermal and chemical causes. Histologic findings in the distal lung parenchyma may assist in determining that the victim was alive or deceased before the start of a fire and document the pathophysiological alterations based on the rapidity and the degree of involvement of the respiratory tract. The histologic findings in humans of fire-death lungs are: bronchiolar dilatation, ductal over-insufflation, alveolar over-insufflation, and alveolar hemorrhage (de Paiva et al. 2008).

Thermal injury

Thermal damage may be seen if the animal breathes in hot gases resulting in edema and/or burns as discussed above. This can cause damage to the oral mucosa, nasopharynx, pharynx, and possibly the lower respiratory tract. Thermal injuries can cause edema of the larynx, which may or may not be obstructive. It also can cause severe laryngospasm resulting in suffocation (Saxon and Kirby 1992). At any point in the first twenty-four hours the injury to the upper airway may cause upper airway obstruction (Tams 1989). The heat-damaged mucosa lining the airways sloughs into the lumen causing further airway obstruction in the first two to six days after the insult (Saxon and Kirby 1992) and impairing surfactant production (Jutkowitz 2005). Furthermore, systemic inflammation from the burn wounds or from sepsis may indirectly cause acute lung injury or acute respiratory distress syndrome (ARDS) (Jutkowitz 2005).

Smoke toxicity

Smoke toxicity refers to direct injury from the inhalation of smoke and poisoning resulting from the inhalation of toxic chemicals. These noxious chemicals are the by-products of incomplete combustion of natural and synthetic material in the fire. Chemical injury is caused by the inhalation of toxic gases attached to carbon particles that are deposited in the deep lower airway. These poisonous gases include carbon monoxide; nitrous oxide; chlorine; sulfur dioxide; aldehydes; hydrogen cyanide; hydrogen chloride; and acrolein from the burning of room furnishings, clothing, plastics, and other materials. The combustion of some plastics may produce benzene, whose anesthetic effects may allow easier passage of noxious particles into the lungs (Tams 1989).

All of these chemicals cause injury to the lungs, producing pulmonary edema. The chemicals cause injury at the endothelial–epithelial interface, bronchociliary damage, inactivation of ciliary movement, and decreased production of surfactant causing alveolar collapse (Saxon and Kirby 1992, Di Maio and Di Maio 2001). A mushroom of thick, white foam at the nostrils or mouth indicates breathing while the fire was in progress. This is due to pulmonary edema and heart failure due to the asphyxiating effect of carboxyhemoglobin and its direct toxicity on the heart muscle (Spitz 2006). In addition, macrophage function is impaired because of smoke poisons. In animals that survive the initial insult, pneumonia is the biggest life-threatening risk in the first week because of the denuded mucosal surfaces, impaired macrophage function, and loss of ciliary function and surfactant protection.

Carbon monoxide poisoning

Carbon monoxide (CO) is a colorless, odorless, poisonous gas weighing lighter than air that is a result of the incomplete combustion of hydrocarbon fuels (Carson 1986). It acts by competing with oxygen for binding sites, primarily on hemoglobin. Carbon monoxide has an affinity for hemoglobin that is 240 times higher than that of oxygen (Tams 1989). When CO binds with hemoglobin it forms carboxyhemoglobin (COHb), which inhibits its ability to carry oxygen. Furthermore, it causes the oxygen dissociation curve to shift to the left, which decreases oxygen release into the tissues. The ultimate result is hypoxia to the tissues of the body. The brain and the heart are the most sensitive tissues to hypoxia. COHb causes a bright cherry-red or bright pink discoloration to the skin or in areas of lividity.

The symptoms of CO poisoning are based on the percentage of carboxyhemoglobin in the body. The symptoms may be gradual as the CO in the air increases. Animals build up fatal COHb levels faster than adult humans due to their higher metabolic rate (Spitz 2006). At 10%–20% carboxyhemoglobin levels, clinical signs of mild dyspnea, shortness of breath, and confusion appear. The animal becomes more disoriented and loses the will and capability to escape as CO levels increase. With higher levels increased irritability, nausea, vomiting, loss of coordination, and convulsions may be seen. Respiratory failure and death may occur at levels greater than 50%–60% (Tams 1989). Death may occur quickly with sudden high levels. This is thought to result from cardiac arrest because cardiac dysfunction usually occurs prior to central nervous system effects.

In CO poisoning the postmortem exam findings may include dilated bronchi and distension of the major blood vessels. The ventricles of the heart may be dilated, especially the right ventricle, which may result from the sudden increase in central venous pressure sometimes seen in CO toxicity. The cherry red color of the blood may or may not be present (Carson 1986). Brain changes may be seen related to anoxia, including necrosis in the cortex and white matter of the cerebral hemispheres, globus pallidus, and brainstem. Edema, demyelination, and hemorrhage in the brain and necrosis in the Ammon's horn of the hippocampus may occur (Carson 1986).

Tests for carboxyhemoglobin may be run at a human hospital laboratory. Venous blood should be used and transported on ice. The results are reported as the percentage of saturation of hemoglobin in the carboxyhemoglobin state (Tams 1989). The timing of sample collection is important and should be done as soon as possible. The COHb levels decrease over time during blood sample storage with saturation levels dropping up to 20% over three months in frozen blood samples (Spitz 2006). Once the animal is no longer exposed to CO, the carboxyhemoglobin level may return to normal levels within three to four hours of when the animal breathes fresh air (Carson 1986). If the animal breathes 100% oxygen the levels drop more rapidly. This improves tissue oxygenation, especially for the brain and myocardium, and accelerates the elimination of the COHb. The half-life of carboxyhemoglobin is four hours at room air and thirty minutes at 100% oxygen (Tams 1989).

Cyanide gas poisoning in fires

Cyanide gas is produced in a fire by the burning of many common synthetic substances. It is also produced when hydrogen cyanide salts come into contact with an acid. It is rare to be a contributory cause of death in human fire victims due to the relatively low amount of gas produced in a fire.

Cyanide binds to and inhibits the cellular respiratory enzyme mitochondrial cytochrome oxidase, disrupting the ability of cells to use oxygen. It most severely affects the brain and heart. In most cases, death rapidly follows the onset of symptoms. The body may appear pink or cherry red, similar to carbon monoxide poisoning, which is caused by fully oxygenated blood due to the inability of the tissues to extract oxygen from the blood. It is possible for the victim to be cyanotic. The victims of cyanide gas poisoning may have a distinctive aroma of bitter almonds or musty. The ability to smell the aroma is a genetic trait and a significant portion of the human population lack it (Dix et al. 2000).

Diagnostic testing for cyanide gas poisoning can be difficult. Decomposition causes the production of cyanide in the blood, whether in the body or in a test tube artificially increasing the levels. The testing for cyanide is also problematic in that other substances in the blood (sulfides) can react like cyanide, which causes falsely elevated cyanide levels (Di Maio and Di Maio 2001).

REFERENCES

Akyldiz, E., I. Uzun, M.A. Inanici, and H. Baloglu. 2009. Computerized Image Analysis in Differentiation of Skin Lesions Caused by Electrocution, Flame Burns, and Abrasion. *Journal of Forensic Sciences.* 54(6):1419–1422.

Bleetman, A., R. Steyn, and C. Lee. 2004. Introduction of the Taser into British Policing. Implications for UK Emergency Departments: An Overview of Electronic Weaponry. *Emergency Medicine Journal.* 21:136–140.

Carson, T.L. 1986. Toxic Gases. In: *Current Veterinary Therapy IX Small Animal Practice*, R.W. Kirk, ed. pp. 203–205. Philadelphia: W.B. Saunders.

Cattaneo, C. 2012. Fires, Flies, and Wasps: PMI Estimation of Burned Remains. Presented at the American Academy of Forensic Sciences Annual Scientific Meeting, 20–25 February, Atlanta, Georgia.

de Paiva, L.A.S., E.R. Parra, Da.C. da Rosa, C. Farhat, C. Delmonte, and V.L. Capelozzi. 2008. Autopsy-Proven Determinants of Immediate Fire Death in Lungs. *The American Journal of Forensic Medicine and Pathology.* 29(4):323–329.

Di Maio, V.J. and D. Di Maio. 2001. *Forensic Pathology*, Second edition. Boca Raton, FL: CRC Press.

Dix, J., M. Graham, and R. Hanzlick. 2000. *Asphyxia and Drowning: An Atlas*. Boca Raton, FL: CRC Press.

Fraser, C.M. 1986. Physical Influences. In: *The Merck Veterinary Manual*, Sixth edition, C.M Fraser, ed. pp. 611–621. Rahway: Merck and Co., Inc.

Gerdin, J. 2011. Necropsy for the Forensic Veterinarian. Presented at the 4th Annual Veterinary Forensic Sciences Conference of the International Veterinary Forensic Sciences Association, 2–4 May, Orlando, Florida.

Hargis, A.M. and T.P. Lewis. 1999. Full-thickness cutaneous burn in black-haired skin on the dorsum of the body of a Dalmatian puppy. In *Veterinary Dermatology*. 10(1):39–42.

Hedlund, C.S. 2002. Surgery of the Integumentary System. In: *Small Animal Surgery*, Second edition, T.W. Fossum, ed. pp. 134–228. St. Louis: Mosby.

Jutkowitz, L.A. 2005. Care of the Burned Patient. In: *Proceedings of the Eleventh International Veterinary Emergency and Critical Care Symposium*. Atlanta, GA, September 7–11, 2005. pp. 243–249.

Knight, B. 2004. Electrical Fatalities. In: *Knight's Forensic Pathology*, Third edition, pp. 326–338. London: Arnold Publishing.

Levy, A.D., H.T. Harcke, J.M. Getz, and C.T. Mallak. 2009. Multidetector Computed Tomography Findings in Deaths With Severe Burns. *The American Journal of Forensic Medicine and Pathology.* 30(2):137–141.

Munro, H.M. and M.V. Thrusfield. 2001. Battered Pets: Non-Accidental Physical Injuries Found in Dogs and Cats. *Journal of Small Animal Practice.* 42:279–290.

Munro, R. and H. Munro. 2008. Thermal Injuries. In: *Animal Abuse and Unlawful Killing: Forensic Veterinary Pathology*, pp. 47–54. Edinburgh: Elsevier.

Pahor, K. 2012. Detection of Gasoline From Lung Tissue and Heart Blood for Use in Determining Victim Status at the Time of a Fire. Presented at the American Academy of Forensic Sciences Annual Scientific Meeting, 20–25 February, Atlanta, Georgia.

Perper, J.A. 2006. Microscopic Forensic Pathology. In: *Spitz and Fisher's Medicolegal Investigation of Death: Guidelines for the Application of Pathology to Crime Investigation*, Fourth edition. W.U. Spitz and D.J. Spitz, eds. pp. 1092–1134. Springfield: Charles C. Thomas Publisher, Ltd.

Platt, M.S., D.J. Spitz, and W.U. Spitz. 2006. Investigation of Deaths in Childhood, Part 2: The Abused Child and Adolescent. In: *Spitz and Fisher's Medicolegal Investigation of Death: Guidelines for the Application of Pathology to Crime Investigation*, Fourth edition. W.U. Spitz and D.J. Spitz, eds. pp. 357–416. Springfield: Charles C. Thomas Publisher, Ltd.

Saxon, W.D. and R. Kirby. 1992. Treatment of Acute Burn Injury and Smoke Inhalation. In: *Kirk's Current Veterinary Therapy XI Small Animal Practice*, R.W. Kirk and J.D. Bonagura, eds. pp. 146–154. Philadelphia: W.B. Saunders.

Sinclair, L. and R. Lockwood. 2006. Cruelty Toward Cats. In: *Consultations in Feline Internal Medicine*, J.R. August, ed. pp. 693–699. St. Louis: Elsevier Saunders.

Smith, M.M. 1995. Oral and Salivary Gland Disorders. In: *Textbook of Veterinary Internal Medicine: Diseases of the Dog and Cat*, vol. 2, Fourth edition. S.J. Ettinger and E.C. Feldman, eds. pp. 1084–1097. Philadelphia: W.B. Saunders.

Spitz, W.U. 2006. Thermal Injuries. In: *Spitz and Fisher's Medicolegal Investigation of Death: Guidelines for the Application of Pathology to Crime Investigation*, Fourth edition. W.U. Spitz and D.J. Spitz, eds. pp. 747–782. Springfield: Charles C. Thomas Publisher, Ltd.

Tams, T.R. 1989. Pneumonia. In: *Kirk's Current Veterinary Therapy XI Small Animal Practice*, R.W. Kirk and J.D. Bonagura, eds. pp. 376–384. Philadelphia: W.B. Saunders.

8
Firearm Injuries

Melinda D. Merck

Missiles often attain more curious places by accident than they could by design.

Sir John Bland-Sutton

INTRODUCTION

Most animal gunshot victims have a common history of being outside and unattended. A gunshot study of animals revealed that most gunshot wounds involved animals that were allowed to wander outdoors unsupervised. In urban areas, dogs were more likely to be shot in the evening and early morning hours. Handguns were the most common firearm documented in urban areas, with high-velocity rifles and shotguns most common in rural areas. Air-powered firearms, including BB and pellet guns, were more prevalent in suburban areas (Pavletic 1985). In the study by Munro and Thrusfield, the veterinarians surveyed reported air gun injuries in a disproportionately higher number of cats than dogs. In fact, all firearm injuries were reported in a higher number of cats than dogs (Munro and Thrusfield 2001).

To properly interpret gunshot injuries, veterinarians need to understand wound ballistics. Gunshot wounds can be very complex and a large amount of information must be analyzed and documented. Veterinarians must be able to classify the gunshot wounds as entrance or exit, recognize what can affect their appearance, and determine the gunshot range that caused them. They also should recognize wound patterns associated with specific weapons and ammunition and properly collect ballistic evidence. The trajectory of the projectile through the body must be determined and compared with investigation findings.

Finally, the veterinarian must properly record the injuries and prepare the forensic report. Most of the following information on gunshot wounds comes from human gunshot victims with the same principles and guidelines applicable to animals.

OVERVIEW OF FIREARMS

A basic knowledge of firearms is necessary to properly interpret gunshot wounds. There are five categories of small arms: handguns, rifles, shotguns, submachine guns, and machine guns. Military firearms and ammunition are not covered in this chapter. Firearms also can be classified by their velocity, which has a direct impact on the amount of damage inflicted to the victim. High-velocity firearms include high-powered handguns and rifles. They fire a projectile at the speed of 2,500 feet/second or higher, which creates tremendous kinetic energy. Low-velocity firearms include handguns and air-powered guns, which can fire a projectile at the speed of 1,000 feet/second.

Handguns

The four most common types of handguns are single-shot pistols, derringers, revolvers, and auto-loading pistols (automatics). Handguns have rifled barrels (see Rifling). The most common handgun in the United States is the revolver. These have a revolving cylinder that contains several chambers, which hold a single bullet cartridge. This cylinder rotates to align each chamber successively with the barrel and firing pin. The auto-loading pistol is also referred to as automatic pistol, automatic, or pistol. The automatic term comes from the auto-loader, which requires

Veterinary Forensics: Animal Cruelty Investigations, Second Edition. Edited by Melinda D. Merck.
© 2013 John Wiley & Sons, Inc. Published 2013 by John Wiley & Sons, Inc.

the trigger to be pulled for every shot fired. Each time the gun is fired, the pistol uses the forces from the fired cartridge to extract and eject the empty case, load a fresh cartridge, and then return the mechanism to the ready position to fire the new cartridge (Di Maio 1999). These cartridges usually are stored in a removable magazine, also called the clip, which is stored in the grip of the pistol.

Rifles

A rifle is a firearm with a rifled barrel that is made to be fired from the shoulder. The minimum barrel length requirement in the United States is 16 inches (Di Maio 1999).

Shotguns

A shotgun is a firearm with a smooth or rifled barrel that is made to be fired from the shoulder. The smooth bore is designed to fire multiple pellets but also can fire a single projectile. Rifled shotgun barrels are used to fire slugs. Most have a degree of choke, which refers to the partial constriction of the bore at the muzzle to control shot patterns. The choke is usually expressed in shot percentages that fall within a 30-inch circle at 40 yards: 67%–75% full choke, 55%–65% modified, 45%–55% improved cylinder, and 35%–45% cylinder bore (Spitz 2006). The minimum required barrel length in the United States is 18 inches (Di Maio 1999).

Caliber nomenclature

The caliber of the weapon is intended to refer to the inside diameter of the barrel before any rifling is cut into the metal, which also matches the caliber of cartridge used for that particular gun. However, this does not apply to all firearms and their munitions, and caliber designations vary greatly (Di Maio 1999). The term gauge for shotguns is used to describe their caliber, and refers to the number of lead balls, or pellets, of a bore diameter that can make up a pound. A 12-gauge would take twelve lead balls to make up a pound. The exception is the .410, which refers to the bore diameter of 0.410 inches (Di Maio 1999).

Rifling

Rifled barrels are found in handguns, rifles, submachine guns, and machine guns. This rifling is comprised of spiral grooves cut along the length of the interior (bore) of the barrel. The rifling marks are the grooves and the metal between the grooves is called the lands. These marks are unique "fingerprints" to that individual gun. No two barrels are exactly alike, even when cut with the same tools. These rifling marks are imparted to the projectile as it travels down the barrel, allowing ballistic comparisons to identify the weapon from which it was fired.

Decomposition can affect the rifling marks on the bullet, depending on the composition of the bullet and location in the body. Each model of gun has a specific type of rifling and the model of the gun may be determined by examining the projectile. Attempts may be made to modify the rifling by physically altering the muzzle end of the bore. This will rarely damage the entire length and the original rifling may be retrieved by casting the bore.

Rifling causes a rotational spin to the bullet along its longitudinal axis, which stabilizes the bullet's air flight. The term twist refers to the number of inches or centimeters for one complete spiral (Di Maio 1999). When the twist is clockwise, it is referred to as a right twist; when counterclockwise it is called a left twist. Another type of rifling, introduced by Heckler and Koch, is when the bore has a rounded rectangular profile called polygonal boring. This type of rifling makes ballistic comparisons challenging (Di Maio 1999).

Ammunition

The small arms cartridge consists of a cartridge case, primer, propellant (gunpowder), and the bullet or other projectile. The cartridge case is usually made of copper and zinc. It is designed to expand and seal the chamber to prevent the gases from escaping to the rear when fired. The base of the cartridge cases have a head stamp containing letters, symbols, numbers, and/or trade name for identification (Di Maio 1999).

Small arms cartridges contain a primer at the base that explodes through the flash hole and ignites the gunpowder. The cartridge is classified as centerfire if the primer is located in the center, or rimfire if the primer is located around the rim. In the United States, the primer is composed of chemical ingredients: lead stryphnate, barium nitrate, and antimony sulfide. Most primers contain all three chemicals, although some primers contain only two of the components. Gunpowder residue tests detect these compounds (Di Maio 1999).

The weapon used to fire the cartridge may impart unique class characteristics to the cartridge case or primer, which can be used for ballistic comparisons to identify the firing weapon. These markings may be caused by the magazine, firing pin, extractor, ejector, and breach face of the weapon. Propellants used in cartridges may be smokeless powder, Pyrodex (a synthetic black powder), or a combination of both. Smokeless powder may have chemical or graphite coating which may be lost after discharge from a weapon. Uncoated powder grains are pale green or beige and may be found on the fur, skin, or wounds of the victim (Di Maio 1999).

The bullet is located at the tip of the cartridge and leaves the muzzle of the firearm when the cartridge is discharged. Two types of bullets may be used: lead and metal-jacketed. Jacketed ammunition has a lead or steel core covered by a jacket of gilding metal (copper and zinc), gilding metal-clad steel, cupro-nickel (copper and nickel), or aluminum. The bullets may be full metal–jacketed or partial metal–jacketed. Centerfire rifle ammunition used for hunting is partial metal–jacketed. Ammunition for revolvers and automatics may by full or partial metal–jacketed. The two most common forms of partial metal–jacketed bullets are semi-jacketed soft point and hollow point (Di Maio 1999). Both of these forms of ammunition are designed for greater mushrooming of the bullet when it strikes the target.

Bullet distortion may occur on impact or when the bullet is fired from a weapon not appropriate for that caliber of ammunition. Bullets that are severely distorted or fragmented may be analyzed and linked to other ballistic evidence. Quantitative compositional analysis may be conducted using scanning electron microscopy with energy dispersive X-ray (SEM-EDX) (Di Maio 1999). Frangible bullets are growing in popularity because they are lead free, composed of a copper particulate, and non-jacketed. They are designed to dissipate on impact and fragment the target surface yet reduce ricochet and fragmentation when penetrating a hard target. A study on the frangible bullets when penetrating pig heads found bullet fragmentation occurred with 5.56 mm and no fragmentation of smaller ammunition. The 5.56 mm created the expected fragmentation snowstorm on radiographs and the fragment size was insufficient for ballistic comparison (Downs 2012).

The exited bullet may contain tissue or hair evidence related to where the bullet penetrated the body. This is especially useful when multiple bullets are found at the scene to determine which bullet perforated the body. Obvious tissue and hair should be collected (Chapter 2). Tissue may be too small to be identified and may be retrieved through a washing process of the bullet by the forensic lab. A low-velocity bullet usually has greater tissue adherence (Di Maio 1999).

The shotgun cartridge, also called shotgun shell, is comprised of a tube (brass, paper, or plastic); a thin brass or brass-coated steel head; a primer; powder; paper, cardboard, or composition wads; and lead shot. Some may have plastic or felt wads. Buckshot and birdshot shells have granular white polyethylene or polypropylene filler, which can cause stippling marks that extend out a greater distance than the powder tattooing. Birdshot is used for birds or small game and buckshot is used for large game. The smaller the shot size number, the larger the pellet diameter. Buckshot is labeled by the number of pellets per shell (Di Maio 1999).

Shotgun slugs are used for deer and bear hunting in heavily populated areas. The slug rapidly loses velocity, providing protection from shooting accidents. The Brenneke slug is solid lead with a pointed nose, felt and cardboard wads screwed to the base, and twelve angled ribs on the surface. The Foster slug by Winchester is made of soft lead with a round nose, deep concave base, cup wad and cardboard filler wads, and twelve to fifteen angled, helical grooves on the surface. It also can be made with a hollow point. The Remington Foster slug may have a plastic insert on the tip and uses a combination of plastic and cardboard wads. The Federal Foster slugs have a one-piece plastic wad. The Sabot slug has an hourglass configuration with a hollow base with a plastic insert. This slug is enclosed in a Sabot made of two halves of high-density polyethylene plastic. Once the unit exits the muzzle, the Sabot falls away. Depending on the manufacturer, the slug may have a hollow point, a cup wad, cardboard filler wad, and a nose section that separates on impact, which can produce four additional wound tracks (Di Maio 1999).

Firing of a weapon

The firing of a weapon starts with pulling the trigger, which releases the firing pin. The firing pin strikes the primer, crushing it and igniting the primer composition and producing an intense flame. The flame flows through the flash hole in the primer and ignites the powder in the cartridge, producing a large quantity of gas and heat. This heated gas increases the pressure on the base of the projectile and sides of the cartridge case, propelling it down the barrel with some of the gas leaking past and ahead of the projectile and the majority following after it exits the muzzle. As the bullet emerges it is accompanied by a jet of flame, gas, powder, soot, primer residue, metallic particles stripped from the bullet, and vaporized metal from the bullet and cartridge case. The flame is from incandescent superheated gases, which can sear the skin in contact and near-contact wounds. A ball of fire, also called muzzle flash, accompanies the exit of the projectile. This is caused by superheated oxygen-deprived gases reacting to atmospheric oxygen. Revolvers have a cylinder-barrel gap in which soot and powder can exit, causing blackening and powder tattooing of the skin in contact wounds. If the cylinder does not completely line up with the barrel, the bullet may be shaved and fragments cause stippling of the skin.

WOUND BALLISTICS

The amount of damage caused by the gunshot is directly related to the amount of kinetic energy from the projectile that is absorbed by the tissues. The greater the energy transferred to the tissues, the greater the tissue damage. Kinetic energy refers to the energy possessed by a moving object. The kinetic energy is measured by the following equation:

$$\text{Kinetic energy} = \text{mass} \times \text{Velocity}^2/2$$

This equation shows that if the mass of the projectile is doubled, the kinetic energy is doubled, but if the velocity is doubled, the kinetic energy is quadrupled (Kraus 1992).

In gunshots, the projectile causes tissue to balloon outward, stretching and tearing in a process known as cavitation. Cavitation also creates a vacuum affect as it passes through the target, pulling debris and hair deeper into the wound track (Pavletic 2006). This shearing, compression, and contraction process continues as it travels through the body, causing injury to the surrounding tissue, sometimes distant from the bullet's path. Depending on the kinetic energy of the projectile, this may cause rib fractures without a direct impact from the bullet.

In addition to the kinetic energy of the projectile, the degree of injury depends on the characteristics of the tissue through which it travels. If a high-velocity bullet passes through a leg without impact to the bone, the amount of damage depends on the kinetic energy transferred to the surrounding tissue. The thicker and denser the tissue, the more energy is absorbed. The lung and muscle are more resilient and elastic and able to able to absorb a portion of the cavitation process, resulting in less damage (Pavletic 2006).

A bullet can penetrate or perforate bone depending on the velocity, construction, angle of impact, type of bone, its thickness, and its surface configuration. Fracture patterns depend on the type of bone and angle of impact. Cancellous bone is softer and tends to absorb more of the energy, causing less fragmentation. Cortical bone tends to fracture and shatter. The angle of the bullet impact (such as 90° vs. tangential) and the weight and position of long bones also can affect the fracture pattern. Tests were conducted by Vincent Di Maio using fresh human bone and 9-mm Parabellum ammunition loaded with 125 g round nose lead bullets. Using flat bone (4–6 mm thick), bullet penetration with depressed fractures started at 250 feet/second with perforation at 290–300 feet/second. Using bone 7–9 mm thick, perforation started at 350 feet/second. Using bone 10 mm thick, there was no perforation at velocities up to 460 feet/second. Using human femurs, there was no perforation until 552 and 559 feet/second, respectively (Di Maio 1999).

When a bullet penetrates bone, it can cause fragmentation and a temporary cavity which propels bone fragments resulting in additional injury. In the absence of skin surface characteristics, these secondary missiles may contain the only information needed to determine gunshot range, i.e., soot deposits (Spitz 2006). With the undulation of the cavity some of the fragments return to the center. The direction of the bullet can be determined by the appearance of the wound in the bone with outward bone beveling indicating the direction of travel.

Secondary fractures of the skull occur due to intracranial pressure waves generated by the gunshot. These most commonly occur in the thinner bone areas. In contact wounds, the gas produced from the weapon discharge enters the cranial cavity and expands. The more gas that is produced, the more likely there will be secondary fractures. Distant wounds cause secondary fractures by the increased pressure produced by the temporary cavity formation. This is directly related to the kinetic energy lost by the bullet as it passes through the skull (Di Maio 1999).

Gunshot wounds, tissue damage, and the bullet path are affected by the characteristics of the ammunition. The caliber of the bullet, presence of an outer jacket, and design of the jacket directly affect the injuries. The design of the projectile may be for greater tissue damage, such as for bullet fragmentation (frangibility) and partial or complete flattening upon impact (mushrooming). In shotgun wounds, the degree and type of injuries is related to the ammunition and the gunshot range (see Determining Gunshot Range).

Backspatter is the ejection of blood and tissue from an entrance gunshot wound. This may be found on the shooter, the weapon, and nearby objects. Backspatter is more likely to occur with contact wounds to the head than a distant wound to the body. A study was conducted of hard and loose head gunshots using calves. The backspatter was categorized as macrospatter (stain diameter 0.5 mm) and microbackspatter (less than 0.5 mm). Macrospatter was found with every shot with the stains' maximum traveling distance 72–119 cm, the majority 0–50 cm. Microbackspatter was found with every shot with the stains' maximum traveling distance of 69 cm; the majority were 0–40 cm. The microbackspatter stains were more numerous than the macrospatter. The micro-stains were circular or oval and the macro-stains were variable, from circular to exclamation marks. Both stains showed exiting direction of all angles, creating a 180° semi-circle spray, although the individual droplets were uneven and asymmetrical (Di Maio 1999).

DETERMINING ENTRANCE AND EXIT WOUNDS

General characteristics

The type of bullet and the presence, separation, or fragmentation of the jacket affects the appearance of entrance wounds. Entrance wounds are typically smaller than exit wounds. A distant gunshot wound to the head may have a stellate or irregular appearance. This is most often seen over a bony prominence and may be confused with a contact or exit wound. The animal's hair may be pulled inward into the opening of entrance wounds. Dirt, debris, and hair may be dragged further into the wound track.

Most entrance wounds have a zone of reddish to reddish-brown flattened, abraded skin called the abrasion ring, which occurs where the bullet rubbed the edges of the wound as it penetrated the skin (Figures 8.1 and 8.2). An abrasion ring may appear moist or dried. Some bullets do not tend to cause abrasion rings such as centerfire rifle and jacketed/semi-jacketed handgun bullets (Di Maio 1999). The width of the abrasion ring varies depending on the caliber of the weapon, anatomical site of entrance, and angle of entrance. It may appear concentric (90° angle) or eccentric due to entering the skin at an oblique angle. The zone of abrasion is wider in the direction from which the bullet came if the skin surface is flat. Curves and depressions on the body can make this determination difficult (Figure 8.3).

A gray coloration to the abrasion ring, called a bullet wipe, may be seen with entrance wounds. A bullet wipe consists primarily of soot, and sometimes lubricant, from the surface of the bullet that is imparted as it penetrates the skin. This should not be confused with soot and searing found in contact wounds (Di Maio 1999).

Soot is produced by the combustion of gunpowder as it emerges from the muzzle. It contains carbon and vaporized metals from the primer, bullet, and cartridge case. The size, intensity, and appearance of the soot pattern around an entrance wound and the maximum range from which it can occur depend on several factors. These include the gunshot range, propellant, barrel length, angle of the muzzle, weapon caliber, type of weapon, target material, and whether or not the target is bloody (Di Maio 1999). If the muzzle is at a 90° angle to the body, the soot pattern is concentric around the entrance hole. At other angles, the soot pattern is eccentric. Soot may be accidentally removed by wiping or washing the wound depending on the gunshot range (see protocol under Examination of Gunshot

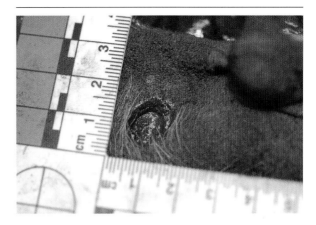

Figure 8.1 Gunshot entrance wound with eccentric abrasion.

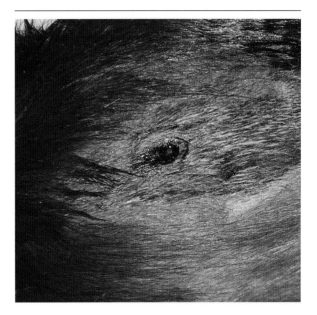

Figure 8.2 Gunshot entrance wound caudal to the right shoulder. (Photo courtesy of Diane Balkin.)

Victims). In cases when there is difficulty determining entrance injuries and associated soot and searing, the area may be excised and submitted for scanning electron microscopy with SEM-EDX analysis (Di Maio 1999).

The muscle around the entrance may have a cherry red color because of carboxyhemoglobin and carboxymyoglobin formed from the carbon monoxide in the muzzle gas. However, perforation of the lung may also cause a bright red discoloration of the surrounding muscle (Spitz 2006). These levels may be detected on chemical analysis of the

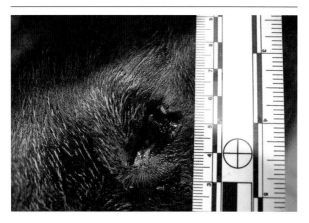

Figure 8.3 Gunshot entrance wound through the right eye.

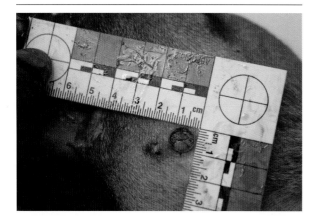

Figure 8.4 Gunshot entrance wound.

muscle, submitting a control sample from another area (Di Maio 1999).

High-velocity projectile entrance wounds may lack abrasion rings and cause micro-tears at the edges that radiate outward from the perforation edges, which may partially or completely involve the circumference (Di Maio 1999). Entrance wounds without abrasion rings have a round to oval punched-out appearance with clean margins (Figure 8.4). Depending on the ammunition, velocity, and tissues impacted, the associated exit wound can appear the same on perforated gunshot wounds. Determination can be accomplished by examining for hair directionality and wound track characteristics (see Determining Trajectory).

In bones, the entrance tends to be round to oval, have clean edges, and have a punched-out appearance. Super-

ficial chips of bone may flake off the edges of an entrance hole. The exit wound is excavated out and appears funnel shaped. Skull entrance wounds are associated with internal beveling of the bone with external beveling more typical of exit wounds. Entrance and exit wounds in thin bone can be difficult to determine (see below) (Di Maio 1999). There may be lead deposits on the bone edges of entrance wounds.

Gunshot wounds to the head in which the bullet does not enter the cranial cavity can cause severe cerebral injury, usually contusions, resulting in death. Tangential gunshot wounds to the skull (gutter wounds) may be classified as first degree when only the outer table of the skull is grooved by the bullet and small bone fragments are carried away. In second-degree gutter wounds, pressure waves created by the bullet fracture the inner table. In third-degree wounds, the bullet perforates the skull in the center of the tangential wound, the outer table of the skull is fragmented, and there are depressed fragments of the internal table. There may be comminution and pulverization of both tables at the wound track and fragments of bone may penetrate the brain. The last classification is superficial perforating wounds in which there are separate entrance and exit holes in the skull (Di Maio 1999).

A keyhole wound can be produced when a bullet strikes the skull at a shallow angle. The bullet begins to penetrate, causing an entrance hole, then part of the bullet shears off and travels under the scalp with the remaining bulk of the bullet entering the skull. At one end of this wound there is a typical entrance wound into the bone with the opposite end having the external beveling associated with the exit (Di Maio 1999).

The tumbling of the bullet, flattening, fragmentation, and kinetic energy absorbed by the body affect the appearance of the exit wounds. Exit wounds are usually larger and more irregular than entrance wounds. They may appear stellate, slit-like, circular, crescent-shaped, or completely irregular (Figure 8.5). Exits through tight skin usually cause larger, irregular, often stellate, wounds. Exits in loose skin can be small and slit-like. Shored exit wounds have abraded margins and are created when the skin is next to a hard surface when the bullet exits, abrading the everted wound margins. The imprint pattern of the surface may be present and there may be wide abrasion collars that may resemble entrance wounds when dry. It is possible for exit wounds to be smaller than the entrance wound and smaller than the diameter of the bullet because of the elastic nature of skin. The shape of the exit wound does not correlate with the type of bullet used (Di Maio 1999).

It is possible for a bullet to have enough velocity to create an exit hole yet not exit the body due to the elastic

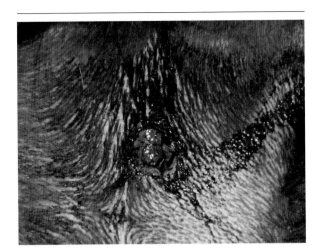

Figure 8.5 Gunshot exit wound associated with Figure 8.2 at the right thoracic inlet, confirming the dog was shot while running away. (Photo courtesy of Diane Balkin.)

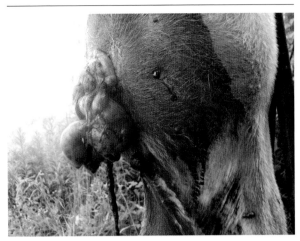

Figure 8.6 Projectile still visible inside exit wound.

nature of the skin or blockage by an object or surface (which will also cause shored margins). The bullet may be found partially protruding from the exit hole or it may have rebounded back into the wound track (Figure 8.6). With the use of semi-jacketed ammunition, the lead core may exit the body while the jacket, which has greater ballistic importance than the lead core, remains in the body. The jacket may be found adjacent to the exit site and only be visible on radiographs. It is important to note that the bullet path of the exiting projectile is not necessarily a straight line. The bullet may be tumbling or deformed and aerodynamically unstable. It can go off in any direction and veer from its projected trajectory. The shorter the path traveled through the body, the more stable the bullet may be upon exiting.

A graze wound is an abrasion created when a bullet strikes the skin at a shallow angle without perforating or tearing the skin. If the injury extends to the subcutaneous tissue, it is called a tangential wound. The entrance end has a partially abraded margin and the exit end is split. Any tears along the margin point in the direction of travel. There may be a bunching of tissue at the end of both graze and tangential wounds (Di Maio 1999).

Shallow perforating wounds in which the entrance and exit are close together are called superficial perforating wounds. The entrance usually has an abrasion ring and the exit usually has only a partial abrasion, which indicates the direction of travel. When a bullet passes through one part of the body (intermediary target) then re-enters another, it is called a re-entry wound. This wound usually is large and irregular with ragged edges and a wide irregular abrasion ring (Di Maio 1999).

Intermediary targets

When a bullet passes through an intermediary object before hitting the body, it can cause significant changes in the wound appearance or number of wounds. For shotgun pellets, the intermediary object may cause wider dispersal of the pellets, making gunshot range determination more difficult. The object may fragment and create stippling. These fragments also may be found embedded in the tip of the bullet. The bullet may become unstable and deformed after passing through the object, creating a larger and more irregular entrance wound with a wider and irregular abrasion ring. A semi-jacketed bullet passing through an intermediary object may become separated from the jacket and both may strike the body. Because of its light weight, the jacket may or may not impact or penetrate the body. The lead from the separated core can be deposited on the entrance wound of the body, simulating soot. This can cause the wound to be misinterpreted as a contact or similar close-range wound (Di Maio 1999).

Caliber determination

The caliber of the bullet that caused the entrance wound cannot be determined by the size of the skin wound. In addition to the diameter of the bullet, the size of the wound is affected by the elasticity of the skin and location of penetration. An entrance in bone cannot be used to determine the caliber, but it can exclude certain calibers. Typically a bullet larger than the diameter of the entrance hole could not have been used. However, bone does have some elasticity and a 9-mm bullet can produce an 8.5-mm hole. The type of bullet can affect the caliber determination in bone. Lead bullets tend to expand on impact, creating larger entrance holes (Di Maio 1999).

Ricochet bullets

Depending on the construction of the bullet, a bullet may strike an object at an angle and ricochet rather than penetrate. Round nose, full metal–jacketed, or low-velocity bullets are more likely to ricochet than flat-nosed, lead, or high-velocity bullets. The bullet may fragment on impact, causing the fragments to spray out in a fan paralleling the plane of the ricochet surface. The surface may fragment with the impact of the bullet causing secondary missile wounds. These may be confused initially with powder tattoo marks but they are larger and more irregular. Ricocheted or deflected bullets may have trace evidence inclusions that survive the wound production process (Haag 2007).

The ricocheting bullet usually tumbles and has an unpredictable trajectory which results in larger, irregular entrance wounds with ragged edges and large, irregular abrasions surrounding the hole. These bullets tend to be penetrating rather than perforating because of the loss of energy from the ricochet. Destabilized full metal-jacketed bullets typically penetrate less than direct strikes by the same bullet. Destabilized jacketed hollow-point bullets often fail to expand and subsequently penetrate more deeply than direct shots with the same bullet (Haag 2007). Sometimes a lead bullet may have a flattened surface on one side that may appear like a ricocheted bullet. This flattening can actually be caused when the bullet strikes a heavy bone such as a femur or humerus. This usually involves a small-caliber low-velocity lead bullet such as the .22 rimfire (Di Maio 1999).

Stippling

Stippling refers to multiple punctate abrasions of the skin caused by the impact of small fragments of foreign material which may be embedded. Powder tattooing, also called powder burns, is stippling caused by gunpowder. These abrasions cannot be wiped away. The powder may be identified by the shape such as ball, cylinder, or flake (thick disks). All embedded particles should be collected for analysis. If the powder is unburned or partially burned, it can be analyzed to identify the material as gunpowder (Di Maio 1999). Powder tattooing is truly an antemortem phenomenon. Its appearance depends on the form of the powder. Flake and cylindrical powder cause irregular-shaped marks of variable size and are reddish-brown in color. They are usually sparse compared with ball powder. Flake powder also can cause slit-like marks when striking on their side. If they penetrate the dermis there may be hemorrhage associated with the sites. Spherical (true) ball powder causes more dense, numerous, fine, circular, and bright red marks. The initial impression is that of an area of petechiae. Flattened ball powder is similar to true ball powder but the marks are fewer in number (Di Maio 1999). On postmortem examination the tattooing can appear gray or yellow.

The pattern of powder tattooing depends on the type of powder, range, barrel length, caliber, and intermediary objects. The greater the gunshot range, the less dense the pattern. A shorter barrel has more unburned particles of powder than a long barrel. The hair coat density of an animal may reduce stippling or the particles may be on the hair surface. Ball powder readily perforates hair at close and medium range. Flake powder may penetrate at close range (Di Maio 1999).

Pseudo-powder tattooing is caused by non-gunpowder fragments as previously discussed and can be easily differentiated from powder tattooing. The markings usually are larger, more irregular, and sparse compared with powder tattoo marks. Larger pieces of the object may be found embedded in the skin.

Insect feeding can resemble powder stippling. These marks often have a linear pattern indicating the feeding path of the insects. They may appear dry, red, or yellow, or have dark brown or black crusts. In humans, gunshot wounds located in hair-dense areas can produce hemorrhage in the surrounding hair follicles that can resemble stippling.

DETERMINING GUNSHOT RANGE

General characteristics

Gunshot range is defined as the range from the muzzle to the target. There are four categories of gunshot range: contact, near-contact, close-range, and distant. Characteristic findings of gunshot wounds that help define the distance from which the animal was shot are affected by the wound location, type weapon, angle of fire, and the ammunition used. The surface characteristics are not affected by decomposition until the skin is degraded in the late active or advanced decay stages of decomposition. Until then, the gunshot wounds can maintain the characteristics unique to each gunshot range. Changes to bullet wound diameter are minimal with decomposition. Insect activity did not produce pseudo-gunshot wounds in one study despite extensive maggot activity (MacAulay, Barr, and Strongman

2009a). Wounds that are covered with ice and snow become desiccated but the characteristics are not altered to the extent that would lead to misinterpretation. Desiccated muzzle impressions from contact wounds and desiccated gunpowder patterns from close-range wounds can still be present (MacAulay, Barr, and Strongman 2009b).

All contact wounds are defined by a tight zone of soot and/or searing of the skin. Subcutaneous hemorrhage around the entrance wound may appear purple to black and be mistaken for soot initially. The dried edges of a gunshot entrance wound may appear blackened, similar to soot. In addition to soot, all contact wounds have powder, carbon monoxide, and vaporized metals from the bullet, primer, and cartridge case deposited in the injury and along the wound tract (Di Maio 1999). Careful layer dissection is required to reveal burned and unburned gunpowder granules and soot deposit within the wound track tissues or bone (see Examination of Gunshot Victims). Soot may be differentiated from a bullet lead deposit by close examination of the bone defect and documenting the location. Soot is distributed circumferentially and lead deposits are localized (Spitz 2006). In contact wounds, the explosive gases entering the body can propel the skin or body toward the muzzle, leaving an imprint of the muzzle on the skin.

Contact wounds may be further characterized as hard contact, loose, angled, and incomplete. In hard contact wounds, the muzzle is pressed firmly to the skin, indenting the skin to envelop the muzzle. The edges of the wound are blackened by the soot and seared by the hot gases of combustion. This soot is embedded in the skin and cannot be removed by wiping or washing the wound.

In loose contact wounds, the muzzle is placed lightly against the skin and is in complete contact. The gas indents the skin, creating a temporary gap through which it can escape. This soot can be wiped away easily. A few unburned powder grains may be found deposited in the zone of soot.

Angled contact wounds are caused by the barrel being held at an acute angle to the skin. The muzzle has incomplete contact with the skin, allowing gas and soot to radiate outward and creating an eccentric pattern of soot. A few powder grains may be found deposited in the zone of soot. The eccentric zone points to the direction in which the gun was directed. If the angle decreases, more material is allowed to escape, producing powder tattooing. Incomplete contact wounds are caused by the curvature of the body. The muzzle is held against the skin, but there is a gap that allows escape of the gas. This produces an elongated zone of soot and searing. Powder tattooing may be seen. In near-contact wounds the muzzle of the gun is held a short distance away from the skin but close enough to prevent

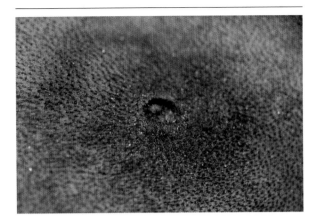

Figure 8.7 Near-contact gunshot entrance wound with visible soot and embedded gunpowder grains.

powder tattooing. The zone of soot is wider and overlying the seared and blackened skin. The soot in the seared zone is embedded and cannot be wiped away. There may be a few clumps of unburned powder grains in the seared area (Figure 8.7). In near-contact angled wounds, two zones are created by the soot: a blackened seared zone on the same side as the muzzle and a light gray fan-shaped zone. This is the opposite of angled contact wounds. To differentiate the two, the bullet path must be correlated to the soot pattern. If both the bullet and soot zone point in the same direction, then it is an angled contact wound. If the bullet points one way and the zone another, it is an angled near-contact wound. As the angle increases, the entrance hole moves toward the center, making it difficult to differentiate between the two types of wounds.

Close-range gunshot wounds are caused when the gun is fired from farther away but close enough to deposit gunpowder residue and produce powder tattooing of the skin. This occurs at distances of 18–24 inches for most handguns and several feet for rifles, depending on the weapon and type of ammunition used (see below) (Spitz 2006). The transition between near-contact and close-range is determined by the presence of distinct, individual tattoo marks. When the muzzle is at an angle, the area on the same size of the muzzle shows denser gunpowder residue and tattooing than on the opposite side. As the distance increases between the muzzle and the target, the density of particle dispersion decreases. For handguns, no soot is usually visible on the target surface beyond 6–7 inches (Spitz 2006). Dense hair may partially or completely filter powder particles. With revolvers, soot and powder may escape from the cylinder gap, producing tattooing of the skin. This pattern is usually sparse and may include fragments from shearing of the bullet. The length of the barrel of a firearm is an important factor on the diameter of the gunpowder pattern deposited on the skin surface. A rule of thumb used for handguns is that gunpowder residue may be identified by naked-eye examination of the target at a distance double the length of the barrel, with barrel length defined as from the cylinder to the muzzle (Spitz 2006).

Distant gunshot wounds typically are characterized by having only the mark of the bullet perforation. Small amounts of soot may be seen along with occasional powder grains. Gunshot residue may be detected on the bone surface or under the periosteum in gunshot wounds where the gunshot range is up to six feet (Berryman, Kutyla, and Davis 2010).

Handgun gunshot wounds

Handguns are low-velocity, low-energy weapons with muzzle velocity below 1,400 feet/second. Hard contact wounds to the head from .22 Short or .32 Smith and Wesson Short cartridges can be difficult to interpret because of the small amount of powder in these cartridges. They may appear to be distant wounds because of the apparent lack of soot or unburned powder grains. A dissecting microscope is needed to examine the wound. The maximum distance for soot deposition of most handguns is 20—30 cm (Di Maio 1999).

A contact wound to skin overlying bone tends to be stellate or cruciform in appearance. This rarely occurs in contact wounds to the trunk. This is caused by the gas of discharge, which expands the subcutaneous tissue, lifting and distending the skin, which often creates tears radiating from the entrance hole. This tearing and its extent depend on the caliber of the weapon, amount of gas produced, firmness with which the muzzle was held to the skin, and elasticity of the skin. The margins can be re-approximated to reveal the original entrance hole. Less powerful calibers may cause very large, circular wounds with blackened, seared margins. Occasionally this is seen with more powerful cartridges (Di Maio 1999).

Contact wounds of the head tend to have soot deposited on the outer table of the skull located at the entrance wound. It also may be found on the inner table and dura. A wound caused by either a .22 Short or .32 Smith and Wesson Short cartridge usually does not have soot on the bone (Di Maio 1999).

Muzzle imprints with contact wounds from handguns can occur in the chest and abdomen and in places where there is a thin layer of skin overlying the bone. These imprints may be larger than the actual dimensions of the muzzle. A zone of abraded skin may be seen from the skin sliding against the muzzle and flaring back to envelop the muzzle. This may be confused as a zone of searing from the hot gases which contains soot, whereas this zone of abraded skin does not (Di Maio 1999).

Contact wounds to the head, chest, or abdomen from handguns do not cause the massive injuries seen with rifles or shotguns because of the smaller gas explosion from the barrel. The exceptions are Magnum-caliber, or high-velocity, high-energy cartridge loadings of medium-caliber weapons.

Near-contact wounds may have small clumps of unburned powder on the edges of the entrance injury and the seared zone of skin. This is most evident in wounds created by .22 Magnum handguns with cartridges containing ball powder. Near-contact wounds from handguns usually occur at ranges less than 10 mm (Di Maio 1999). The searing or burning of hair is rarely seen in humans. This is thought to result from the gas emerging and blowing the hair away.

Close- or distant range gunshots can cause irregular, cruciform, or stellate entrance wounds. This occurs in areas in which the skin is over a bony prominence or in places where the bone is curved with a thin, tightly stretched layer of skin. Close-range wounds may have blackening of the skin in addition to powder tattooing. This soot is absent beyond 30 cm. The pattern of powder tattooing may indicate the range, depending on the weapon. From experiments on animals, the .38 Special revolver with a 4-inch barrel and cartridges with flake powder produce powder tattooing out to 18–24 inches, with flattened ball out to 30–36 inches with true or spherical powder out to 36–42 inches. These maximum ranges should be used as a rough guide. Pseudo-gunpowder stippling has been reported due to the fragmentation of a plated bullet during the gun barrel transit. This can result in misclassification of the gunshot range or improper conclusions regarding ricochet or interposed target (Prahlow et al. 2003).

Distant gunshot wounds from handguns begin beyond 24 inches for cartridges with flake powder and beyond 42 inches for ball powder. Further range determination is not possible.

.22 Caliber rimfire weapon gunshot wounds

The .22 rimfire cartridge is the most commonly fired cartridge in the United States and may be used in handguns or rimfire rifles. The four types of ammunition are the .22 Short, .22 Long, .22 Long Rifle, and .22 Winchester Magnum rimfire.

Contact wounds from the .22 Short have a no tears, little deposition of soot or powder, and some blackening and searing of the edges. The absence of soot and powder is more pronounced with rifles. There may be a muzzle imprint with hard contact wounds. Head contact wounds usually have no skull fractures. The bullet ricochets within the cranial vault and does not exit (Di Maio 1999).

Hard contact wounds to the head from the .22 Long Rifle can range in appearance from a circular perforation with a narrow band of blackened, seared skin to a larger, circular wound with ragged, blackened, seared edges. Soot, powder, and searing are evident and muzzle imprints are common. The bullet may perforate the body. Secondary fractures of the skull are seen with the bullet exiting (Di Maio 1999).

Contact wounds with the .22 Magnum cartridge are more destructive, resulting in stellate wounds. Ball powder can be found at the exit wounds. Extensive secondary fractures of the skull may be seen and the bullet usually exits. Muzzle imprints are common and the bullet may perforate the body (Di Maio 1999). In close-range wounds, the powder tattoo pattern depends on the type of powder and barrel length. In tests conducted on rabbits, a .22 caliber rimfire revolver with a 2-inch barrel firing .22 Long Rifle cartridges with flake powder produces powder tattooing out to 18–24 inches and absent at 30 inches, with ball powder out to 12–18 inches. The flake powder extends farther than the ball powder because the balls are so light and small (Di Maio 1999).

Distant gunshot wounds are usually circular and can measure 5 mm in diameter, including the abrasion ring. They may be 3 mm where the skin is very elastic and be misinterpreted as puncture wounds. The .22 hollow-point bullets do not usually mushroom on impact when fired from a handgun. They may mushroom when fired from a rifle because of greater velocity. The .22 Long Rifle bullets can produce linear fractures of the skull in distant-range wounds.

Centerfire rifle gunshot wounds

Wounds from centerfire rifles are significantly different than those from handguns or .22 rimfire rifles. The muzzle velocity of centerfire rifles ranges between 2,400 and 4,000 feet/second. The muzzle kinetic energy ranges from 1,000 to 5,000 feet pound. A centerfire rifle gunshot wound can result in injuries distant from the wound track (Di Maio 1999).

The bullets for centerfire rifles have either full or partial metal jacketing. The full metal-jacketed bullet is used by the military. Soft-point rifle bullets have a partial metal-jacketing with the lead core exposed to facilitate expansion when the bullet strikes. Hollow-point rifle bullets are partial

metal-jacketed hunting bullets with a lead core and cavity at the tip to facilitate expansion when it strikes. The last category of bullets is a miscellaneous group of controlled expansion projectiles (Di Maio 1999).

Contact wounds of the head produce a bursting rupture of the head. The entrance wounds have large, irregular tears radiating from the site. There is usually soot and searing at the entrance. The entrance may be difficult to identify because of the destruction. The large quantities of gas produced emerge from the muzzle, delivering an explosive effect. If the rifle is discharged in the mouth, massive wounds to the mouth and face are seen (Di Maio 1999).

Contact wounds to the chest and abdomen usually have a circular and large injury. There is usually no tearing of the skin. Soot is found in and around the wound, although there is usually less than that found in handgun wounds. The imprint of the muzzle is common, and it may include the front sight or the end of the magazine (in lever-action weapons). The internal injuries produced usually are massive, including organ destruction. The musculature around the entrance and exit may have cherry red coloration from the large amount of carbon monoxide gas (Di Maio 1999).

Powder tattooing is present in close-range wounds. The range for tattooing depends on the type of powder. Ball and cylindrical powder are used in centerfire bullets. Powder tattooing extends farther out with ball powder than with flake in centerfire cartridges because of the aerodynamic form of the ball powder. Tests were conducted on rabbits with different powder forms. With the .30-30 rifle and cartridges located with cylindrical powder there was heavy powder tattooing with soot deposition at 6 inches, by 12 inches there were only a few scattered tattoo marks, by 18–24 inches there were none. With ball powder, tattooing extended out to 30 inches with moderate density; at 36 inches there were no tattoo marks. With the .223 rifle and cartridges loaded with cylindrical powder, there was rare tattooing out to 12 inches; at 18 inches there were no marks. With ball powder there was heavy tattooing at 18 inches, scattered at 36 inches, and absent at 42 inches. These findings may serve as a guide to the maximum distances at which powder tattooing can occur (Di Maio 1999).

The severity of the head wound with close and distant wounds depend on the style of bullet and entrance site. Bullets entering through thicker bone cause greater injuries. Expanding bullets can cause as much destruction as contact wounds. The location of the entrance and exit wounds can require skull reconstruction. Distant and close-range entrance wounds over bone can appear stellate because of temporary cavity formation and tearing of the skin (Di Maio 1999).

Distant wounds to the trunk may appear as round, punched-out holes with micro-tears with abrasion rings. The internal injuries are massive with severe organ tissue destruction. The chest or abdominal wall may be propelled outward and have an imprint of an adjacent object (Di Maio 1999).

Exit wounds for all ranges are larger and more irregular than entrance wounds. They are usually 25 mm or less in diameter but can be as large as 40 mm (Di Maio 1999).

Radiographs of victims shot with hunting ammunition show a typical pattern called a lead snowstorm or lead shower. Fragments of lead break off the lead core and are propelled into the surrounding tissues. The X-ray shows hundreds of small radiopaque fragments along the wound track. They can vary from dust-like to large, irregular pieces. Pieces of the jacket may be seen. This phenomenon does not require the bullet to hit bone. The absence of the lead snowstorm does not rule out centerfire hunting ammunition. The bullet may be traveling at low velocity because of an extreme range or from passing through an intermediary target. A similar finding can be seen with head wounds from a .357 Magnum. However, the breakup of the bullet requires perforation of the bone and the fragments usually are larger and fewer in number with the absence of lead dust (Di Maio 1999).

Hunting or medium- and large-caliber bullets exit the body. The .222 or .22-250 varmint cartridges tend to stay in the body. With other ammunition, the ability to perforate the body depends on the weight of the bullet, the body location penetrated, and length of the wound path (Di Maio 1999).

Shotgun gunshot wounds

Shotguns are the most destructive of all small arms. The severity and lethality of birdshot and buckshot loads depends on the number of pellets that enter the body, organs struck, and amount of tissue destruction. There is no temporary cavity injury associated with pellet wounds. Shotgun slugs produce direct wounds as well as injury from temporary cavity formation.

As the range increases, there is a decrease in the number of pellets that strike the victim and a rapid decline in velocity of the pellets. The larger shot retains its velocity better than small shot. The maximum effective hunting range for birdshot is 45–65 yards. The maximum traveling range for lead birdshot is 110 yards for number 12 shot and 396 yards for BB shot. The maximum range for buckshot is 528 yards for number 4 Buck and 726 yards for number 00 Buck. The effective range is much less because of the velocity needed to penetrate skin (Di Maio 1999).

The general rule for all shotgun wounds and range of fire is: circular wound: contact to 2 feet; scalloped margins on wound: 3 feet; pellet marks only: 6 to 7 feet (de Jong 2011). The entrance wound of a shotgun slug is circular with a diameter measuring that of the slug, although the gauge cannot be determined. The wound edge is abraded. The wads may enter through the entrance wound or strike adjacent skin, causing circular, oval, or elliptical contusions or abrasions. With the Sabot slug, the two halves of the Sabot may enter the body or impact the skin; or, depending on the manufacturer, there may be wounds or tracks created by four different components (see Ammunition). With the Brenneke slug, the wadding enters the wound because it is screwed into the base. Slugs produce massive internal injuries similar to those of centerfire rifle hunting bullets. They tend to flatten and remain in the body. Comma-like pieces may break off of the disk (Di Maio 1999).

Wounds from buckshot and birdshot depend on the gunshot range. A contact wound is circular and the diameter the same as the bore of the gun. The wound edges are abraded and seared. Soot may be deposited in loose contact wounds. Powder tattooing appears when the range increases beyond a few centimeters. In 12-gauge shotguns, this extends out to a maximum of 90–125 cm for ball powder and 60–75 cm for flake. The diameter of the entrance wound increases as the range increases. For buckshot ammunition at a distance of 3 feet, the wound edges have a scalloped shape; at 4 feet the buckshot pellets separate to produce a large gaping wound with a few satellite wounds; by 9 feet there are individual pellet wounds.

The wad follows the buckshot into the wound at close range but as this range increases, the wad usually impacts the skin, causing a circular, oval, or elliptical contusion or abrasions. This may be found among or adjacent to the pellet wounds. Cork filler wads may fragment on firing, causing irregular abrasions on the skin (Di Maio 1999). Injuries associated with large numbers of small projectiles are due to their dispersion as they strike one another upon penetration into the body, or a billiard ball effect. This does not usually apply to 00 buck shot due to its larger mass. The pellets can become emboli in live victims. It is possible to see lead marks from the pellets inside the cranium. For birdshot injuries, the firing distance can be estimated by using the following guideline: measure the diameter of the largest cluster of skin injuries in inches and multiply by 3 to obtain the number of feet for the firing distance (Spitz 2006).

In general, contact shotgun wounds cause massive, mutilating damage. Large fragments of the skull and brain may be ejected from the head. This is caused by the charge

Table 8.1 Linear regression analysis for shotguns.

Shotguns	Shot size	a	b
12-gauge (full choke)	2	−60.4	94.1
	5	−45.1	84.3
12-gauge (cylinder bore)	2	−7.8	51.7
	5	11.5	39.0
16-gauge (cylinder bore)	2	−44.8	66.4
	5	−27.5	53.6

Note: Modified from original table. Overall data adjusted $R^2 = 0.82$.

Source: Arslan, M.M., H. Kar, B. Üner, and G. Çetin. 2011. Firing Distance Estimates with Pellet Dispersion from Shotgun with Various Chokes: An Experimental, Comparative Study. *Journal of Forensic Sciences*. 56(4):988–992.

of the shot, which directly fractures the skull, shreds the brain, and produces pressure waves. The gas expands, adding to the pressure waves, which shatters the skull. The entrance wound has large quantities of soot and the edges are seared and blackened. The pellet exit site may be difficult to determine because of the large amount of missing tissue and bone (Di Maio 1999).

Close range wounds to the head cause similar mutilation seen with contact wounds due to the pellets traveling in a single mass. There are large gaping tears at the entrance, which when re-approximated have an abrasion ring. The pellet exit site may be difficult to determine (Di Maio 1999).

Contact wounds to the trunk have a circular entrance and a diameter measuring approximately that of the bore of the gun. The edges are seared and blackened without soot in hard-contact wounds. A muzzle imprint is common, including the front sight. The wound may be surrounded by a wide zone of abraded skin from the skin flaring against the muzzle. In loose-contact or near-contact wounds there is a circular area of soot that increases in diameter but reduces in density as the distance increases. Soot deposition continues out to approximately 30 cm. The muscle at the entrance may be cherry red from the carbon monoxide gas. This can spread 15 cm or greater from the entrance and may follow the path of the shot through the body (Di Maio 1999).

Powder tattooing occurs at ranges beyond 1–2 cm. This tattooing is less dense than that found with handguns. Testing on rabbits, conducted using a 12-gauge shotgun with a 28-inch barrel and flake powder in the shells, showed powder tattooing out to 24 inches and absent by 30 inches; with ball powder the tattooing was present at 30 inches, few marks at 36 inches, and absent by 40 inches (Di Maio 1999). In addition to powder tattooing, petal marks (four petals) may be seen from plastic shot cups 1–3

feet with 12-, 16-, and 20-gauge shotguns. In .410 shotguns, the petal marks (three petals) appear at 3–5 inches and are absent at 2 feet.

Wadding may be found inside the shotgun wound or it may create a separate, typically circular, entrance wound. It can impact the skin surface causing abrasions or bruising. It may impact the edge of the entrance wound, causing an irregular abraded margin on one side. If the shell contains an over-the-shot wad and a plastic cup, there may be two sets of wad markings. As the distance increases, the wad loses energy and fails to mark the skin. It is not usually found in the body at gunshot distances of greater than 6 feet (de Jong 2011). With filler wads, marks may be seen out to 15 feet and plastic wads out to 20 feet (Di Maio 1999).

With distant wounds, the circular wound diameter increases until the pellet mass separates, producing individual pellet wounds. Photographs should be taken and the spread pattern measured for comparison of test shots. Individual pellets also should be measured. Range determination is usually made using the actual weapon and same brand of ammunition to conduct a series of test shots, though some studies have provided guidelines. A 2011 study determined firing distance estimates using pellet dispersion from 12- and 16-gauge shotguns with various chokes (Table 8.1). The study produced a formula to determine firing distance (FD) using linear regression analysis based on the radius of pellet dispersion with an R-value of 82% (Arslan et al. 2011):

$$FD = a + b \times R$$

(FD : firing distance; a and b :
fixed values for each shotgun;
R: radius of largest circumscribed circle of
pellet dispersion as centimeter)

At 2 feet, birdshot (regardless of gauge) produced a 0.75- to 1-inch wound; at 3 feet the wound had scalloped margins and measured 7/8 inch for modified choke and 1.25 inches for a cylinder bore; at 4 feet, the wound was 1 inch for modified choke and 1.75 inches for cylinder bore with scattered satellite pellet wounds; at 6–7 feet there was a cuff of satellite pellet wounds around an irregular wound for a modified choke; the wound was ragged with a prominent cuff of pellet wounds; at greater distances there was large variation in the size of the pellet pattern depending on the ammunition, choke of the gun, and range (Di Maio 1999).

Air weapon gunshot wounds

Animals are often the target of air-powered guns and these low-velocity firearms can cause severe and even fatal damage. Air-powered guns range from toy BB guns to expensive and highly sophisticated air rifles. Some air weapons have smooth bores and others have rifled bores which can impart rifling marks on certain types of ammunition. The models are constantly changing with variable muzzle velocities due to manufacturer enhancements.

A steel BB gun can have a muzzle velocity of 275–350 feet/second. In pneumatic type guns, the air is pumped into a storage chamber and can produce a maximum velocity of 770 feet/second. The spring-air compression system uses a powerful spring compressed by manual action that produces velocities of 1,000 feet/second or higher. The air rifle has a rifled barrel and uses compressed air or gas to propel the projectile. Carbon dioxide is used for gas-compression systems, which have the same muzzle velocity of spring rifles. The minimum velocity required for eye penetration of 4.5-mm steel BB in pigs and rabbits is 56–66 meters/second (184–217 feet/second). The minimum velocity required for eye penetration of a 6-mm plastic projectile in pigs is 99 meters/second (325 feet/second) (Marshall, Dahlstrom, and Powley 2011).

The calibers used are 0.177, 0.20, and 0.22 inches. The most common ammunition for air-powered guns is the Diabolo pellet, an hourglass shaped, soft-lead missile. The rifling of the barrel is on the front edge. These pellets lose velocity rapidly and are harmless at less than 100 yards. Pointed conical bullets are made for air rifles.

Captive-bolt gun gunshot wounds

Captive-bolt guns are most commonly used as weapons for humane slaughtering of animals by placement of the gun against the animal's forehead. It is used in the meat industry and may be used by farmers, especially in areas where firearm licensure is an issue. The gun consists of a simple cylindrical metal barrel with a heavy flange muzzle from which a metal bolt is launched upon discharge of a blank powder gun cartridge. The bolt is usually 15–17 cm long and 1 cm wide. The tip of the bolt is concave with very sharp edges similar to a circular punching tool.

After launching, the bolt is pulled back into the barrel by a withdrawal spring. Around the central barrel there are two lateral round openings as diverging smoke conduits, 0.3-cm diameter with 2.2-cm distance between them, which serve as outlets for the explosion gases while the bolt seals the wound, preventing soot or gas entrance into the wound. Wounds caused by captive-bolt guns have specific morphological features that distinguish these wounds than those made by other handguns. Depending on the angle and distance of the muzzle, these wounds have a punched round entrance wound and double pattern smoke soiling on either side of the wound. The entrance hole and soot appearance can identify the weapon, direction of discharge, angle, and distance of the muzzle (Simic et al. 2007).

When the gun is placed perpendicularly to the animal forehead the wound created is a central round defect of the skin and underlying soft tissue. The entrance wound edges are smooth and flat without contusions and the diameter is the exact size or smaller than the bolt diameter. On either side of the entrance wound there are eccentric oval zones of blackening from the smoke conduits. Hair or fur may act as a filter and lessen the soot deposition. The entrance wound on the outer plate of the skull is round with sharp edges, approximately the same diameter as the bolt and without soot deposits. The inner table of the skull has beveling resembling a gunshot wound defect. Radiating bone fractures are not common with captive bolt wounds. When the gun is placed at an oblique angle it may produce an incomplete, semicircular entrance wound, similar to a flap, with associated contusions. The powder discharges tend to produce two elongated eccentrically blackened areas which decrease in intensity as angle of firing decreases and the zone radiates outward and wider. Near-contact firing displays larger and even less intensive soot or blackening patterns (Simic et al. 2007).

The brain injury tends to be less than that from standard contact gunshot wounds because there is no intracranial gas pressure associated with captive-bolt guns due to the sealing by the bolt. The wound track is due to the bolt and associated bone projectiles. The brain lesions around the track are similar to those from low-velocity projectiles (less than 300 meters/second) even though the captive-bolt gun has an even lower impact velocity of less than 50 meters/second. This is thought to be due to kinetic energy transfer from the bolt and bone fragments to the soft tissue. There are no associated indirect lesions from the impact such as skull fractures, intracerebral hemorrhages, or cortical contusions (Simic et al. 2007).

Stud gun (nail gun) gunshot wounds

Stud guns are common tools used in construction work that are similar to firearms in that they fire metal studs into concrete, steel, or wood. They have tremendous penetrating power with caliber capacities ranging from .22– .38. There are no distinguishing marks on the missiles that can be used for matching to a particular stud gun. If there is a missile still present in the body it should be carefully removed to protect any associated evidence on the object (Chapter 6). Testing was conducted on human cadavers at close and distant ranges in different body areas. At 3 inches, a 1-inch diameter wound was created in the thigh and produced extensive skull fractures. At 27 inches, 6 feet, and 9 feet, the missiles perforated the body and the wounds showed no marginal abrasions (Spitz 2006).

EXAMINATION OF GUNSHOT VICTIMS

Gunshot injuries may easily be mistaken for puncture wounds, bite wounds, or lacerations. Any animal with unexplained wounds should have full body radiographs taken. Additional examination findings may be an indicator of a gunshot injury including pneumothorax, pneumomediastinum, cardiac tamponade, dyspnea, lethargy, limping, fractures, peritonitis, hemoabdomen, and hemothorax. The animal also may present with symptoms of lead poisoning from a retained projectile in the body. This is commonly seen when a projectile is inside the joint, where the synovial fluid dissolves the lead with slow systemic absorption.

As discussed in Chapter 3, it is important to have all the investigation information and crime scene investigation findings, especially with regard to weapon and ammunition, prior to examining a gunshot victim. All gunshot victims should have full body radiographs to locate the projectile and injuries. It is important to consider that the animal may have suffered additional injuries such as blunt force trauma and the skin should be reflected on deceased animals to look for evidence of injury (Chapter 3).

Each gunshot wound should be photographed *in situ*, then shaved to reveal wound characteristics and any skin surface evidence and re-photographed. Any surface, wound, or wound tract evidence should be collected (see below). The sequence of multiple gunshot wounds may be difficult to determine. Assessment of the associated wound hemorrhage can provide clues to their sequence and detect postmortem injuries. The wound findings should be compared to witness and suspect statements. Layer dissection of the wound track should be performed on necropsy. This can be done in a flap-by-flap method which allows documentation of the wound track, wounds linked with the temporary and permanent cavity, associated ballistic evidence, and determination of trajectory (Freminville et al. 2011).

In decomposed bodies where the wound morphology is significantly modified, antimony can still be detected using gunshot residue analysis testing. This includes situations where the body has almost reached skeletonization, confirming a questioned wound is due to gunshot (Gibelli et al. 2010). Other components of gunshot residue, barium and lead, also may be detected is decomposed tissue. The detection in blowfly larvae was found only on days three and four postmortem (LaGoo et al. 2010). Firearms detection field kits may be used to detect lead from wounds. This can help confirm gunshot injury where the wound characteristics are unclear. These detection kits have been used on skulls that have been buried for several years.

Collection of gunshot residue

Gunshot residue (GSR) is the result of the discharge of a firearm through gases or particles leaving the end of the barrel or escaping through openings in the weapon. GSR may be comprised of primer, powder, and/or projectile material, and the products of their combustion. The composition of ammunition varies based on type and manufacturer.

GSR may be deposited around the wounds and found on the hands of the shooter. It is analyzed at a crime lab and its presence and location can assist with gunshot range determination. Gunshot wounds should be examined for evidence of GSR, and samples collected prior to cleaning the wound. Blood may obscure its presence; the blood can be removed with spraying of hot water or hydrogen peroxide to dissolve it. GSR may be found on the skin surrounding the entrance wound, inside the opening, and in the wound track. Primer-derived GSR may be found on the bone surface and under the periosteum. This may be useful in cases where the gunshot wound is atypical or for differentiating bone fracture from blunt force trauma (Berryman, Kutyla, and Davis 2010). These areas should be swabbed or scraped to collect the residue (Chapter 2). Any gunpowder grains should be collected and described (flake, ball, or cylinder). The animal may have licked the wound, potentially removing evidence.

In charred bodies, cellulose nitrate, a main component of gunpowder, may be identified in the wound track by Fourier transform infrared (FT-IR) microscopy.

Gunpowder has a variable microscopic appearance depending on the extent to which it has been burned. Nearly completely burned gunpowder appears as dark, nearly opaque granular carbonaceous material. Less severely burned gunpowder appears as slightly larger pieces of granular to polygonal, variably translucent material. Less burned or unburned gunpowder appears as large, ovoid, translucent particles. Detection of gunpowder in the wound track of charred remains can assist with the determination of direction and range of the gunshot (Dolinak, Wise and Jones 2008).

Collection of projectiles and wadding

The location of all bullets and fragments must be determined to retrieve the projectile. Full body radiographs should be taken to identify the presence of projectiles and related injuries. The presence of an exit wound does not necessarily indicate the bullet fully exited (see Determining Entrance and Exit Wounds). Careful handling and packaging of the body at the scene is required to prevent loss of ballistic evidence. Previous gunshot wounds typically are surrounded by fibrous tissue without associated hemorrhage or corresponding skin wounds (Figure 8.8). Bullet emboli are possible, causing the projectile to travel distances from the wound track through the bloodstream. Projectiles that enter the airways may be coughed up and swallowed, locating in the stomach.

The bullet and all the fragments must be removed carefully, avoiding the creation of additional surface marks. The rifling marks on the bullet surface are crucial for ballistic comparisons. Removal may be performed using gloved fingers or protected instruments covered with cotton, tape, or plastic IV tubing. For multiple projectiles, the bullet should be identified with a number or letter on the base using a soft marking pencil. For pelleted shotgun wounds, a representative sample of the projectiles should be collected and packaged (Chapter 2). The entrance wound should be examined for the presence of the wadding associated with shotgun wounds which may be composed of plastic, cork, or cardboard. Forensic examination of the wad can determine the gauge of the shotgun and make of the ammunition. Plastic wads and Sabots may retain scratch marks important for ballistic comparisons.

Manufacturers of ammunition make up a large batch of molten lead to make thousands of bullets to which they add a certain amount of trace elements that are unique to that batch. For gunshot injuries where only fragments are present, the lab can run an elemental analysis that can be compared to other ammunition associated with the investigation.

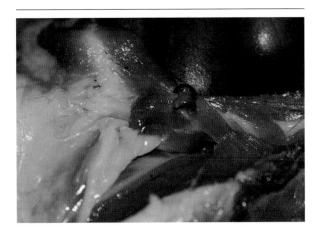

Figure 8.8 Older gunshot injury. Note the lack of associated hemorrhage and fibrous covering.

Collection of casings

Casings are usually found at the crime scene. Infrequently, casings may be found in the body. The casings contain important forensic evidence, including potential fingerprints, and should be carefully collected and packaged (Chapter 2). The end of the casing typically has marks created by the firearm (see Ammunition). The firing pin has unique characteristics that are transferred to the casing when the cartridge is fired, which can be used for ballistic comparisons. After the bullet is fired, the casing moves backward and contacts the breech face of the gun. This marking has unique and distinctive marks from the manufacturer of the gun. When a shotgun is fired the firing pin will leave a distinctive mark on the shell casing.

Determining trajectory

The projectile directory through the body is important to interpret crime scene findings, determine the location and position of the shooter and the victim, and support or refute witness or suspect statements. To evaluate the trajectory, it is important to determine all the injuries and tissue destruction from the projectile (Figure 8.9). Considerations should be given to the dynamic actions and motion of the victim and/or shooter and their expected behaviors, especially in multiple gunshot case. Interpretation of the examination findings, crime scene, forensic analyses, and investigation information can be used to recreate the crime.

Certain exam findings can assist with the determination of the projectile pathway (Figures 8.10–8.12). Blood clots and hemorrhage are associated with injury to major vessels or severe tissue injury. Bone fracture characteristics, beveling, lead deposits, and embedded projectile fragments can

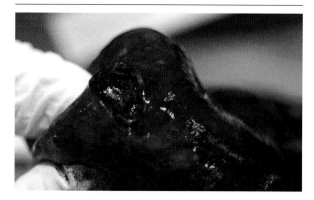

Figure 8.9 Gunshot wound through the lung with projectile still attached. (Photo courtesy of Dr. Doris Miller.)

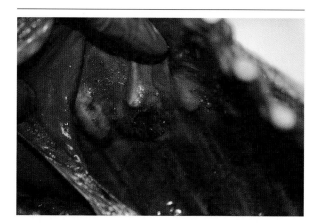

Figure 8.10 Gunshot wound inside thorax with everted, irregular edges indicating direction of projectile travel into the chest.

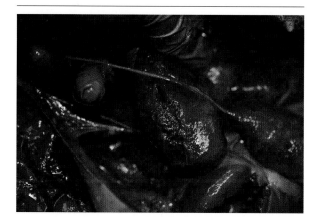

Figure 8.11 Wound track on surface of lung.

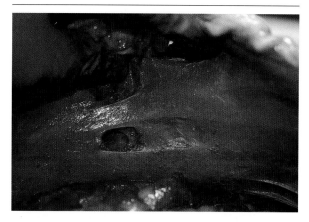

Figure 8.12 Wound track abrasion on interior surface of abdominal wall.

be seen in bone fractures, indicating direction of travel (see above). The embedded fragments may not be grossly visible and only detected with magnification. A projectile does not usually veer off the trajectory path after striking or perforating bone unless it has lost all of its forward velocity. In this case, the bullet may be found within a short distance of the impact site.

To visualize the bullet path, care should be taken to preserve the evidence of injury using flap dissection as discussed above. Radiographs can provide trajectory information. The track may be carefully probed, avoiding dislodging the missile or creating false tracks. Special trajectory rods are available from evidence collection supply companies. Other rods may be used such as metal or plastic rods from a craft store or rifle cleaning rods. Rods with some elasticity allow easier manipulation with probing. Establishing the wound track and trajectory may involve direct or retrograde probing of the entrance wounds, exit wounds, or from within body cavities.

Documentation of examination findings

All ballistic evidence and injuries should be photographed and recorded with written and diagram documentation. The Evidence of Injury section in the report templates maybe used to document the gunshot wounds and associated injuries (Chapter 3). An identification system that corresponds to associated wounds can be used. Because numbers are normally used to identify other lesions or wounds on a body, a different system may be used to eliminate confusion, especially in gunshot cases where there are additional injuries. A letter-number system can be used where letters designate the gunshot wound and numbers designate entrance vs. exit: the number one (1) is used for entrance and number two (2) is used for exit wounds. For example: A1=entrance wound A, A2=exit wound associated with A1.

The wound's location should be described using location references (e.g., dorsal, caudal) and taking measurements from a nearby physical landmark. The appearance of the wound and surrounding features should be described (wound measurements, estimated gunshot range). Multiple gunshot wounds, such as from shotguns, may be handled as groups. For stippling patterns, abrasion rings, burns, or muzzle imprints, measurements should be taken using a clock reference, making the midline of the body 12:00. The trajectory through the body should be described using estimated angles from physical reference planes. The injuries should be described including all tissues penetrated or perforated. The appearance of any recovered ballistic evidence should be described and its location documented.

REFERENCES

Arslan, M.M., H. Kar, B. üner, and G. Çetin. 2011. Firing Distance Estimates with Pellet Dispersion from Shotgun with Various Chokes: An Experimental, Comparative Study. *Journal of Forensic Sciences.* 56(4):988–992.

Berryman, H.E., A.K. Kutyla, and J.R. Davis, II. 2010. Detection of Gunshot Primer Residue on Bone in an Experimental Setting—An Unexpected Finding. *Journal of Forensic Sciences.* 55(2):488–491.

de Jong, J.L. 2011. Gunshot Wounds. Presented at the 63rd Annual Scientific Meeting of the American Academy of Forensic Sciences, 21–26 February, Chicago, Illinois.

Di Maio, V.J.M. 1999. *Gunshot Wounds: Practical Aspects of Firearms, Ballistics, and Forensic Techniques.* Boca Raton, FL: CRC Press.

Dolinak, D., S.H. Wise, and C. Jones. 2008. Microscopic and Spectroscopic Features of Gunpowder and its Documentation in Gunshot Wounds in Charred Bodies. *The American Journal of Forensic Medicine and Pathology.* 29(4):312–319.

Downs, S.J. 2012. Shooting Euthanized Pig Heads to Determine Penetration Capabilities of Frangible Bullets and the Impact on a Forensic Investigation. Presented at the American Academy of Forensic Sciences, 20–25 February, Atlanta, Georgia.

Freminville, H., F. Rongieras, N. Prat, and E.J. Voiglio. 2011. The Flap by Flap Dissection in Terminal Ballistic Applied to Less Lethal Weapons. *The American Journal of Forensic Medicine and Pathology.* 32(2):149–152.

Gibelli, D., A. Brandone, S. Andreola, D. Porta, E. Giudici, M.A. Grandi, and C. Cattaneo. 2010. Macroscopic, Microscopic, and Chemical Assessment of Gunshot Lesions on Decomposed Pig Skin. *Journal of Forensic Sciences.* 55(4):1092–1097.

Haag, L. 2007. Wound Production by Ricocheted and Destabilized Bullets. *The American Journal of Forensic Medicine and Pathology.* 28(1):4–12.

Kraus, K.H. 1992. Acute Management of Open Fractures, Including Gunshot, Shearing, and Degloving Wounds. In: *Kirk's Current Veterinary Therapy XI Small Animal Practice,* R.W. Kirk and J.D. Bonagura, eds. pp. 154–158. Philadelphia: W.B. Saunders.

LaGoo, L., L.S. Schaeffer, D.W. Szymanski, and R. Waddel Smith. 2010. Detection of Gunshot Residue in Blowfly Larvae and Decomposing Porcine Tissue Using Inductively Coupled Plasma Mass Spectrometry (ICP-MS). *Journal of Forensic Sciences.* 55(3):624–632.

MacAulay, L.E., D.G. Barr, and D.B. Strongman. 2009a. Effects of Decomposition on Gunshot Wound Characteristics: Under Moderate Temperatures with Insect Activity. *Journal of Forensic Sciences.* 54(2):443–447.

MacAulay, L.E., D.G. Barr, and D.B. Strongman. 2009b. Effects of Decomposition on Gunshot Wound Characteristics: Under Cold Temperatures with No Insect Activity. *Journal of Forensic Sciences.* 54(2):448–451.

Marshall, J.W., D.B. Dahlstrom, and K.D. Powley. 2011. Minimum Velocity Necessary for Nonconventional Projectiles to Penetrate the Eye. *The American Journal of Forensic Medicine and Pathology.* 32(2):100–103.

Munro, H.M. and M.V. Thrusfield. 2001. Battered Pets: Features that Raise Suspicion of Non–Accidental Injury. *Journal of Small Animal Practice.* 42:218–226.

Pavletic, M.M. 1985. A Review of 121 Gunshot Wounds in the Dog and Cat. *Veterinary Surgery.* 14:61–62.

Pavletic, M.M. 2006. Managing Gunshot Wounds in Small Animals. *Veterinary Technician.* 27(1):36–44.

Prahlow, J.A., S.B. Allen, T. Spinder, and R.A. Poole. 2003. Pseudo-Gunpowder Stippling Caused by Fragmentation of a Plated Bullet. *American Journal of Forensic Medicine and Pathology.* 24(3):243–247.

Simic, M., D. Draskovic, G. Stojiljkovic, R. Vukovic, and Z. M. Budimlija. 2007. The Characteristics of Head Wounds Inflicted by "Humane Killer" (Captive-Bolt Gun)—A 15-Year Study. *Journal of Forensic Sciences.* 52(5):1182–1185.

Spitz, W.U. 2006. Injury by Gunfire. In *Spitz and Fisher's Medicolegal Investigation of Death: Guidelines for the Application of Pathology to Crime Investigation,* Fourth edition. W.U. Spitz and D.J. Spitz, eds. pp. 607–746. Springfield: Charles C. Thomas Publisher, Ltd.

Voiglio, J. 2011. The Flap by Flap Dissection in Terminal Ballistic applied to Less Lethal Weapons. *The American Journal of Forensic Medicine and Pathology.* 32(2):149–152.

9
Asphyxia

Melinda D. Merck and Doris M. Miller

Just as life depends on the equal functioning of the tripod of life, i.e., heart, lung, and brain, so also a successful investigation of crime depends on equal functioning of forensic medicine, forensic science, and police investigation.

> *Professor L. Fimate, President of the Indian Academy of Forensic Medicine*

OVERVIEW OF ASPHYXIA

Death resulting from asphyxia in the forensic context is defined as forensic situations where a body does not receive or utilize oxygen (Sauvageau and Boghossian 2009). This can result from partial oxygen deprivation (hypoxia) or total oxygen deprivation (anoxia). Asphyxia can be categorized into suffocation, strangulation, mechanical asphyxia, and drowning (Table 9.1). In each of these categories there are subcategories that define the anatomical site and the nature of the force used to cause the asphyxia. Chemical asphyxia falls under vitiated atmosphere in the suffocation category and is covered in Chapter 7 under Smoke Inhalation.

Asphyxiation, specifically strangulation, is the most common cause of death in human sexual assaults. Any animal victim of asphyxia should be examined for possible sexual abuse. Several forms of asphyxia require the assailant to be in close proximity to the victim with the likely transfer of evidence and the potential for infliction of injury by the victim. There may be evidence of sphincter incontinence at the scene of the assault.

GENERAL FINDINGS IN ASPHYXIA

The different categories of asphyxia can produce similar gross and histological findings. The findings that are considered classic signs of asphyxia in humans are visceral congestion, petechiae, cyanosis, and fluidity of the blood (Di Maio and Di Maio 2001). Unfortunately, these classic signs are non-specific and can be associated with other causes of death. Other findings associated with each category of asphyxia along with additional testing can assist with the determination of asphyxia as the cause of death. In some cases, the diagnosis of asphyxia may be based on the circumstances surrounding death and the exclusion of other causes of death. It is important to have a complete history to support the gross and microscopic findings suggestive of suffocation, strangulation, mechanical asphyxia, or drowning. Resuscitative efforts involving intubation may cause injuries to the pharynx and larynx which can mimic similar injuries produced by strangulation or neck holds.

Visceral congestion is caused by obstructed venous return and capillovenous congestion, which are more susceptible to hypoxia. This produces dilation of the vessels and blood stasis (Di Maio and Di Maio 2001). Congestion also may be seen in the face. Visceral petechiae result from the sudden over-distention and rupture of small vessels, primarily the venules. They are commonly seen in the epicardium and visceral pleura (Di Maio and Di Maio 2001). Petechial hemorrhages on the surface of the lung are caused by small ruptures of blood vessels resulting from pressure changes in the lungs when air flow is obstructed through the nose and mouth.

Veterinary Forensics: Animal Cruelty Investigations, Second Edition. Edited by Melinda D. Merck.
© 2013 John Wiley & Sons, Inc. Published 2013 by John Wiley & Sons, Inc.

Table 9.1 Forensic classification and definitions of asphyxia.

Term	Definition
Suffocation	A broad term encompassing different types of asphyxia associated with deprivation of oxygen
Smothering	Asphyxia by obstruction of the air passages above the epiglottis, including the nose, mouth, and pharynx
Choking	Asphyxia by obstruction of the air passages below the epiglottis
Confined spaces/ entrapment/ vitiated atmosphere	Asphyxia in an inadequate atmosphere by reduction of oxygen, displacement of oxygen by other gases, or by cases causing chemical interference with the oxygen uptake and utilization
Strangulation	Asphyxia by closure of the blood vessels and/or air passages of the neck as a result of external pressure on the neck
Ligature strangulation	A form of strangulation in which the pressure on the neck is applied by a constricting band tightened by a force other than the body weight
Hanging	A form of strangulation in which the pressure on the neck is applied by a constricting band tightened by the gravitational weight of the body or part of the body
Manual strangulation	A form of strangulation caused by an external pressure on the structures of the neck by hands, forearms, or other limbs
Mechanical asphyxia	Asphyxia by restriction of respiratory movements, either by the position of the body or by external chest compression
Positional or postural asphyxia	A type of asphyxia where the position of an individual compromises the ability to breathe
Traumatic asphyxia	A type of asphyxia caused by external chest/abdomen compression by a heavy object
Drowning	Asphyxia by immersion in a liquid

Source: Sauvageau, A. and E. Boghassian. 2010. Classification of Asphyxia: The Need for Standardization. *Journal of Forensic Sciences*. 55(5):1259-1267.

The location of the petechiae also may depend on the mechanism of asphyxia. It should be noted that petechiae are nonspecific findings and may be seen in other conditions, such as bleeding disorders and septicemia. In humans, they may be found in the reflected scalp or the epiglottis and are considered unremarkable (Di Maio and Di Maio 2001). Petechiae also can develop postmortem in dependent areas in which the gravitational setting of blood overwhelms the vessels resulting in mechanical rupture. These areas can enlarge to areas of ecchymoses. Cyanosis also is a non-specific finding. The increased fluidity of the blood is due to the absence of postmortem clotting (W. Spitz 2006). This is caused by an increased rate of fibrinolysis that is seen in rapid deaths and is thought to result from high agonal catecholamine levels. It is considered a nonspecific finding and may be seen with other causes of rapid death (Di Maio and Di Maio 2001).

SUFFOCATION

Suffocation refers to death caused by oxygen deprivation. The microscopic findings for suffocation may include areas of over-insufflation of the alveoli and alveolar collapse. Reports in humans indicate alveolar collapse, congestion, and edema were histologic determinants associated with suffocation, which can be used to discriminate from fire lung injury (bronchiolar dilatation, ductal over-insufflation, alveolar over-insufflation, and alveolar hemorrhage) (de Paiva et al. 2008). The three categories of suffocation are smothering; choking; and confined spaces, entrapment, and vitiated atmosphere (see Chapter 7 for chemical asphyxia).

Smothering

Smothering is caused by the mechanical obstruction or occlusions of the air passages above the epiglottis including the nose, mouth, and pharynx (Sauvageau and

Boghossian 2010). This may be associated with a plastic bag secured over the animal's head, placing the animal inside a plastic bag, live burial, or placing a conforming object (e.g., pillow) on top of the face and pressing down.

The physical findings are consistent with the expected struggle including abrasions and/or contusions on the external and internal surfaces of the face, mouth, and lips, with possible torn frenula. There may be trace evidence inside the mouth or nasal air passages, or embedded in the nails from the object or method used. If a bag was secured around the neck, there may be evidence of claw marks on the neck where the animal struggled to get it off. The object used may not be found still attached or in proximity to the body. In humans, petechiae may be found on the face, sclerae, conjunctivae, or gingiva, but they are often absent. There may be non-specific findings of petechiae on the epicardium and pleural surface of the lungs. Diagnosis usually is made by exclusion of other causes of death and the circumstances surrounding death.

Any recovered object may be linked to the perpetrator(s) and victim. The brand and manufacturer of plastic bags can be identified and if torn from a roll the bottom edge can be linked to the original roll. DNA from the animal's saliva, blood, or urine may be found on the surface of the object used. There may be fingerprints on the bag from the perpetrator or other unique identifiers of the victim such as nose prints (Chapter 4).

When an animal is buried alive more than one type of asphyxia may cause death. Depending on the depth and weight of the fill on the body, compression of the chest can contribute to the asphyxia. In live burials, soil or burial material may have been inhaled or swallowed. Visible soil may be found in the upper and/or lower airways. Depending on the circumstances and conditions of burial, the presence of soil in the outer nares and a small amount in the mouth may be due to soil settling. Soil found in the nasal cavities, trachea, esophagus, stomach, or deeper airways is consistent with respiratory effort and/or ingestion of soil and not passive seepage (Figure 9.1) (Munro and Munro 2008). Soil particles may be found microscopically in the deeper airways. The soil also may lodge in the airway, causing an obstruction (see Choking). The animals may have frayed or broken nails on their feet with embedded soil. Other evidence may be found in the grave (see Chapter 2).

Choking

Choking is caused by an obstruction in the air passages below the epiglottis including the larynx, trachea, or the bronchi. Choking deaths may be related to accidental ingestion or aspiration of foreign material, forcible

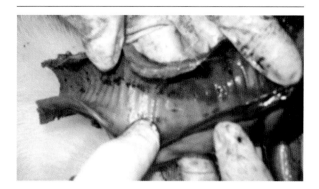

Figure 9.1 Soil in trachea associated with live burial.

introduction of foreign material, or inhalation of blood from head trauma or throat cuts. Findings of blockage of the airway by foreign material are diagnostic of choking. If the object was removed during resuscitative efforts, the diagnosis can be made only through the medical history. Histologic findings in the lungs include congestion, intra-alveolar flooding and hemorrhage, alveolar over-distension, and possible particles of the foreign material.

Asphyxia may occur by severe airway swelling that obstructs the passage of air due to a number of causes. It may involve the larynx and surrounding tissues, bronchi, or bronchioles. Anaphylaxis can cause swelling in the larynx and surrounding tissues, leading to obstruction. Infection and neoplasia, either within or adjacent to the airways, can lead to obstruction. There are several thermal and chemical causes of swelling obstruction (Chapter 7). Irritating agents such as pepper can cause the lining of the airway to swell and result in obstruction, which is further complicated by the accumulation of mucus, inflammatory debris, and airway spasm. A blow to the neck can cause severe swelling of the larynx and surrounding tissue resulting in airway occlusion which can take minutes to hours to develop.

Confined spaces/entrapment/vitiated atmosphere

Confined spaces, entrapment, and vitiated atmosphere asphyxia is due to an inadequate atmosphere by reduction of oxygen, displacement of oxygen by other gases, or by gases causing chemical interference with the oxygen uptake and utilization. A vitiated atmosphere most commonly occurs when an animal becomes entrapped in a small space such as a refrigerator or similar closed spaces. With entrapment, initially there may be sufficient oxygen but as the animal continues to breathe, the oxygen supply is exhausted, displaced by carbon dioxide, and is followed by asphyxiation. The necropsy findings include dark fluid blood and congested organs, and the brain may be dusky and edematous. Carbon dioxide rapidly accumulates after death making blood analysis for CO_2 poisoning inaccurate for diagnosis (W. Spitz 2006). Diagnosis of entrapment suffocation due to carbon dioxide poisoning is made by the circumstances surrounding death and exclusion of other causes of death.

STRANGULATION

Overview

Strangulation is defined as the closure of the blood vessels and/or air passages of the neck as a result of external pressure on the neck (Sauvageau and Boghassian 2010). The causes include ligature strangulation (garroting), hanging, and manual strangulation (throttling).

The cause of death in strangulation is cerebral hypoxia caused by the compression and occlusion of the arteries supplying the brain, which include the carotids and vertebrals. Venous drainage is primarily through the jugular veins. The carotid arteries are easily compressed, in contrast with the vertebral arteries, which are resistant to direct pressure. The vertebral arteries can be occluded by severe lateral flexion or rotation of the neck, as is seen in hanging (Di Maio and Di Maio 2001). When there is compression of the carotid and jugular vessels, the vertebral arteries continue to supply blood to the head. This increases the pressure in the capillovenules, causing them to rupture and producing petechiae. Petechiae associated with strangulation are indicative of local venous congestion (Di Maio and Di Maio 2001). If there are compression and release or partial compression of the vessels, the pressure may be altered and petechiae may be absent or reduced. If the compression of the neck vessels is sudden and complete, as with some incidents of hanging, no petechiae may be found. The presence of petechiae is associated with other conditions and is not diagnostic of strangulation.

General findings

The features of strangulation in animals are similar to those found in humans. There were two reported cases of attempted strangulation with detailed descriptions of their findings in the study by Munro and Thrusfield. In one case a dog, less than two years old, presented with evidence of a crushing injury to the trachea, severe laryngeal edema, lingual swelling, and fractures of the hyoid bone seen on radiographs. There were also edema of the lips and eyelids, subconjunctival hemorrhages, and small internal eye hemorrhages. In the second case a dog, more than two years of age, presented with swelling and edema of the neck,

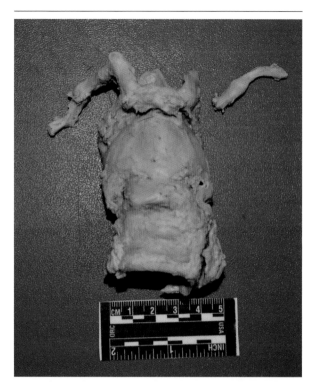

Figure 9.2 Manual strangulation case with fractures of the hyoid apparatus: the right epihyoid bone has visible fracture with palpable fractures at the junctional area of the right basihyoid and the ceratohyoid. (Photo courtesy of Dr. Doris Miller.)

breathing difficulties, edema around the eyes, and bruising around the head and lips (Munro and Thrusfield 2001).

Hyoid fractures may be difficult to see on radiographs and more easily identified on necropsy examination (Figure 9.2). This fracture caused by strangulation is more common after bone ossification, which occurs two to three months after birth in carnivores (Liebich and König 2009). In dogs, the stylohyoid, thyrohyoid, and epihyoid are ossified at birth; the basihyoid ossifies one month postpartum and the ceratohyoid at two months postpartum; the tympanohyoid does not ossify (Evans 1993). Antemortem fractures of the hyoid bone, thyroid, or cricoid cartilage are usually associated with hemorrhage at the fracture site and/or surrounding tissues.

The tongue may have findings of petechia on the sublingual surface or intramuscular hemorrhage. On necropsy exam, multiple crosswise slices into the tongue should be made to look for internal hemorrhage within the tissue. Middle ear hemorrhage is reported in humans. The mechanism is thought to be due to increased pressure from compression of the jugular vein impeding venous blood flow return and/or tympanic barotrauma due to breathing effort against a closed glottis (Duband et al. 2009). Microscopic findings may include areas of over-insufflation of the alveoli, alveolar collapse, and intra-alveolar hemorrhage.

Ligature strangulation (garroting)

Ligature strangulation results from a constricting band applying pressure on the neck that is tightened by a force other than the body weight. This ligature applies pressure to the neck, causing occlusion of the carotid arteries and depriving oxygen to the brain. A variety of ligatures may be used including leashes, electrical cords, telephone cords, rope, plastic lock-ties, neckties, sheets, scarves, hose, and towels. The ligature mark appearance depends on the nature of the ligature, amount of force used by the assailant, and resistance of the victim (Figures 9.3 and 9.4). The mark may reflect the configuration of the ligature used, such as the weave of the rope or an imprinted pattern. Evidence of a ligature may be the presence of indentation of hair and/or skin. Alternatively, the mark may be faint or absent, especially if the ligature was soft or removed immediately after death. The more narrow and firm the ligature, the more distinct the mark. The ligature should be removed only during necropsy and retained as evidence. Any knot or fastening should be preserved intact by cutting the ligature on the opposite side and taping the ends.

Typically, a ligature mark encircles the neck, creating a furrow; initially it has a yellow parchment-like appearance on the skin surface in humans and turns dark brown over time (Di Maio and Di Maio 2001). The ligature marks may be more visible on reflected skin in the dermis or subcutaneous tissues of animals where vital reaction may be more apparent (Figure 9.5). There may be a break in the furrow where the assailant grasped the ends of the ligature and tightened. There are usually no abrasions or contusions unless the victim clawed at the neck. If two loops were wrapped around the neck, there may be skin contusions in the area that was compressed between the loops (Di Maio and Di Maio 2001). There may be multiple marks on the neck or atypical marks due to repeated attempts to apply the ligature on the neck. Decomposition does not typically affect the appearance of a ligature mark which is thought to be due to the compression preventing access to the area by putrefying bacteria (Di Maio and Di Maio 2001). The ligature marks and furrow should be described in detail, including the direction, depth, width, color, ligature patterns, area of neck involved, and its relation to local landmarks (Di Maio and Di Maio 2001).

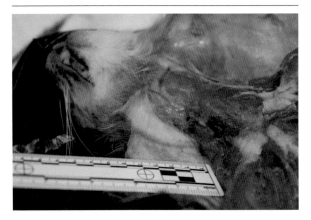

Figure 9.3 Cat hanged with a beaver snare. Ligature marks are seen on skin reflection of the ventral neck and indentation on right neck musculature.

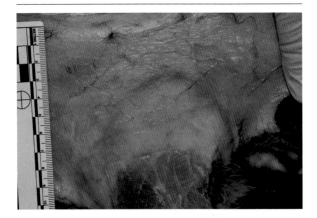

Figure 9.4 Ligature marks apparent on dorsal skin reflection of the neck from Figure 9.3.

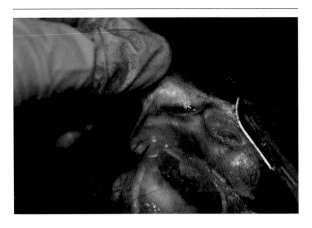

Figure 9.5 Ligature mark with hemorrhage.

The face and neck above the ligature are usually congested and edema fluid may be present in the nostrils. Scleral hemorrhage along with petechiae on the face, the periorbital region, conjunctivae, and gingiva may be seen. In ligature strangulation there is complete compression of the jugulars but incomplete compression of the arteries so that blood continues to the head through the vertebral arteries but cannot flow out, causing increased intravascular pressure, congestion, and rupture of the vessels (Di Maio and Di Maio 2001). Injuries to the neck may or may not be present. Fractures of the thyroid cartilage may occur but hyoid bone fracture is rare. There may be minimal to severe soft tissue hemorrhage within the neck (Dix et al. 2000).

Hanging

General findings

In hanging, the neck structures are compressed by a constricting band that is tightened by the gravitational weight of the body, or part of the body, resulting in asphyxia. There may be complete suspension of the body or partial suspension, with part of the body touching the ground or floor. Hanging can cause compression or constriction of the blood vessels. In partial suspension hangings, the weight of the head can be enough to cause occlusion of the neck vessels.

Obstruction of the airway may or may not occur in hanging. The airway obstruction may be caused by compression of the trachea, or through the elevation and posterior displacement of the tongue and floor of the mouth when the noose is above the larynx (Di Maio and Di Maio 2001). This obstruction of the airway usually results in a violent struggle, a condition called air hunger. This condition generates tremendous fear of impending death along with violent attempts to open the airway (W. Spitz 2006).

Cervical soft tissue emphysema was reported in just over 50% of human hanging cases, which is thought to be due to trauma to the cervical airways or as a result of an alveolar rupture secondary to high intra-alveolar pressure (Nikolić et al. 2012). Cervical vertebral displacement, dislocation, or fractures may be seen with hangings. Compression of the ligature may cause fractures of the transverse processes. The struggle of the animal while suspended creates extreme hyperextension, hyperflexion, and rotational forces. This can result in a fracture of the proximal dens on C2 vertebra and/or brainstem or spinal cord injury (Figure 9.6). The pressure applied to the thyroid gland can cause leakage of thyroglobulin and free T3 where high postmortem levels may be an indicator of vital reaction in hanging cases (Şenol et al. 2008). Hyoid fractures may be seen.

The pathophysiology, or mechanism, of death due to hanging is thought to be respiratory asphyxia, interruption

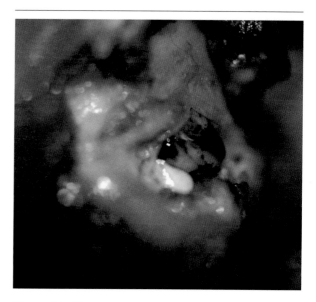

Figure 9.6 Hemorrhage on proximal spinal cord and brain stem associated with hanging.

of cerebral blood flow due to occlusion of neck vessels, or cardiac inhibition secondary to nerve stimulation (Clément, Redpath, and Sauvageau 2010). The stimulation of the baroreceptors in the carotid sinuses and the carotid body can cause a reflex vagal inhibition. A review was conducted of published studies using animal models on the respiratory, circulatory, and neurological responses to hanging which included cats, dogs, rabbits, and rats. The study found that cessation of blood flow, rather than airway obstruction, is responsible for the loss of respiratory function. It found that occlusion of the airways did not accelerate the decline of respiratory movements (Boghossian et al. 2010).

These studies were divided into groups: ligation of carotid and vertebral arteries with airway open (cats and dogs); ligation of carotid and vertebral arteries, vagus nerves, internal jugular veins, and trachea (dogs); and external ligature (rabbits and rats). The loss of respiratory movements occurred in less than two minutes with cats and ranged from less than two minutes to eight minutes in dogs for both groups. Respiratory rest occurred in 6–6.3 minutes in rabbits and 120–197 seconds in rats.

In the cat studies convulsions occurred early (under one minute), sometimes preceded by clonic movements of one foot or rigidity of the whole body, followed by a brief period of tetanic convulsions and then gross clonic convulsions of the whole body. Loss of EEG waves occurred 10–120 seconds with highest brain areas failing first.

In the dog studies there was loss of muscle movement in 1.5–2 minutes, convulsions, urination (frequently in the first minute), and complete medullary paralysis in eight to fourteen minutes. Loss of EEG waves occurred in 1.5–2 minutes with convulsive waves during the terminal respirations.

The rat showed loss of muscle movement in 1.8–3.5 minutes and erection of tail, and urination frequently occurred. No neurological component was assessed in rabbits.

The circulatory component in the cat studies showed immediate increase in pulse rate; the heart slowed with cessation of respiration and then briefly became rapid again between two and four minutes later with failure of vagus center. In the dog studies the heart rate increased after two to three respiratory movements until circulatory collapse in four to six minutes. The blood pressure increased (1.5 times) for 1–1.5 minutes until apnea occurred, then gradually decreased. In rabbits, the cerebral blood flow dropped immediately then rose suddenly and gradually dropped after three to four minutes with terminal hypotension in 6.5–8.5 minutes. In rats, the absence of the heartbeat occurred in 4.5–6 minutes (Boghossian et al. 2010).

In dogs and pigs the vertebral arteries supply the majority of the cerebral circulation due to less developed internal carotids. In cats the internal carotids are atrophied at birth and the important epidural vessels are from the arterial cerebral circle. Death due to hanging may be slower than in humans due to these anatomic differences, depending on the location and amount of compression of the ligature. There may be a prolonged period of consciousness or semi-consciousness that may initially include violent struggling movements that eventually subsides and eventual death occurs. In cats this violent struggle can last for more than a minute before cessation (Chester 2010).

The ligature or noose used in hangings may be constructed from anything that is handy and available. It may be comprised of rope, wire, electrical cords, leashes, belts, phone cords, or from something softer such as strips of cloth. The point of suspension varies in location around the neck and is usually from the knot.

The ligature causes a furrow on the neck but does not completely encircle it, producing an inverted V-pattern which can be misinterpreted as manual strangulation.

Initially the furrow may be light, with a congested rim, and then change to darker brown as it dries out. The furrow is deeper and darker in color opposite the point of suspension and becomes lighter where it angles upward toward the point of suspension.

As with ligature strangulations, the furrow may reflect the configuration of the ligature. With a thin, firm ligature, the groove is more distinct and well demarcated. There may be abrasions from the surface of the material or contusions. Nooses from softer material tend to cause a poorly defined groove or no marks at all. The upper margin may be red caused by postmortem congestion of the vessels and the lower margin may be pale (Di Maio and Di Maio 2001). There may be two furrows if the noose was composed of two loops. These furrows may be parallel, overlap, or have two different paths and compress the skin between them, causing tissue hemorrhage. If a belt is used it may produce two parallel marks on the neck from where each edge dug into the skin. The longer the body is suspended, the more prominent the mark will be because of vessel congestion (Di Maio and Di Maio 2001). Ligature marks and patterns may be more visible on skin reflection in animals. Occasionally, the ligature marks are horizontal, depending on the position of the body. It is possible that an animal was first killed by ligature strangulation then suspended using the ligature. In this case the markings on the neck are more horizontal rather than the inverted V pattern seen in hanging. However, it is possible to have noose marks if the victim was deceased when hanged. In humans, these marks can be seen if the victim was hanged within two hours after death (Di Maio and Di Maio 2001).

Judicial hanging

Judicial hangings involve a sudden drop of the body with complete suspension. In humans, death is caused by the fracture and dislocation of the upper cervical vertebrae and transaction of the spinal cord. If the body falls an insufficient distance, death is caused by strangulation. If the body falls too far, the victim may be decapitated. The classic hangman's fracture in humans, which is associated with cord injury at C2-C3, is caused by hyperextension and distraction. The fracture is through the pedicles of C2, where the caudal aspect remains fixed with C3 and the cranial aspect remains fixed with C1 (Di Maio and Di Maio 2001).

Other injuries to the cervical vertebrae may occur instead of the hangman's fracture. There may be fractures of the transverse processes of C1-C3 and C5, the cervical body of C2, the occipital bones, or the styloid processes in humans. There may be separation of C2 and C3 with complete transection of the cord, fractures of the thyroid cartilage and the hyoid bone, and hemorrhage into the cervical muscle. There may be bilateral vertebral artery lacerations with basilar subarachnoid hemorrhage or bilateral internal carotid tears with subdural hematomas

(Di Maio and Di Maio 2001). In animals, these injuries may or may not be seen based on the thicker neck musculature associated with certain species or breeds.

Examination of hanging victims

The body should be photographed prior to being cut down, preserving any knots. The ligature should only be removed during necropsy examination. The nature, composition, width, location, type of knot, and mode of application should be documented prior to removal of the ligature. It may be slipped over the head without alteration of the knot or cut on the side opposite the knot and the ends taped together. The ligature marks should be photographed and documented as discussed in ligature strangulation.

The skin under the ligature should be examined for hemorrhage within the skin and underlying tissue layers which is indicative of active blood flow at the time of hanging (W. Spitz 2006). The neck and body should be examined for other marks and injuries including claw marks and abrasions on the neck and face from the struggle.

It is not uncommon for hanging victims to have suffered other injuries prior or after hanging such as from blunt force trauma or dragging. In non-judicial hangings, there are often no internal neck injuries. Occasionally, fractures of the thyroid cartilage, hyoid bone, and cervical spine may be seen. Hemorrhage around laryngeal fractures, which indicate that the victim was alive at hanging, may be minute and require meticulous dissection (W. Spitz 2006). Findings may include hemorrhage of the strap muscles of the neck and blood-tinged fluid in the nostrils (Di Maio and Di Maio 2001). Tears in the carotid artery may be seen due to trauma by the ligature. These frictional intimal tears of the carotid arteries with subintimal dissection and hemorrhage are additional evidence that the animal was alive at the time of hanging (W. Spitz 2006).

The victims of hanging often have protrusion of the tongue caused by the noose pushing the larynx upward, forcing the tongue out of the mouth. The tongue may be red, red-black, or black caused by drying (Dix et al. 2000). If the jugular veins were compressed for a period of time prior to compression of the carotid arteries, the face may appear congested. Petechiae may be found on the conjunctivae, periorbital regions, and gingiva. The density of petechiae found on the skin and head can be an indicator for the duration of the process with a higher density seen with slow, protracted asphyxia (W. Spitz 2006). Petechiae may be minimal or absent in cases of hanging where the compression of the neck occludes both the jugular and carotid vessels. A retrospective study in humans found that the presence of petechiae in hanging deaths was higher

(50%) with incomplete hanging than complete suspension (29%) (Clément et al. 2011). The face is usually pale except for lividity (Dix et al. 2000). In hangings there is gravitational blood pooling to the dependent portion of the body. The large amount of blood can overwhelm the vessels, causing them to rupture and producing areas of pseudo-hemorrhage, also called Tardieu spots.

Hemorrhages into the anterior aspect of the intervertebral disks in the lumbar region of the spine have been described in human cases of death by hanging. These hemorrhages, known as Simon's hemorrhage, appear as dark red to violet lines between the vertebral bodies of the lower thoracic and lumbar spine. They do not penetrate into the vertebral bodies and are limited to the area of the anterior ligament of the intervertebral disks. Simon's hemorrhage occurs in hanging due to a combination of agonal convulsions and traction of the body as a result of gravity. It is more common in humans under fifty years of age, with minimal degenerative changes in the lumbosacral region of the spinal cord and in cases with free body suspension. It is reported that these hemorrhages and putrefactive changes cannot be differentiated histologically. Simon's hemorrhage was reported in 37% of human hanging deaths but it may also be seen with drowning, hypothermia, blunt trauma situations such as traffic accident injuries, and falls from heights. It is not seen in natural deaths. It is considered a valid diagnostic autopsy sign of pre-mortem hanging but is not specific for hanging. The absence of these hemorrhages does not exclude death by hanging. It has greatest diagnostic significance when there is minimum amount of findings in the cervical region (Hejna and Rejtarová 2010).

One variation of hanging is the suspension of an animal upside down. Death can result if the animal is suspended for a sufficient period of time. The mechanism of death is thought to be acute respiratory and/or cardiac failure. In humans, the length of time for death depends on the health of the victim, ranging from a few hours to a day or longer (Di Maio and Di Maio 2000). Expected injuries are related to the apparatus of suspension and its attachment to the body. Congestion of the head and petechiae on the face may be seen due to postmortem lividity. There may be other injuries to the body if additional physical trauma was inflicted while the victim was suspended.

Manual strangulation (throttling)

Manual strangulation is caused by the external pressure on the structures of the neck by hands, forearms, or other limbs. This compression of the internal structures causes occlusion of the blood vessels to the brain. There is usually compression of the carotids and jugulars, but the vertebral arteries

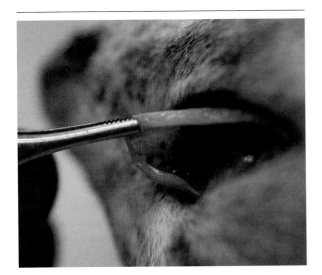

Figure 9.7 Petechiae on nictitating membrane from manual strangulation.

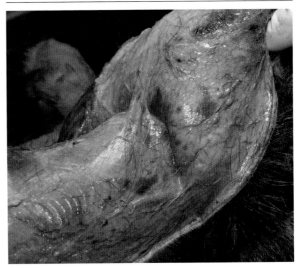

Figure 9.8 Circular bruising under the mandible and lateral neck from manual strangulation.

continue to supply blood to the head. The face is usually congested and may appear cyanotic (Di Maio and Di Maio 2001). Petechiae may be seen on the face, conjunctivae, nictitating membranes, sclerae, or gingiva (Figure 9.7). Petechiae found on the mucosa of the larynx or epiglottis is not exclusively diagnostic of strangulation or asphyxia. Pulmonary edema may be seen, with foamy edema fluid found in the nostrils (Di Maio and Di Maio 2001).

There may or may not be visible injuries to the external and internal structures of the neck with manual strangulation. There may be abrasions, contusions, finger contusions, and fingernail marks on the skin or visible on skin reflection and in deeper tissues (Figures 9.8 and 9.9). Fingernail marks are usually from the fingers and not the thumb because the thumb pad is used to apply pressure. These marks can appear as linear or semi-linear, or scratches or scrapes. Fingertips can cause erythematous impression marks or contusions. They appear curved, oval, triangular, dashed, rectangular, or similar to an exclamation mark (Di Maio and Di Maio 2001).

The animal may struggle and claw at the assailant's hand, arm, or limbs, retaining evidence on the feet and nails. There is often significant hemorrhage of the strap muscles of the neck and the surrounding soft tissue caused by the large amount of force used and the movement between the victim and assailant. Mild or absent hemorrhage may be seen if there is a large disparity of size between the assailant and victim with minimal movement (Dix et al. 2000).

Fractures of the thyroid and cricoid cartilage may occur. Fractures of the hyoid bone may be found if ossification

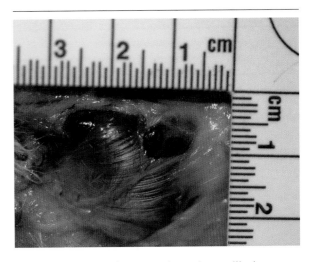

Figure 9.9 Hemorrhage on the submandibular lymph node from manual strangulation.

has occurred. The U-shape of the hyoid makes it susceptible to compression fractures which are primarily seen with manual strangulation, though it is also associated with other types of asphyxia (Di Maio and Di Maio 2001).

A choke hold refers to compression of the anterior neck using an object or arm. Yoking refers to the compression of the neck by the forearm, usually from behind the victim. Because the forearm is a broad, soft object, there may little to no external injury to the neck. If a large amount of force is applied and there is significant movement between the

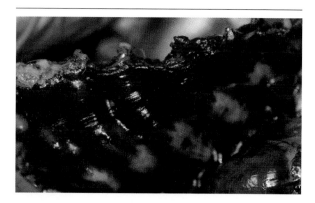

Figure 9.10 Intercostal muscle hemorrhage from chest compression asphyxia.

victim and assailant, there may be contusions on the neck, especially when an object is used. The damage to internal neck structures is variable and may include fractures of the larynx or hyoid. The presence of petechiae on the face, sclerae, conjunctivae, and gingiva may be found but is variable (Dix et al. 2000).

MECHANICAL ASPHYXIA

Mechanical asphyxia is caused by the restriction of respiratory movements, either by position of the body or by external chest/abdomen compression. Positional or postural asphyxia occurs when the position of the individual compromises the ability to breathe. Traumatic asphyxia is due to compression by a heavy object. Compression applied to the chest or upper abdomen can prevent breathing, resulting in asphyxia. When extreme pressure is exerted on the chest, there is a sudden increase in intrathoracic pressure. This affects the cardiac hemodynamics, causing an increase in venous pressure. In humans, findings include marked dusky congestion of the head, neck, and upper torso. Petechiae are found in the face, sclerae, conjunctivae, periorbital skin, neck, and upper torso. There may be external marks on the torso from the compressing agent, more visible on skin reflection, or there may be no evidence of trauma. Internally, there may be small hemorrhages in the neck and chest muscle attachments, rib fractures, and internal organ damage (Figure 9.10).

DROWNING

Overview

Drowning is defined as death secondary to hypoxemia due to asphyxia while immersed in a liquid, most commonly water. Submersion can be the total body or just enough to cover the external airway openings. Although there are several physiological responses in the process of drowning, such as cardiac changes, the most important consequence is asphyxia. Drowning of animals as a form of cruelty may be under-reported due to lack of body detection and reluctant witnesses. In the study by Munro and Thrusfield, there were three reported cases of drowning or attempted drowning. It is interesting to note that two of the three cases happened inside the home (Munro and Thrusfield 2001).

The behavior of animals and humans during the drowning process can be divided into several stages. It usually begins with a struggle to stay above water with a period of panic and hyperventilation. When the head is submerged breath holding occurs, usually for one to two minutes, until the accumulation of carbon dioxide concentrations build up causing an involuntary respiratory effort. This results in the inhalation of the water into the lungs, which may be small or large in volume. A large volume of water may be swallowed, which can be found in the stomach. This can cause the animal to vomit and possibly aspirate the gastric contents. Coughing, swallowing, and vomiting of water is followed by convulsions and spasmodic inspiratory effort. Consciousness is progressively lost over two to three minutes followed by cardiopulmonary arrest and subsequent death (D. Spitz 2006). Following submersion death usually occurs in five to ten minutes (D. Spitz 2006, Rohn and Frade 2006).

There is a range of pathophysiologic changes related to death by drowning, and they differ between fresh and saltwater drowning. Several previous animal studies have been conducted which found that fresh or brackish (0.5% NaCl) water drowning causes hemodilution due to increased intravascular volume. The hypotonic fresh water and hypertonic plasma cause an osmotic gradient resulting in large amounts of water crossing from the alveoli into the vasculature. Fatal cardiac dysrhythmias, usually ventricular fibrillation, were caused by profound hyponatremia and hypokalemia (D. Spitz 2006). Fresh water also dilutes and damages the lung surfactant resulting in alveolar collapse and reduced lung compliance. The hypertonicity of saltwater (3%–5% NaCl) actually draws water from the interstitial space into the alveoli resulting in hemoconcentration (D. Spitz 2006) and increases alveolar filling known as secondary drowning (Hawkins 1995).

Another factor to consider is the possibility of neurogenic pulmonary edema caused by brain hypoxia. This may be a primary factor when minimal water is inhaled (D. Spitz 2006). The amount of water inhaled is found to be more significant than the type of water in causing significant electrolyte changes (Dix et al. 2000). A study in dogs using fresh water found that significant hyponatremia and ventricular fibrillation were seen after aspiration of 20 cc of water/pound of body weight, while 10 cc of water/pound had little effect on sodium concentration (D. Spitz 2006). For both fresh and saltwater drowning the mechanism of death is similar, i.e., cerebral hypoxia.

Based on animal and clinical research studies it is estimated that in approximately 10%–15% of drownings there is no inhalation of water. The theories for this finding include dry-drowning and sudden cardiac death occurring while in water (D. Spitz 2006). The term dry-drowning has been used to describe victims of drowning in which the lungs do not have the typical heavy, boggy, and edematous appearance seen in drowning lungs. The theory is that in some cases of drowning there is sudden laryngospasm through a vagal reflex when water enters the larynx or trachea. There may be the development of thick mucous, foam, and froth that forms a physical plug, preventing water aspiration. The cause of death is the same, from cerebral hypoxia. There is debate regarding this theory due to the fact that the physical plug has not been identified postmortem and laryngospasm cannot be demonstrated after death because of the relaxation of the musculature. Instead the argument is that these lung findings are just one of a spectrum of the changes seen in drowning with the opposite end being wet drowning with the heavy, boggy lungs that contain massive amounts of edema fluid (Di Maio and Di Maio).

Cold water immersion may result in death due to hypothermia or drowning. The events in humans are well documented. Initially pain ensues after immersion followed by intense shivering. Immersion in 43°F (6°C) water causes severe vasoconstriction of the peripheral blood vessels resulting in severe pain over the entire body. This pain is transient and disappears as the skin temperature reaches the water temperature. The temperature of deeper tissues declines linearly but behind the skin temperature. The physiologic responses to cold water immersion are initially increased blood pressure, respiratory rate, and heart rate (D. Spitz 2006). Confusion and disorientation occur as the core temperature drops (82°–90°F or 28°–32°C in dogs and cats) and semiconsciousness occurs around 68°–82°F (20°–28°C) in dogs and cats. Death occurs at temperatures below 68°F (20°C) in dogs and cats (Chapter 11). Drowning is more likely to occur in cold water even without generalized hypothermia due to local muscle cooling which decreases muscle strength and impairs swimming performance (D. Spitz 2006).

In near-drowning incidents the animal survives submersion in water. Depending on the circumstances, these also may be classified as attempted drowning or inflicted submersion injury. The injuries seen usually are caused by hypoxemia and aspiration of the water. The water aspirated is usually small in quantity but enough to cause pulmonary damage. The amount of damage depends on several factors including whether it is fresh or salt water and the presence of debris, sand, or chemicals in the water. Any water purged by the animal should be saved for analysis. Aspiration pneumonia may result from the debris and chemicals in the water, or the aspiration of the animal's own vomit. The bacteria present in the water can cause secondary bacterial pneumonia. Hypoxemia injuries can include cerebral edema, herniation, and death. Acute respiratory distress syndrome can occur as a result of near-drowning and patients should be hospitalized and monitored for worsening symptoms (Hawkins 1995). In humans, hematuria may be seen within two to three days following near-drowning in freshwater (D. Spitz 2006).

Effect of submersion on deceased victims

Submersion in water, as with any moisture contact, can obscure visible findings of injury. Abrasions and contusions may not be visible until the body is dried. Prolonged submersion in water causes the skin to wrinkle, which may be most evident on animal foot pads. Epidermal sloughing, similar to decomposition changes, can occur due to submersion. There may be mud or aquatic debris in the nares or mouth. When a body is placed in water, the remains are subject to several actions, depending on the type and characteristics of the water. The temperature, depth of water, salinity, oxygenation, current, shores, bottoms, and life forms present within the water all affect what happens to the body (Haglund and Sorg 2002). The body may be subjected to abrasions or buried in sediment. The floating limbs are more subject to abrasions and disarticulation caused by their movement. The mandible may disarticulate before or after the limbs (Haglund and Sorg 2002). Aquatic and marine life may consume the internal viscera. Bones may be subject to modifications, such as encrustation by marine life and dissolution (Chapter 3).

The body may initially float or sink, depending on the fat content and the density and viscosity of the water. In animals, fur or feathers increase the body's buoyancy. The finding of heavy weights attached to the body is indicative of body dumping and may be associated with cruelty (Figure 9.11). The body may sink over time, and as decomposition progresses, the gaseous build-up within body cavities and interstitial spaces may overcome external water pressure, causing the body to resurface. If the body has sunk to sufficient depth, the decomposition gas will not

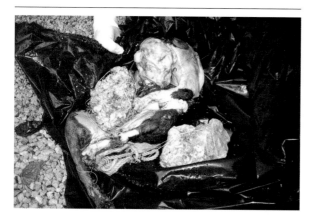

Figure 9.11 Cat found inside a plastic bag that had been found in water. There are weights attached to the body and noticeable skin slippage. Subsequent radiographs revealed gunshot wounds to the head from an air gun. (Photo courtesy of Dr. Doug Mader.)

cause the body to resurface (Haglund and Sorg 2002). In cold water, the decomposition is delayed and it may be weeks to months before the body resurfaces. When the body is floating, the exposed surface area is subject to insect infestation and bird scavenging. The submerged portion of the body is subject to water life scavenging.

Determining the time of death is difficult in aquatic death investigations though it may be possible to determine the postmortem submersion interval (PMSI) using decomposition scoring and entomology (Chapters 14 and 15). New areas of research include aquatic or marine bacteria, how it affects decomposition, and the presence of successive bacterial species that may provide a PMSI. The onset of rigor is variable due to antemortem struggling, which can deplete ATP (adenosine triphosphate), and water temperature. The pattern of lividity reflects the position of the body when it was submerged; it may be pink in cold water drowning.

Decomposition in the water is affected by a variety of factors, including the temperature, salinity, pH, and bacterial content (Haglund and Sorg 2002). It is slower in saltwater than fresh water because high salinity retards bacterial growth and is faster in stagnant water where bacteria are abundant. Algae growth on the body can slow decomposition due to their antibacterial properties (D. Spitz 2006). It is generally slower in water than on land due to the cooler water temperatures than air. Decomposition also is slower in cold water than in warm. Decomposition accelerates once the body is out of the water, resulting from the proliferation of bacteria in the body; therefore, a necropsy

should be performed as soon as possible. The rule of thumb for putrefaction of a body is one week in air equals two weeks in water equals eight weeks in the ground (D. Spitz 2006). The formation of adipocere may occur in bodies that are submerged in cold water (Chapter 14), which hinders decomposition and also may interfere with postmortem estimates (Haglund and Sorg 2002).

Gross and microscopic examination findings

There are no pathognomonic necropsy findings to diagnose drowning. It is a diagnosis of exclusion based on the circumstances of death and nonspecific necropsy findings. It should be noted if the external body is wet and samples of the liquid collected. In wet drowning, as opposed to the findings in dry-drowning, there is white or hemorrhagic foam in the nostrils, mouth, and airways. This foam is produced in the lungs due to the mixing of albumin with water and air. Rupture of alveolar capillaries causes the foam to be blood-tinged (D. Spitz 2006). This foam can continue to form when wiped away. Compression of the chest can cause this foam to flow out. This pulmonary edema fluid is nonspecific and can result from other causes. This foam cone is the most suggestive indicator that a victim was alive when in the water (Dix et al. 2000). The absence of foam does not rule out drowning or that the victim was deceased when submerged. Studies of pediatric drowning in humans found that attempted resuscitation can decrease the incidence of frothy exudates. In addition, as the time interval between the drowning and autopsy increases, the incidence of this foam decreases significantly. This increased time interval also decreases the incidence of pleural effusion findings (Somers et al. 2006).

The lungs are usually large and bulky, and may bulge from the open thoracic cavity caused by the presence of water and entrapped air. The lungs are heavy due to pulmonary edema and the aspirated liquid within the lungs. The lungs are usually dark red-blue, congested, and markedly edematous. On cut section, large quantities of frothy edema fluid may flow out or can be expressed from the cut surface by compression of the tissue (D. Spitz 2006). On microscopic exam there is often proteinic reddish to light pink material in the lumen of alveoli of animals. The right ventricle of the heart may be dilated. The brain may show nonspecific varying degrees of edema, with flattening of the gyri (Di Maio and Di Maio 2001) and red-brown discoloration of the cerebral cortex in saltwater drownings due to the osmotic shifts and hemoconcentration (D. Spitz 2006).

Fluid from the drowning medium may be found in the paranasal sinuses, the frontal sinuses, of animals. This fluid may be aspirated and examined for foreign material and submitted for diatom testing (see below). Additional findings reported in humans include clear or bloody fluid within the sphenoid sinus and middle ear or mastoid air cell hemorrhage (Alexander and Jentzen 2011). Hemolytic staining of the proximal portion of aortic root intima without staining of the proximal pulmonary artery has been reported in 5% of freshwater drowning cases. This staining of vascular intima can occur where red cell lysis has occurred such as hemodilution, putrefaction, thermal injuries, sepsis, and coagulopathies. It is not found associated with saltwater drowning (Tsokos, Cains, and Byard 2008).

Neck, conjunctival, and scleral hemorrhage also have been reported. Fascial neck muscle congestion and hemorrhage has been reported in 8.1%–51.3% of human drowning cases, conjunctival petechial hemorrhages in 4.1%–15.8%, and scleral hemorrhage in a recent case (Alexander and Jentzen 2011). The hemorrhage in the neck musculature and eye structures is believed to be due to elevated cephalic venous pressure associated with drowning-related coughing, gagging, vomiting, and forceful abdominal and thoracic contractions. Hemorrhage found throughout the neck musculature not confined to the fascial surface requires further investigation into the possibility of traumatic injury (Alexander and Jentzen 2011).

Findings of water and/or foreign material, such as sand/silt, or flora from the water in the upper airways are nonspecific due to their possible passive entrance when the body is submerged. Passive entrance into the distal airways is highly significant due to the length of the trachea in most animals (Munro and Munro 2008). Foreign material found in the deep airways is suggestive of active respiratory effort while in the water (D. Spitz 2006). In addition, if these findings are present in a body that was not found in water they are indicative that the body was submerged at some time prior to discovery. The aspiration of gastric contents commonly occurs during the unconscious gasping phase of drowning (D. Spitz 2006). Samples of all water and debris found should be collected for testing which can also help identify the location of drowning (see Diatoms).

The body should be examined for evidence of perimortem injury and other contributing factors or causes of death and radiography performed. Forcible drownings may have associated bruising from where the animal was held or restrained. The location depends on the method used and if compressed against a firm surface such as in a bathtub. Bruising may be found on the head, neck, torso, distal legs, and over bony prominences. If the body has been immersed in water for a prolonged period of time, the blood from external injuries can be leached out by the water resulting in the appearance of a postmortem injury.

Diagnostic testing

There are additional tests which may be conducted to determine drowning depending on the type of water where it occurred. The analysis of the pericardial fluid and cardiac and peripheral blood is performed in humans. In one study, the pericardial calcium was significantly higher than the clinical reference range in saltwater drownings when compared to other cause of death groups of freshwater drowning, blunt/sharp force injury, fire fatalities, pneumonia, intoxication, mechanical asphyxia, acute cardiac death, hyperthermia, and hypothermia. The pericardial magnesium level also was significantly higher with saltwater drownings and elevated in sharp force injury cases. The Mg/Ca ratio was higher for saltwater drowning and sharp force injury (Li 2009).

In humans there does not appear to be a significant rise in serum Ca or Mg in the cardiac or peripheral blood. In a human study, the Ca and Mg levels were significantly higher in saltwater drownings than the groups of freshwater drowning, asphyxiation, blunt/sharp force injury, fire fatalities, methamphetamine poisoning, delayed death due to trauma, and acute myocardial infarction/ischemia. This is most likely due to the aspiration of saltwater. The Ca was significantly elevated in freshwater drownings and fire fatalities, most likely from peripheral skeletal muscle. The Mg level was significantly elevated in asphyxia and fatal methamphetamine poisonings, most likely from myocardial and/or peripheral muscle (Zhu 2005).

The vitreous sodium levels may help determine drowning deaths, including the drowning medium. A study in humans found that the vitreous humor sodium levels were elevated in saltwater drownings ranging from 145–184 mM (mean 160.2±9.9 mM). In fresh water drowning cases the vitreous humor sodium levels were decreased, ranging from 73–148 mM (mean 129.8 ± 17 mM). These changes may be due to hemodilution or hemoconcentration following inhalation of water or diffusion across the eye external membranes in contact with the water. Because in humans the sodium levels in serum may decrease postmortem at the average rate of 0.9 mEq/L, the finding of increased vitreous sodium levels may be of significance (Byard and Summersides 2011).

Diatoms

Overview

Diatoms are microscopic unicellular algae with a uniquely extracellular coat composed of silica. There are more than 10,000 morphologically distinct varieties of diatoms that range in size from 5 to greater than 500 mm.

They are present in every naturally occurring body of water, from a puddle to the ocean. They are generally in small numbers in tap water but have large concentration in swimming pool water. They also may be found in moist soil and the atmosphere. The type of diatoms found in a certain location is unique and specific to that area. The season also affects what type is found. The diatom populations have monthly fluctuations in their concentrations in a particular body of water (Pollanen 1998). In one body of water, several types of diatoms may be found, but all are located in a separate and specific area. These characteristics can help identify the location and even season of death. Because of the presence of diatoms in all types of water, the analysis for diatoms has been developed as a conclusive test for drowning.

Diatoms can enter the body in three different ways: through inhalation of airborne diatoms, ingestion of material containing diatoms, and aspiration of water containing diatoms. This last route is the foundation for forensic diatom testing, which in conjunction with other findings provides a diagnosis of drowning. When water enters the lungs, either through aspiration if the victim was alive or by postmortem submersion, diatoms may enter the lung tissue passively where they remain and do not disseminate unless the heart is beating. When the diatoms perforate the alveolar-capillary barrier they enter the bloodstream and are disseminated to various organs, including the bone marrow. The detection of diatoms in the bone marrow is then compared with the water that was aspirated into the airways or stomach, from the surface of the body, or from the site at which the body was recovered. A positive match indicates that drowning was the cause of death and the victim was breathing upon entry into the water (Pollanen 1998).

A negative test may be seen with dry-drowning, i.e., when there is no aspiration of water. However, a negative test does not rule out drowning. Diatom testing may be used (a negative test) to determine if the body was dumped in the water postmortem, especially when presented with dismembered limbs (Gruspier and Pollanen 2000). A study in Taiwan also found negative results on non-drowning cases (Lin et al. 2012). Putrefaction, embalming, or burial appear to have no effect on the detection of diatoms in the bone marrow in drowning cases (Chandrasiri 2001).

The testing of soil for diatoms also has been used to determine cause of death or site of death in severely decomposed or skeletonized bodies found on land. If a body was submerged, presumably drowned, subsequently removed from the water, and then dumped on land or buried, the diatoms from the outside of the body and within the lungs are deposited in the soil underneath the body.

Because diatoms may be found in moist soil, samples from underneath and adjacent to the body are tested and compared to soil samples farther away but near the body. These samples also may be compared to water diatoms from nearby bodies of water to determine the site of submersion. A higher concentration of diatoms in the soil associated with the body than the surrounding soil can be indicative that the victim died by drowning.

Diatom testing

The acceptance of diatom testing has been questioned because of the ubiquitous nature of diatoms in the environment. The validity of this test is supported by the criterion of concordance, which demands that the diatoms recovered from tissue be comparable to the diatoms in the alleged drowning medium (Pollanen 1998). The concentration of diatoms in bone marrow and other tissues is directly proportional to the concentration found in the drowning medium. Aquatic diatoms are diagnostically different that those living in other environments. Any contamination is detected by the investigator when comparison is made with the putative drowning medium. This removes the ambiguity of the origin of the diatoms and proves the diatoms were introduced during the drowning process. New testing modalities may further increase the sensitivity and reliability of the diatom test (Rohn and Frade 2006). A study using a quantitative diatom-based reconstruction technique was able to confirm drowning as the cause of death and the site of drowning (Horton et al. 2006).

The diatom test may be conducted on bone marrow or from other tissue in the body. It has been found that the sternum may be the best source for diatoms because the depositional interval for diatoms is shorter than for the femur (Rohn and Frade 2006). The testing of other tissue may provide additional confirmation to bone marrow findings; however, caution must be used when testing other tissues to prevent contamination. The body must not be decomposed and the body cavities must not have been damaged while submerged.

Collection and preparation of samples for diatom testing should be done in such a manner as to prevent contamination from other water supplies. This includes changing gloves when touching or handling a single area and limiting contact of samples to only triple-distilled water (Di Maio and Di Maio 2001). A sample of the drowning medium should be collected from the scene at the site where the body was recovered for comparison testing. Approximately 500–1,000 ml should be collected in a clean container. Additional samples should be taken of the water in the stomach, sinus, or airways. All water samples should be kept separate from the body, stored in separate containers to prevent contamination, and refrigerated to prevent microbe growth. The tissue test for diatoms is usually conducted on the femoral or sternal bone marrow. Tests also may be performed on other tissue from closed organ systems such as an encapsulated kidney from a non-decomposed body.

The body and chest/leg should be cleaned prior to the removal of the bone to prevent contamination with exogenous diatoms. Before removing the bone from the body, it is important to change gloves to prevent contamination of the surface. The bone should be washed in distilled water then placed in a sealed plastic bag and frozen prior to submission to the laboratory for testing (Pollanen 1998).

Strontium testing

Strontium is a trace metal found in the crust of the earth and is widely present in sea water. It is found in smaller quantities in fresh and domestic water. Blood strontium quantification has been used as a supportive test for the diagnosis of drowning and can be performed at most medical laboratories. The foundation for the use of this test is that strontium has a naturally low level in plasma. Elevated levels in the blood are supportive of drowning. The water strontium content affects blood levels, with salt water containing higher levels than fresh water. Decomposition in the water also reduces the detectable blood levels of strontium (Pollanen 1998).

REFERENCES

Alexander, R.T. and J.M. Jentzen. 2011. Neck and Scleral Hemorrhage in Drowning. *Journal of Forensic Sciences.* 56(2):522–525.

Boghossian, E., R. Clément, M. Redpath, and A. Sauvageau. 2010. Respiratory, Circulatory, and Neurological Responses to Hanging: A Review of Animal Models. *Journal of Forensic Sciences.* 55(5):1272–1277.

Byard, R.W. and G. Summersides. 2011. Vitreous Humor Sodium Levels in Immersion Deaths. *Journal of Forensic Sciences.* 56(3):643–644.

Chandrasiri, N. 2001. Detection of Diatoms in the Marrow of Thigh Bones as Evidence of Death by Drowning. *Ceylon Medical Journal.* 46(4):145–146.

Clément, R., J.-P. Guay, M. Redpath, and A. Sauvageau. 2011. Petechiae in Hanging: A Retrospective Study of Contributing Variables. *American Journal of Forensic Medicine and Pathology.* 32(4):378–382.

Clément, R., M. Redpath, and A. Sauvageau. 2010. Mechanism of Death in Hanging: A Historical Review of the Evolution of Pathophysiological Hypotheses. *Journal of Forensic Sciences.* 55(5):1268–1271.

de Paiva, L.A.S., E.R. Parra, D.C. da Rosa, C. Farhat, C. Delmonte, and V.L. Capelozzi. 2008. Autopsy-Proven Determinants of Immediate Fire Death in Lungs. *The American Journal of Forensic Medicine and Pathology.* 29(4):323–329.

Chester, A. 2010. Personal communication regarding video of cat hanging.

Di Maio, V.J. and D. Di Maio. 2001. *Forensic Pathology*, Second edition. Boca Raton, FL: CRC Press.

Dix, J., M. Graham, and R. Hanzlick. 2000. *Asphyxia and Drowning: An Atlas.* Boca Raton, FL: CRC Press.

Duband, S., A.P. Timoshenko, A.L. Morrison, J.-M. Prades, M. Debout, and M. Peoc'h. 2009. Ear Bleeding: A Sign Not to be Underestimated in Cases of Strangulation. *The American Journal of Forensic Medicine and Pathology.* 30(2):175–176.

Evans, H.E. 1993. Prenatal Development. In: *Miller's Anatomy of the Dog*, Third edition, H.E. Evans, ed. pp. 32–97. Philadelphia: W.B. Saunders Company.

Gruspier, K.L. and M.S. Pollanen. 2000. Limbs Found in Water: Investigation Using Anthropological Analysis and the Diatom Test. *Forensic Science International.* 112(1):1–9.

Haglund, W.D. and M.H. Sorg. 2002. Human Remains in Water Environments. In: *Advances in Forensic Taphonomy*, W.D. Haglund and M.H. Sorg, eds. pp. 201–218. Boca Raton, FL: CRC Press.

Hawkins, E.C. 1995. Diseases of the Lower Respiratory System. In: *Textbook of Veterinary Internal Medicine: Diseases of the Dog and Cat*, Vol. 1, Fourth edition, S.J. Ettinger and E.C. Feldman, eds. pp. 767–811. Philadelphia: W.B. Saunders.

Hejna, P. and O. Rejtarová. 2010. Bleedings into the Anterior Aspect of the Intervertebral Disks in the Lumbar Region of the Spine as a Diagnostic Sign of Hanging. *Journal of Forensic Sciences.* 55(2):428–431.

Horton, B.P., S. Breham, and C. Hillier. 2006. The Development and Application of a Diatom-Based Quantitative Reconstruction Technique in Forensic Science. *The American Journal of Forensic Medicine and Pathology* 51(3):643–650.

Li, D.-R., L. Quan, B.-L. Zhu, T. Ishikawa, T. Michiue, D. Zhao, C. Yoshida, J.-H. Chen, Q. Wan, A. Komatsu, Y. Azuma, and H. Maeda. 2009. Evaluation of Postmortem Calcium and Magnesium Levels in the Pericardial Fluid with Regard to the Cause of Death in Medicolegal Autopsy. *Legal Medicine.* 11(1):276–278.

Liebich, H.-G. and H.E. König. 2009. Axial Skeleton (skeleton axiale). In: *Veterinary Anatomy of Domestic Mammals, Textbook and Colour Atlas*, Fourth edition, H.E. König and H.-G. Liebich, pp. 49–112. Stuttgart: Schattauer.

Lin, C.-Y., T.-Y. Huang, C.-C. Huang, F.-C. Chung, and H.-C. Shih. 2012. Diatom Analysis From Suspected Drowning Cases. Presented at the American Academy of Forensic

Sciences Annual Scientific Meeting, 20–25 February, Atlanta, Georgia.

Munro, H.M. and M.V. Thrusfield. 2001. Battered Pets: Non-Accidental Physical Injuries Found in Dogs and Cats. *Journal of Small Animal Practice* 42:279–290.

Munro, R. and H. Munro. 2008. Asphyxia and Drowning. In: *Animal Abuse and Unlawful Killing: Forensic Veterinary Pathology*, pp. 65–69. Edinburgh: Elsevier.

Nikolić, S., V. Živković, Babić, and F. Juković. 2012. Cervical Soft Tissue Emphysema in Hanging—A Prospective Autopsy Study. *Journal of Forensic Sciences*, 57(1):132–135.

Pollanen, M.S. 1998. *Forensic Diatomology and Drowning*. Amsterdam: Elsevier Science.

Rohn, E.J. and P.D. Frade. 2006. The Role of Diatoms in Medicolegal Investigations I: The History, Contemporary Science, and Application of the Diatom Test for Drowning. *The Forensic Examiner* 15(3):11–15.

Sauvageau, A. and E. Boghassian. 2010. Classification of Asphyxia: The Need for Standardization. *Journal of Forensic Sciences*. 55(5):1259–1267.

Şenol, E., B. Demirel, T. Akar, ö. Gülbahar, C. Bakar, and N. Bukan. 2008. The Analysis of Hormones and Enzymes Extracted from Endocrine Glands of the Neck Region in Deaths Due to Hanging. *The American Journal of Forensic Medicine and Pathology*. 29(1):49–54.

Somers, G.R., D.A. Chiasson, and C.R. Smith. 2006. Pediatric Drowning: A 20-Year Review of Autopsied Cases: II. Pathologic Features. *The American Journal of Forensic Medicine and Pathology* 27(1):20–24.

Spitz, D.J. 2006. Investigation of Bodies in Water. In: *Spitz and Fisher's Medicolegal Investigation of Death: Guidelines for the Application of Pathology to Crime Investigation*, Fourth edition, W.U. Spitz and D.J. Spitz, eds. pp. 846–881. Springfield: Charles C. Thomas Publisher, Ltd.

Spitz, W.U. 2006. Asphyxia. In: *Spitz and Fisher's Medicolegal Investigation of Death: Guidelines for the Application of Pathology to Crime Investigation*, Fourth edition. W.U. Spitz and D.J. Spitz, eds. pp. 783–845. Springfield: Charles C. Thomas Publisher, Ltd.

Suárez-Peñaranda, J.M., T. álvarez, X. Miguéns, M.S. Rodríguez-Calvo, B.L. de Abajo, M. Cortesão, C. Cordeiro, D.N. Viera, and J.I. Muñoz. 2008. Characterization of Lesions in Hanging Deaths. *Journal Forensic Sciences*. 53(3):720–723.

Tsokos, M., G. Cains, and R.W. Byard. 2008. Hemolytic Staining of the Intima of the Aortic Root in Freshwater Drowning. *The American Journal of Forensic Medicine and Pathology*. 29(2):128–130.

Venker-van Haagen, A.J. 1995. Diseases of the Throat. In: *Textbook of Veterinary Internal Medicine: Diseases of the Dog and Cat*, Vol. 1, Fourth edition, S.J. Ettinger and E.C. Feldman, eds. pp. 567–575. Philadelphia: W.B. Saunders.

Zhu, B.-L., T. Ishikawa, L. Quan, D.-R. Li, D. Zhao, T. Michiue, and H. Maeda. 2005. Evaluation of Postmortem Serum Calcium and Magnesium Levels in Relation to the Causes of Death in Forensic Autopsy. *Forensic Science International*. 155(1):18–23.

10
Poisoning

Sharon M. Gwaltney-Brant

In a sense, the victim shapes and moulds the criminal.

Hans von Hentig

OVERVIEW OF INTENTIONAL POISONINGS

Incidence

For a variety of reasons the actual incidence of intentional animal poisonings cannot be accurately determined. Perhaps most importantly, many intentional poisonings are never actually witnessed by animal owners, which may result in a poisoning case being mistaken for an infectious, metabolic, or other condition. It may be mistakenly assumed that an intentional poisoning has occurred when animals are accidentally exposed to toxic agents in their environment. Many toxicoses manifest as non-specific signs (e.g., vomiting and depression) that can make the diagnosis of an unwitnessed poisoning challenging. Additionally, a nationwide means of reporting animal poisonings does not exist. Animal and (some) human poison control centers maintain databases on the animal poisoning cases they receive, but there is no central reporting agency to which animal poisonings can be compiled so that accurate accounting of intentional poisonings can be made. In most cases, animal poisonings reported to poison control centers are done so for real-time treatment recommendations, so if an animal has died there is little incentive to report to a poison control center. Even if a central reporting center did exist, animal owners or veterinarians might be reluctant to report suspected intentional poisonings because of lack of sufficient evidence or, in the case of veterinarians, time.

Intentional poisonings include abuse or misuse of products and malicious intent. Abuse may include intentional intoxication of an animal as a "joke" (e.g., intentionally blowing marijuana smoke into a pet's face), whereas in cases of misuse of an agent, the actual intent generally was not to cause harm to the animal (e.g., giving acetaminophen to an ill cat). Rare instances of attention seeking by means of factitious illness (i.e., Münchausen syndrome by proxy) involving poisoning of pets have been reported (Munro and Thrusfield 2001b). Malicious poisonings may be aimed at destroying animals that the poisoner considers pests, occasionally with unfortunate consequences for non-target animals that also may be exposed, or the poisoning may be done in retaliation against the animal or its owners. Rarely, malicious poisoning is done strictly for the sadistic pleasure it brings the poisoner.

Because of these limitations, one can assume that the incidence of intentional animal poisonings reported to poison control centers (animal and human) very likely greatly underestimates the actual incidence. In spite of this, poison control data can show some trends that may be of interest in evaluating intentional animal poisonings. Based on information from human and animal poison control centers, intentional exposures comprise less than 1% of all exposures of animals to potentially toxic agents, and malicious poisonings account for less than 0.5% of all poisonings reported (Hansen et al. 2001). Of intentional exposures, abuse/misuse of agents accounts for approximately one-half of feline exposures, with the majority of these being off-label use of dog flea control products on cats (ASPCA 2011). Malicious exposures in cats account

Veterinary Forensics: Animal Cruelty Investigations, Second Edition. Edited by Melinda D. Merck.
© 2013 John Wiley & Sons, Inc. Published 2013 by John Wiley & Sons, Inc.

for approximately one-third of intentional exposures, whereas in dogs more than one-half of intentional exposures to potentially toxic agents are reported as malicious in nature (Hornfeldt 1997; ASPCA 2011).

When considered as a subset of injuries that occur in instances of animal abuse or cruelty, poisoning still is relatively uncommonly reported. In surveys of practicing veterinarians in the United Kingdom and the Republic of Ireland, poisonings accounted for 4.1% and 12.1% of non-accidental injuries reported, respectively (Munro and Thrusfield 2001a; McGuinness et al. 2005).

Demographics

Although intentional poisonings can occur in any species, such poisonings are most commonly reported in dogs and cats. Dogs account for more than 75% of malicious poisoning cases, cats account for approximately 15%, and other species, including wildlife, comprise the remainder of reported malicious poisonings. Of the malicious canine poisonings reported to the American Society for Prevention of Cruelty to Animals (ASPCA) Animal Poison Control Center between 2002 and 2005, 22% involved either Labrador retrievers or German shepherds (ASPCA 2006) (Table 10.1). German shepherds and their mixes appear to be over–represented in malicious poisonings, as they account for just 4.2% of all toxicoses (Gwaltney-Brant 2006), although they were involved in 11% of malicious poisonings. Conversely, pure- and mixed-breed Labrador retrievers appear to be under-represented in malicious intent (11%) compared with overall poisonings (17.6%) and their relative popularity (15%). These trends are similar to those found in an earlier study of malicious poisonings in dogs during 1999 and 2000, with the exception that in the previous study Rottweilers and their mixes accounted for 6% of malicious poisonings compared with 3% in the more recent study (Hansen et al. 2001). These breed trends also mirror the breed trends identified in cruelty cases involving other forms of non-accidental physical injury (Munro and Thrusfield 2001a, McGuinness et al. 2005). No specific breed trends have been reported in feline malicious poisonings.

Index of suspicion

Unfortunately, it is not uncommon for animal owners to assume that an ill animal has been poisoned and present it to the veterinarian as a poisoning. It is important that the veterinarian in this type of situation not allow the client's opinion to cloud medical judgment. In the majority of poisoning cases, whether intentional or accidental, it is usually the acute onset of significant clinical signs that appear to have no obvious cause that triggers suspicion of

Table 10.1. Top ten dog breeds involved in malicious poisonings.

Breed	Percent
German shepherd	11%
Labrador retriever	11%
Mixed breed, unspecified	8%
Chihuahua	6%
American pit bull terrier	5%
Great Dane	5%
Golden retriever	3%
Great Pyrenees	3%
Jack Russell/Parson Russell	3%
Rottweiler	3%

Source: ASPCA. 2006. AnToxTM Database, 2002–2005. ASPCA Animal Poison Control Center: Urbana, IL.

poisoning. Less commonly, insidious illness resulting from chronic exposure to a toxicant may occur. In all cases, it is important to consider all potential differentials before settling on a diagnosis of poisoning, and lacking direct evidence of exposure to a potential toxicant, poisoning should be considered a diagnosis of exclusion.

EVIDENCE AND HISTORY

Occasionally, an animal owner may witness the exposure of the pet to a potential toxicant or find evidence of the toxicant on the animal's coat or fur, or the animal may quickly vomit up the agent, making it evident that an ingestion has occurred. More frequently, animal poisonings are not witnessed, and diagnosis of poisoning relies on other observations.

Historical information is essential to determine as much as possible the events leading up to the poisoning of the patient. Whether the animal was indoors or outdoors prior to development of clinical signs, the number and status of other animals in the same environment, the rapidity of onset and progression of clinical signs, and the presence of children or adolescents in the environment are all factors that may provide clues to the source and intent of a poisoning.

The patient's prior health history, including any current medications, should be obtained to determine if any pre-existing conditions are present that may alter the patient's response to therapy, exacerbate signs of toxicosis, or confound toxicological testing.

Clinical findings

Very few toxicants produce definitively diagnostic clinical signs, although in many cases the clinical signs provide valuable clues as to the class of potential agents involved

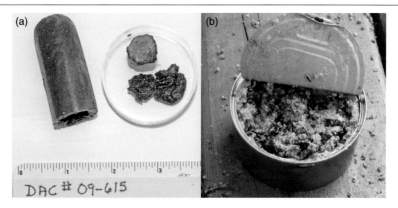

Figure 10.1. Evidence of malicious tampering with food. (a) A hot dog that had been cored out and filled with blue-green granules then sealed at the end with a plug of hot dog was found in the yard of a dog that presented to the veterinarian with seizures. A similar piece of hot dog was vomited up by the dog; the granules were later identified as aldicarb, a carbamate insecticide. (b) Cat food adulterated with an anticoagulant rodenticide (green) and strychnine (red). (Photos courtesy of T. Brant and M.K. McLean, respectively.)

(e.g., central nervous system [CNS] depressant vs. CNS stimulant). As with any emergent patient, the potential poisoning patient should be examined thoroughly and any life-threatening issues dealt with immediately. After the patient has been stabilized, abnormalities in vital signs and cardiovascular, hematological, neurological, musculoskeletal, and gastrointestinal (GI) function should be recorded in detail. Examination of skin, eyes, and oral mucosa for ulceration or inflammation should be performed. Blood should be drawn for baseline clinical chemistry and hematological analysis; at this time, evaluation for defects in hemostasis may be performed. Ancillary clinical procedures that may aid in narrowing down the potential agent involved in a poisoning include radiography, ultrasonography, and endoscopy.

Olfactory clues to poisonings include the garlicky odor associated with toxicants such as arsenic, thallium, and zinc phosphide or the bitter almond odor of cyanide. Many pesticides, especially insecticides, have a hydrocarbon odor. Bleaches, alcohols, and ammonia-based products leave their distinctive odors on the coat or breath of the animal.

Response to therapy also may yield clues as to the type of toxicant involved. Animals presenting with agitation or tremors from sympathomimetic drugs such as amphetamines frequently become even more agitated if treated with diazepam, but tend to respond well with low doses of acepromazine. Similarly, cats with tremors from exposure to concentrated formulations of pyrethroids (e.g., permethrin) frequently do not respond well to diazepam but tremors often quickly resolve upon administration of methocarbamol.

Animals found dead should be examined externally for evidence of antemortem clinical signs. Vomit or diarrhea staining of the hair coat indicates antemortem GI dysfunction, whereas rapid onset of rigor mortis can be suggestive of antemortem seizures or hyperthermia. Samples of residues on the hair coat should be taken, and any vomitus or diarrhea should be collected, carefully labeled and sealed, and saved for future analysis. Once external examination and sample collection is complete, a necropsy should be performed.

Environmental and physical evidence

Evaluation of the environment in which the animal lives may aid in detecting potential sources of poisonings. This is especially important when malicious poisoning is suspected, because potential sources of accidental poisoning need to be identified and eliminated as potential causes to add weight to the case for intentional poisoning. Indoor environments should be evaluated for potential exposure to items such as plants, pharmaceuticals, illicit drugs, cleaning and other household products, lead-containing items, pesticides, and potentially toxic foods. Outdoor habitats should be similarly evaluated for the above-mentioned items as well as mushrooms, lawn care and pool products, poisonous and venomous animals, water-borne toxicants (e.g., blue-green algae), compost piles, mulches, automotive materials, and garbage containers.

Environmental clues to intentional poisonings might include the unexpected presence of scattered food products (Figure 10.1), product containers, or granular or pelleted materials in the animal's habitat. Open gates or doors to areas where potential toxicants are stored may indicate the recent presence of an uninvited person to the animal's environment.

DIAGNOSTICS

Investigation of intentional animal poisonings requires close attention to detail in evaluation of history and clinical findings, accurate and appropriate sample collection, maintenance of chain of custody of evidence, and judicious use of analytical testing. The veterinarian's role in evaluating a suspected malicious poisoning encompasses all of these requirements, as well as appropriate contact with the necessary public authorities (animal control and/or law enforcement) to ensure that adequate evidence is collected to provide for successful prosecution should the perpetrator be found.

Necropsy considerations

Forensic necropsy of suspected malicious poisoning victims ideally should be performed by a board-certified pathologist at a veterinary diagnostic laboratory; this is especially important if the case is expected to be pursued by the legal system. Although most veterinary practitioners have been trained to perform a basic necropsy, cases of malicious poisoning may have few or subtle lesions that may be overlooked. Additionally, forensic necropsies require detailed record keeping, documentation in full detail with photographs, and accurate animal identification so that accurate testimony can be given, often years after the necropsy was performed. Veterinary diagnostic laboratories have the facilities required for secure, possibly long-term, storage of biological evidence. Finally, veterinary diagnostic laboratories compile data that can be useful as references for future cases and epidemiological studies of animal poisonings.

If referral of a body to a diagnostic laboratory is not possible, the veterinary practitioner should perform a thorough and complete necropsy, maintaining numerous records. A tape recorder may be used to dictate findings, which later can be transcribed into a written report. Initial examination should include photographs of the body and any external abnormalities. Foreign material on the haircoat or in the oral cavity should be swabbed and saved for possible future analysis.

Once the external examination is complete, a thorough examination of internal organs (including brain) should be performed. It is important that the prosecutor not jump to conclusions or make assumptions during the necropsy. Each organ system should be examined thoroughly and samples collected methodically. Epidermis, subcutaneous tissue, and muscle associated with any identified injection sites should be excised and saved. For exclusionary purposes, samples may be submitted for non-toxicology–related tests (e.g., microbiology) based on lesions found at necropsy. Stomach contents should be examined closely for evidence of foreign objects, such as granules and pellets, plant material, foods, pill casings, tablet fragments, or illicit drugs. Samples of all major organs should be taken and preserved in fixative for histopathological examination. For large organs, such as liver, sections should be taken from multiple areas rather than a single site.

Toxicology testing

Sample collection and submission

When investigating potential malicious poisonings, sample collection is essential for confirmatory tests to be performed. When collecting samples, it is always best to err on the side of taking too many samples, because one can always throw away unneeded samples but it is not possible to resurrect material that has been discarded (Table 10.2). Live animal samples include stomach contents from lavage and/or vomitus, urine, feces, whole blood, serum or plasma, and hair. The patient's oral cavity should be inspected for agents lodged in the teeth or trapped in mucosal folds; these items should be collected and saved for future analysis. Because some analytes may be damaged by contact with red blood cells, it is best to collect both whole blood and serum or plasma.

In general, glass containers are preferred over plastic because plastic can leach contaminants into samples over time. If plastic containers must be used, harder plastics pose less risk of sample contamination. Never store samples in syringes, because leakage may occur and syringes with needles are hazardous to receiving personnel. For toxicological analysis, serum and plasma may be frozen prior to shipping, whereas whole blood should be refrigerated, never frozen. Urine may be refrigerated or frozen. Vomitus, gastric contents, and feces should be stored in glass or hard plastic and may be frozen prior to shipping. Hair samples are most useful for topical exposures and they may be stored in paper envelopes or hard plastic or glass vials. Damp hair should be allowed to thoroughly air dry before being placed in sealed containers.

For necropsy specimens, samples of heart blood, liver, kidney, urine, stomach/intestinal contents, hair, and feces should be saved for toxicological analysis. If exposure to anticholinesterase agents (organophosphates or carbamates) is suspected, samples of brain and retina (submit entire eyeball) may be evaluated for cholinesterase activity.

Table 10.2. Sample collection for toxicology.

Sample	Amount	Storage	Analysis
All major organs	Multiple small samples	10% buffered neutral formalin (or other fixative)	Histopathology
Liver	300 grams	Chilled, frozen	Heavy metals, pesticides, pharmaceuticals
Kidney	300 grams	Chilled, frozen	Heavy metals, ethylene glycol, pharmaceuticals, plant toxins
Brain	One–half (remainder for histopathology and infectious disease)	Chilled, frozen	Sodium, cholinesterase, pesticides
Fat	300 grams	Chilled, frozen	Organochlorines, PCBs, bromethalin
Ocular fluid	Entire eye	Chilled	Potassium, nitrates, magnesium, ammonia
Lung/spleen	100 grams	Chilled, frozen	Paraquat, barbiturates
Injection site	100 grams	Chilled	Some drugs
Whole blood	5–10 mL	Chilled	Heavy metals, cholinesterase, insecticides
Serum	5–10 mL	Chilled	Some metals, pharmaceuticals, alkaloids, electrolytes
Urine	5–100 mL	Chilled	Pharmaceuticals, heavy metals, alkaloids
Milk	30 mL	Chilled	Organochlorines, PCBs
Ingesta/feces	Up to 500 grams	Chilled	Metals, plants, mycotoxins, other organic toxicants
Hair	3–5 grams	Dry, store in paper	Pesticides, some heavy metals
Feed	1 kg composite	Dry: store in paper, wet: freeze	Ionophores, salt, pesticides, heavy metals, ionophores, mycotoxins, nutrients, botulism
Plant	Entire	Dry; press between sheets of newspaper	Alkaloids, glycosides, pesticides
Water	1–2 liters	Glass containers	Pesticides, heavy metals, salt, nitrates, blue–green algae
Soil	500 grams	Glass containers	Pesticides, heavy metals

It is important to remember that there is no single toxicology screen that can detect all known toxic agents, and testing at random can prove to be expensive and futile. Determining which toxicant to look for in a chemical analysis is based on the clinical, historical, and environmental findings in the case, which hopefully provide the clinician with a list of potential rule-outs to consider. In a 2003 outbreak of suspected malicious poisonings of dogs in a public park in Portland, Oregon, the clinical signs shown by the affected dogs (oral ulcerations, gastrointestinal signs, progressive respiratory distress) allowed veterinarians to suspect paraquat and request the appropriate analysis; paraquat poisoning was confirmed in several of the dogs (Cope 2004).

Some laboratories offer specific screening tests based on clinical findings. For instance, Michigan State University's diagnostic laboratory (Appendix 37) offers a convulsant screen that analyzes for toxicants frequently associated with seizures or convulsions, including bromethalin, metaldehyde, organophosphate insecticides, carbamates, strychnine, and tremorgenic mycotoxins. In general, however, one needs to have an idea of what toxicant is suspected to request the appropriate analysis. In these situations, consultation with a veterinary toxicologist can frequently provide the most cost-effective and efficient means of determining which toxicological tests should be performed.

An important aspect in the interpretation of toxicology results is to realize that exposure to a potential toxicant does not necessarily indicate that a toxicosis has occurred. With all toxic agents, there is a threshold below which signs will not develop (i.e., "The dose makes the poison"). This is especially important to remember as our ability to analyze and detect agents in samples improves, and our ability to measure the presence of agents at minute levels means we will at times detect the presence of agents at levels consistent with casual exposure but not toxicosis. Close attention should be paid to the normal background levels indicated by the testing laboratory that accurate interpretation of analytical results occurs. Again, consultation with a veterinary toxicologist can provide the appropriate interpretation of laboratory results.

Finally, once a diagnosis of toxicosis has been confirmed through evaluation of clinical findings and laboratory results, the determination of malicious intent still can be difficult to establish. This is especially true in cases of malicious animal poisonings, because the victims cannot testify that they saw the perpetrator expose them to the poison. Ancillary trace evidence should be collected and retained, including any potentially poisoned foods materials (e.g., cans of tuna or pet food mixed with rodenticides or ethylene glycol) along with their containers. The food materials can be analyzed for the presence of the toxic agent, and fingerprints or trace evidence on the containers may provide sufficient evidence that the suspected perpetrator was in possession of the tainted material at some time.

Chain of custody

Maintaining chain of custody of collected evidence entails complete documentation of sample collection (date/time of collection, condition of sample, type of storage); witnesses to sample collection; and the name of parties responsible for sample during collection, storage, and transit (Galey 1995). Courier services with tracking capabilities should be used when transporting samples to maintain chain of custody (Chapter 3).

Human laboratories

Human hospital laboratories may be of assistance in determining exposure to agents commonly associated with toxicosis in humans. The currently available bench-top tests for ethylene glycol can result in both false positives and false negatives under a variety of circumstances (e.g., using isopropanol on the skin prior to venipuncture). Because of the questionable accuracy of these tests, samples from patients in which malicious ethylene glycol poisoning is suspected should be sent to a human hospital or veterinary diagnostic laboratory.

When a rapid diagnosis is needed in the emergent patient, human hospitals can generally perform ethylene glycol testing on a STAT basis. Human hospitals use a quantitative test that gives the actual serum level rather than a positive or negative result. Other tests that can be performed by human hospitals include serum iron levels, total iron binding capacity, acetaminophen levels, and salicylate levels. Additionally, most hospitals use ToxiLab® as a quick screening test for a variety of commonly abused human drugs, including opioids, marijuana, amphetamines, barbiturates, antidepressants, and cocaine. These tests also may be beneficial in determining exposure of animals to these agents, with the caveat that most of these tests have not been validated in species other than humans.

Over-the-counter testing kits

Over-the-counter (OTC) home testing kits for a variety of illicit drugs (opioids, marijuana, amphetamines, barbiturates, cocaine, and benzodiazepines) have become readily available in most human pharmacies and via the Internet. These kits are easy to use, affordable, and are frequently used in veterinary emergency clinics with varying success for diagnosing cases of animal poisonings with these agents (Figure 10.2).

A study of one such test revealed that it correctly identified the presence of metabolites of barbiturates, benzodiazepines, opiates, amphetamine/methamphetamine, cocaine, and phencyclidine in canine urine, but did not detect metabolites from marijuana or methadone, a synthetic opioid (Teitler 2009). Although these tests can be valuable screening tests for suspected toxicosis of certain drugs in clinical settings, their accuracy has not been validated in non-humans. Therefore, in a potential legal case, samples from an OTC kit-positive patient should be sent to an accredited diagnostic laboratory for confirmation.

AGENTS USED IN ANIMAL POISONINGS

Introduction

There are virtually an unlimited number of agents that might potentially be used to maliciously poison animals, making diagnosis of malicious poisonings challenging.

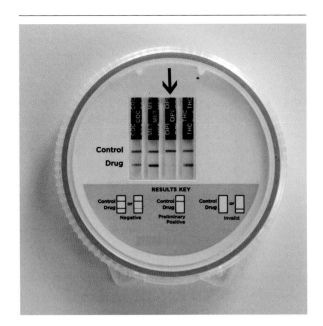

Figure 10.2. Over–the–counter multidrug urine test kits can be helpful in diagnosing cases of suspected drug ingestion in animals. In this test, a positive result is indicated by a lack of development of a line in the "Drug" row, indicating exposure to opioids (arrow), while cocaine, methamphetamine and marijuana columns are negative. For legal cases, results of this type of test should be confirmed through additional testing by a validated diagnostic laboratory. (Photo courtesy of T. Brant.)

However, in spite of the wide variety of agents available, most poisoners tend to use a narrow range of agents. An informal survey by the author of toxicologists at veterinary diagnostic laboratories across the country indicated that the primary poisons of choice in intentional poisonings are anticoagulant rodenticides and ethylene glycol. Other commonly reported poisons involved in malicious poisonings included organophosphate insecticides, carbamates, strychnine (particularly in the northwestern United States), caffeine, and methylxanthines.

Ethylene glycol

Sources

Ethylene glycol (EG) is most commonly found in automotive antifreezes and windshield de-icers, but it is also present in brake fluids, inks, and some paints. Automotive antifreeze is 95% EG, although it is usually diluted to 50% in automobile radiators. EG is inexpensive, easily obtained, and palatable, although the attractiveness of the taste of EG to dogs has been exaggerated (Marshall and Doty 1990). EG can be mixed readily with other foods to entice target animals to ingest it and is fairly well known for its toxicity to animals, all of which may contribute to the fact that it is one of the most commonly used malicious poisons.

Cats are very sensitive to EG. Less than a teaspoon of undiluted EG is fatal to most cats. Dogs are about three to four times less susceptible than cats to EG.

Mechanism of action

The toxicity of EG is primarily caused by its conversion to highly toxic metabolites (Bischoff 2009). Parent EG is an alcohol, which accounts for the initial inebriation that develops. As EG is converted to acidic metabolites, severe metabolic acidosis ensues. The metabolite oxalic acid binds with serum calcium to form calcium oxalate crystals, which collect in the renal tubules. The renal damage likely results from a combination of metabolic derangement of the tubular epithelium caused by the toxic metabolites as well as mechanical injury caused by the presence of calcium oxalate crystals in the kidney.

Clinical signs and clinical laboratory findings

EG toxicosis is characterized by three stages: inebriation, acidosis, and renal failure. These stages may overlap, the animal may appear to recover from one or more stages, or death may occur during any of these stages. The inebriation stage occurs within thirty minutes of exposure and may persist up to twelve hours. The primary signs are central nervous system (CNS) depression, ataxia, disorientation, tremors, muscle fasciculations, hypothermia, polyuria, and gastrointestinal (GI) irritation. In dogs ingesting lower dosages of EG, signs may subside and apparent recovery may occur, whereas cats tend to remain markedly depressed.

Acidosis develops within twelve to twenty-four hours after exposure and is characterized by deepening CNS depression, tachypnea, tachycardia, pulmonary edema, metabolic acidosis, high anion gap, and high osmolal gap. Hypocalcemia occurs in approximately one-half of EG intoxicated patients, although hypocalcemic tetany is uncommon. Calcium oxalate crystalluria can be seen as early as three hours postexposure in cats and six hours in dogs, but the absence of crystalluria does not rule out an ethylene glycol toxicosis. Elevations in blood urea nitrogen (BUN) and serum creatinine may occur as early as twelve hours in cats and twenty-four hours in dogs. Oliguric or anuric renal failure subsequently develops, accompanied by vomiting, depression, anorexia, renal pain, oral ulceration, and seizures.

Diagnostics

Diagnosis of ethylene glycol toxicosis can be challenging, because the signs of toxicosis vary depending on the stage in which the patient is presented. Early stages of inebriation can resemble intoxication by alcohol or marijuana. Because many automotive antifreezes contain fluorescent dye, examination of a suspected EG victim's fur, paws, face, mouth, vomitus, and urine with a Wood's lamp may reveal fluorescence, indicating exposure. Fluorescence may be detectable in urine up to six hours after ingestion, but the absence of fluorescence does not rule out the possibility of EG exposure.

The newer enzyme-based bench-top EG test kits have the advantages of ease of use and speed when compared to the previously available in-house test kit; additionally, these tests are sensitive enough to allow for EG testing in cats. Unfortunately, these tests have proven to be less than ideal, because there are quite a few compounds that can cause them to give false positive results, including other alcohols (e.g., isopropanol used on skin prior to venipuncture), other glycols (e.g., propylene glycol from activated charcoal formulations), and glycerin (e.g., soft-moist pet foods). False negatives appear to be less of a concern other than in patients treated with fomepizole, so for most patients, a negative result can be believed.

When absolute confirmation of EG levels is required it is recommended that quantitative analysis be done. Most human hospitals are able to do this on a STAT basis. Blood EG levels over 20 mg/dL in cats and 50 mg/dL in dogs are indicative of toxic levels and merit aggressive treatment. It is important that blood samples be taken at least an hour after exposure to EG.

Other confirmatory laboratory changes associated with EG exposure include increased osmolality with high osmolal gap, high anion gap, elevated BUN, elevated creatinine, and hyperglycemia. Hyperkalemia, hypocalcemia, hyperphosphatemia, and isosthenuria or hyposthenuria are present variably. Calcium oxalate crystalluria is strongly suggestive of exposure, but absence of crystalluria does not rule out EG intoxication.

Ultrasonography of kidneys in later stages of EG toxicosis may reveal a halo sign, with areas of higher echogenicity within the cortical and medullary regions surrounding an area of lower echogenicity at the corticomedullary junction and central cortical areas. The halo sign is most often associated with the onset of anuria (Thrall et al. 2006).

Trace mineral analysis of kidneys generally reveals renal calcium concentrations greater than 8,000 ppm and a calcium:phosphorus ratio of greater than 2.5 (Rumbeiha 2006).

Lesions

Gross lesions of EG toxicosis may be absent in animals that die of acidosis or hypothermia prior to the onset of renal injury. Animals dying of renal failure may have pale, soft, swollen kidneys that can be gritty on cutting. An impression smear made with the cut surface of kidney can reveal the presence of numerous birefringent crystals. Other potential lesions in animals dying of renal failure include uremia-associated oral and gastric ulceration, mineralization of gastric mucosa (gritty on cutting), and ulcerative colitis (especially in cats). In uremic animals surviving several days, mineralization of the endocardium, lungs, and intercostal muscles may be evident as white, gritty plaques (Maxie 1985). Histopathological lesions in the kidney reveal the presence of birefringent crystals within the renal tubules associated with renal tubular degeneration and necrosis. Mineralization of the tubular basement membrane often is present. In cases that survive more than a few days, evidence of tubular regeneration may be evident. Calcium oxalate crystals may be found in other areas occasionally, including the liver and meninges. Evidence of metastatic mineralization may be found in the gastric mucosa, media of arteries and arterioles, pulmonary interstitium, epicardium, myocardium, and meninges.

Differential diagnoses for ethylene glycol are many and they vary with the stage at presentation of the animal. The initial inebriation seen in EG toxicosis is similar to that seen with ingestion of other alcohols or glycols (e.g., methanol, propylene glycol) as well as marijuana and some medications affecting CNS function (e.g., baclofen). Other alcohols can produce acidosis and high serum osmolality, and ethanol may cause transient hypocalcemia). Differential diagnoses for acute renal failure include nonsteroidal anti-inflammatory drug (NSAID) toxicosis, aminoglycoside ingestion, grape/raisin ingestion, Lilium or Hemerocallis ingestion (cats), and ingestion of vitamin D or its analogues (e.g., calcipotriene). Non-toxicologic rule-outs to consider for renal failure include leptospirosis, borreliosis, hemolytic uremic syndrome, hemoglobin/myoglobin nephropathy, renal dysplasia, and acute decompensation of chronic renal failure.

Anticoagulant rodenticides

Sources

Anticoagulant rodenticides include a large number of different compounds, including warfarin, pindone, brodifacoum, bromadiolone, chlorphacinone, difethiolone, and diphacinone. First-generation anticoagulants include warfarin and pindone, whereas second-generation anticoagulants encompass most of the other agents.

Second-generation anticoagulants were developed to poison warfarin-resistant rats and mice. Anticoagulant rodenticides are available as grain-based pellets, paraffin-based blocks, meal baits, tracking powders, grains, and dusts (Murphy and Talcott 2006). Rodenticides are not color coded, so identification of a particular rodenticide can be difficult if the packaging is not available.

Mechanism of action

Anticoagulants are vitamin K antagonists as they inhibit the recycling of vitamin K epoxide hydroxylase, thereby inhibiting the recycling of vitamin K in the body. This ultimately results in decreased synthesis of vitamin K–dependent clotting factors II, VII, IX, and X. As these factors become depleted, a process that usually takes three to five days to become clinically evident, evidence of coagulopathy develops.

Clinical signs and clinical laboratory findings

The clinical signs seen with anticoagulant rodenticide toxicosis depend on the site of hemorrhage. Frank hemorrhage may occur from the oral cavity, nose, rectum, vulva, or prepuce, or from minor skin lesions that fail to stop bleeding. Internal hemorrhage into the lungs, mediastinum, thymus, or trachea may present as acute dyspnea, whereas hemorrhage into muscle or subcutis may present with large hematomas. Lameness may occur because of bleeding into joint cavities and neurological signs may develop if bleeding into the brain or spinal cord occurs. Hemorrhage into the abdomen may manifest as weakness, lethargy, anorexia, and pallor. Failure of blood to clot may be noted upon venipuncture for blood collection.

Laboratory abnormalities may include decreases in hematocrit and plasma protein levels secondary to hemorrhage as well as elevations in coagulation parameters. Prothrombin times tend to elevate first in all animals except horses, in which partial thromboplastin time (PTT) can elevate first within twenty-four hours of exposure to anticoagulants (McConnico et al. 1997).

Diagnostics

Elevations in coagulation parameters with associated hemorrhage are highly suspicious for exposure to anticoagulant rodenticides, especially in otherwise healthy animals. Reduction in coagulation parameters in response to vitamin K1 therapy within twelve to twenty-four hours of initiation of treatment is supportive of anticoagulant rodenticide toxicosis. Pre-existing liver disease may be a non-toxic cause of coagulopathy; therefore, a complete serum chemical profile should be obtained. Unlike anticoagulant rodenticide-induced coagulopathy, coagulopathy secondary to hepatopathy tends to be poorly responsive to vitamin K1.

Anticoagulant rodenticides can be detected in plasma, serum, liver, and other tissues. Many veterinary diagnostic laboratories perform a rodenticide screen to detect the major rodenticides, including all of the anticoagulants. Because of the varying half-life of anticoagulant rodenticides and the fact that the initial dose ingested is rarely known in an intentional poisoning, the concentrations of anticoagulant found in the liver or serum often do not correlate well with the severity of the clinical syndrome seen. However, detection of anticoagulant in tissues of an animal with a coagulopathy is highly supportive of anticoagulant toxicosis.

When intentional poisoning with anticoagulant rodenticides is suspected, it is important that investigators be informed that the exposure would have been anywhere from three to seven days prior to the patient presenting with coagulopathy.

Lesions

Lesions are related to hemorrhage, either externally or into a variety of bodily sites, including meninges, thymus, larynx, renal or perirenal tissue, thoracic cavity, abdominal cavity, liver, pericardial sac, GI tract, nasal cavity, joints, muscles, and mediastinum. On necropsy, blood clots poorly, and usually there is a generalized pallor to tissues.

Differential diagnoses for anticoagulant rodenticide toxicosis include coagulopathies secondary to disseminated intravascular coagulopathy, congenital clotting factor deficiencies, von Willebrand's disease, paraneoplastic syndromes, liver disease, platelet defects, and infectious disease (e.g., ehrlichiosis).

Bromethalin

Sources

Bromethalin is a neurotoxic rodenticide that is occasionally mistaken for an anticoagulant because of similarity of its name with the anticoagulants bromadiolone and brodifacoum. Bromethalin is formulated in pellets or block forms for residential use and 2%–10% solutions are available for use by licensed pest control operators (Dorman 2006).

Mechanism of action

Bromethalin requires activation to desmethyl bromethalin to exert its toxic effect. Interestingly, as guinea pigs are deficient at desmethylation, they are highly resistant to the effects of bromethalin (Dunayer 2003). Desmethyl bromethalin is thought to uncouple oxidative phosphorylation in the CNS, resulting in decreased adenosine triphosphatase (ATP) production and failure of ATP-dependent ion pumps. Dissociation of fluid into myelinated areas of the brain and spinal cord results in edema of myelin sheaths and interference with nerve conduction. Some of the adverse effects of bromethalin within the CNS may also result from lipid peroxidation of cerebral membranes (Dorman 2006).

Clinical signs and clinical laboratory findings

Clinical signs associated with bromethalin are dose dependent in onset and severity. Very large ingestions result in onset of severe CNS signs within twenty-four hours of exposure; they are characterized by muscle tremors, hyperexcitability, hyperesthesia, hyperthermia, and focal motor or generalized seizures. Death generally occurs within twenty-four to thirty-six hours after ingestion. Ingestion of lower doses results in a syndrome characterized by delayed onset (three to six days) of neurological signs, including hindlimb ataxia, paresis or paralysis, and depression. Cats may show abdominal distention secondary to enlarged bowel loops. Other potential signs include behavior changes, nystagmus, abnormal posturing, opisthotonos, muscle tremors, vomiting, and anorexia. Signs may progress over a one- to two-week period to end in death, or signs may stabilize with gradual improvement possible over days to weeks.

Clinical laboratory findings with bromethalin toxicosis are expected to be unremarkable. Alterations in electrolyte status secondary to dehydration and anorexia are possible.

Diagnostics

There is no specific antemortem test to confirm bromethalin exposure, so diagnosis is based on history and clinical findings. Postmortem evaluation of fat, liver, kidney, and brain can detect the presence of bromethalin.

Differential diagnoses for bromethalin toxicosis include head trauma, neoplasia, cerebral vascular disorders, infectious encephalitides (including rabies), and other toxic agents such as antifreeze, metaldehyde, zinc phosphide, and psychotropic drug ingestion.

Lesions

Gross necropsy findings usually are unremarkable. Histopathological evaluation of animals succumbing to bromethalin toxicosis reveals extensive vacuolation of the white matter within the CNS. The presence of typical lesions along with analytical evidence of bromethalin within tissues is confirmatory for bromethalin toxicosis.

Cholecalciferol rodenticides

Sources

Cholecalciferol rodenticides, such as anticoagulant rodenticides and bromethalin, come in a variety of formulations and colors, making identification of unpackaged baits often impossible. Most cholecalciferol baits contain 0.075% of the active ingredient, which equates to 23.4 mg of cholecalciferol per ounce of bait. With toxic dosages for dogs and cats of greater than 0.5 mg/kg, toxicosis can occur with 3 grams (just over one-half teaspoon) in a 5-kg (11-lb) animal.

Mechanism of action

Cholecalciferol enhances absorption of phosphorus and calcium from the GI tract and distal tubules of the kidney and enhances the mobilization of calcium from bone. The end result is increased serum calcium and phosphorus levels, which can persist up to several weeks after exposure (Rumbeiha 2006). Sustained elevations in serum calcium and phosphorus result in soft-tissue mineralization, most notably within the kidney, but the CNS, myocardium, GI tract, and lung also may have extensive mineralization. Most animals that die from cholecalciferol die because of renal failure; however, death secondary to cardiac arrhythmia, seizure, or pulmonary hemorrhage is possible.

Clinical signs and clinical laboratory findings

Initial signs of toxicosis generally develop about thirty-six to forty-eight hours after ingestion and are characterized by depression, weakness, and anorexia. Vomiting, constipation, polyuria, polydipsia, and dehydration occur as renal injury develops. GI ulceration caused by uremia and gastric mucosal metastatic mineralization is possible and the presence of hematemesis is considered a grave prognostic indicator (Rumbeiha 2006).

Serum phosphorus tends to rise early within the first twelve hours of exposure, with serum calcium levels rapidly following suit. Elevations in BUN and serum creatinine occur as renal failure develops. Urine specific gravity is usually low (1.002 to 1.006), and calciuria may be noted early in toxicosis.

Diagnostics

Live animal testing may include serum intact parathyroid hormone, which is expected to be depressed in cholecalciferol toxicosis. Ionized calcium 25-hydroxycalciferol (23(OH)D3) levels in serum are elevated above fifteen times normal in cholecalciferol toxicosis.

In the dead animal, bile and kidney can have 25(OH)D3 levels measured. Alternatively, trace mineral analysis of the kidney may reveal renal calcium levels at 2,000 to 3,000 ppm with a calcium:phosphorus ratio of 0.4 to 0.7, which is strongly suggestive of cholecalciferol toxicosis (Rumbeiha 2006).

Differential diagnoses for cholecalciferol intoxication include ingestion of other vitamin D3 analogues (calcipotriene, calcitriol), paraneoplastic hypercalcemia syndromes (especially lymphoma and anal sac apocrine gland adenocarcinoma), acute or chronic renal failure, hypercalcemia of granulomatous diseases, and hyperadrenocorticism.

Lesions

Gross lesions in animals dying from cholecalciferol may be minimal, but may include gastric ulceration, oral uremic ulcers, and mineralization (gritty on cutting) in the kidney, lung, and heart. Histological examination confirms mineralization of multiple organs, but these lesions also are seen in other conditions, such as uremia and hypercalcemia of malignancy.

Strychnine

Sources

Strychnine is available for use as a rodenticide, and is frequently used to poison coyotes, particularly in the northwestern United States. Most baits are 0.5%–1% strychnine sulfate and the baits are frequently formulated as red- or green-colored grains such as wheat, milo, corn, and oats.

Mechanism of action

Strychnine exerts its toxic effect by inhibiting the release of the inhibitory neurotransmitter glycine from the Renshaw cells on the anterior horn of the spinal cord. Inhibition of inhibitory nerve transmission results in uncontrolled neuronal activity, producing exaggerated reflexes and marked muscle spasms. Extensor muscles are more severely affected, resulting in hyperextension that can progress to tetanic convulsions.

Clinical signs and clinical laboratory findings

Onset and severity of clinical signs are dose dependent, with severe signs developing within ten minutes after large ingestions (Talcott 2006). Lower levels of exposure may result in delayed onset of mild ataxia and muscle stiffness within two hours of exposure. Initial signs may include anxiety, apprehension, tachypnea, and hypersalivation followed by ataxia, muscle spasms, and stiffness. Muscular signs generally begin in the face and progress to the neck and limb muscles. Violent generalized tonic-extensor convulsions may follow, accompanied by impairment of respiratory efforts. Animals may be hyperesthetic with convulsions worsening on exposure to sensory stimuli (light, sounds, touch). Convulsions can be continuous or intermittent with periods of depression between convulsive episodes. Death is caused by respiratory compromise.

Diagnostics

There are no consistent clinical pathological abnormalities associated with strychnine that would aid in diagnosis of the acutely ill patient.

Strychnine can be identified via analysis of vomitus, gastric contents, serum, or urine. Although strychnine may be found in liver, bile, or kidney, generally these samples are considered less likely to yield positive results than stomach contents (Talcott 2006).

Differential diagnoses for strychnine toxicosis includes other toxicants that can cause tremors and seizures such as metaldehyde, tremorgenic mycotoxins, 4-aminopyridine, methylxanthines, *Clostridium tetani* toxin, cocaine, amphetamine, organophosphorus and carbamate insecticides, organochlorines, and pyrethroids (especially in cats).

Lesions

Because strychnine toxicosis results in a biochemical lesion, no specific gross or histopathological lesions are associated with strychnine toxicosis.

Zinc phosphide

Sources

Zinc phosphide (and similar compounds, aluminum and magnesium phosphides) is a metallophosphide rodenticide available as pastes, tracking powders, or grain-based pellets.

Mechanism of action

Zinc phosphide is corrosive to the GI tract, and in the acidic environment of the stomach zinc phosphide is converted to phosphine gas. Phosphine gas also is corrosive and it complexes with metal ions, interfering with cellular respiration and producing reactive oxygen species that damage cellular structures. The phosphine gas is eructated and inhaled, resulting in pulmonary injury. Systemic absorption of phosphine results in damage in tissues with high oxygen demand, such as heart, brain, kidney, and liver (Knight 2006).

Clinical signs and clinical laboratory findings

Initial signs after ingestion of zinc phosphide include emesis within the first hour of ingestion resulting from the strong emetic effect. Other signs may have a delay of up to four to twelve hours and include vomiting (may contain blood), depression, and anorexia. A garlicky or rotten fish odor may be noted in the vomitus or on the patient's breath. Care should be taken to avoid exposure of veterinary personnel to the odor, because phosphine gas poses a risk to humans if inhaled. Pain from the GI injury may result in behavior changes. As systemic absorption of phosphine occurs, anxiety, pacing, weakness, ataxia, dyspnea, convulsions, and collapse may take place. Other signs that might be seen include persistent retching, vocalization bruxism, urinary and bowel incontinence, fasciculations, disorientation, recumbency, and convulsions. Cardiac arrhythmias, hypotension, and shock may occur. Evidence of renal or liver injury may develop as late as one to two weeks after acute exposure.

Clinical chemistry abnormalities may include elevations of hepatic and renal values, metabolic acidosis, and a variety of electrolyte disorders. Hematological alterations may include methemoglobinemia, hemolysis, and coagulopathy.

Diagnostics

There is no specific diagnostic antemortem test to detect zinc phosphide exposure. Suspicion of exposure may be aroused by the garlicky or rotten fish odor that may be detected on the animal's breath or in vomitus. Because of the hazards of inhalation of phosphine gas, necropsy should only be performed in a well-ventilated area and personnel should take measures to avoid inhalation of the gas. Samples taken for toxicological analysis should be placed in airtight containers and frozen promptly, because phosphine gas rapidly dissipates. Zinc phosphide toxicosis can be associated with elevated zinc levels in gastric contents, liver, and kidney.

Differential diagnoses for zinc phosphide toxicosis include strychnine, metaldehyde, tremorgenic mycotoxins, organophosphate and carbamate insecticides, 4-aminopyridine, sodium monofluoroacetate, and CNS stimulant medications.

Lesions

Gross lesions of zinc phosphide toxicosis may include pulmonary edema and generalized hyperemia of viscera and the gastrointestinal tract. Histopathological lesions reported include generalized congestion, vacuolar degeneration and interstitial edema of the brain, and edema of the myocardium (Knight 2006). None of these findings is specific or, by itself, diagnostic of zinc phosphide toxicosis.

Sodium monofluoroacetate (1080)

Sources

In the United States, sodium monofluoroacetate (1080) is currently registered only for the use of livestock protection collars for sheep and goats, but at one time it was used as a rodenticide; therefore, unlicensed persons still may have access to the agent for the intentional poisoning of other species (Parton 2006).

Mechanism of action

The proposed mechanism of action of 1080 is related to its effects on the tricarboxylic (TCA; Kreb's) cycle of cellular respiration (Parton 2006). Fluoroacetate combines with acetyl coenzyme A, forming fluoroacetyl coenzyme A, which in turn combines with oxaloacetate to produce fluorocitrate. Fluorocitrate is converted to 4-hydroxy-trans-aconitate, which binds to and inhibits aconitase. This results in inhibition of the oxidation of citric acid, essentially shutting down the TCA cycle and resulting in energy depletion, an accumulation of lactic and citric acid, and acidosis. High citrate levels inhibit phosphofructokinase, further impairing cellular energy metabolism (Goh et al. 2005). Organs most susceptible to 1080 are those with high metabolic rates, such as brain, kidneys, and heart. Accumulated citric acid also binds to serum calcium, resulting in a decrease in ionized calcium.

Clinical signs and clinical laboratory findings

Clinical signs occur thirty minutes to two hours after ingestion. Carnivores show CNS excitation characterized by agitation, hyperesthesia, frantic behavior, vocalization, and tonoclonic convulsions (Goh et al. 2005). GI signs include hypersalivation, vomiting, defecation, and tenesmus. Urinary incontinence and hyperthermia may also occur. Late signs include convulsions, collapse, dyspnea, and cardiorespiratory arrest. Death occurs from cardiopulmonary failure within two to twelve hours after the onset of clinical signs.

Clinical pathological abnormalities associated with 1080 toxicosis include hyperglycemia, acidosis, hypokalemia, and hypocalcemia. Cats may show decreases in ionized rather than total calcium (Goh et al. 2005).

Diagnostics

Gastric contents, bait, or vomitus may be evaluated for 1080 analysis; in most cases a minimum of 50 g of material is required for analysis. Very low levels of sodium monofluoroacetate may be found in urine, serum, plasma, and fat tissues using high power liquid chromatography (Goh et al. 2005).

Differential diagnoses for 1080 toxicosis include other agents capable of causing acute onset of CNS stimulation and convulsions, including amphetamines, strychnine, methylxanthines, organochlorines, hypocalcemic tetany, acute head trauma, and lead.

Lesions

No specific gross or histological lesions are expected with 1080 exposures.

Metaldehyde

Sources

Metaldehyde is a molluscicide commonly used to control snails and slugs on horticultural and home garden crops. Baits are available as powders, liquids, pellets, and granules. Many formulations contain bran or blackstrap molasses to attract the molluscs, making these products appealing to pets, especially dogs. The pelleted forms can resemble dry dog kibble. Most formulations of metaldehyde contain 1.5%–5% metaldehyde and some are combination products containing insecticides such as carbaryl.

Mechanism of action

The exact mechanism of action of metaldehyde is not fully elucidated. Metaldehyde may act by affecting g-aminobutyric acid (GABA) neurotransmission in the CNS, resulting in decreased levels of GABA within the CNS. Reduced GABA levels result in decreased inhibitory neurotransmission leading to stimulation. Depletion of other neurotransmitters, such as serotonin and norepinephrine, also has been associated with the decreased seizure threshold seen in metaldehyde toxicosis (Puschner 2006).

Clinical signs and clinical laboratory findings

Signs of metaldehyde toxicosis occur within three hours of ingestion. Initial signs are related to CNS stimulation, including agitation, anxiety, diarrhea, hyperthermia, muscle rigidity, cyanosis, tremors, and seizures. Later signs may include profound CNS depression, narcosis, and respiratory depression. Evidence of liver injury may develop over two to three days after exposure. The syndrome in cats can be somewhat different; signs include dyspnea, ataxia, hyperthermia, muscle spasms, mydriasis, nystagmus, and opisthotonos; sensory stimuli may trigger seizures (Puschner 2006). A formaldehyde odor may be noticed in the vomitus or on the animal's breath.

Diagnostics

Laboratory abnormalities associated with metaldehyde include profound acidosis. Chemical analysis of stomach contents, serum, urine, and liver can detect metaldehyde. Samples should be kept frozen prior to analysis.

Differential diagnoses of metaldehyde toxicosis include other CNS stimulants such as strychnine, 1080, zinc phosphide, bromethalin, organophosphorus and carbamate insecticides, pyrethrins (cats), 4-aminoppyridine, and tremorgenic mycotoxins.

Lesions

No specific gross or histopathological lesions are found in metaldehyde-intoxicated animals. The stomach contents may have a distinct formaldehyde odor and rapid onset of rigor mortis may be noted.

Organophosphorus insecticides

Sources

Organophosphates (OPs) are widely used insecticides, many of which are declining in use with the availability of less toxic insecticides. OPs are available in a variety of forms including powders, dusts, granules, emulsions, sprays, dips, shampoos, flea and tick collars, and foggers. As a class OPs include agents with very minimal potential for mammalian toxicity (e.g., tetrachlorvinphos) and those that are highly toxic to mammals (e.g., disulfoton).

Mechanism of action

OPs act through the inhibition of acetylcholine esterase (AChE), an enzyme that breaks down the neurotransmitter acetylcholine within synapses of the autonomic nervous system, parasympathetic system, neuromuscular junctions, and cholinergic synapses within the CNS. Inhibition of AChE results in accumulation of acetylcholine at these synapses, resulting in overstimulation of the postsynaptic neurons and muscles. Some OPs have the ability to "age" on the AChE molecule, resulting in permanent disability of that molecule. This accounts for the prolonged effects that can be seen with OPs when compared with carbamates.

Clinical signs and clinical laboratory findings

Clinical signs of OP toxicosis are classically described as those resulting from overstimulation of nicotinic, muscarinic, and central receptors. Nicotinic signs include muscle tremors, tetany, and stiffness followed by weakness, paresis, and paralysis because of depolarizing neuromuscular blockade. Muscarinic signs include salivation, lacrimation, urination, defecation, miosis, increased bronchial secretions, dyspnea, bradycardia, abdominal pain, and emesis. Central signs are related to cholinergic overload and include anxiety, restlessness, depression, seizures, respiratory depression, and coma. Not all signs are present in an individual animal and signs vary with the toxicity, dose, and route of exposure to the OP, as well as the species involved and stage of toxicosis. In dyspneic animals, sympathetic effects (e.g., tachycardia, mydriasis) may override the expected parasympathetic effects (bradycardia, miosis).

Clinical laboratory findings generally are unremarkable, although animals that have had extended seizure activity may have acid-base, electrolyte, or fluid imbalances.

Diagnostics

Measurement of cholinesterase activity can aid in the diagnosis of OP toxicosis but laboratory turnaround times generally are too long to be of use in acute toxicosis. Heparinized whole blood samples should be kept refrigerated to maintain cholinesterase activity.

For the emergent animal, an atropine test dose may be used in cases in which OP toxicosis is suspected but not confirmed. A dose of 0.02 mg/kg of atropine is administered intravenously and the animal monitored for resolution of hypersalivation or for an increase in heart rate. If hypersalivation resolves or the heart rate increases more than five beats per minute, the cause of the signs is not an OP, because it would require at least ten times that dose of atropine to override the effects of an OP. Stomach contents, vomitus, hair, and suspected baits can be submitted to a veterinary diagnostic laboratory for an OP screen. Brain and retina may be submitted for cholinesterase levels. These are especially important in cases in which animals have died quickly after developing signs, because blood cholinesterase may not have had a chance to become depressed.

Differential diagnoses for OP toxicosis include carbamates, tremorgenic mycotoxins, ethylene glycol, organochlorines, metaldehyde, strychnine, and zinc phosphide.

Lesions

No specific gross lesions are expected in animals that have died from OP toxicosis. Hair or stomach contents may have a petroleum, sulfur, or garlicky odor. Histopathologically, pulmonary edema and pancreatitis may be seen.

Carbamate insecticides

Sources

Carbamates are widely used insecticides, many of which are declining in use in the United States with the availability of less toxic insecticides. However, carbamates are still widely used in other countries, where the availability makes it a common compound for malicious animal poisonings. In South America, carbamates are considered a public health concern due to their use as agents of human suicide (Paulo Maiorka 2011, written communication). Carbamates are available in a variety of forms including powders, dusts, granules, emulsions, sprays, dips, shampoos, flea and tick collars, and foggers (Figure 10.3). As a class, carbamates include agents with very minimal

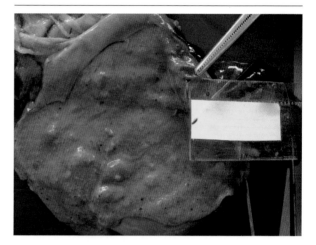

Figure 10.3. Malicious carbamate poisoning in a cat with typical findings of black granules in the gastric contents. (Photo courtesy of Dr. Paulo Maiorka.)

potential for mammalian toxicity (e.g., carbaryl) and those that are highly toxic to mammals (e.g., methomyl).

Mechanism of action

Carbamates act through the inhibition of AChE, an enzyme that breaks down the neurotransmitter acetylcholine within synapses of the autonomic nervous system, parasympathetic system, neuromuscular junctions, and cholinergic synapses within the CNS. Inhibition of AChE results in accumulation of acetylcholine at these synapses, resulting in overstimulation of the postsynaptic neurons and muscles. Unlike OPs, carbamates do not age and are rapidly broken down in the body. For this reason, signs generally are of shorter duration than those of OP toxicosis.

Clinical signs and clinical laboratory findings

Clinical signs of carbamate toxicosis are classically described as those resulting from overstimulation of nicotinic, muscarinic, and central receptors. Nicotinic signs include muscle tremors, tetany, and stiffness, followed by weakness, paresis, and paralysis caused by depolarizing neuromuscular blockade. Muscarinic signs include salivation, lacrimation, urination, defecation, miosis, increased bronchial secretions, dyspnea, bradycardia, abdominal pain, and emesis. Central signs are related to cholinergic overload and include anxiety, restlessness, depression, seizures, respiratory depression, and coma.

Not all signs are present in an individual animal and signs vary with the toxicity, dose, and route of exposure, as well as the species involved and stage of toxicosis. In dyspneic animals, sympathetic effects (e.g., tachycardia, mydriasis) may override the expected parasympathetic effects (bradycardia, miosis). Pancreatitis has been reported as a potential complication during acute carbamate toxicosis (Bradberry 2005). Clinical laboratory findings generally are unremarkable, although animals that have had extended seizure activity may have acid-base, electrolyte, or fluid imbalances. Changes indicative of pancreatitis (e.g., elevation of pancreatic enzymes) may be present, and leukopenia secondary to bone marrow necrosis may occur in some animals that survive acute intoxication (Paulo Maiorka, 2011, written communication).

Diagnostics

Measurement of cholinesterase activity is less helpful in carbamate toxicosis, because carbamates tend to rapidly dissociate from the AChE molecule and depressed AChE levels may not be found. Heparinized whole blood samples should be kept refrigerated to maintain cholinesterase activity.

For the emergent animal, an atropine test dose may be used in cases in which OP toxicosis is suspected but not confirmed. A dose of 0.02 mg/kg of atropine is administered intravenously and the animal monitored for resolution of hypersalivation or for an increase in heart rate. If hypersalivation resolves or the heart rate increases more than five beats per minute, the cause of the signs is not a carbamate, because it would require at least ten times that dose of atropine to override the effects of a carbamate. Stomach contents, vomitus, hair, and suspected baits can be submitted to a veterinary diagnostic laboratory for a carbamate screen. Given the inconsistency of cholinesterase levels in carbamate toxicosis, this may be the best means of confirming exposure to carbamates. Brain and retina may be submitted for cholinesterase levels. These are especially important in cases in which animals have died quickly after developing signs, because blood cholinesterase may not have had a chance to become depressed.

Differential diagnoses for carbamate toxicosis include organophosphates, tremorgenic mycotoxins, ethylene glycol, organochlorines, metaldehyde, strychnine, and zinc phosphide.

Lesions

No specific gross lesions are expected in animals that have died from carbamate toxicosis. Hair or stomach contents may have a petroleum, sulfur, or garlicky odor. Histopathologically, pulmonary edema may be seen.

Paraquat

Sources

Paraquat is a restricted use pesticide that has been associated with outbreaks of suspected malicious poisonings of dogs in the Pacific Northwest in 2003 and 2004 (Cope 2004). Paraquat was once widely used for agricultural purposes and outdated stocks tend to be readily available.

Mechanism of action

Concentrated paraquat is highly corrosive to tissues, and ingestion results in marked oral, esophageal, and GI ulceration. The systemic toxicity of paraquat stems from the extensive cyclic oxidation–reduction reactions it undergoes in tissues resulting in the formation of oxygen-derived free radicals that bind cellular macromolecules and cause tissue injury. Paraquat preferentially isolates to the lung, where progressive tissue injury develops, leading to respiratory compromise. Dermal exposures can result in localized dermal irritation and ulceration, whereas ocular exposure can result in severe corneal injury.

Clinical signs and clinical laboratory findings

The signs seen with paraquat toxicosis are dose dependent, with higher doses resulting in fulminant respiratory compromise, pulmonary edema, and multi-organ failure. Moderate doses result in slower onset of pulmonary, hepatic, and renal failure with death generally resulting from hepatic failure. Low doses result in progressive pulmonary fibrosis, with death occurring in days to weeks from pulmonary fibrosis. Initial signs in oral paraquat toxicosis are vomiting, anorexia, lethargy, oroesophageal ulceration, abdominal pain, and oral pain. Within three days after ingestion, evidence of renal failure and hepatocellular necrosis develop with vomiting, diarrhea, polyuria, and polydipsia becoming apparent. Within several days of ingestion, evidence of pulmonary injury becomes apparent. Animals are tachypneic, dyspneic, and cyanotic. Death is caused by respiratory compromise.

Clinical laboratory findings are not specific to paraquat. Elevation in hepatic enzymes and renal values may be seen in animals developing hepatic and renal insufficiency. Elevations in serum lipase can be seen after exposure to paraquat (Cope 2004).

Diagnostics

The development of acute GI upset followed within days by progressive respiratory compromise is highly suggestive of exposure to paraquat. Radiographic changes to the lungs include bilateral ground-glass pulmonary shadows, diffuse consolidation, and pneumomediastinum; the latter change is considered one of the earliest changes in paraquat-poisoned dogs (Oehme and Mannala 2006). Paraquat can be measured from the stomach contents, vomitus, or bait from an acute exposure or from urine up to forty-eight hours after ingestion. Measurement of paraquat in tissues is best done using lung and kidney, but by the time pulmonary fibrosis has developed tissue levels of paraquat may be below the range of detection.

Lesions

Gross lesions of paraquat poisoning include ulcerative stomatitis and esophagitis. Pulmonary lesions include edema and hemorrhage in acute cases, and shrunken and fibrotic lungs in chronically affected animals. Histopathological changes in the lung include hyperplasia of type II pneumocytes with fibroplasia. Evidence of proximal renal tubular degeneration and midzonal hepatic degeneration also may be present.

Acetaminophen
Sources

Acetaminophen is an analgesic and antipyretic that is widely available in a wide variety of formulations, both as a single drug and in combination with other drugs, such as hydrocodone and pseudoephedrine. Cats may be at increased risk for malicious poisoning by acetaminophen because many lay people are aware that cats are highly sensitive to acetaminophen and it is readily available and inexpensive.

Mechanism of action

The mechanism of toxicity of acetaminophen stems from the formation of toxic metabolites that deplete cellular glutathione, resulting in oxidative injury to cell components. Oxidative injury to red blood cells results in methemoglobinemia and possibly hemolysis. Cats are highly susceptible to methemoglobinemia because of deficiency in methemoglobin reductase and the fact that feline red blood cells have eight sulfhydryl groups to which the toxic metabolites can bind. Ferrets appear to be approximately as sensitive to acetaminophen as cats. In most other animals, the primary effect of acetaminophen is hepatotoxicity resulting from oxidative damage to hepatocytes. Methemoglobinemia can occur in these species but generally only at very high acetaminophen doses.

Clinical signs and clinical laboratory findings

Methemoglobin formation can occur within a few hours of ingestion and is characterized by cyanotic to muddy mucous membranes, chocolate brown blood, respiratory distress, facial and/or paw edema, depression, hypothermia, and vomiting. Evidence of hepatic injury may take more than twenty-four hours to develop. Animals may develop vomiting, anorexia, diarrhea, icterus, and depression.

Clinical laboratory abnormalities reported with methemoglobinemia include hemolysis, hemoglobinemia, and hemoglobinuria. Increases in hepatic enzymes, particularly serum alanine transaminase (ALT), generally are apparent within twenty-four hours in animals at risk of developing acute hepatic failure. As hepatic failure develops, BUN, cholesterol, and albumin levels drop, whereas serum bilirubin increases.

Diagnostics

In cats and dogs, the presence of methemoglobinemia should raise suspicion of acetaminophen exposure. The concomitant presence of facial and paw edema are highly suggestive of acetaminophen toxicosis. Most human hospitals can determine serum, urine, or plasma levels of acetaminophen in a timely manner and may be useful in diagnosing the acutely ill patient.

Differential diagnoses for methemoglobinemia include other agents, such as nitrites, naphthalene, phenols, phenazopyridine, and skunk spray (Zaks et al. 2005). Differential diagnoses for acute hepatic insufficiency include leptospirosis or other infectious hepatitis, and hepatopathy induced by other toxic agents such as hepatotoxic mushrooms, aflatoxin, iron, blue-green algae, and cycad palms.

Lesions

Gross lesions of acetaminophen toxicosis include generalized icterus, methemoglobinemia, and mottled or swollen liver. Histopathological lesions include centrilobular hepatocellular degeneration and necrosis with congestion. Degeneration of renal tubular epithelium has been described in dogs with acetaminophen toxicosis.

Ibuprofen
Sources

Ibuprofen is an NSAID available in a large number of OTC and prescription products in various formulations, both alone and in combination with other medications, such as pseudoephedrine or hydrocodone.

Mechanism of action

Ibuprofen is thought to inhibit the conversion of arachidonic acid to prostaglandins by blocking the action of cyclooxygenase (COX) enzymes. The pharmacological effects of ibuprofen (analgesic, antipyretic, anti-inflammatory) result from inhibition of COX-2 enzymes, whereas the adverse effects of ibuprofen are largely caused by inhibition of COX-1 enzymes. COX-1 enzymes are responsible for producing prostaglandins that allow for the maintenance of normal gastric mucosal barriers, renal blood flow, and platelet aggregation. Adverse effects of COX-1 inhibition include GI ulceration and renal tubular injury. Sensitivity to adverse effects of ibuprofen is species- and individual-specific, and in general cats and ferrets are about twice as sensitive as dogs.

Clinical signs and clinical laboratory findings

Clinical effects from ibuprofen are dose dependent. At lower dosages, GI ulceration may develop one to five days after acute exposure characterized by vomiting, abdominal pain, hematemesis, melena, and diarrhea. Severe cases may manifest with acute hypovolemic shock, pallor, and anemia; perforation of GI ulcers may result in signs of peritonitis. As dosages increase (.175 mg/kg in dogs), renal injury develops manifested by vomiting, anorexia, depression, polyuria, and polydipsia. At very high doses (.400 mg/kg in dogs) acute CNS signs may be present, including depression, seizures, and coma. Ferrets are especially sensitive to the CNS effects of ibuprofen, and depression, ataxia, and coma are seen frequently.

Clinical laboratory abnormalities expected in animals with GI hemorrhage include decreased hematocrit and serum protein. Severe ulcers may be associated with elevations in white blood cell counts, whereas severe sepsis secondary to peritonitis may result in hypoglycemia and leukopenia secondary to sequestration of white blood cells. Animals developing renal failure secondary to ibuprofen toxicosis have elevations in BUN and serum creatinine, hyposthenuric urine, glucosuria, and proteinuria; numerous cellular casts may be present in urinary sediment.

Diagnostics

There is no readily available screening test for ibuprofen. Although levels can be determined from blood collected during acute toxicosis, long turnaround times generally preclude these tests as being useful for diagnosing the acute patient.

Differential diagnoses for ibuprofen overdosages resulting in GI signs include hemorrhagic gastroenteritis, hypoadrenocorticism, GI foreign body, inflammatory bowel disease, GI neoplasia, and anticoagulant rodenticides. Differentials for renal injury secondary to ibuprofen toxicosis include other leptospirosis, borreliosis, aminoglycoside antibiotic toxicosis, grape/raisin ingestion, Lilium or Hemer ocallis ingestion (cats), and other NSAID intoxicants. Differentials for acute CNS effects include trauma, infectious encephalitis, CNS depressant or stimulant medication, alcohols, marijuana, ivermectin and other macrolides, and ethylene glycol.

Lesions

GI lesions of ibuprofen toxicosis may include ulcers within the stomach, duodenum, or colon. Oral ulcers may develop in severely azotemic animals with renal insufficiency from ibuprofen toxicosis. Histopathological examination of affected kidneys reveals proximal renal tubular degeneration and necrosis with intraluminal casts. Papillar necrosis is a less common finding in animals with ibuprofen toxicosis. No specific CNS lesions have been described in animals with CNS signs from ibuprofen.

Amphetamine

Sources

The amphetamine family contains a large number of products, including amphetamine, dextroamphetamine, fenfluramine, methamphetamine, pemoline, and phentermine. These drugs have been used to manage human conditions such as obesity, attention deficit disorder, and narcolepsy, and some of these products are being used in veterinary medicine for various behavioral disorders. All members of this class of drugs are controlled substances and there is high potential for abuse. Illicit production of amphetamines, especially methamphetamine, occurs in clandestine laboratories.

Mechanism of action

The exact mechanism for the effects of amphetamines on the CNS is not fully elucidated. It is known that amphetamines stimulate the cerebral cortex, reticular-activating system, and medullary respiratory center. Amphetamines also stimulate release of norepinephrine from adrenergic terminals and directly stimulate both a- and b-adrenergic receptors. Other actions of amphetamines include monoamine oxidase inhibition and dopamine excitatory receptor stimulation.

Clinical signs and clinical laboratory findings

Most formulations of amphetamines have the potential to cause rapid onset of clinical signs. Signs of amphetamine toxicosis include agitation, restlessness, anxiety, mydriasis, hypersalivation, vocalization, hyperthermia, tachypnea, ataxia, tachycardia and other arrhythmias, tremors, and seizures. Late in toxicosis animals may become depressed, weak, and bradycardic.

Clinical laboratory abnormalities may include acidosis, electrolyte abnormalities, and hypoglycemia, although none of these is specifically diagnostic for amphetamine toxicosis.

Diagnostics

Amphetamines can be detected in blood, urine, and saliva. OTC test kits can detect amphetamine metabolites in urine and anecdotally have been used to diagnose amphetamine toxicosis in dogs. Other sympathomimetics with similar metabolites (e.g., pseudoephedrine) cross react with these tests.

Differential diagnoses for amphetamines include other CNS stimulants such as pseudoephedrine; phenylpropanolamine; cocaine; methylxanthines; metaldehyde; concentrated permethrin (cats); organophosphorus and carbamate insecticides; organochlorines; tremorgenic mycotoxins; lead; and herbal supplements containing ma huang, ephedra, or guarana. Non-toxic differentials include head trauma, hepatic encephalopathy, and infectious encephalitis (e.g., rabies).

Lesions

No specific lesions are expected in animals that succumb to amphetamine toxicosis. Rapid onset of rigor mortis and generalized congestion of major organs may be noted.

Marijuana

Sources

Marijuana is composed of the dried leaves, stems, seeds, and flowers of *Cannabis sativa*. The primary active component in marijuana is d-9-tetrahydrocannabinol (THC), the concentration of which varies depending on growing conditions such as temperature, light, moisture, soil pH, and trace elements.

Recreational use of marijuana by humans is generally through inhalation of smoke, although ingestion is also popular.

Recently synthetic "designer" chemicals that bind to cannabinoid receptors and have similar clinical effects to THC have emerged (Fattore and Fratta 2011). These products, sold as herbal mixtures with names such as "Spice," "Silver," "Aroma," "K2," "Genie," and "Dream" were originally sold as "herbal highs" or "legal highs." However, several U.S. states passed laws making these products illegal, and in November 2010 the U.S. Drug Enforcement Administration used its emergency power to classify these drugs as Schedule I controlled substances. Although the clinical effects are similar, anecdotally these drugs appear to have higher potency than natural cannabis.

Mechanism of action

THC and other cannabinoids in marijuana bind to cannabinoid receptors within the nervous system (Volmer 2006). Two cannabinoid receptors, CB1 and CB2, have been identified. CB1 is widely distributed throughout the brain, especially in areas controlling memory, perception, and movement. Cannabinoids stimulate dopamine release, enhance GABA turnover, and may enhance the release of norepinephrine, dopamine, and serotonin (Donaldson 2002). CB2 is found in peripheral nerves where stimulation by THC may provide an analgesic effect.

Clinical signs and clinical laboratory findings

Signs of marijuana toxicosis include depression, ataxia, vomiting, mydriasis, weakness, disorientation, hypersalivation, hypothermia, bradycardia, and tremors. Other signs that may occur include nystagmus, stupor, apprehension, hyperesthesia, hyperexcitability, urinary incontinence, and tachycardia. Anecdotally, "medical marijuana" and synthetic cannabinoids appear to be much more potent than the street drug, and clinicians report more significant clinical signs, including seizures and hyperthermia, with these agents when dogs and cats are exposed (Karen Bischoff, written communication, 2011). Clinical laboratory abnormalities are not expected with marijuana intoxication.

Diagnostics

Stomach contents and urine may be analyzed for the presence of cannabinoids and levels in urine can be elevated for several days after an acute exposure. OTC test kits include marijuana and can be considered but at least one brand was unable to detect cannabinoid metabolites in one study (Teitler 2009), and anecdotal reporting from veterinary emergency clinicians indicate that testing for cannabinoids with this type of test yields inconsistent results. It is also not known whether the newer designer cannabinoids are detected by these kits.

Differential diagnoses of cannabinoid intoxication include alcohols, ethylene glycol, propylene glycol, CNS depressant drugs, centrally acting skeletal muscle relaxants, macrolide parasiticides, and hallucinogenic mushrooms. Non-toxic differentials include head trauma, hepatic encephalopathy, and infectious encephalitides (e.g., rabies).

Lesions

No specific lesions are expected in animals with marijuana toxicosis. Fortunately, deaths from marijuana exposures in animals are uncommon.

Cocaine

Sources

Cocaine is an alkaloid derived from the shrub *Erythroxylum coca* (Volmer 2006). Cocaine is a schedule II drug but is widely available as an illicit street drug. Cocaine comes as a powdered hydrochloride salt or free base form consisting of flakes, crystals, or rocks. The hydrochloride salt is readily dissolved in water and can be taken intravenously or intranasally. Free base cocaine may be smoked or taken orally.

Mechanism of action

Cocaine has strong sympathomimetic properties and it blocks the reuptake of norepinephrine and serotonin at adrenergic nerve endings, resulting in excessive stimulation of adrenergic receptors (Volmer 2006). Cocaine also sensitizes sympathetic effector cells, resulting in exaggerated response to endogenous catecholamines. Cocaine also may have a direct cytotoxic effect on the myocardium.

Clinical signs and clinical laboratory findings

Clinical signs may occur within ten to fifteen minutes of exposure and include hyperactivity, ataxia, mydriasis, vomiting, hypersalivation, hyperthermia, tachycardia, tachypnea, tremors, and seizures.

No specific clinical laboratory abnormalities are expected with cocaine, although severely symptomatic animals may have alterations in fluid, electrolyte, and acid-base status. Additionally, prolonged hyperthermia may predispose to disseminated intravascular coagulopathy, whereas prolonged seizure activity may result in rhabdomyolysis, myoglobinuria, and renal injury.

Diagnostics

Cocaine can be detected in serum, plasma, gastric contents, and urine. Many readily available and affordable OTC test kits are on the market and may prove useful in diagnosis of cocaine toxicosis.

Differential diagnoses for cocaine toxicosis include other CNS stimulants such as amphetamines; pseudoephedrine; methylxanthines; metaldehyde; concentrated permethrin (cats); organophosphorus and carbamate insecticides; organochlorines; tremorgenic mycotoxins; lead; and herbal supplements containing ma huang, ephedra, or guarana. Non-toxic differentials include head trauma, hepatic encephalopathy, and infectious encephalitides (e.g., rabies).

Lesions

No specific gross or histopathological lesions are expected with cocaine toxicosis.

Phencyclidine

Sources

Phencyclidine (PCP) was originally developed as a human anesthetic but was withdrawn because of adverse side effects during use. Because of its emergence as a drug of abuse, PCP was later removed from the veterinary market as well (Volmer 2006). PCP is a schedule II drug, but it is easily and inexpensively synthesized in illicit laboratories and is a popular recreational drug. Ketamine is an analogue of PCP with about 1/10 to 1/20 the potency of PCP.

Mechanism of action

The exact mechanism of action of PCP is not known, but the overall effect is to dissociate the somatosensory cortex from higher cortical centers (Volmer 2006). The binding of PCP to N-methyl-D-aspartate (NMDA) receptors results in noncompetitive blockade of glutamate receptors, blocking excitatory neurotransmission within the cortex and limbic structures in the brain. PCP may block reuptake of norepinephrine and dopamine, inhibit GABA, and stimulate opiate receptors.

Clinical signs and clinical laboratory findings

Phencyclidine can result in rapid onset of behavior abnormalities in animals, including jaw snapping and blank staring. Muscular rigidity, hypersalivation, hyperthermia, and seizures also may be seen.

No specific clinical laboratory abnormalities are expected with phencyclidine toxicosis, although acidosis and electrolyte abnormalities resulting from muscle activity and/or dehydration may be seen in some case.

Diagnostics

Some OTC drug test kits for home use screen for PCP, although in legal cases, confirmation of positive results via an accredited diagnostic laboratory is recommended. Patients administered ketamine may show false positives to PCP when using OTC kits. Some veterinary diagnostic laboratories are not equipped to analyze for PCP, so samples may need to be sent to human laboratories if PCP exposure is expected. Veterinary clinicians should contact their veterinary diagnostic laboratory to verify whether the lab is able to analyze the sample. PCP can be detected in urine, serum, and stomach contents. It may be detectable in urine up to two weeks after exposure.

Differential diagnosis for toxicosis from PCP includes exposure to hallucinogenic mushrooms, marijuana, LSD, antipsychotic and antidepressant medication, and hops.

Lesions

As with most other psychotropic drugs, no specific gross or histopathological findings are expected in animals with PCP intoxication.

Alcohols

Sources

Alcohols most commonly associated with animal poisonings include ethanol, methanol, and isopropyl alcohol. Ethanol is most often found in alcoholic beverages but also may occur as solvents in paints and disinfectants as well as carriers in some liquid medications. Significant ethanol exposures can occur through ingestion of fermenting fruit and raw yeast bread dough. Isopropyl alcohol is most commonly used for first aid and as a carrier for a variety of spray-on products, especially flea sprays for pets. Methanol is most commonly found in windshield washer fluids for automobiles, but also can be found in gasoline line antifreezes, household products, and paint removers.

Mechanism of action

All alcohols act as general CNS narcotics and may act through the inhibition of cyclic guanosine monophosphate (cGMP) in the brain and slowing of nerve conduction. In humans and some other primates, metabolites of methanol can cause blindness and neuronal necrosis. This is not an issue in non-primates because of differences in metabolism.

Clinical signs and clinical laboratory findings

Clinical signs of alcohol intoxication generally begin within thirty to forty minutes of ingestion and include CNS depression, narcosis, ataxia, disorientation, coma, and hypothermia. Vomiting and diarrhea also may be seen. Clinical laboratory abnormalities include increased serum osmolality, hypoglycemia, and acidosis.

Diagnostics

Most human hospitals are able to determine blood ethanol levels on a STAT basis. Whole blood methanol and isopropanol levels can be determined, although turnaround time makes these tests less useful for immediate diagnosis of acutely ill patients.

Differential diagnoses for alcohol ingestion include ingestion of ethylene glycol, propylene glycol, ivermectin and other macrolide antiparasitic agents, benzodiazepines and other CNS depressant drugs, and amitraz.

Lesions

No specific lesions are expected with ingestion of alcohols by non-primate animals. In primates with methanol toxicosis, retinal and optic disk edema may be seen, with associated neuronal necrosis in the cerebrum.

Caffeine

Sources

The methylxanthine caffeine is found in wide variety of products, including OTC stimulants, caffeinated beverages, coffee beans, teas, cocoa products, and herbal supplements containing guarana. In addition to caffeine, cocoa products also contain high levels of theobromine, another methylxanthine that can contribute significantly to the effects produced by caffeine.

Mechanism of action

Methylxanthines inhibit cyclic nucleotide phosphodiesterases and inhibit the receptor-mediated activity of adenosine. The net result is stimulation of the CNS and cardiovascular system, and diuresis. Caffeine triggers synthesis and release of catecholamines, such as norepinephrine. High doses of caffeine stimulate medullary, vasomotor, vagal, and respiratory centers within the brain.

Clinical signs and clinical laboratory findings

Clinical signs generally occur within one to two hours of ingestion and are characterized by agitation, hyperactivity, restlessness, behavior abnormalities, and vomiting. Panting, tachycardia (heart rate above 200 bpm with ventricular premature contractions), ataxia, diuresis, hyperexcitability, hyperthermia, hypertension, muscle tremors, and convulsions are possible. Late stages include coma, cardiac arrhythmias, respiratory failure, and death.

Hypokalemia and metabolic acidosis may be present.

Diagnostics

Caffeine levels can be measured in stomach contents, serum, urine, and liver. Levels may be detectable up to three days after initial exposure.

Differential diagnoses for caffeine toxicosis are other stimulants, including 4-aminopyridine, strychnine, nicotine, amphetamine, organochlorines, metaldehyde, 1080, and tremorgenic mycotoxins.

Lesions

No specific lesions have been associated with caffeine toxicosis. Non-specific GI irritation and generalized congestion have been described in dogs killed by caffeine intoxication.

SUMMARY

Collecting evidence for suspected malicious animal poisonings requires attention to detail, meticulous record keeping, appropriate sample collection, maintaining chain of custody, selection of appropriate diagnostic tests, and accurate interpretation of test results in light of the patient's clinical syndrome.

REFERENCES

ASPCA. 2011. AnTox™ Database 2010. Urbana, IL: ASPCA Animal Poison Control Center.

ASPCA. 2006. AnTox™ Database 2002–2005. Urbana, IL: ASPCA Animal Poison Control Center.

Bischoff, K.A. 2009. Automotive Toxins. In: *Kirk's Current Veterinary Therapy XIV*, J.D. Bonagura and D.C. Twedt, eds. pp. 130–135. St Louis: Saunders.

Blodgett, D.J. 2006. Organophosphate and Carbamate Insecticides. In: *Small Animal Toxicology*, Second edition, M.E. Petersen and P.A. Talcott, eds. pp. 941–955. St. Louis: Saunders.

Carson, T.L. 2006. Methylxanthines. In: *Small Animal Toxicology*, Second edition, M.E. Petersen and P.A. Talcott, eds. pp. 845–852. St. Louis: Saunders.

Cope, R.B. 2004. Helping Animals Exposed to the Herbicide Paraquat. *Veterinary Medicine* 99(9):755–762.

Donaldson, C.W. 2002. Marijuana Exposure in Animals. *Veterinary Medicine* 97(6):437–439.

Dorman, D.C. 2006. Bromethalin. In: *Small Animal Toxicology*, Second edition, M.E. Petersen and P.A. Talcott, eds. pp. 609–618. St. Louis: Saunders.

Dunayer, E.K. 2003. Bromethalin: The Other Rodenticide. *Veterinary Medicine* 98(9);732–736.

Fattore, L., W. Fratta. 2011. Beyond THC: The New Generation of Cannabinoid Designer Drugs. *Frontiers in Behavioral Neuroscience* 5:60.

Galey, F.D. 1995. Diagnostic and Forensic Toxicology. *Veterinary Clinics of North America: Equine Practice* 11(3):443–454.

Goh, C.S.S., D.R. Hodgson, S.M. Fearnside, J. Heller, and N. Malikides. 2005. Sodium Monofluoroacetate (Compound 1080) Poisoning in Dogs. *Australian Veterinary Journal* 83(8):474–479.

Gwaltney-Brant, S.M. 2011. Epidemiology of Animal Poisonings. In: *Veterinary Toxicology: Basic and Clinical Principles*, Second edition, R.C. Gupta, ed. San Diego: Elsevier Academic Press.

Hansen, S.R., L.A. Murphy, S.A. Khan, and C. Allen. 2001. An Overview of Malicious Animal Poisonings. North American Congress of Clinical Toxicology. October 4–9, 2001. Montreal, Quebec, Canada.

Hornfeldt, C.S. and M.J. Murphy. 1997. Poisonings in Animals: The 1993–1994 Report of the American Association of Poison Control Centers. *Veterinary and Human Toxicology* 39(6);361–365.

Knight, M.W. 2006. Zinc Phosphide. In: *Small Animal Toxicology*, Second edition, M.E. Petersen and P.A. Talcott, eds. pp. 1101–1118. St. Louis: Saunders.

Marshall, D.A., Doty, R.L. 1990. Taste Responses of Dogs to Ethylene Glycol, Propylene Glycol, and Ethylene Glycol-Based Antifreeze. *Journal of the American Veterinary Medical Association* 197(12):1599–1602.

Maxie, M.G. 1985. The Urinary System. In: *Pathology of Domestic Animals*, Vol. 2, Third edition, K.V.F. Jubb, P.C. Kennedy, and N. Palmer, eds. p. 375. San Diego: Academic Press.

McConnico, R.S., K. Copedge, and K.L. Bischoff. 1997. Brodifacoum Toxicosis in Two Horses. *Journal of the American Veterinary Medical Association* 211(7): 882–886.

McGuinness, K., M. Allen, and B.R. Jones. 2005. Non-Accidental Injury in Companion Animals in the Republic of Ireland. *Irish Veterinary Journal* 58(7):392–396.

Munro, H.M.C., M.V. Thrusfield. 2001a. Battered Pets: Non-Accidental Physical Injuries Found in Dogs and Cats. *Journal of Small Animal Practice* 42:385–389.

Munro, H.M.C., M.V. Thrusfield. 2001b. Battered Pets: Münchausen Syndrome by Proxy (Factitious Illness by Proxy). *Journal of Small Animal Practice* 42:385–389.

Murphy, M.J. 2009. Small Animal poisoning: Additional Considerations Related to Legal Claims. In: *Kirk's Current Veterinary Therapy XIV*, Bonagura, J.D. and D.C. Twedt, eds. pp. 105–108. St Louis: Saunders.

Murphy, M.M. and P.A. Talcott. 2006. Anticoagulant Rodenticides. In: *Small Animal Toxicology*, Second edition, M.E. Petersen and P.A. Talcott, eds. pp. 563–577. St. Louis: Saunders.

Oehme, F.W. and S. Mannala. 2006. Paraquat. In: *Small Animal Toxicology*, Second edition, M.E. Petersen and P.A. Talcott, eds. pp. 964–977. St. Louis: Saunders.

Parton, K. 2006. Sodium Monofluoroacetate (1080). In: *Small Animal Toxicology*, Second edition, M.E. Petersen and P.A. Talcott, eds. pp. 1055–1062. St. Louis: Saunders.

Puschner, B. 2006. Metaldehyde. In: *Small Animal Toxicology*, Second edition, M.E. Petersen and P.A. Talcott, eds. pp. 830–839. St. Louis: Saunders.

Rumbeiha, W.K. 2006. Cholecalciferol. In: *Small Animal Toxicology*, Second edition, M.E. Petersen and P.A. Talcott, eds. pp. 629–642. St. Louis: Saunders.

Talcott, P.A. 2006. Strychnine. In: *Small Animal Toxicology*, Second edition, M.E. Petersen and P.A. Talcott, eds. pp. 1076–1082. St. Louis: Saunders.

Teitler, J.B. 2009. Evaluation of a Human On-Site Urine Multidrug Test for Emergency Use With Dogs. *Journal of the American Animal Hospital Association* 45:59–66.

Thrall, M.A., H.E. Connally, G.F. Grauer, and D. Hamar. 2006. Ethylene Glycol. In: *Small Animal Toxicology*, Second edition, M.E. Petersen and P.A. Talcott, eds. pp. 702–726. St. Louis: Saunders.

Volmer, P.A. 2006. Recreational Drugs. In: *Small Animal Toxicology*, Second edition, M.E. Petersen and P.A. Talcott, eds. pp. 273–311. St. Louis: Saunders.

Zaks, K.L., Tan, E.O., Thrall, M.A. 2005. Heinz Body Anemia in a Dog That Had Been Sprayed With Skunk Musk. *Journal of the American Veterinary Medical Association* 226(9):1516–1518.

11
Neglect

Melinda D. Merck, Doris M. Miller, and Robert W. Reisman

There is a principle which is a bar against all information, which is proof against all arguments and which cannot fail to keep a man in everlasting ignorance—that principle is contempt prior to investigation.

Herbert Spencer

INTRODUCTION

Neglect can be generally defined as the failure to provide for an animal's mental and physical well-being (Chapter 4). Criminal neglect implies that an animal's health has been so severely compromised by the neglect of its mental and physical well-being that the person responsible may be subject to criminal charges and prosecution under the animal cruelty statute. Criminal neglect is the most common form of animal abuse.

Different circumstances can result in neglect of an animal's well-being and compromise of the animal's health. These include inadequate food, water, and shelter; inappropriate restraint such as unrestricted (extended or continuous length of time) and/or inappropriate tethering (short tie-outs, heavy chains, embedded collars); unsanitary, unsafe, or unhealthy living conditions (e.g., isolation without sunlight); failure to maintain the animal's hair coat and nails; failure to provide necessary medical care for health problems, also called failure to treat; and sometimes failure to take necessary actions to prevent medical issues or harm that are expected as a minimum standard of care.

The Five Freedoms For Animal Welfare have been established as a guideline for the welfare of animals: freedom from hunger or thirst; freedom from discomfort; freedom from pain, injury, or disease; freedom to express normal behavior; and freedom from fear or distress (Chapter 4 and Appendix 37). It is the veterinarian's responsibility to evaluate and document the health of the animal. At presentation the full extent of the effect of the neglect on the animal's health may not be clear based on physical examination alone. Ancillary diagnostic tools such as blood, urine, and fecal tests along with radiographs are often necessary to complete the animal evaluation. Observation and evaluation should continue after the initial exam as the full extent of the medical problems may become more apparent.

Some state and local laws have broad language defining neglect that are open for interpretation, whereas others have clear, detailed definitions of what constitutes neglect. In states where there is no endangerment clause in the animal cruelty statute, which is the majority of states, it is generally necessary for the neglect of an animal to have compromised an animal's health. A "reasonable person" standard is often applied when making legal decisions on neglect cases regarding charges or sentencing. This standard refers to what a reasonable person would know, how he or she would act or not act, and what he or she would expect as an outcome. This is a very important aspect to consider when evaluating neglect cases.

Neglect can be an act of omission or commission. It is often a continuum of action or lack of action by the owner over a prolonged period of time. The legal issue, which may be used to prove intent, is at what point in this continuum the owner had to have knowledge of the problem and still failed to take appropriate action. It is important to

Veterinary Forensics: Animal Cruelty Investigations, Second Edition. Edited by Melinda D. Merck.
© 2013 John Wiley & Sons, Inc. Published 2013 by John Wiley & Sons, Inc.

note what would have been obvious to the owner, such as any discharge, foul odor, and animal behavior. Any detected odors should always be described in physical exam findings. Abnormal odors are evidence of an unclean haircoat (e.g., feces and urine soiling), bacterial wound infection, and/or tissue necrosis. The animal's health may have continuously deteriorated over the period during which the animal was neglected. The veterinarian may be able to describe the sequence of events and the signs of deterioration of the animal's health.

One of the authors (Reisman) was asked at trial to describe the sequence of signs that were ignored by the owner in a small breed dog with a strangulating hair mat of its paw where loss of blood supply to the paw resulted in soft tissue necrosis of the metacarpus. The sequence of signs would have initially been noticeable lameness of the affected limb and/or vocalization (the dog cried when the affected paw was handled during examination), which are both evidence of pain. As the problem progressed the odor of tissue necrosis would have become evident followed by discoloration of the hair mat becoming apparent. The veterinarian's assessment of the animal's condition and environmental findings are the foundation for a criminal prosecution of animal cruelty.

Questions arise regarding clients who decline treatment or procedures. Each case is unique and should be evaluated considering all aspects. Client education and communication is the imperative to achieve the best outcome for all veterinary patients. Reasonable alternatives should be offered and documented when financial issues prohibit the owner's ability to comply with recommended treatment. However, the owner has an obligation to provide basic care for the animal, including preventing or eliminating suffering, and financial excuses do not alleviate that responsibility. Basic care may be defined in the laws or subject to interpretation by enforcement authorities who may rely on the veterinarian's opinion. The owner's personal beliefs cannot extend to the level at which they become a detriment for the health and welfare of the animal. Medical conditions in which the animal is in pain or otherwise suffering and the owner refuses reasonable options to remedy the situation may rise to the level of abuse.

Request for euthanasia of an apparent healthy animal may be an indicator that the animal has been abused and is usually a warning sign of deeper, hidden issues with the owner or within the home. These situations require an intensive effort by the veterinarian to determine the true reason for the request and work toward finding an alternate solution to euthanasia. Initially, a physical exam should be performed to determine if there are any indicators of abuse.

Based on the exam and discussions with the owner, reporting to authorities may be indicated. If the animal was originally obtained from a shelter or rescue organization, that organization may be willing to take the animal or it may be discovered that the owner has a history of adopting animals that cannot be legitimately accounted for (ran away, accidental death, multiple euthanasias). In all of the above situations, viable options for the pet should be discussed with the owner to prevent animal suffering and ensure the animal is not at risk for abandonment.

ENVIRONMENT EXAMINATION

The animal's environment, which contains valuable information in neglect cases, is required by the veterinarian to accurately and objectively analyze the physical examination findings in the proper context and determine what additional testing may be indicated. As discussed in Chapter 3, when the veterinarian is not present at the crime scene certain information should be obtained from the investigating officer, and the use of an Intake Questionnaire can be useful (Appendices 8–9).

Often multiple issues are found at the scene; these commonly include overcrowding, inappropriate tethering, and inappropriate housing. Several issues can be related to housing: lack of protection from environmental elements including weather conditions and full sun and unsanitary or inappropriate flooring; failure to provide an area free of urine and feces for the animal; failure to secure water containers to prevent over-turning; housing construction that retains heat such as plastic enclosures; and overcrowding with issues of competition for resources, mating, and age mixing of adults and juveniles.

Some jurisdictions have laws governing the minimum length of the tether based on the animal body length, the maximum time allowed on a tether which may be further regulated based on seasons and time of day, and the weight maximum as a percentage of the animal's body weight (BW). Legal restrictions regarding tethering as a BW percentage are usually found in local or municipal ordinances; they have included: no more than 5% of BW, no more than 1/18 of BW, and no more than 1/10 of BW. Tethers should be measured and compared to the length of the animal and chains should be weighed and compared to the weight of the animal.

Commonly there is a lack of potable water or lack of containers or containers that the animal cannot fully access (e.g., 5-gallon buckets with food or water only at the bottom), inappropriate food for the size of the animal or life stage (e.g., adult dog food for puppies, large kibble for recently weaned juveniles), and food unfit for consumption. It should be noted that a starved animal can become so debilitated it may not eat even with the presence of food.

The environment is often unsanitary and cluttered with hazardous debris, with urine and feces covering most surfaces. The level of ammonia in the environment can cause or contribute to eye and respiratory problems. It is important to look for evidence of illness such as vomitus, diarrhea, and blood due to hemorrhage. Groups of neglected or starved animals housed together may have bite wounds due to fighting over resources. Significant environmental flea infestations should be noted because they can result in severe anemia.

A general time period should be estimated for conditions noted at the crime scene to have been present. Several findings can assist with this determination including the conditions of feces (fresh, dried, or moldy), debris covering the front of pen/cage doors, moldy food, or the presence of algae in the water container. The amount of feces present can provide a minimum time frame to the last time the feces were removed based on the digestibility of the food provided and normal appetite/defecation patterns for the species and age of the animal. For example, on highly digestible food a cat will defecate on average once daily and dogs one or two times daily with a normal appetite; on lower digestible food, defecation may be four to six times a day. There may be significant botany evidence, such as vines growing over pens and the absence of grass or vegetation around a dog tether. Entomology evidence may be present on deceased animals, food, dirty containers, litter boxes, or trash, which can provide time estimates (Chapter 15).

MALNUTRITION: IMPROPER FEEDING

The issue of improper feeding resulting in malnutrition may be considered an act of animal cruelty. For the purposes of this section, improper feeding refers to feeding an unbalanced diet that results in medical problems for the animal and feeding an animal in such a way to result in gross obesity. Veterinarians are expected to handle these situations with client education and developing appropriate medical, nutritional, and exercise plans for the health of the animal. It is when the owner refuses to follow these guidelines or otherwise take steps to remedy the problem that it becomes a legal issue of cruelty.

Certain aspects must first be considered before such situations rise to the level of animal cruelty. From the legal aspect the first questions to be answered regard the owner's knowledge of the animal's condition and how to correct or treat it. It must be documented that the owner has been fully educated on the current medical issues, nutritional

cause(s), prognosis, and risk for future medical problems. A complete written treatment plan for the animal should be signed and dated by the owner and a copy retained as part of the medical record. This plan should outline the medical problems, nutritional causes, prognosis, medical treatment, diet, exercise, follow-up veterinary visits, and any other expectations of the owner. Part of the plan should include monitoring progress and an established communication conduit to address any issues or questions the owner may have. These documentation steps are recommended for general veterinary practice but are especially important when failure to comply for any medical condition may result in criminal charges.

The next legal issue is defining how the animal suffered as a result of the improper feeding. Finally, it must be determined if and how the owner failed to take action to remedy the situation by evaluating several things such as the reasonableness of the treatment plan, appropriateness of the plan, reasonableness of the time allotted to implement and comply with the plan, ensuring the owner fully understood the plan, any mitigating factors affecting owner compliance, and any other factors with the animal that would affect the success of the plan.

Obesity in animals is the most common form of malnutrition in western societies (Toll et al. 2010). Obesity may be defined by comparing the relative body weight (RBW) to the ideal weight. RBW is the current body weight divided by the optimal weight. For dogs and cats, obesity is characterized by RBWs greater than 20% (Toll et al. 2010).

The health and longevity of companion animals is compromised with obesity. Numerous diseases and conditions are caused or exacerbated by obesity. Adipocytes produce fat-derived peptides that are pro-inflammatory and can affect many body systems, with obesity potentially causing a chronic, low-grade inflammation (Toll et al. 2010). Obesity also increases oxidative stress which is linked to cancer, diabetes mellitus, heart disease, liver disease, and urinary tract disease (Toll et al. 2010). Animals suffering from obesity are predisposed to insulin resistance, diabetes mellitus, cardiac disease, hypertension, congestive heart failure, traumatic and degenerative orthopedic disorders, exacerbation of osteoarthritis, oral disease, urinary tract disease (cats), urolith formation, idiopathic hepatic lipidosis (cats), dermatologic problems, neoplasia, transitional cell carcinoma, dyslipidemia, heat intolerance, exercise intolerance, dyspnea/respiratory distress, dystocia, anesthesia complications, and decreased immune function (Toll et al. 2010).

The other common malnutrition issue is feeding an unbalanced diet. Different species of animals have certain requirements in their diets to prevent medical problems. Over-supplementation also may have detrimental effects on the animal's health. Exclusive feeding of all boneless-meat diets, which is severely low in calcium, can lead to nutritional secondary hyperparathyroidism. The body compensates for the low calcium intake through bone resorption resulting in osteopenia and spontaneous, patho-logic fractures. Animals suffering from this condition typi-cally have severe bone pain. They predictably resist being touched, and have difficulty with ambulation, holding their head up, and masticating.

MALNUTRITION: STARVATION

Overview

Starvation is the result of inadequate nutrition which can be caused by food deprivation, poor quality food, inappro-priate food, intermittent feeding, or a lack of appetite which is often due to an underlying disease process. It is imperative that all causes of starvation be investigated through diagnostic testing and full postmortem examina-tion, including histopathology. Blood, urine, and fecal tests should be performed due to the severe detrimental effects of starvation and dehydration on the body systems. Radiographs can provide supporting evidence of emacia-tion/starvation (narrow abdominal waist, loss of abdominal detail, ingested foreign material) and evidence of addi-tional abuse (e.g., recent and old rib fractures).

The animal's hydration status and presenting weight should be recorded and progressively monitored with changes documented. Prior medical history of the animal can provide information about pre-existing medical condi-tions and/or the animal's healthy body weight. Food and water should be offered to demonstrate appetite and thirst. Videography should be considered to document the ani-mal's response. It cannot be assumed that an emaciated animal has been starved. Many medical conditions can result in an emaciated body condition (e.g., cancer, under-lying gastrointestinal disease). It is necessary for a criminal prosecution to have a definitive diagnosis of starvation. Starvation can be proved by showing an animal's body condition increases from an underweight condition with minimal or no medical intervention. For starvation cases involving multiple animals there may be varying degrees of underweight body conditions among the group.

A body condition score (BCS) should be given for every underweight animal (Chapter 3). For thick- or long-coated breeds it is helpful to shave the coat to show the loss of fat and/or muscle mass for photography. There are actually

two times to record the animal's body condition score: (1) at presentation, and (2) after the animal has reached an ideal weight. It is the latter determination that can be used to calculate weight gain relative to the animal's ideal weight which provides conclusive evidence of starvation. The presenting weight also can be used to calculate the estimated weight loss based on medical history informa-tion with the animal's previous weight or an estimation made for ideal weight based on the species or breed:

$$\text{Ideal weight} \left(\text{confirmed or estimated}\right) - \text{presenting weight} = X$$

$$X \div \text{presenting weight} = \% \text{ weight gain}$$

$$X \div \text{ideal weight} = \% \text{ weight loss from ideal weight}$$

Another method for estimating weight loss at presenta-tion is the Purina BCS (Appendices 13–14). Each step in the Purina BCS represents a 5% loss of tissue weight, so an emaciated animal has experienced a minimum 20% tissue weight loss from the ideal body condition. The percentage weight loss does not include water weight loss due to dehy-dration which must be excluded from the determination of percentage weight loss. The body tissue weight loss from 5 (Ideal) to 3 (Thin) is due to the loss of body fat; from 3 (Thin) to 1 (Emaciated) is due to loss of fat and muscle (Table 11.1).

The veterinarian may be asked to provide an estimate for how long it took the animal to reach a specific body condi-tion score or to die from starvation. This can be difficult without knowing the initial body condition. The animal may have been fed or had access to nutritional sources intermittently which would prolong, not cease, the pro-gressive deterioration of starvation. A study was conducted on obese dogs under total caloric restriction measuring the weekly percent weight loss which found the weight loss was higher in the first two weeks and then leveled off at 3%–4%/week (Table 11.2) (Anderson and Lewis 1980). Depending on the circumstances and case information, the time estimate that can usually be provided is a broad range of weeks to months.

There can be issues related to choosing a single body condition score at presentation by the initial underestima-tion of the animal's weight loss, which can compromise the criminal prosecution. It may be better to choose two body condition scores at presentation: the BCS believed to rep-resent the actual weight loss from ideal, and the next higher BCS score. It is preferable to overestimate than underesti-mate the weight loss. After the animal has gained weight back to an ideal BCS a calculation should be performed to

Table 11.1. Underweight scores in Purina Body Condition Scale.

Purina 9-point scale	% Decrease body tissue weight	% Body fat	% Decrease body fat	% Decrease body muscle	Example: ideal weight 100 lbs.
5 Ideal		20–24			100 lbs.
4 Lean	5	15–19	5		95 lbs.
3 Thin	10	10–14	10		90 lbs.
2 Very thin	15	6–9	14	1–5	85 lbs.
1 Emaciated	More than 20	Less than or equal to 5	More than 15	More than 5	

Source: Lusby, A.L. and C.A. Kirk. 2009. Obesity. In: *Kirk's Current Veterinary Therapy XIV*, Fourteenth edition, J.D. Bonagura and D.C. Twedt, eds. pp. 191–195. St. Louis: Saunders Elsevier.

Table 11.2. Weight loss during total caloric restriction in obese dogs.

	Weight loss (%BW)
Week 1	8%
Week 2	5%
Week 3	3%–4%
Week 4	3%–4%
Week 5	3%–4%
Week 6	3%–4%

Source: Anderson, G.L. and L.D. Lewis. 1980. Obesity. In: *Current Veterinary Therapy VII*, pp. 1034–1039. Philadelphia: W.B. Saunders Company.

Table 11.3. Basal caloric requirements of dogs and cats.

Large-breed dog	40 kcal/kg/day
Medium-breed dog	50 kcal/kg/day
Small-breed dog	60 kcal/kg/day
Cat	70 kcal/kg/day

Source: M.A. Labato. 1992. Nutritional Management of the Critical Care Patient. In: *Kirk's Current Veterinary Therapy XI Small Animal Practice*, R.W. Kirk and J.D. Bonagura, eds. pp. 117–125. Philadelphia: W.B. Saunders Company.

determine if the difference in ideal weight and the presenting weight supports the original BCS. For example, if the animal was originally scored as very thin (2 on the Purina scale), then the weight gain should be at least 15%–20% of the ideal weight.

The feeding of a starved animal should be conducted carefully to prevent re-feeding syndrome. These animals present with starvation metabolism which can take weeks to convert back to normal. Significant weight gain is not necessary during the first two weeks. The animal should be fed based on the calculation of the daily energy requirement (DER), using a target weight of slightly more than the intake weight.

Process of starvation and the physical effects

Starvation, also referred to as protein-calorie malnutrition (PCM), causes the gradual loss of lean body mass (muscle) and adipose tissue due to the lack of intake of protein and calories, increased demand, or both (Table 11.3). It should be noted that an animal can succumb to starvation during the progressively deteriorating process, including prior to consuming all of the body fat stores. It is important to place the state of starvation in context with the animal's life stage. Young animals with the demanding nutritional needs of growth can be more profoundly affected than adults. Starvation causes weight loss and stunted growth in young growing animals, where radiographs may show growth arrest lines in the long bones (Munro and Munro 2008a). Pregnant starving animals may give birth to weak neonates or dead fetuses.

A variety of clinical abnormalities of the skin result from nutritional deficiencies, including starvation (Hand 2011). A common finding is a sparse, dry, dull, and brittle haircoat with hairs that epilate easily. There can be associated abnormal skin scale accumulation (seborrhea sicca). Loss of hair occurs due to anagen defluxion and/or telogen defluxion. In the anagen or growth phase of the hair cycle there can be loss and/or abnormal growth of hair resulting in broken hair shafts. With telogen defluxion there is widespread loss of hair in the quiescent phase of the hair cycle due to large numbers of hair follicles being synchronized in this phase. Loss of normal hair color and hair keratinization abnormalities can occur. In cats there is decreased melanin deposition in hair due to amino acid deficiencies and the haircoat takes on a reddish cast, sometimes called red coat. There also may be erythema or crusting in areas of friction or stretching such as the distal extremities. Decubital ulcers can be a serious and painful result of starvation. Poor wound healing also occurs with starvation. Secondary bacterial or yeast skin infections of the skin are common.

The nutritional status of an animal can be reflected in the levels of certain isotopes in hair, feathers, and other tissues. The hair is resistant to degradation and any isotope changes correlate to those found in tissues. The analysis of anagen hair has been used to study the nutritional history of animals in modern and ancient populations. The levels and ratios of stable isotopes are measured. Research studies in horses have shown that a one-day change of diet is reflected in the hair. Other studies have been conducted on bats, rattlesnakes, lizards, chickens, crows, quail, lemurs, and llamas, which found changes in eating habits and nutritional stress were recorded in hair and tissues. The hair information is held chronologically and is limited by the length of the hair. The lack of abundant anagen hairs and potential shorter length in some animals can be a factor (Tran 2010).

Starvation causes a slowly progressive decrease in the metabolic rate. In a well-nourished animal, carbohydrate serves as an immediate energy source. Carbohydrate stored as glycogen provides a short-term energy reserve, i.e., provides for energy needs for about one day. Excess carbohydrate is converted to lipid or fat, which is the animal's long-term energy reserve. The energy needs of the animal are met, at least initially, primarily through the oxidation of fats, which spares body protein breakdown. In the liver there is a loss of amino acids for glucose production (Labato 1992). The stored lipid in the body is the primary source of energy and varies from animal to animal. The fat content of a healthy dog or cat is approximately 20%–24% (Lusby 2009). Because amino acids are not stored in the body, the protein of the body must be maintained by intake. The protein content of a healthy animal is approximately 14%–20% of the lean body weight, although in a well-muscled animal such as an American Staffordshire Terrier this percentage may be higher. Of an animal's total body protein, only about one-third is available as a potential energy source (Labato 1992).

The body's response to inadequate nutritional intake varies from when disease is present (i.e., illness, injury), resulting in stressed starvation, relative to when the animal's body is in a healthy state, or simple starvation (Chan 2006). During periods of healthy state starvation the body uses fat as its preferential energy supply, saving protein as the final source. In the process of starvation, this protein source is broken down into amino acids, which can then be oxidized as a direct energy source, stripped of nitrogen, and converted to glucose, or the amino acid can be put back together as a protein to maintain crucial organs. Cats are unique (vs. dogs) because during starvation they are capable of down-regulating their energy requirements and increase the use of fat for energy, but their need for protein remains unchanged. Therefore, their body protein is not conserved.

When an animal has been subjected to trauma or is suffering from a severe illness or sepsis, the metabolic rate increases. When this increased metabolism is associated with starvation, the body rapidly uses up its fat stores, resulting in the early use of body protein (Labato 1992). When an animal is in a hyper-metabolic state of starvation due to injury or illness, which is compounded by a lack of nutritional intake, the animal experiences certain deleterious effects including immune dysfunction and decreased wound healing. The compromised immune system increases the animal's susceptibility to infection and sepsis and the lack of protein intake slows down wound healing. Starvation affects the immune system in several different ways. The cell-mediated immunity becomes impaired in as little as three to five days of anorexia. There is often decreased lymphocyte activation. Other immune system effects are seen, including impaired antibody and interferon production, and decreased T lymphocytes, immunoglobulin A (IgA), and inflammatory response.

There may be decreased leukocyte function because leukocyte products are proteins such as lymphokines, immunoglobulins, and bacteriocidal enzymes. Findings also may include atrophy of the thymus, spleen, and peripheral lymph nodes. However, the lymph nodes of young animals may be enlarged and edematous (Munro and Munro 2008a). There may be T-cell dysfunction, which can cause decreased immunoglobulin production. The total lymphocyte count may be decreased or normal, with the T-cell proportion decreased. Although total immunoglobulin levels may be normal or even increased, their binding affinity is decreased compared with normal animals. The IgA levels may be decreased in the lacrimal, salivary, and mucosal secretions. Lastly, the bacteriocidal activity of neutrophils and macrophages, in addition to the concentration of complement proteins, are reduced. The amount of this reduction is directly related to the severity of the starvation (Labato 1992).

Starvation has several adverse effects on the body and numerous organ systems. Reduced elasticity of the lungs may develop (Labato 1992). There is impairment of the respiratory defense system, thereby predisposing the animal to secondary pneumonia. Dehydration is believed to increase mucus viscosity in the respiratory tract, which decreases or stops mucociliary movement (López 2001).

There is a substantial decrease in the size of organs in starvation. In the heart, there is reduced cardiac contractility in addition to reduced mass of the ventricles (Miller and Bartges 2000). The cardiac muscle is less able to use lactic acid (Labato 1992). Starvation also results in reduced cardiac output, contractile force, and ventricular compliance (Allen and Toll 1995).

Under the conditions of starvation, the kidney functions as a gluconeogenic organ (Labato 1992). Acute starvation may increase uric acid production because of the increased catabolism of nucleic acids, purines, and amino acids. Increased uric acid levels in the urine may result because of hyperuricemia, which increases the risk of urate urolith formation (Allen and Toll 1995).

The gastrointestinal tract can have profound changes, such as prolonged gastric emptying and gastrointestinal transit times. Gastric erosions and ulcerations may be seen, especially if the animal has ingested non-nutritive substances (see below). The intestinal villi flatten because of the lack of local trophic and nutritional factors, which reduces the absorptive area. With starvation, fat and carbohydrate digestion are impaired (Labato 1992). Hepatic lipidosis may or may not be seen in cats suffering from chronic starvation. Liver and pancreatic atrophy may be seen (Munro and Munro 2008a). In addition to the reduction of the basal metabolic rate, there is decreased insulin secretion. There is also increased fluid and sodium retention, which can cause hypertension, although the causes are unknown (Miller and Bartges 2000).

Animals suffering from starvation, especially if they are hypoproteinemic, may have ulceration of the lingual or buccal mucosa. This is because the oral cell turnover is the fastest in the entire body. The cause of the ulceration may be due to the lack of protein for cell regeneration resulting in sloughing of the epithelial cells. In addition, decreased IgA secretion in stressed and debilitated animals allows bacterial and fungal growth in the mouth (Burrows, Batt, and Sherding 1995) which also can contribute to increased dental disease.

Dehydration

Dehydration is often found in starved animals, and the estimated percentage should be recorded. Even if water loss is not part of the final calculation of weight loss, dehydration is a sign of neglect. Dehydration can result due to the lack of access to water, lack of potable water, or the animal becoming too weak to drink. The length of time for death to occur due to dehydration can be influenced by increased water needs such as high ambient temperature and medical conditions. It also can be affected by intermittent access to water sources such as rain or food sources. Complete water deprivation can lead to death within days, whereas animals may survive for weeks with water but without food. Severe dehydration can cause profound life-threatening electrolyte imbalances. Large water deficits of 15%–20% of body weight can lead to death.

Dehydration is not easy to determine in an emaciated animal. Many of the tools a veterinarian uses to assess hydration in a recently healthy animal cannot be used in an emaciated animal. Skin turgor cannot be used to assess hydration. Pre-renal azotemia (i.e., elevated BUN) may not be present in a dehydrated emaciated animal where there is reduced muscle mass and nitrogen metabolism is reduced resulting in less urea production and less creatinine production. Because urea also contributes to urine specific gravity, concentrated urine may not be seen in a dehydrated emaciated animal. Mucous membrane moisture is really the only reliable way to assess dehydration in an emaciated animal. It is not unreasonable to make a basic assumption that a weak, emaciated animal is also dehydrated.

Behavior

Abandonment issues

Abandonment of animals creates a serious problem that can often result in charges under local or state criminal statutes. These may be based on laws specific to abandonment, loose animal, damage to property, or dangerous dog. They also can be based on resulting neglect issues such as starvation, injuries, and death. The legal issue applied can be a "reasonable person" standard, in which a reasonable person knows that all living things, including plants, require nutrition and water. Abandonment of an animal without providing for its nutrition or water violates this standard. This also includes when animals are unable to obtain their own water or food due to physical limitations or a lack of skills and knowledge as a result of socialization and human dependency.

The expected behavior of abandoned animals should be considered and addressed when evaluating the scene and animal exam findings. The environmental conditions, physical restrictions, available resources, previous husbandry, species, socialization, and age and health of the animal are all factors in the assessment. Insect evidence is commonly present and can provide timelines to establish time of death (Chapter 15). The cause of death may be difficult to determine in abandonment cases but a reasonable conclusion

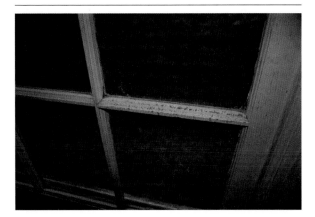

Figure 11.1. Cat hoarding case. Evidence of cats scratching at window to get out.

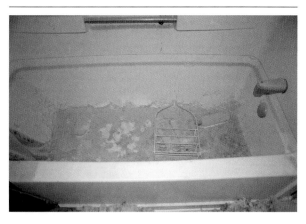

Figure 11.3. Evidence of dog activity searching for water in an abandonment case.

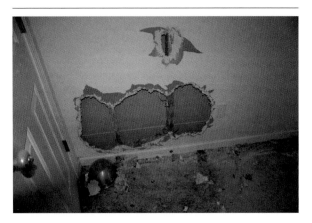

Figure 11.2. Dog abandonment case in which the animal was confined in a room within the home. Evidence of attempted efforts to escape the room.

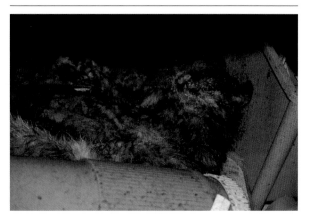

Figure 11.4. A cat that had crawled into a cabinet before death. Note the insect evidence around the head.

may be reached based on the resources available, the length of abandonment, and environmental conditions. Nutrition and water are required to sustain life. If one of these critical resources becomes unavailable, a reasonable deduction may be made as to the cause and/or contributing cause of death. If food was present and the water resource became unavailable, then dehydration may be considered as the primary cause of death. If water was present and the food resource became unavailable, then starvation becomes the primary consideration. If both food and water were unavailable, then dehydration would be the primary factor.

The scene findings provide information about the progression of the animal's health. As a consideration for all abuse cases, it is important to find evidence to establish the animal was alive at the time of abandonment. Evidence of life may

include the presence of feces, urine, torn food packages, scavenging of trash, and paw prints. There may be evidence of attempts to escape or searching for food or water such as scratches, biting, or tearing of surfaces surrounding doors, windows, cabinets, refrigerators, and any caged enclosure; or paw prints around tubs, sinks, or toilets (Figures 11.1–11.3). The location of the deceased animal may provide clues to the cause of death or suffering. If confined outside, the animal may have dug a hole in an attempt to escape sunlight and heat. The animal may be found close to the once available water resource such as a faucet or bathroom. Animals typically seek a dark, cubby-hole type area when close to death and in enclosed environments may be found under or between furniture or inside cabinets (Figure 11.4).

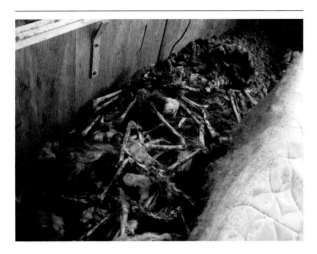

Figure 11.5. Cannibalism in cat hoarding case in which the cats were suffering from starvation. (Photo courtesy of Diane Balkin.)

Animals that are abandoned with access to the outdoors may still succumb to starvation or dehydration. Socialized animals that have become dependent on human beings for food and water do not necessarily possess the skills to forage and hunt for these resources. In addition, they may not have developed appropriate self-preservation skills and instincts, making them much more prone to animal attacks or motor vehicle accidents. Some animals may have physical limitations or medical conditions that prevent them from obtaining food and water. Cats have very strong homing instincts and become entrained to daily routines. They become instinctively programmed to stay at home and rely on the routine feeding by their owners. There are cases in which cats have been abandoned inside a home with the windows open and then subsequently died from starvation. Abandonment of an animal in a strange environment does not mean the animal can survive. Novel environments can invoke severe stress responses. Even feral cat colonies, when relocated, may disperse due to their homing instincts.

Cannibalism

Cannibalism may be seen with mothers of puppies or kittens. This behavior, usually brought on or exacerbated by a stressful environment, often involves a mother that is extremely nervous or anxious. Situations in which there is a lack of adequate resources (i.e., food, water, shelter) or a perceived threatening environment may cause the mother animal to cannibalize her young whereas she otherwise may not. Cannibalism also may be a natural behavior and not one of maternal neglect, such as when a newborn is sickly.

Cannibalism is not just limited to maternal animals. This behavior may occur with young or adult animals in neglect situations. In cases of starvation in which one of the animals has died, it is not uncommon for the surviving animals to eat the recently deceased animal when there is no other food source available (Figure 11.5). In cases in which there are a number of sexually intact adult animals of both sexes housed together, the absence of newborn or juvenile animals may be a result of cannibalism, especially in situations where the adult animals are suffering from malnutrition, starvation, and overcrowding. Other possible explanations for the lack of juvenile animals include unsuccessful breeding due to age or disease, or the owner could have disposed of the animals through selling, giving them away, or killing them.

Cannibalistic behavior may be restricted to the feet and lower extremities of the deceased animal, which is not a normal predatory feeding pattern, demonstrating an animal's reluctance to feed on its own species. In other cases, it may involve feeding on the entire body except for the head and tail. Often there are intact or disarticulated skeletal remains found at the scene of starvation cases. It is important to identify the species of animal (Chapter 3). Evidence of scavenging is common regarding the location of the remains and on the bone surfaces. If the bones are located in an enclosed structure without access to other scavengers, then a reasonable deduction can be made that the animals present are the source of the scavenging marks.

Eating non-nutritive substances

A starving animal may eat anything in an effort to stay alive. Generally these substances, such as plastic, glass, wire, rocks, dirt, debris, and items discarded as garbage have no nutritive value. This behavior is most commonly seen in dogs. Pica, a craving for non-nutritive substances, also may be seen with stress or boredom in animals but is typically associated with mild ingestion of these substances.

The items ingested may cause injury to gastric mucosa and/or intestinal mucosa, which has already been compromised by the effect of starvation. The mucosal injury can present as erosions, ulceration, or perforation, all with the resulting clinical sign of melena (upper gastrointestinal bleeding). If the items pass through the gastrointestinal tract, they will be present in the feces. Gastric ulceration and melena is commonly seen in animals that have starved to death. Melena seen in a live animal indicates a severely compromised animal that warrants intensive care. For starvation and neglect victims, it is very important to examine the feces of the animal for the first twenty-four to seventy-two hours. Radiography is also helpful in determining if a starving animal has ingested non-nutritive substances.

Laboratory testing

Underlying disease considerations

Emaciation is not always the result of starvation and it is necessary to make a definitive diagnosis. It is important to identify any underlying diseases. There may be primary medical issues or secondary issues related to the compromised immune system. Any underlying disease process must be identified because it may be a contributing cause to the health problems or death. Complete laboratory diagnostics can help determine underlying medical problems. Based on case information and individual clinical presentations, screening for infectious diseases such as parvovirus, panleukopenia, feline leukemia, and feline immunodeficiency virus should be considered. In large scale cases this may be cost prohibitive and the medical protocol adjusted to conduct diagnostics on representative population samples based on the circumstances of the case (Chapter 4). Postmortem, the bone marrow may be tested for feline leukemia; the spleen and small intestine may be used for parvovirus and panleukopenia testing. In addition to starvation, the animal is often suffering from stress and inflammation caused by concurrent disease and the environmental conditions. Stress and inflammation can affect the laboratory results (Chapter 3).

Starvation effects on laboratory test results

Starvation has a profound effect on the entire body, affecting several laboratory results. The albumin level is a good indicator of prolonged starvation, reflecting a prolonged negative nitrogen balance. In early starvation, the levels are normal because the serum concentrations are slow to change. The albumin results must be interpreted in light of other conditions that may affect the levels, such as dehydration, over-hydration, blood loss, hemodilution, and liver disease. The half-life of albumin in dogs is 8.2 days (Labato 1992). A presenting normal albumin level may fall below normal range once an emaciated/starved animal is rehydrated. A presenting normal albumin level may be much higher once the animal has been rehydrated and gained weight. Presenting low normal albumin levels generally represent hypoalbuminemia for an emaciated/starved animal.

Transferrin is a glycoprotein that binds and transports iron. It has a smaller body pool and shorter half-life than albumin and more accurately reflects acute changes in body protein content. The level of serum transferrin should be measured using radioimmunodiffusion. However, an estimate can be reached through the total iron-binding capacity measurement (Labato 1992).

Hypoglycemia may not be present in a starving animal. The gluconeogenic mechanisms in animals can be very effective in maintaining normal blood glucose levels. Hypoglycemia is more likely to be seen in juvenile animals or adults that have decreased or depleted hepatic glycogen and fat stores (Leifer 1986).

In starvation, the body struggles to maintain serum electrolyte concentrations. As starvation persists, the total body potassium, magnesium, and phosphate are depleted. The serum concentrations actually may be normal and do not reflect the total body stores (Miller and Bartges 2000). Blood magnesium is bound to albumin, so presenting low blood magnesium cannot be separated from presenting low blood albumin (Wortinger 2011). It is difficult to know the true presenting body store of magnesium.

Creatine kinase (CK), also called creatine phosphokinase (CPK) is a skeletal muscle enzyme that becomes elevated with skeletal muscle injury or starvation. The half-life is approximately two hours, and depending on the cause, peaks in six to twelve hours, returning to normal in hours to a few days. In starvation, the CPK may be significantly elevated due to increased muscle catabolism, in some cases greater than 8,000 U/L. This elevation is caused by the consumption of muscle protein for energy. If the animal is severely emaciated, the CPK may be normal due to the depletion of available skeletal muscle protein stores and subsequent lack of protein breakdown for energy use. Elevated CPK may not be solely due to protein catabolism and may be a result of muscle trauma which may be the cause or contributing cause. Repeat measurements based on the half-life may help differentiate the causes.

The urine specific gravity is usually low and the urine volume increased with starvation. Polyuria and polydipsia have been reported in a study of dogs. This may be caused by the decrease in protein intake or serum urea nitrogen; therefore, less urea is filtered by the glomerulus and reabsorbed by the renal medulla (Allen and Toll 1995). The serum creatinine may be artificially increased when measured using the Jaffe method. Non-creatinine chromogens, such as acetoacetate, which is produced during starvation, interfere with the Jaffe method. Measurements of creatinine and serum urea nitrogen using the enzyme method are unaffected by the non-creatinine chromogens (Allen and Toll 1995).

Non-regenerative anemia is commonly seen in animals suffering from starvation. The anemia may be caused by parasites such as hookworms and fleas, certain diseases or toxins, or any chronic disease state, including starvation (anemia of chronic disease).

The animal's immune status may be evaluated by measuring the total lymphocyte count. In dogs and cats, a total lymphocyte count of less than 800/ml is indicative of immune suppression (Labato 1992). Ketogenesis occurs if an animal does not eat for forty-eight hours or longer. Dogs and cats use ketones efficiently so ketoacidemia usually does not occur. If ketonuria or ketoacidemia is present, then diabetes mellitus or liver failure may be the underlying cause, though starvation causes should still be a consideration. The serum bilirubin, alanine transaminase (ALT), aspartate transaminase (ASP), and sulfobromophthalein retention time (BSP) may be increased because of liver gluconeogenesis. Blood urea nitrogen, urine specific gravity, glomerular filtration rate, and serum phosphorus may be decreased because of decreased protein consumption. Plasma potassium may be decreased because of the increased aldosterone secretion that occurs with food deprivation (Bartges and Osborne 1995).

For intermittent starvation (inanition), i.e., going without food for four to five days at a time, supportive laboratory changes may be seen of slightly increased total bilirubin which may be accompanied by slightly decreased calcium and/or slightly increased AST.

Dehydration effects on laboratory test results

Dehydration can cause several changes in laboratory values depending on the severity of dehydration and the degree of emaciation (see above). These include increased total protein, hematocrit, urine specific gravity, and blood urea nitrogen. It is important to factor in the effects of starvation, such as decreased total protein, albumin, hematocrit, and blood urea nitrogen, which dehydration can falsely increase. Once a starving and dehydrated animal is rehydrated, the laboratory tests should be repeated for more accurate results. Postmortem chemistries can be performed to diagnose perimortem dehydration (Chapter 3).

Bone marrow fat analysis

During the process of starvation, the body consumes its own fat stores and muscle protein for nourishment, with fat being the primary source. The body uses its fat stores in a sequential manner, using the most expendable fat stores first and the more vital areas last. The external fat stores are used first, then the internal thoracic and abdominal cavity fat, followed by the deep organ fat (heart and kidney). The very last place the body consumes body fat is the bone marrow.

A bone marrow fat analysis can be performed postmortem to determine if the animal was suffering from the final stages of starvation. A histopathology analysis may be performed to assess the bone marrow fat and a determination made on the amount present. A bone marrow fat percentage analysis may be conducted at a laboratory (Appendix 37). A study at Purdue University reported a normal bone marrow fat percentage of greater than 80% in canine, bovine, and equine samples with a range of 63%–101%. In cases of severely emaciated animals the mean value was less than 20%, indicating severe malnutrition with the lower range extending to less than 1% (Meyerholtz et al. 2011). It is important to note that a normal bone marrow fat percentage does not rule out starvation. An animal can succumb to starvation prior to the consumption of all the fat stores. A low bone marrow fat percentage should be interpreted with consideration of case and animal examination findings.

Because this is a percentage analysis, and not a quantitative analysis, it is possible for the test to be performed on animals that are decomposed. With cool, cold, or freezing environmental conditions, including with buried remains, the bone marrow fat may be preserved for a longer period of time postmortem. Significant decomposition and drying may prohibit testing or affect the results, which should be discussed with the laboratory. Results should be interpreted in context of the living or postmortem body condition score with consideration of the postmortem environment effects.

A study was conducted on fresh, removed bones (i.e., without skin or tissue protection or external wrappings) from cows, horses, and dogs. Researchers found that refrigeration or freezing of fresh bone did not affect bone marrow results for up to thirty to sixty days. Exposure to ambient temperatures (9.9°C–34.4°C or 50°F–94°F) had minimum effect on cow and horse bones. In dogs, it had a significant effect on initial bone marrow fat percentages greater than 60% and moderate to no effect on those below 60% (Lamoureaux et al. 2011).

The bone marrow fat percentage test requires a minimum quantity of bone marrow to get an accurate result. Studies on cows, horses, and dogs found that the all four proximal limb bones are equally useful (Lamoureaux et al. 2011). If the amount of available bone marrow is in question or the animal is small, then several, if not all, of the long bones should be submitted for testing. Blood and tissue should be removed prior to submission. The bones should be refrigerated prior to transport to preserve the bone marrow and shipped on ice overnight. Consideration should be given to collection of samples which may be held frozen until testing decisions are made.

Some cases of animal starvation may be similar to anorexia nervosa in humans, in which the animal may have been intermittently fed with food that was inadequate in quantity or nutritional value. MRI has been used to document bone marrow changes. A study of bone marrow changes, biopsy, and aspirates in human patients with anorexia nervosa found there was an excellent correlation between cytological and histological findings. The primary cytohistological changes seen were bone marrow focal or diffuse hypoplasia to aplasia with partial or focal gelatinous degeneration, or atrophy of the bone marrow. Gelatinous degeneration of the bone marrow, identified histochemically as hyaluronic acid, is an extreme condition often associated with bone marrow necrosis. There was no consistent correlation of peripheral blood changes associated with bone marrow changes, making it a poor predictor of the degree of bone marrow involvement. Severity of bone marrow changes were correlated to the amount of weight loss, not the length of the condition of the anorexia nervosa. The study found that anorexia nervosa patients initially have an increased bone marrow fat tissue fraction because of a relative increase in the size and number of adipocytes as the hematopoietic tissue disappears. Eventually, the adipocytic tissue collapses as gelatinous degeneration of the bone marrow develops (Abella et al. 2002).

Gross and microscopic findings in live and deceased animals

In addition to the physical effects already discussed, other findings associated with starvation are seen in necropsy examinations and may be detected in live animals. The most common gross finding in starvation is the lack of fat. This may be external fat, internal fat, omental fat, and/or deep organ fat. Body condition scoring is possible in fresh cadavers. The perceived body condition is affected with progression of decomposition. In some cases of starvation, the animal will still have an adequate amount of body fat which does not necessarily contradict other positive starvation findings. The animal may have initially had a high body condition score and may succumb to starvation prior to the depletion of the body fat stores.

Serous atrophy of fat occurs rapidly in animals suffering from starvation. It has a gray gelatinous appearance compared with the normal white or yellow color. Although this may be seen around any deep organ, such as the perirenal fat, it is most readily seen around the heart, especially in the coronary groove and around the auricles. Microscopically, the lipocytes are atrophied and there is edema in the interstitial tissues (Van Vleet and Ferrans 2001). Fat drops in the myocytes and loops of Henle in the kidney may be seen (Munro and Munro 2008a).

There is a substantial decrease in organ sizes in starvation. In dogs, starvation causes gross cardiac edema, myofibrillar atrophy, and interstitial edema of the myocardium. There is reduced glycogen content, decreased protein synthesis, proteinase activation, and mitochondrial swelling (Allen and Toll 1995).

Muscle atrophy is seen in malnutrition and starvation because of the metabolism of protein for nutrients. Therefore, rigor mortis may not develop in emaciated animals (Munro and Munro 2011). Except for cachexia resulting from febrile disease, this atrophy occurs gradually, affecting the entire body's muscles to different degrees. The postural muscles are initially spared and in some cases the type I fibers may have hypertrophied. This is compensatory hypertrophy resulting from the increased workload. In atrophied muscles, some of the muscle nuclei disappear as the volume of muscle decreases (McGavin and Valentine 2001). In starvation, the loss of muscle occurs after twenty-four hours. The visual appearance of muscle atrophy begins in the back and thigh muscle progressing to all muscle groups (Munro and Munro 2011). Diffuse muscle atrophy is one reason why live emaciated/starved animals are weak at presentation. Their posture is that of a weak animal with its head and tail hanging down. Photographs of the animal at presentation compared to photographs when the animal is an ideal weight will frequently show this contrast in posture and strength.

On gross postmortem examination, the muscles appear flabbier, thinner, smaller, and darker than normal muscle and devoid of fat. In muscles with lipofuscinosis, the muscle has brownish discoloration. The pigment, lipofuscin, is also referred to as the "wear and tear" pigment. It is a yellow-to-brown, granular, iron-negative lipid pigment found in skeletal muscle, myocardium, neurons, liver, kidney, and adrenal cortex. This pigment accumulates in secondary lysosomes and is later converted to small, dense aggregates known as residual bodies in electron microscopy. These tissues accumulate lipofuscin with age or past or present episodes of cachexia or starvation (McGavin and Valentine 2001).

In addition to the haircoat and skin changes previously discussed, the epidermis and dermis may show atrophy with reduced muscle, subcutaneous fat, and hyperkeratosis. Peripheral edema is found if the animal is subjected to prolonged, severe protein deficiency (compared with calorie intake) because of low serum albumin (Hargis and Ginn 2001). The gastrointestinal tract should be examined for the presence of ingesta and the quantity estimated. The stomach and intestines may be empty after three or more days of food deprivation. The gastrointestinal tract may be less malodorous than normal (Munro and Munro 2011).

The presence of food in the stomach demonstrates the presence of perimortem appetite. Small intestinal crypt ectasia is a common finding in animals with chronic anorexia or starvation. Villous atrophy may be seen. The stomach may contain gastric erosions or ulcers which, if bleeding, will result in melena. A combination of starvation and hypothermia (see Hypothermia section) may cause gastric ulceration due to reduced perfusion of the gastric mucosa (Munro and Munro 2011). The liver may have signs of hepatic lipidosis. The gall bladder may be full but after a period of time postmortem may spontaneously empty. The lymph nodes may show lymphoid depletion. Diffuse hemosiderosis may be seen in cachexia.

Anemia is commonly associated with starvation cases. If the animal had perimortem anemia, the gums and tongue may appear pale postmortem. The liver may show centrilobar hepatic necrosis due to anoxia caused by the anemia. Microscopically, extramedullary hematopoiesis is indicative of antemortem anemia due to chronic blood loss such as bleeding gastric ulcers, severe flea infestations, and hookworms. This may be found in the lung, liver, and kidney tissue. With antemortem non-regenerative anemia, the bone marrow may show increased hemosiderin deposits because of an inadequate bone marrow response from a bone marrow disorder (Searcy 2001). If the animal also had a chronic suppurative infection, the bone marrow may show granulocytic hyperplasia (Searcy 2001). Gross changes that suggest dehydration include decreased skin turgor (not accurate with emaciation), sunken eyes (which can be due to loss of retrobulbar fat from starvation), and dry or tacky mucous membranes. There are no specific microscopic lesions found with dehydration. Papillary necrosis in the kidneys has been observed in racing greyhounds with dehydration.

ANIMAL HOARDERS AND ANIMAL SANCTUARIES

Overview

Animal hoarding is a complex behavior resulting from a variety of psychological and behavioral deficits which may limit a person's ability to care for themselves or others. There has been a tremendous amount of research and publications on the subject of animal hoarding. In 1997, the Hoarding of Animals Research Consortium (HARC) was established at Tufts University to study and increase awareness of this issue. The consortium posts continuous updates on their website: http://vet.tufts.edu/hoarding/.

Animal hoarders are animal abusers whose actions are the result of a complex and poorly understood mental condition (Sinclair, Merck, and Lockwood 2006). Animal hoarding is about the need to accumulate and control animals, which supersedes the needs of the animals. In addition, animal hoarders usually hoard other items, such as newspapers, magazines, clothes, videos, and so on. The onset of animal hoarding is usually sudden, triggered by the loss of a significant, stabilizing relationship or a highly stressful, dramatic change in status, health, or lifestyle conditions (Nathanson and Patronek 2012). Animal hoarding behavior may be typified by several characteristics: failure to provide minimum standards of space, sanitation, nutrition, and veterinary care for the animals; inability to recognize the effects of this behavior on the welfare of the animals, human members of the household, and the environment; denial or minimization of problems and living conditions for people and animals; and obsessive attempts to accumulate or maintain a collection of animals in the face of progressively deteriorating conditions (Patronek 1999).

Hoarding is not limited to any socioeconomic class or education level. Hoarders may be otherwise highly functioning individuals with professional careers. Women are more likely than men to be involved with animal hoarding cases. The average age of animal hoarders is 52.6 years for women and 48.7 years for men (Lockwood 2004). Diogenes syndrome is a syndrome described in the clinical literature in elderly individuals. It is characterized by extreme squalor, poor personal hygiene, and social isolation. These individuals hoard physical material and may have a small to large number of pet animals (Byard and Tsokos 2007).

Animal hoarders seem to have issues of impaired judgment and actions, or failures to act, which may arise from a variety of factors. These factors include difficulties understanding relevant information about animals' needs, inaccurate appreciation of a situation and its consequences, inability to reason about treatment options and alternative courses of action, faulty self-governance, psychological defenses and behaviors in response to stress, as well as magical thinking, lack of insight, and other cognitive distortions. When these impairments become associated with functional deficits, such as the failure to provide adequate food, water, proper sanitation, necessary medical care, and failure to recognize and attend to fundamental behavioral and mental needs of animals, incompetent care occurs and animal suffering results (HARC 2010).

Hoarders have a tremendous impact on the animals, the people, and the community. Although hoarding may start out as a seemingly altruistic mission to save animals, eventually the resulting compulsive caregiving is pursued in the attempt to fulfill unmet human needs, while the needs of the animals are ignored or disregarded. Hoarders may be found acting as individuals or masquerading as animal rescue activities, such as animal sanctuaries. Animal rescuer-hoarders demonstrate pathologic altruism (Nathanson and Patronek 2012). In contrast to legitimate rescue organizations, these hoarders will not take appropriate action in response to deteriorating conditions to increase staff, increase resources, stop animal intake, or increase adoptions (HARC 2010).

Hoarding constitutes cruelty to animals and is often accompanied by elder or child abuse. One of the major problems with animal hoarders is they do not believe they are doing anything wrong. They fail to acknowledge the deteriorating conditions of the animals or environment. They also do not recognize the adverse effect on their own or other household members' health and well-being. Animal hoarding is considered a pathology, not a conscious lifestyle choice. A proposed model to explain animal hoarding has been developed by Nathanson and Patronek (see the Tufts website). Because animal hoarders do not see the harm of their actions, they are not motivated to get treatment. Even in hoarders of inanimate objects, of those who seek treatment only 15% show sustained improvement (Lockwood 2006). Animal hoarders have nearly a 100% recidivism rate. This becomes an issue that the courts must address by including home monitoring (the right of inspection) as part of sentencing. It is important to share this burden of monitoring with other agencies, including animal control, adult protective services, police, and the health department.

The following are hallmark signs of animal hoarding (Lockwood 2006):

- Will not let visitors see their facilities
- Will not say how many animals they have
- Make little effort to adopt out the animals; the main focus is on animal acquisition
- Continue to acquire the animals in the face of declining health for the existing animals
- Claim to be able to provide excellent lifetime care for animals with special needs, such as feline leukemia–positive cats or paralyzed animals
- The number of staff and/or volunteers is inconsistent with the number of animals
- Only receive animals at a remote location rather than on-site

Additional warning signs of hoarding among veterinary clients follow:

- There is a constant change in pets, with few, if any, repeat visits (Patronek 2004).
- There are recurrent illnesses that can be related to a stressful or unsanitary environment.

- The veterinarian rarely sees the same animal to old age or for geriatric problems.
- The veterinarian rarely sees the animals for preventative health care; instead, he or she only sees the animals for injury or infectious disease (Patronek 2004).
- Hoarders tend to use multiple veterinarians, come at odd hours, and travel great distances to the veterinary practice (Patronek 2004).
- Hoarders may seek great heroics in futile cases, especially for a recently acquired animal (Patronek 2004).
- Hoarders are unwilling to say how many animals they have.
- Hoarders refuse home veterinary visits.
- There is a foul odor from the owner, the carrier, or the animal and the possible use of perfume to mask the odor.
- Hoarders may bring in an animal that is in a severe state of neglect and claim they just rescued the animal (Patronek 2004).
- Hoarders show an interest in acquiring more animals.

Crime scene findings

Ideally, the veterinarian should be at the scene of all hoarding cases, especially to assist with emergency triage. Most cases of animal hoarding involve a large number of animals and the scene should be processed as described in Chapters 2 and 4. An important initial consideration involves taking ammonia readings prior to personnel entrance as additional evidence for the case and for protection of the personnel. This should be done prior to opening up any windows or doors, which rapidly reduces the levels. Ammonia is considered a toxic gas at certain levels. The pungent odor may be detected by humans at approximately 10 ppm or less. The Occupational Safety and Health Administration standard for ammonia states that levels of 50 ppm or higher are considered an extreme irritant. The ammonia gas acts as a chronic stressor to animals at levels less than 100 ppm (Carson 1986). Anything equal to or greater than 300 ppm is considered a direct threat to health and life.

This gas is water soluble and reacts to the moist membranes of the eyes and respiratory tract. Symptoms of toxicosis include epiphora, tachypnea, and clear or purulent nasal discharge. Ammonia causes irritation to the mucosal lining of the entire airway system, from the nose to the deep lung tissue. This in turn causes increased secretion of mucus from the respiratory epithelium, tachypnea, bronchiolar constriction, and hyperplasia of the alveolar and bronchiolar epithelium (Carson 1986).

General observations of the animals and environmental findings should be documented and may be assessed using the Tufts Scale (Appendix 30). The scene documentation should include the number of live and deceased animals, obvious signs of disease seen on the animal or in the environment, the conditions of care, any timeline evidence, and the behavior of the animals. The availability and conditions of any food and water should be documented. The veterinarian should evaluate all medications found, including the indication for their use, whether they are stored correctly, the date of the prescription, the expiration, the name of the veterinarian and hospital, the animal prescribed for, and the amount that has been used. There may be paperwork that provides information about the origination of animals, their names, or medical history. Animal sanctuaries may have records of contracts with people who transferred their animal to the sanctuary. Investigation into these records may result in the discovery of financial or fraud crimes.

The environment can directly impact what is found on the physical examination of the animals. They are usually suffering from starvation, dehydration, parasites, and infectious diseases. The findings commonly associated with these issues have been previously discussed.

Deceased animals are frequently present, in 59% of reported cases (Patronek 1999), and they may be found around the property, in cages or bags, or buried. The lack of deceased animals should prompt further investigation to determine the location or if they were removed by the owner.

The environmental conditions usually are extremely unsanitary for humans and animals. Precautions should be taken to wear appropriate personal protective equipment when investigating the scene. Cockroaches and rodent activity may be present. There is usually a tremendous amount of feces and urine present on the floors and other surfaces of the home or facility. The presence of feces and rotting food can be a source of infection and spread of disease. This includes intestinal parasites, viruses, Salmonella, and other bacterial infections. The odor and unsanitary conditions are often overwhelming and can cause irritation and injury to animals and humans. This includes injury to the skin, eyes, and respiratory tract. At the scene, a towel or fresh piece of carpet should be laid at the entry to the home for investigators to walk on as they go in and out. When the investigation is complete, this towel or carpet should be bagged in an airtight container to preserve the odor as potential evidence for court.

Psychological harm

There is psychological harm to hoarded animals both while in the hoarding environment and after removal. In the hoarding environment the animals suffer harm from overcrowding, noise, competition conflict, deprivation of human companionship, long-term confinement (especially in small spaces), noxious environment, extreme boredom, and unnatural light cycles. This causes emotional distress, which impacts their physical health (Chapter 4). There is psychological harm after the animal is removed. This is a result of the animal being unfamiliar with the stimuli and events which may be perceived as threatening and may or may not diminish over time. These stimuli and events may be nothing encountered in the prior hoarding environment or in the animal's history. Another source of harm after removal and placement may come from expressed behaviors. The behavior may have been normal in the hoarding environment but may be undesirable in the "normal" pet environment, which can result in the animal being resented and punished by the caregiver and socially ostracized.

The major contributor to post-removal harm is due to inadequate socialization with humans. The can result in fearful responses where even a gentle touch or approach can cause severe fear and stress (Chapter 4). The animal can be withdrawn, attempt to escape, freeze, shut down, or become fear aggressive. A study by McMillan (2012) on cats removed from a hoarding case found that they were more social after removal, even to unfamiliar people. They purred, rubbed, rolled over, and laid in laps more than the control group. When cats go through human deprivation, they tend to be more social. The cats showed more fear to loud noises and vacuum cleaners than the control cats. There were not statistical differences in behavior problems between the hoarded cats and the controls one year after removal.

Exam findings

Hoarded animals most commonly suffer from neglect. They have been subjected to severe stress from overcrowding, lack of adequate food and water, and unsanitary conditions. This stress compromises their immune system, which makes them more susceptible to disease. The presence of a large number of animals also increases the risk of infectious diseases commonly seen in communal situations. The unsanitary environment increases the risk of re-infection among the animals.

When examining the animals, it is important to note what would have been readily apparent to the owner. These animals are usually suffering from prolonged malnutrition, starvation, and dehydration. A body condition score should be recorded. The animal should be scanned for a microchip. It is not uncommon to find stolen animals in hoarding cases. Malnutrition and eating rotting food can cause severe dental disease. This is very common in hoarded cats. It is common for hoarded to cats to have lost most if not all of their

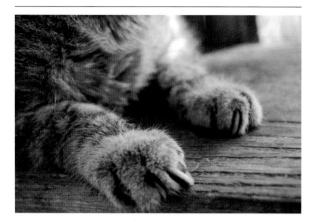

Figure 11.6. Embedded claws on a cat.

teeth. Chronic upper respiratory disease, common in cat hoarding situations, and the decreased oral immunity associated with starvation can contribute to poor dental health.

Hoarded cats frequently have severe infectious upper respiratory disease. Cats may present with phthisic eyeballs as a result of chronic untreated upper respiratory infections which may require surgical enucleation. Commercial veterinary laboratories can perform upper respiratory pathogen identification by PCR testing which can help direct further medical care. One major concern is virulent calicivirus, which will evolve in the hoarding environment. Because cats in that environment are constantly exposed to this evolving calicivirus, mortality due to the virus may not be very great. However, if these cats are brought to another animal facility, other cats at that facility may be extremely susceptible to this evolved calicivirus and mortality among this group may be very high.

Hoarded animals are often infested with external and internal parasites, including ear mites. They may have severe ear infections with secondary ear polyps. They may have skin conditions secondary to the external parasites and the unsanitary conditions can predispose them to pyoderma. Demodicosis and dermatophyte infections may be seen, especially in severely stressed, immunocompromised animals. Ringworm or dermatophytosis is another common infectious disease problem present in hoarding situations.

Animals may have extremely long nails that may be embedded (see Chapter 3 for nail growth rates) (Figure 11.6). They may have scars, wounds, or abscesses from fighting among themselves. There may be evidence of alopecia because of stress-induced allogrooming. Their coats may be severely matted with feces and urine around the perineum, causing skin scald. Severe matting can compromise the

animal's ability to walk, see, defecate, and urinate. This should be documented, preferably with videography. Any significantly matted fur that is shaved off should be photographed and the fur mat saved as evidence.

The genital area should be examined on every animal. The male animals (cats and dogs) may have infections within the penile sheath and females may have vaginitis or vaginal plugs (cats) composed of fur and feces. Hoarding situations involving a large number of intact cats living in a confined area can produce forced mating injuries to the females. Female cats that are in heat may cause arousal of the males and incite them to breed other females regardless of their heat status. The female cats may be weak and unable to get away from the males, regardless of whether or not the female is in heat. Examination may reveal vulva and/or vaginal trauma such as abrasions.

As previously discussed, full laboratory diagnostics should be considered, especially for animals with obvious illness or low BCS. Another consideration is on-site testing to determine any infectious diseases that need to be addressed by the receiving animal facility. These animals often have abnormal blood work related to starvation, inanition, and dehydration (see Starvation). They often have urinary tract infections related to the unsanitary conditions and fur soiling. It should be noted that there is a risk of disease outbreak in these animals after they are removed from the hoarding environment. Initially, the animals may be free of severe infectious disease, even though they are carrying disease, because the colony of animals has reached a state of stability. Any additional stressor, such as removal from the environment, can cause instability and precipitate a disease outbreak.

The treatment for each condition should be documented in the report including any routine prevention measures the owner could have taken (e.g., heartworm preventative). The veterinarian should address the physical and mental stress and the medical and behavioral effects on the animals living in that environment.

PUPPY MILLS

Puppy mill cases have similar characteristics of hoarding cases in regard to the psychological harm and the findings of neglect at the scene and on animal examinations. The people involved often have similar behaviors of hoarders except their goal is profit. Protocols for large scale investigations are covered in Chapter 4.

As with hoarding cases, investigation of paperwork may reveal additional financial or fraud crimes. The crime scene findings may include a large amount of medical supplies which may or may not have been used, or a lack of adequate medical supplies for the number of animals. There may be surgical supplies or instruments which may be indicative of illegal unlicensed veterinary practice activities. The housing is often inadequate and inappropriate for the large number of animals with overcrowding and ventilation problems. Overcrowding issues increase the animals' stress and can result in physical injuries from fighting (especially with intact males and females), increased disease, and malnutrition due to competition for resources.

The housing flooring often varies with different negative effects on the animals. The most common issues with flooring are inadequate cleaning, inadequate drainage, and cold surfaces without bedding or other options for the animal to stand or lay on. The result is animals are forced to live in unsanitary conditions which cause skin, coat, and feet problems. Wire flooring can result in hyperextension of feet and ligaments and extreme nail growth (Chapter 3).

The housing is usually segregated to facilitate breeding and whelping. These may be poorly designed or regulated, resulting in accidental cross-breeding. The offspring of these undesired matings may be killed or sold as "designer" breeds. The finding of only a single individual of a particular breed at the scene, whether female or male, should initiate further investigation. Puppy mills are by definition a breeding operation and there should be a minimum of a breeding pair representative of each breed found. A single animal may indicate that the breeding mate is at another location for the purposes of breeding, whelping, or to hide the animal; the animal was just acquired (legally or illegally) with plans to obtain a breeding mate; or the breeding mate has died.

With a large scale breeding operation, there will be a higher than normal death rate of the puppies due to the increased stress and disease associated with these cases and the sheer numbers which prohibit adequate monitoring. Maternal cannibalism is not uncommon. The dogs and puppies are often poorly socialized, which presents unique challenges that require special considerations for handling to prevent injury to the animal and human and prevent reinforcement of the animals fear (Chapter 4). Additional examination findings are the same as with hoarding cases and any neglect.

HEAT STROKE

Overview

Heat stroke is a severe pathological state in which the body temperature is extremely elevated. This is considered non-pyrogenic hyperthermia vs. pyrogenic hyperthermia, which is caused by a fever (Ruslander 1992). Elevated body temperatures may be associated with cerebral damage, hypoxia, or violent deaths in humans. Severe psychologic stress can produce abnormally high body temperatures in animals and humans (Demierre et al. 2009). In animal cruelty cases, hyperthermia may be caused by leaving an animal inside a hot vehicle or building, or outside without any protection from high environmental temperatures and direct sunlight. The environmental temperature is influenced by relative humidity. As humidity increases, the heat index is actually higher than the recorded temperature.

There are two general causes of heat stroke:

- Exertional: Heat stroke that results from physical exertion in a warm/hot environment. Muscular activity from physical exertion causes the generation of significant heat internally and in a warm/hot environment the body can fail to adequately dissipate the internally generated heat.
- Environmental: Heat stroke can result from a dog being placed in an environment where the dog's ability to dissipate heat is compromised or overwhelmed. This can occur when the dog's ability to moderate the environment is compromised as might occur with a dog in a hot environment on a tether with no access to water, shade, or a cool surface. It can occur when a dog is placed in a contained, extremely hot environment such as a locked car on a warm or hot day.

Heat stroke is commonly seen in animals left in a vehicle. A dog can die in as little as twenty minutes in a car parked in direct sun (Gregory 2004). Several studies have been conducted on the internal heating of automobiles under different conditions. In 85°F (29°C) ambient temperature, the temperature inside a car, even with the windows left slightly open, can reach 102°F (39°C) in ten minutes and 120°F (49°C) in thirty minutes (API 2005). A study using a dark blue sedan with medium gray interior was conducted under ambient temperatures ranging between 72°F and 96°F (24°C and 36°C). The study found that the average temperature rose 3.2°F (1.8°C) per five-minute interval: 3.4°F (1.9°C) with the windows closed; 3.1°F (1.7°C) with the windows open 1.5 inches. The interior temperature reached its maximum in sixty minutes with 80% of the rise within the first thirty minutes regardless of the outside temperature. Even at the lowest ambient temperature the internal vehicle temperature reached 117°F (47°C) with an average maximum increase of approximately 41°F (5°C) (McLaren, Null, and Quinn 2005).

Another study was conducted using a dark colored sedan and light colored minivan. The conditions were 93°F (34°C) ambient temperature, partly cloudy, and 53%

relative humidity. The study found that within twenty minutes both cars exceeded 125°F (52°C) and reached approximately 140°F (60°C) in forty minutes (Gibbs, Lawrence, and Kohn 1995). The exterior color of the vehicle does not seem to make a difference to the internal temperature in the passenger compartment, but darker-colored cars have a higher temperature in the trunk (Di Maio and Di Maio 2001). The heating of dark colored interior components can reach 180°F (82°C) to more than 200°F (93°C), which heats the adjacent air by conduction and convection (McLaren, Null, and Quinn 2005). Shade vs. direct sun can make a difference on the inside temperature. None of the studies found that lowering the windows had any significant effect on the inside temperature unless they were fully open.

Heat stroke is not commonly reported in cats, which may be due to lack of detection. When heat stroke is seen, it is usually caused by the cat being subjected to a sudden change in temperature or the cat being confined in an area in which it cannot escape the extreme temperatures. Cats that are debilitated are more susceptible to heat stroke.

A dog's body normally maintains the body temperature within a very narrow range called the set-point. When the body's internal temperature deviates from the set-point physiologic processes are activated to elevate or decrease body temperature. When a dog's internal body temperature reaches 106°F (41°C), the dog is in danger of heat-related illness. If the dog's body temperature reaches 110°F (43°C), there is a complete breakdown of cellular processes and the dog will die within a short period (five to fifteen minutes) (Flournoy, Wohl, and Macintyre 2003; Fluornoy, Macintyre, and Wohl 2003).

The body obtains heat from two sources: internal (metabolism or muscle activity, such as shivering or seizures) and external (environmental) sources. A dog's body dissipates heat through four methods:

- Conduction (direct contact of the body with a cooler surface), which is enhanced by cutaneous vasodilation
- Radiation (direct radiation of infrared heat into environment), which is enhanced by cutaneous vasodilation
- Convection (air blowing over body, removing warmed air layer next to body), which is enhanced by postural changes and cutaneous vasodilation
- Evaporation

Dogs typically use the first three methods when the environmental temperature is at or below 89.6°F (32°C). More than 70% of the total body heat loss in dogs is dissipated through radiation and convection from body surfaces. The fourth method (i.e., evaporation) comes into play as the environmental temperature gets closer to body temperature. It is not known how significant conduction is as a method of heat dissipation in dogs. Dogs dissipate heat by evaporation by panting. They do not sweat as humans do to dissipate heat by evaporation. The oral cavity and nasal passages provide a large surface area for the loss of water from the moist mucous membranes. Heat stroke occurs when the heat dissipating mechanisms cannot compensate for the rising body temperature such as occurs with exposure to high extreme environmental temperatures.

It is important to document the ambient temperature in the location where the animal died. Climate data for every region of the United States is available from the National Weather Service website (www.nws.noaa.gov/climate). A measure of risk caused by environment for human heat related illness is predicted by the heat index. The heat index, sometimes referred to as the apparent temperature and given in degrees Fahrenheit, is a measure of how hot it really feels when relative humidity is factored with the actual air temperature. The basis for including humidity as a significant factor in the effect on human heat related illness is that as the humidity increases, the heat-dissipating benefit of evaporation (sweating) is decreased. Because dogs increasingly benefit from evaporation (panting and evaporation of moisture from the oral and nasal cavities) as temperatures greater than 89.6°F approach body temperature (101°–102.5°F), it can be assumed that the combined effect of environmental temperature and humidity is applicable to dog health and heat related illness. The National Weather Service Heat Index provides a heat index table showing environmental temperature, humidity, and calculated heat index (in degrees Fahrenheit).

Dogs with heat stress start to pant. Then they begin to salivate and their tongue hangs out of their mouth. When the rectal temperature reaches 40.5°C (105°F), there is loss of equilibrium, and uncontrolled hyperpyrexia may occur. The dog becomes excited and starts to bark. At 42.8°C (109°F) the dog becomes ataxic with possible abdominal swelling from aerophagia, and collapses (Gregory 2004).

Cats have a limited ability to sweat and primarily sweat in their pads. The cat will first pant through its nose. When the rectal temperature reaches 39.4°C (103°F), the cat starts open-mouthed panting. The cat may groom to spread saliva for evaporation cooling (Gregory 2004).

Several factors may predispose an animal to suffer heat stroke, including a confined space with a high ambient temperature, high humidity, lack of water, obesity, increased exercise, lack of acclimation to the environment, certain drugs, central nervous disease, brachycephalic breeds, animals with upper airway disease, and previous episodes of heat stroke (Ruslander 1992). Dehydration exacerbates the negative effects of heat stroke. Heat stress in conjunction with dehydration causes conflicting needs. With heat stress, the body needs to vasodilate the peripheral blood vessels for heat dissipation. With dehydration, the body needs to vasoconstrict these vessels to maintain blood volume. These conflicting processes can cause cerebral hyperthermia (Gregory 2004).

Exam findings

There are clinical signs during life that occur with heat stroke. These are not the same in all dogs, because there are physiologic differences among dogs and the causes of heat stroke vary. For example, there are muscle changes that occur with exertional heatstroke that do not occur with cases of environmental heat stroke. A dog that is exposed to extremely high temperatures in a locked car on a sunny day will die more quickly than one that dies from other causes of heat stroke. Because these dogs die more quickly, the range of clinical signs may be more limited than in dogs that are not exposed to this environmental extreme.

The range of clinical signs that occurs in dogs with heat stroke includes: rapid breathing, excessive panting, severe respiratory distress, dehydration, vomiting which may become bloody, diarrhea which may become bloody, collapse, mental depression, coma, and/or seizures. Seizures occur less frequently than mental depression and coma.

The severe, complex pathological consequences of heat stroke result from direct thermal injury to body tissues. Diagnosis of heat stroke should be considered when the temperature of the dog is 106°F (41°C). The critical temperature considered to consistently cause multi-organ deterioration is 109°F (43°C).

The animal may present in a stupor or coma. The central nervous system is affected by the high body temperature. Neuronal injury, neuronal death, cerebral edema, and localized areas of intraparenchymal hemorrhage can lead to seizures, coma, or death (Ruslander 1992). The cerebellum may be permanently affected, even in surviving animals. The hypothalamus also may be destroyed or damaged permanently, causing dysfunction of the thermoregulatory center. This dysfunction will subsequently predispose the animal to future heat stroke episodes (Ruslander 1992).

The heart is affected by hyperthermia. The cardiac output is increased. The development of tachyarrhythmias and cardiogenic shock is common, which is likely caused by myocardial ischemia, hemorrhage, and necrosis. There is tissue hypoxia resulting from increased metabolic demand, decreased vascular resistance, and hypovolemia caused by dehydration (Ruslander 1992).

The animal may have acid-base abnormalities such as respiratory alkalosis caused by excessive panting and severe metabolic acidosis caused by excessive muscular activity and shock. The gastrointestinal tract may develop ulceration and present early with bloody vomiting and diarrhea. This is unrelated to disseminated intravascular coagulation, which may develop later on. Often, the animal subsequently develops endotoxemia.

The liver may have severe and even fatal damage to the parenchyma caused by thermal injury. The kidney may be severely affected from the high temperatures causing acute renal failure, especially in the face of dehydration. Severe thermal injury to the muscle can cause muscle necrosis, resulting in rhabdomyolysis. The urine may be dark brown in color. Rhabdomyolysis may cause further kidney damage resulting from dehydration, hypoperfusion, and pigment deposition (Ruslander 1992).

Hemoconcentration may be seen as a result of dehydration, leukocytosis caused by catecholamine release, anemia from blood loss, and clotting abnormalities. High body temperatures can cause decreased clotting factor synthesis with liver damage and destruction to the clotting factors. Thrombocytopenia is often seen early on; it is caused by increased consumption resulting from gastrointestinal bleeding. The megakaryocytic line is also highly sensitive to thermal damage, causing decreased production, the effects of which may not be seen for a few days. Disseminated intravascular coagulation may be seen early on or within several days of the incident. This may be seen because of the consumption and destruction of clotting factors, lack of platelets, disruption of the vascular endothelium, and sludging of blood secondary to shock (Ruslander 1992).

Gross and microscopic findings

The diagnosis of death resulting from heat stroke is often a diagnosis of exclusion and is based on the circumstances surrounding death, including the crime scene findings. As with all necropsy procedures, it is important to consider and rely on the circumstances surrounding death. Every attempt should be made to rule out other causes or contributory factors to death including radiographs, necropsy, histopathology, and clinical pathology. In a human study of 429 medicolegal autopsies it was reported that an isolated elevation of serum creatinine was found with hyperthermia cases. This is indicative of systemic skeletal muscle damage (Maeda 2008). Pericardial calcium levels were lower than normal in human hyperthermia cases but were also seen in fatal cases of blunt force trauma (Li 2009). Elevated

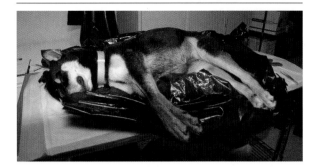

Figure 11.7. Leg rigidity seen in heat stroke.

noradrenaline and low adrenaline levels may be seen (Chapter 3).

Heat stroke can cause a permanent rigidity of the body, in particular one or more legs, which may be mistaken for rigor mortis (Figure 11.7). Rigor mortis is a transient condition that occurs postmortem (Chapter 14). The rigidity caused by heat stroke death is a permanent condition as a result of the coagulation of the muscle proteins which produces muscle shorting and rigidity.

With heat stroke death, there may be generalized tissue autolysis, especially in the internal body cavities. This same autolysis can be seen with advanced decomposition or accelerated decomposition caused by high environmental temperatures. One of the common indicators of heat stroke, depending on the postmortem interval, is advanced internal autolysis that does not correlate with the less advanced decomposition level of the external body. Depending on the level of tissue autolysis it may be difficult to perform microscopic analysis and additional testing. Exceptions include any findings that would show up on microscopic examination despite tissue destruction, such as refractile crystals seen in ethylene glycol poisoning. Viral testing is possible, such as parvovirus on decomposed tissue from the spleen or small intestines.

Examination may reveal gross evidence of disseminated intravascular coagulopathy (DIC) such as scattered petechiae on the skin, internal body cavities, and the surface of the internal organs (Figure 11.8). There may be evidence of cerebral edema and localized areas of intraparenchymal hemorrhage. Stomach ulcerations and bloody intestinal contents may be found. The heart may have gross evidence of myocardial ischemia, hemorrhage, and necrosis.

Microscopic findings can be seen in the peripheral muscles, heart, liver, and brain. The striated muscle findings include evidence of rhabdomyolysis ranging from severe degeneration to necrosis of muscle fibers, reactive proliferation of sarcolemmal nuclei, and dystrophic calcifications.

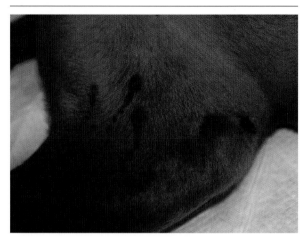

Figure 11.8. DIC development associated with heat stroke.

The myocardium may have focal degeneration and necrosis along with a particular teased or moth-eaten appearance. The liver findings may range from focal degeneration and necrosis to severe and generalized centrilobar necrosis associated with shock. Varying degrees of focal changes may be observed in the brain including focal neuronal shrinkage and necrosis. This is seen especially within Purkinje cerebellar cortical cells which demonstrate a larger selective loss (Perper 2006). There may be microscopic evidence of endotoxemia found on multiple tissue samples. The kidney may contain pigment deposition from rhabdomyolysis. Microthrombi of DIC may not be present postmortem because fibrinolysis continues after death. Most microthrombi are lysed within three hours of death and thus may not be found if the necropsy is delayed.

HYPOTHERMIA

Overview

Hypothermia is present when an animal's core body temperature is below the normal physiologic core temperature. Any situation that causes increased heat loss, decreased heat production, or disruption of normal thermoregulatory function can result in hypothermia. Because an animal's body temperature fluctuates throughout the day, a normal temperature range has been established for cats: 37.5°C–39.2°C (99.5°F–102.5°F), and dogs: 37.8°C–39.5°C (100°F–103.1°F) (Todd 2009).

Hypothermia can be defined as primary or secondary. Primary hypothermia occurs when the body has normal heat production and is exposed to a cold environment. Secondary hypothermia occurs due to altered thermoregulation and

Table 11.4. Classification and clinical signs of primary and secondary hypothermia.

Category	Temperature	Clinical signs
Primary hypothermia		
Mild	32°C–37°C (90°F–99°F)	Shivering, peripheral vasoconstriction, increased metabolic rate, increased cardiac output, piloerection, heat seeking
Moderate	28°C–32°C (82°F–90°F)	Decreased heart rate, decreased respiratory rate, weak pulse, muscle stiffness, hypotension, central nervous system (CNS) depression
Severe	20°C–28°C (68F–82°F)	Peripheral vasodilation, atrial and ventricular arrhythmias, coagulopathies, severe CNS depression or coma, absent pupillary light reflexes (PLRs), absent corneal reflex
Profound	Below 20°C (below 68°F)	Asystole
Secondary hypothermia		
Mild	36.7°C–37.7°C (98°F–99.9°F)	Normal (dogs and cats) to increased (dogs) heart rates, normal mean arterial pressure (MAP), normal respiratory rate, normal level of consciousness
Moderate	35.5°C–36.7°C (96°F–98°F)	Decreased MAP, decreased heart rate (cats), increased heart rate (dogs), mental dullness
Severe	33°C–35.5°C (92°F–96°F)	Decreased heart rate, decreased MAP, respiratory depression, severe CNS depression
Critical	Below 33°C (below 92°F)	Moribund, may appear dead, high mortality rate

Source: Oncken, A.K., R. Kirby, and E. Rudloff. 2001. Hypothermia in Critically Ill Dogs and Cats. *Compendium for Continuing Education*. 23(6):506–521.

heat production due to illness, injury, or drugs. The classification of hypothermia as mild, moderate, severe, or profound is based on the body temperature and the associated clinical signs. Because in secondary hypothermia the clinical signs are seen at higher temperatures than primary hypothermia, the classification system is further separated by the type of hypothermia (Table 11.4) (Oncken, Kirby, Rudloff 2001).

Heat loss can occur through convection, conduction, radiation, or evaporation. Hypothermia is often due to exposure to cold environmental temperatures. The cutaneous heat loss is a function of the exposed body surface area. Immersion in cold water can cause more rapid loss of body heat than exposure to cold air temperatures. The metabolic heat production is a function of body mass. Because of their high surface area to body mass ratio, cats, small dogs, neonates, and cachectic animals are less able to produce heat and are more prone to rapid heat loss (Oncken, Kirby, Rudloff 2001). Decreased body fat also contributes to heat loss due to the loss of this insulation layer. Animals respond behaviorally to hypothermia to reduce heat loss. This includes heat seeking, body curling, and tucking their tail under their nose. An animal will have increased heat loss if its ability to escape or compensate for the cold environment is compromised, such as with geriatric animals, neonates, and animals with severe injuries or debilitating disease (Oncken, Kirby, Rudloff 2001).

Several conditions compromise the body's heat production abilities. Toxins, endocrine diseases, CNS disorders, cardiac disease, severe metabolic disease, shock, immobility, and cachexia are all associated with decreased heat production. Animals are more sensitive to the cold if they are not properly acclimated. Cats are much more sensitive to sudden changes in temperatures than dogs and hypothermia is less commonly reported, most likely due to lack of detection in felines.

Exam findings

Animals can have pain from cold stress. There is limb and body stiffness caused by muscle stiffness and increased viscosity of the joint fluid. In severe cases, this muscle rigidity can inhibit breathing. When animals are ill, they

Table 11.5. Potential complications of hypothermia.

Variables affected	Anticipated change
Clinicopathologic	
Glucose	
Mild hypothermia	Increased glucose level
Moderate hypothermia	Increased glucose level
Severe hypothermia	Decreased glucose level
Potassium	
Mild hypothermia	Decreased potassium level
Severe hypothermia	Increased potassium level
Acid-base	
Metabolic	Acidosis
Respiratory	Acidosis
Coagulation	
Activated partial thromboplastin time/partial thromboplastin time (APTT/PTT)	Prolonged coagulation
Platelets	
Mild hypothermia	Increased aggregation
Severe hypothermia	Decreased aggregation, thrombocytopenia
Metabolic	
Pancreas	Decreased endocrine/exocrine function
Hepatic	Decreased metabolism
Renal	Cold diuresis, acute tubular necrosis
Cardiovascular	
Mild/moderate hypothermia	Increased heart rate (HR) and MAP
Severe/critical hypothermia	Decreased HR, MAP, and cardiac output; vasodilation; conduction disturbances; arrhythmias
Respiratory	Decreased respiratory rate, minute ventilation, and tidal volume; hypoxemia; pulmonary edema; acute respiratory distress syndrome; pneumonia
Neurologic	
Mild/severe hypothermia	Decreased mentation
Critical hypothermia	Central nervous system depression, coma
Immune system	Decreased wound healing, increased incidence of infection

Source: Oncken, A.K., R. Kirby, and E. Rudloff. 2001. Hypothermia in Critically Ill Dogs and Cats. *Compendium for Continuing Education*. 23(6):506–521.

are more sensitive to cold environmental temperatures and have a greater risk of mortality. Cold stress can cause weight loss and immune compromise. With starvation and cold stress there are conflicting demands for energy use (Gregory 2004). The potential complications of hypothermia are listed in Table 11.5. Coagulation tests may miss coagulopathies because they are conducted at 37°C (99°F) (Oncken, Kirby, Rudloff 2001).

The body's initial defense against the cold is vasoconstriction of blood vessels in the skin and muscle to con-serve body heat. There is increased heat production through shivering, piloerection, and chemical thermogenesis, which increases the rate of cellular metabolism (Di Maio and Di Maio 2001). When an animal's body temperature falls below 34°C (94°F) it will cease to shiver or seek heat (Oncken, Kirby, Rudloff 2001). Peripheral vasoconstriction is replaced by vasodilation, facilitating loss of the core body heat. The rate of chemical heat production in cells is depressed due to the decreased metabolic rate; therefore, heat production decreases. Severe hypothermia causes

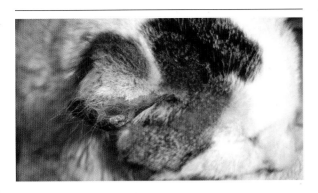

Figure 11.9. Frostbite injury on the ear.

depression of the central nervous system (CNS), resulting in the hypothalamus becoming less responsive to hypothermia. When the body core temperature drops below 31°C (88°F), thermoregulation ceases.

As hypothermia progresses, there is a reduction in respiration and heart rate. When the animal's body temperature drops below 28°C (77°F), respiratory depression can occur. Ventricular fibrillation was seen in 50% of dogs with temperatures below 23.5°C (74°F) and decreased contractility at less than 20°C (68°F). Metabolic acidosis and increased blood viscosity associated with hypothermia contributes to decreased myocardial function. Hypoxia, pneumonia, respiratory distress syndrome, and pulmonary edema may occur (Oncken, Kirby, Rudloff 2001).

In humans, hypothermia can cause hemoconcentration from cold diuresis and leaking of plasma into extracellular spaces (cold edema). In humans and animals, hyperglycemia may be seen in early phases caused by the effects of glucocorticoids and epinephrine on the liver. Eventually, hypoglycemia may develop with possible increased levels of insulin. If a human victim survives for a period of time, he or she may develop hemorrhagic pancreatitis, erosions, and hemorrhage of the gastric mucosa, ileum, and colon. The victim can develop bronchopneumonia, acute renal tubular necrosis, and cardiac muscle degeneration (Di Maio and Di Maio 2001).

In animals, prolonged exposure to cold temperatures or short exposure to severe cold can cause necrosis of the exposed tissue. As in humans, the extremities are the most susceptible to cold damage caused by reduced peripheral circulation and the thin haircoat. The areas most commonly affected in animals include the ears, tail, scrotum, mammary glands, digits, and skin folds in the flank. The affected tissue is pale, hypoesthetic, and cool. It may present as dark or bluish areas with diffuse subcutaneous edema and hemorrhage. Once the tissue is thawed it becomes very painful, hyperemic, and scaly (Figure 11.9). Cell damage

and death occur as a result of ice crystal formation in the intracellular and extracellular spaces. Eventual ischemic necrosis may develop followed by sloughing. The full demarcation of tissue damage may take four to fifteen days (Munro and Munro 2008b). The injury is classified as superficial if it is limited to the skin and subcutaneous tissue, whereas deep injuries extend beyond the subcutaneous tissues (Hedlund 2002).

Gross and microscopic findings

Most gross findings in hypothermia are non-specific and the determination of hypothermia as the cause of death is often based on the circumstances surrounding death, the exclusion of other causes, and the totality of physical exam findings. If an animal dies from uncomplicated hypothermia, there may not be any specific lesions found that are associated with hypothermia. Petechiae may be seen on the surface of the lungs but this is a non-specific finding. Hemorrhages have been reported in humans in the pectoralis minor, intercostal, and iliopsoas muscles. This is thought to be due to intense shivering and/or effort ventilation during the course of lethal hypothermia (Ogata et al. 2007). The liver mortis can have a cherry red color caused by increased amounts of oxyhemoglobin as a result of antemortem binding of oxygen to the hemoglobin. In some cases, the liver mortis can appear white (Di Maio and Di Maio 2001). Analysis of the pericardial fluid may be of value in diagnosing hypothermia. In humans, the magnesium levels are lower than normal. The Mg/Ca ratio is also lower than normal (Li 2009).

In lethal hypothermia, Wischnewsky spots may be seen on the gastric mucosa of humans. These are disseminated, blackish-brown spots ranging in diameter from 0.1–0.4 cm. Reddish fluid may be found in the stomach, although these spots are not gastric erosions. These spots express immunopositivity with anti-hemoglobin antibody. It is thought that the cool temperatures cause hemorrhage of the gastric glands while the victim is alive or in the agonal period. With subsequent autolysis and erythrocyte destruction, hemoglobin is released and hematinized, causing the typical spots (Tsokos et al. 2006).

Microscopic examination findings may include intrapulmonary hemorrhages, acute hemorrhagic pancreatitis, focal pancreatitis with fat necrosis, and small myocardial degenerative foci (Perper 2006). Other findings may be related to the complications of hypothermia such as frostbite. Histologically, areas of frostbite have edema and hyperemia of the dermis with occasional foci of inflammatory cell infiltrates. Postmortem chemistry tests may provide supportive information of hypothermia (Chapter 3).

EMBEDDED COLLARS

Exam findings

Depending on the animal cruelty laws and the degree of injury, embedded collar cases may qualify as felony animal cruelty. Because the collar becomes embedded as the animal grows, younger animals are most affected. Embedded collars can cause severe infection and serious disfigurement of the neck. As the collar grows into the neck, there is pressure necrosis of the skin and underlying tissue. Infection develops that can eventually result in septicemia. The constriction of the collar on the vessels causes tissue swelling and edema. This swelling and pressure of the collar can cause pain and difficulty swallowing, and prevent movement of the head and neck. Many animals with embedded collars also suffer from malnutrition, starvation, and dehydration.

It is important to examine the animal for evidence of additional abuse. When examining the animal it is important to note what must have been obvious to the owner. This includes the odor, purulent discharge, hemorrhage, and physical deformities. Photographs should be taken before and after treatment. The width and depth of the wound should be measured. The collar should be collected as evidence. Gloves should be used to remove the collar which may have to be done under general anesthesia. The collar should be cut away from the fastened area to remove. It should not be untied or unbuckled to prevent loss of any trace evidence. The circumference of the neck, in an area that is not swollen, should be compared with the circumference of the collar as it was fastened.

Establishing timelines

Myiasis, or maggot infestation on live animals, is commonly found with embedded collar injuries and can be used to determine the time since injury (Chapter 15). Samples should be collected for forensic entomology analysis. The wound caused by the embedded collar will haves evidence of healing, i.e., granulation tissue. Bright red, fleshy granulation tissue is formed by new capillaries, fibroblasts, and fibrous tissue. Unhealthy granulation tissue is characterized by a white color and contains an increased fibrous tissue and very few capillaries. Epithelialization commences after a sufficient granulation bed has formed which usually takes four to five days (Hedlund 2002). The granulation bed forms three to five days after injury. It forms at the edge of the wound at a rate of 0.4–1 mm/day (Hedlund 2002). In general, granulation tissue grows at a rate of 1 mm/day and slows as the lesion ages to 1 cm/month (Reisman 2004). A wedge biopsy

perpendicular to the circumferential wound, extending from the haired skin surface through scar tissue to healthy bleeding tissue, can be used for histopathology and measuring scar tissue development. This can be done when the animal is put under general anesthesia to remove the collar and clean the wound.

DEMODICOSIS

Demodicosis deserves special mention because it is often associated with cases of neglect. Demodicosis is usually secondary to a compromised immune system, which occurs in most situations of neglect. When an animal's immune system is suppressed, as seen with starvation, the mites can proliferate and cause skin lesions which can become infected. It is possible for demodicosis to spontaneously resolve once the cause of the immunosuppression is corrected. Generalized demodicosis can be fatal if left untreated. It is important to document the relatively simple treatments that were available to the owner such as oral ivermectin.

UNTREATED INJURIES

Some cases of neglect involve untreated injuries. The veterinarian must document the original injury and the results due to lack of treatment. The degree of pain and the effect on the animal's mobility, appetite, and ability to perform normal functions should be documented. It is important to document the prognosis of regaining full function and the current likely outcome of treatment vs. if it had been initiated when the injury first occurred. It may be helpful to give an estimate of the cost of current treatment and follow-up and compare it to what the cost would have been if treatment had been initiated after the injury.

REFERENCES

Abella, E., E. Feliu, I. Granada, F. Millá, A. Oriol, J.M. Ribera, L. Sánchez-Planell, L. Berga, J.C. Reverter, and C. Rozman. 2002. Bone Marrow Changes in Anorexia Nervosa Are Correlated with the Amount of Weight Loss and Not with Other Clinical Findings. *American Journal of Clinical Pathology* 118(4):582–588.

Allen, T.A. and P.W. Toll. 1995. Medical Implications of Fasting and Starvation. In: *Kirk's Current Veterinary Therapy XII Small Animal Practice*, J.D. Bonagura, and R.W. Kirk, eds. pp. 53–59. Philadelphia: W.B. Saunders.

Anderson, G.L. and L.D. Lewis. 1980. Obesity. In: *Current Veterinary Therapy VII*, pp. 1034–1039. Philadelphia: W.B. Saunders Company.

Anderson, P.J.B., Q.R. Rogers, and J.G. Morris. 2002. Cats Require More Dietary Phenylalanine or Tyrosine For Melanin Deposition in Hair than for Maximal Growth. *Journal of Nutrition*. 132:2037–2042.

API: Animal Protection Institute. Press release 6/15/05, National Call to Save Dogs from Dying in Cars This Summer. www.api4animals.org.

Bartges, J.W. and C.A. Osborne. 1995. Influence of Fasting and Eating on Laboratory Values. In: *Kirk's Current Veterinary Therapy XII Small Animal Practice*, J.D. Bonagura and R.W. Kirk, eds. pp. 20–23. Philadelphia: W.B. Saunders.

Burrows, C.F., R.M. Batt, and R.G. Sherding. 1995. Diseases of the Small Intestine. In: *Textbook of Veterinary Internal Medicine: Diseases of the Dog and Cat*, Vol. 2, Fourth edition, S.J. Ettinger and E.C. Feldman, eds. pp. 1169–1232. Philadelphia: W.B. Saunders.

Byard, R.W. and M. Tsokos. 2007. Forensic Issues in Cases of Diogenes Syndrome. *The American Journal of Forensic Medicine and Pathology.* 28(2):177–181.

Carson, T.L. 1986. Toxic Gases. In: *Current Veterinary Therapy IX Small Animal Practice*, R.W. Kirk, ed. pp. 203–205. Philadelphia: W.B. Saunders.

Chan, D. and L. Freeman. 2006. Nutrition in Critical Illness. In: *Veterinary Clinics of North America—Small Animal Practice, Dietary Management and Nutrition.* 36(6):1225–41, v–vi. Philadelphia: Saunders and Imprint of Elsevier.

Demierre, N., D. Wyler, U. Zollinger, S. Bolliger, and T. Plattner. 2009. Elevated Body Core Temperature in Medico-Legal Investigation of Violent Death. *The American Journal of Forensic Medicine and Pathology.* 30(2):155–158.

Di Maio, V.J. and D. Di Maio. 2001. *Forensic Pathology*, Second edition. Boca Raton, FL: CRC Press.

Flournoy, W.S., D.K. Macintire, and J.S. Wohl. 2003. Heatstroke in Dogs: Clinical Signs, Treatment, Prognosis, and Prevention. *Compendium for Continuing Education.* 25(6):422–431.

Flournoy, W.S., J.S. Wohl, and D.K. Macintire. 2003. Heatstroke in Dogs: Pathophysiology and Predisposing Factors. In *Compendium for Continuing Education.* 25(6): 410–417.

Gibbs, L.I., D.W. Lawrence, and M.A. Kohn. 1995. Heat Exposure in an Enclosed Automobile. *Journal of the Louisiana State Medical Society.* 147(12):545–546.

Gregory, N.G. 2004. *Physiology and Behaviour of Animal Suffering*. Oxford, UK: Blackwell Science.

Hargis, A.M. and P.E. Ginn. 2001. Muscle. In: *Thomson's Special Veterinary Pathology*, Third edition, M.D. McGavin, W.W. Carlton, and J.F. Zachary, eds. pp. 537–599. St. Louis: Mosby.

Hedlund, C.S. 2002. Surgery of the Integumentary System. In: *Small Animal Surgery*, Second edition, T.W. Fossum, ed. pp. 134–228. St. Louis: Mosby.

HARC: Hoarding of Animals Research Consortium. 2010. http://vet.tufts.edu/hoarding/.

Labato, M.A. 1992. Nutritional Management of the Critical Care Patient. In: *Kirk's Current Veterinary Therapy XII Small Animal Practice*, J.D. Bonagura, and R.W. Kirk, eds. pp. 117–125. Philadelphia: W.B. Saunders.

Lamoureaux, J.L., S.D. Fitzgerald, M.K. Church, and D.W. Agnew. 2011. The Effect of Environmental Storage Conditions on Bone Marrow Fat Determination in Three Species. *Journal of Veterinary Diagnostic Investigations.* 23:312–315.

Leifer, C.E. 1986. Hypoglycemia. In: *Current Veterinary Therapy IX Small Animal Practice*, R.W. Kirk, ed. pp. 982–987. Philadelphia: W.B. Saunders.

Li, D.g-R., L. Quan, B.-L. Zhu, T. Ishikawa, T. Michiue, D. Zhao, C. Yoshida, J.-H. Chena, Q. Wang, A. Komatsu, Y. Azuma, and H. Maeda. 2009. Evaluation of Postmortem Calcium and Magnesium Levels in the Pericardial Fluid with Regard to the Cause of Death in Medicolegal Autopsy. *Legal Medicine.* 11(1):276–278.

Lockwood, R. 2004. Cruelty Towards Cats: Who Does What to Whom and Why? Presented at the International Association of Human Interaction Organizations, 6–9 October, Glasgow, Scotland.

Lockwood, R.L. 2006. Hoarding: Psychology and Punishment. Presented at the Animal Cruelty Cases: Investigations and Prosecutions and Animal Law, Institute of Continuing Legal Education in Georgia, May 19, 2006. Atlanta, Georgia.

López, A. 2001. Respiratory System, Thoracic Cavity, and Pleura. In: *Thomson's Special Veterinary Pathology*, Third edition, M.D. McGavin, W.W. Carlton, and J.F. Zachary, eds. pp. 125–195. St. Louis: Mosby.

Lusby, A.L. 2009. Obesity. In: *Kirk's Current Veterinary Therapy XIV, Small Animal Practice*, John D. Bonagura, ed. pp. 191–195. Philadelphia: W.B. Saunders Company.

Maeda, H., B.-L. Zhu, Y. Bessho, T. Ishikawa, L. Quan, T. Michiue, D. Zhao, D.-R. Li, and A. Komatsu. 2008. Postmortem Serum Nitrogen Compounds and C-Reactive Protein Levels with Special Regard to Investigation of Fatal Hyperthermia. *Forensic Science, Medicine, and Pathology.* 4(3):175–180.

McGavin, M.D. and B.A. Valentine. 2001. Muscle. In: *Thomson's Special Veterinary Pathology*, Third edition, M.D. McGavin, W.W. Carlton, and J.F. Zachary, eds. pp. 461–498. St. Louis: Mosby.

McLaren, C., J. Null, and J. Quinn. 2005. Heat Stress From Enclosed Vehicles: Moderate Ambient Temperatures Cause Significant Temperature Rise in Enclosed Vehicles. *Pediatrics.* 116(1):109–112.

McMillan, F.D. 2012. Physical and Mental Issues in Animals Rescued From Hoarding Situations. Presented at the North American Veterinary Conference, 14–18 January, Orlando, Florida.

Meyerholtz, K.A., C.R. Wilson, R.J. Everson, and S.B. Hooser. 2011. Quantitative Assessment of the Percent Fat in Domestic Animal Bone Marrow. *Journal of Forensic Sciences.* 56(3):775–777.

Miller, C.C. and J.W. Bartges. 2000. Refeeding Syndrome. In: *Kirk's Current Veterinary Therapy XII Small Animal Practice*, J.D. Bonagura and R.W. Kirk, eds. pp. 87–89. Philadelphia: W.B. Saunders.

Munro, R. and H. Munro. 2011. Forensic Veterinary Medicine: 2. Postmortem Investigation. *Practice.* 33:262–270.

Munro, R. and H. Munro. 2008a. Neglect. In: *Animal Abuse and Unlawful Killing: Forensic Veterinary Pathology*, pp. 16–29. Edinburgh: Elsevier.

Munro, R. and H. Munro. 2008b. Injuries Associated with Physical Agents. In: *Animal Abuse and Unlawful Killing: Forensic Veterinary Pathology*, pp. 70–74. Edinburgh: Elsevier.

Nathanson, J.N. and G.J. Patronek. 2012. Animal Hoarding: How the Semblence of a Benevolent Mission Becomes Actualized as Egoism and Cruelty. In: *Pathologic Altruism*, B. Oakley, A. Knafo, G. Madhavan, and D.S. Wilson, eds. pp. 107–115. New York: Oxford University Press.

Oncken, A.K., R. Kirby, and E. Rudloff. 2001. Hypothermia in Critically Ill Dogs and Cats. *Compendium for Continuing Education.* 23(6):506–521.

Ogata, M., K. Ago, M. Ago, T. Kondo, K. Kasai, T. Ishikawa, and H. Mizukami. 2007. A Fatal Case of Hypothermia Associated With Hemorrhages of the Pectoralis Minor, Intercostal, and Iliopsoas Muscles. *The American Journal of Forensic Medicine and Pathology.* 28(4):348–352.

Patronek, G.J. 2004. Animal Cruelty, Abuse, and Neglect. In: *Shelter Medicine for Veterinarians and Staff*, L. Miller and S. Zawistowski, eds. pp. 427–452. Ames, IA: Blackwell Publishing.

Patronek, G.J. 1999. Hoarding of Animals: An Under-Recognized Public Health Problem in a Difficult-to-Study Population. *Public Health Reports.* 114(1): 81–87.

Perper, J.A. 2006. Microscopic Forensic Pathology. In: *Spitz and Fisher's Medicolegal Investigation of Death: Guidelines for the Application of Pathology to Crime Investigation*, Fourth edition, W.U. Spitz and D.J. Spitz, eds. pp. 1092–1134. Springfield: Charles C. Thomas Publisher, Ltd.

Reisman, R. 2004. Medical Evaluation and Documentation of Abuse in the Live Animal. In: *Shelter Medicine for Veterinarians and Staff*, L. Miller and S. Zawistowski, eds. pp. 453–487. Ames, IA: Blackwell Publishing.

Ruslander, D. 1992. Heat Stroke. In: *Kirk's Current Veterinary Therapy XII Small Animal Practice*, J.D. Bonagura and R.W. Kirk, eds. pp. 143–146. Philadelphia: W.B. Saunders.

Searcy, G.P. 2001. The Hemopoietic System. In: *Thomson's Special Veterinary Pathology*, Third edition, M.D. McGavin, W.W. Carlton, and J.F. Zachary, eds. pp. 325–379. St. Louis: Mosby.

Sinclair, L., M. Merck, and R. Lockwood. 2006. Forensic Investigation of Animal Cruelty: A Guide for Veterinary and Law Enforcement Professionals. Washington, DC: Humane Society Press.

Todd, J. and L.L. Powell. 2009. Hypothermia. In: *Small Animal Critical Care Medicine*, D.C. Silverstein and K. Hopper, eds. pp. 720–723. Philadelphia: Saunders and Imprint of Elsevier.

Toll, P.W., R.M. Yamka, W.D. Schoenherr, and M.S. Hand. 2010. Obesity. In: *Small Animal Nutrition*, Fifth edition, pp. 501–542. Topeka: Mark Morris Institute.

Tran, H.R.. 2010. Identification of Starvation Events in Pit Bull Terriers Based on Carbon and Nitrogen Stable Isotopes in Hair. Presented the International Veterinary Forensic Sciences Association Annual Conference, 12–14 May, Orlando, Florida.

Tsokos, M., M.A. Rothschild, B. Madea, M. Ribe, and J.P. Sperhake. 2006. Histological and Immunohistochemical Study of Wischnewsky Spots in Fatal Hypothermia. *The American Journal of Forensic Medicine and Pathology.* 27(1):70–74.

Van Vleet, J.F. and V.J. Ferrans. 2001. Cardiovascular System. In: *Thomson's Special Veterinary Pathology*, Third edition, M.D. McGavin, W.W. Carlton, and J.F. Zachary, eds. pp. 197–233. St. Louis: Mosby.

Wortinger, A. 2011. Refeeding Syndrome: Does it REALLY Exist? Presented at the 83rd Western Veterinary Conference, February 20–24, Las Vegas, Nevada.

12
Sexual Abuse

Melinda D. Merck and Doris M. Miller

Legal medicine has been described as the key to the past, the explanation to the present, and, in some measure, as a signpost to the future.

Professor J. Malcolm Cameron,
University of London

OVERVIEW

Sexual abuse may be categorized based on any action involving the genitalia or anus and rectum. The sexual abuse of animals may be disturbing for those involved in the investigation and prosecution, which is unfortunately often met with reluctance or inaction. In veterinary textbooks, sexual abuse does not appear to be included on the differential list for vaginal, anal, rectal, or genitalia lesions (Munro and Munro 2008). This form of abuse involves an extensive species range of animal victims. Depending on the size of the animal and the type of sexual contact it can inflict serious harm which may result in death of the animal. It encompasses a wide arrange of behaviors: vaginal, anal (cloaca in birds), or rectal penile or object penetration; genital fondling or injury; and the injury or killing of an animal for sexual gratification.

Sexual abuse is the eroticization of violence, power, and control (Sinclair, Merck, and Lockwood 2006) involving men and women. A study in the United Kingdom of 448 animal cruelty cases seen by veterinarians found that 6% of the cases were sexual abuse. Of the victims, twenty-one were dogs and five were cats. Physical injuries were present in all the animals, with the exception of two cases (Munro and Thrusfield 2001). A study of 1,000 violent crimes against horses in Germany from 1993–2000 found

injuries associated with the genitalia in 25% of the cases (Schedel-Stupperich 2002).

Sexual acts with animals also can pose a significant risk to the human perpetrator (see Zoonotic Disease). A Brazilian study reported that sex with animals significantly increases the risk of penile cancer (Zequi et al. 2011).

To recognize this type of animal abuse it is important to understand the types of sexual abuse the animal may be subjected to and its significance to society. Sexual abuse of animals has been recognized as one of the early warning signs of psychological dysfunction, including conduct disorder in children and adolescents, and antisocial personality disorder in adults (Beetz 2005a).

Sexual abuse of animals has similar characteristics and distinctions to child sexual abuse. A correlation has been found with childhood sexual abuse in some of the cases of animal sexual abuse. This type of animal abuse also has been linked with violent sex offenders. It is a crime of abuse and cruelty often shrouded in sexual violence (Ascione 2005) with a connection between sexual abuse of animals to sexual abuse of children (Munro and Munro 2008). Investigations of child sex offenders often lead to finding evidence of concurrent animal sexual abuse activities. A connection has been seen between sex with animals and those engaged in sadomasochistic practices (Beetz 2005a).

The type of sexual interaction between a human and the animal includes masturbating the animal, receiving oral sex, performing oral sex, performing vaginal intercourse, performing anal intercourse, receiving anal intercourse, sodomy with objects, and the animal as a surrogate for a

Veterinary Forensics: Animal Cruelty Investigations, Second Edition. Edited by Melinda D. Merck.
© 2013 John Wiley & Sons, Inc. Published 2013 by John Wiley & Sons, Inc.

behavioral fetish such as sadomasochistic practices or sexual murder (Beetz 2005b). Sexual abuse may be conducted alone or in groups. The Brazilian study reported 29.8% acted in groups and 70.2% alone. Several animals were used by 62% of subjects and 38% always used the same animal (Zequi et al. 2011).

In a reported case of child sexual abuse the perpetrator conditioned his male dog to perform anal intercourse on a child. The veterinary examination found the dog became highly sexually aroused and ejaculated with any touch (Ferero Parra 2002). Necrophilic tendencies have been seen with the animal first killed during sexual gratification, then the dead body may be used for masturbation, or may be dissected and mutilated (Beetz 2005a).

Cases have been reported of people sexually assaulting deceased animals found on the side of the road. Depending on the animal cruelty law, charges may or may not be filed in these cases. Charges also may or may not be filed in cases in which the suspect was receiving oral sex or anal intercourse from the animal unless there are medical findings of prior physical harm for training and conditioning the animal to perform these acts. Some jurisdictions have specific "bestiality" laws that include "any contact" as part of the definition of the abuse.

Offenders abuse a wide variety of species of animals including chickens, dogs, cats, horses, cows, sheep, and goats, with either male or female animals involved. There are reported animal-sex farms where people pay to have sex with the animals kept there. On one such farm investigators found horses, large breed dogs, and mice. The patrons may pay more money to have sex with "champion" horses.

Due to greater awareness by the public and law enforcement, more cases of sexual abuse of animals are reported and investigated, requiring the assistance of the veterinarian. Invariably, cases of sexual abuse are seen in veterinary practices. A study in Germany revealed that 36% of surveyed veterinarians had seen animals involved in sexual abuse (Beetz 2005a). The owner may or may not be aware that the animal has been abused and only seek veterinary care if it is injured or has developed an infection. The range of injuries and physical findings of the study by Munro and Thrusfield parallels those found in human sexual assault victims. The findings in dogs and cats from the study include vaginal trauma; vaginal hemorrhage; recurrent or refractory vaginitis; knife wounds in the vagina; uterine tears near the cervix; cervical scarring; uterine or peritoneal hemorrhage; necrotic anal mucosa; anal dilation; anal tears; ligature around the genitalia (penis or scrotum); necrosis of the scrotum or testicles with a ligature no longer

present; castration; and penetrating wounds around the anus, vulva, or perineal area. In addition, intrauterine, intracervical, or vaginal foreign bodies were reported, including a candle, knitting needle, sticks, a broom handle, and a possible tampon (Munro and Thrusfield 2001).

A question of applicable laws is often raised in cases of animal sexual abuse. Some U.S. states have passed special bestiality laws to specifically address the crime. Cruelty laws may require injury be shown and others have to prove pain and/or suffering. Several conclusions can be reached based on the elements of the act regarding pain and suffering, especially using correlations with routine veterinary procedures for the species. Examples may include requirement of sedation/anesthesia for vaginal exams, requirement of restraint and sometimes sedation for digital rectal exams, and how demonstrating how the pain in animals with existing arthritis or spondylosis would be exacerbated by the abuse. It is important that the veterinarian understand his or her animal cruelty laws when examining a case of suspected sexual abuse to understand how the elements may be addressed.

CONSIDERATIONS FOR CRIME SCENE INVESTIGATION

As in all cases of suspected abuse, the circumstances surrounding the incident must be considered along with eliminating other causes of injury which may require diagnostic and specific forensic testing. The crime scene findings may include pornography involving animals, a large amount of pictures/figures of animals copulating, restraints used on the animal, sedatives or tranquilizers (for animal compliance), large amounts of lubricant, and home videos (see below). The use of a UV light or alternate light source (ALS) can help detect biologic and trace evidence at the scene (Chapter 2).

By definition, sexual abuse requires close contact with a high likelihood of evidence exchange between the victim and assailant or the physical items used, including lubricants and foreign objects. Depending on the case, there may be one or more areas where the sexual abuse occurred, including evidence of a violent struggle. The scene and suspected associated items should be searched for stains using UV/ALS, especially the furniture, bedroom, bathroom, pet bedding, restraints or restraint devices, and any towels or cloths that may have been used to clean the assailant or the victim after the incident(s). Consideration should be given to the transfer of semen to other surfaces through dripping or leaking from an orifice or contact such as the victim rubbing or scooting after the sexual penetration. There may be evidence of blood (human or animal) as a result of direct sexual injury, additional inflicted trauma, or defensive actions by the victim. Any evidence that the animal may have defecated or urinated after the sexual assault should be collected for potential DNA or semen testing (see below and Chapter 2). With deceased victims, paper bags should be placed on the feet and the body wrapped in a clean white sheet or body bag prior to transport (Chapter 2).

ASSESSMENT OF VIDEOS

It is not unusual to find personal videos of the sexual abuse on the suspect's computer, phone, or CDs/videotapes. The veterinarian may be asked to review the videos, assess the animal's behavior, and comment on any pain or suffering. Sometimes the unrestrained animal does not appear on video to resist during an assault with rectal or vaginal penetration. This type of assault would be extremely painful (see above) and the lack of resistance could indicate the animal was under the effects of a drug. It also may be an indicator that the animal has been trained and conditioned to accept the assault, an indicator of chronic abuse. The video should be watched at a slow speed to detect subtle signs of pain or resistance. A behaviorist may be consulted to assess the animal's behavior.

GENERAL EXAMINATION FINDINGS

The injuries from animal sexual abuse parallel those found in child abuse and human forensic pathology. There may be minimal to no evidence of physical injury or injuries ranging from mild to fatal. The injuries may involve the anus, perineal area, rectum, colon, vulva, vagina, uterus, scrotum, or penis. Any abuse that involves injuries to the anorectal region or genitalia by definition qualifies as sexual abuse. The injuries found in sexual abuse victims depend on what was used to commit the assault, the type of contact, the size of the penetrating object, and the size of the animal, which may be a factor in the degree of injury.

There may be evidence of acute or chronic abuse which may be related directly or indirectly to sexual abuse. This consideration is especially important in cases where the suspect was receiving oral sex or anal intercourse and there is no obvious physical injury to the animal. The animal may have been stunned using blunt force trauma or physically abused to gain compliance. Findings may include evidence of head trauma and other blunt force injuries to the body (Chapter 5). Violent acts such as stabbings also may have associated sexual abuse. It is possible for animal sexual abuse victims to have peritonitis from rectal or uterine tears. The ears may show acute or chronic injury if the perpetrator restrained the animal by grabbing the ears.

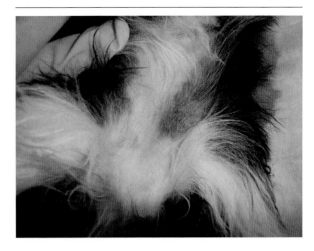

Figure 12.1. Small breed dog (from Figure 12.2) with abdominal bruising from hand-grabbing restraint during the sexual abuse. (Photo courtesy of Dr. Nancy Bradley.)

There may be injuries or physical evidence present resulting from the use of restraints such as ligature bindings and muzzles or grabbing and holding the animal (Figure 12.1).

In human cases of sexual assault the most common mechanism of death is asphyxia, which also may be seen with animal victims, especially if they were surrogates for sexual murder or sadomasochistic practices such as autoerotic asphyxia. With any deceased animal that is thought to be the victim of a sexual abuse, the neck should be carefully examined for evidence of strangulation or attempted strangulation (Chapter 9). The animal's neck may be fractured during the assault or the throat cut (Beetz 2005a). The neck may have evidence of trauma such as swelling or cellulitis from grabbing and/or shaking the animal or use of restraints.

It is possible to see injuries to the tail, which may or may not produce bruising in the perineal region. The perpetrator may pull the tail and force it up or to the side, causing separation or fractures to the coccygeal vertebrae. This usually occurs in the proximal tail region, close to the pelvis. This is not an area of the tail that lends itself to getting caught in something, which is the most common cause of accidental coccygeal fractures and separation and occurs in the distal tail. This injury causes bleeding in the surrounding tissues, which often dissects ventrally around the anus. This looks like bruising to the perianal region.

Ligatures around the genitalia should not be disregarded as just a childish prank. This type of abuse is a common finding in abused male children. In addition to the sadistic injury to the animal, it may be a sign that the child is being abused or witnessing abuse. It should be reported as animal cruelty and investigators can take the appropriate action for the animal and the child (Chapter 1).

EXAMINATION PROCEDURES

In addition to the exam protocols discussed in Chapter 3, there are special considerations and procedures for sexual abuse cases. Prior to examination it is imperative to wear appropriate personal protective equipment to prevent contamination of any evidence and protect against exposure to biological samples that may pose a human health risk. Evidence collection protocols should be followed to prevent contamination and cross-contamination, especially with human DNA, taking precaution to change gloves between collecting and handling evidence samples. The work surface should be cleaned between handling samples and making sure no evidence comes into contact to a surface that contains residue from another biological sample. It is important that the collector not touch his or her body prior to collecting or handling evidence.

In addition to photography, videography should be considered for sexual abuse exams. The animal may demonstrate extreme reactions, behaviors, or clinical signs that are best captured on video. When lifting the tail the animal may show abnormal hyper-reflexivity of the anal tone without any stimulation. There may be pupillary reactions during the exam associated with anxiety, fear, or pain. Another consideration is reproducing the circumstances surrounding the abuse based on case information, such as the environment or certain contact, and observing the animal's reactions. This may be important in chronic abuse cases or whenever the animal appears to be "complying" with the sexual contact. Videography also can detect any avoidance or abnormal arousal behavior of the animal that goes beyond what is expected during a routine examination. These reactions also could be compared to the behavior exhibited during a setting or exam that elicits certain abnormal responses associated with sexual abuse. A behaviorist can be of great value when considering the documentation of behavior reactions to ensure there are minimal outside factors and to evaluate the responses. It is recommended to discuss the conduct of videography with the investigator and/or prosecutor who may or may not want to be present.

The external body should be examined carefully with a UV light or ALS to detect any trace or biological evidence which may be related to the assailant or victim, such as semen, saliva, urine, blood, fibers, or pubic hair. Combing for embedded trace evidence such as pubic hair or fibers should be considered (Chapter 4). Evidence should be properly collected and packaged (Chapter 2). Any wrappings on the body of deceased victims should be examined for obvious evidence and/or the entire item preserved for further examination at a crime laboratory. In human sexual assault crimes it is common for saliva to be transferred to the victim during the assault. For animal sexual abuse consideration should be given to the circumstances surrounding the crime in relation to the injuries to determine where the assailant may have likely deposited saliva on the animal. The saliva may be tested to determine if it is from a human by excluding the animal as the source (Chapter 2). There may be semen found on the animal if the assailant did not wear a condom.

During the abuse, the animal may have transferred DNA or fur to the assailant through contact or resistance; therefore, proper samples should be collected from the animal (Chapter 4). It is important to consider the animal's behavior during the abuse, including pain and fear responses. The victim may have struggled, bit or scratched the assailant during the abuse, and/or been restrained. Radiographs should be performed including the tail. The neck, torso, feet, and legs should be examined for evidence of ligature marks, nail injuries, and trace evidence (Chapter 3). The head and oral cavity may contain evidence of trauma, foreign material, and biological or trace evidence. Depending on the case information and the time elapsed since the incident (see Evaluation section), swabs may be taken from the external lips and canine teeth and along the mucosal regions (Chapter 2). The mouth of an animal contains certain bacteria that may be linked to any bite wound infection present on the suspect including through microbial DNA sequencing (Kennedy 2012).

The assailant's DNA may be present in the vaginal or anorectal region. A human rape kit may be useful for sample collection; it contains sterile swabs, microscope slides, slide holders, labels, gloves, and envelopes for hair evidence. Separate surface swabs should be taken from around the perineal and genital areas even if there is a lack of visible fluids with the UV light source. Swabs should be taken of the vagina and rectum prior to any treatment of the areas or taking a rectal temperature. Several swabs should be taken from the animal for human DNA testing and to look for sperm to increase the chance of sperm detection and to preserve evidence for the defense.

Swabs should be taken in such a manner as to prevent contamination of the anorectal and vaginal areas from fluid dripping during the swabbing process based on the position of the animal's body during sample collection. Multiple swabs should be taken of the vagina, anus, and rectum including the mucosa, any fluids, and secretions. A number of smears should be prepared to search for sperm, retaining separate swab samples for DNA testing. Depending on the case information, the penis of male animals should be swabbed for analysis of human cells and DNA.

A vaginal wash with sterile saline may be performed after initial swabs are collected, taking precautions to avoid human DNA contamination, and the fluid examined for sperm presence and motility. The saline may be infused with a plastic pipette (or syringe with red rubber tube attached that has been cut to shorten), aspirated, infused again, re-aspirated, and then placed in a clean glass tube (Rao, Lew, and Matshes 2005). Centrifuging of vaginal aspirates can result in loss of sperm tails, making identification more difficult (Spitz 2006).

If the rectum is not full of stool, a rectal wash may be performed with sterile saline. If the animal passes stool prior to examination, which may occur during transport, it should be collected for sperm analysis and human DNA testing. The presence of human DNA on any sample may provide proof of contact but not the nature of the contact. It may be possible to determine the location source of the human epithelial cells. In humans, cytoskeleton analysis can discriminate between skin, buccal, and vaginal cells (Schulz et al. 2010). Two slides should be made and air dried. A saline wet mount slide with a fresh specimen may be used to detect live, motile sperm (see Evaluation section). Separate swabs should be saved for DNA, cultures, trace evidence, and any other testing. All swabs should be appropriately packaged and stored based on the type of evidence (Chapters 2 and 4).

It is important to collect a urine sample as soon as possible. In female dogs this should be a voided sample which serves to flush out the vaginal area. The urine is an inhospitable environment for sperm so the sample should be spun, the supernatant decanted, and the sample preserved to examine for evidence of sperm (see Evaluation section). Another consideration for potential evidence is that the animal may have been drugged by the assailant to facilitate the sexual abuse. Blood and urine should be collected for toxicology testing. The drugs used on the animal may include illegal substances, human tranquilizers, or narcotics. The assailant may have given veterinary tranquilizers such as acepromazine, a commonly prescribed drug for animals that have anxiety related to travel, thunderstorms, or fireworks.

There are anatomical considerations in animal sexual abuse. Because the opening of the urethra is inside the vestibule just before the vagina in dogs, there is a chance the assailant's sperm may be in the urethra or bladder. During same species copulation this would not happen because the sperm is deposited cranially at the cervix. In human-to-

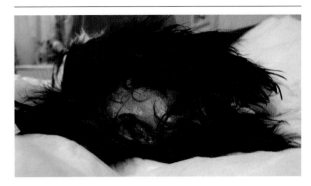

Figure 12.2. Small breed dog with severe anal trauma and anal dilation as a result of sexual abuse. The dog died due to rectal trauma. The littermate suffered the same injuries and later died due to peritonitis. (Photo courtesy of Dr. Nancy Bradley.)

animal sexual abuse, depending on the vaginal size, there may be little to no penile penetration into the vagina and the force of ejaculation at the level of the vulva or vaginal opening could propel the sperm into the urethra.

When examining the genitalia and vaginal and anorectal regions it is important to know what is normal to be able to recognize what is abnormal. An otoscope may be used for vaginal and anal exams, which require sedation or anesthesia. Vaginal speculum attachments are available for use with the otoscope base. Vaginoscopy may be performed with video capture. Colonoscopy may be indicated, especially if blood is found on the fecal swabs or if the animal exhibits painful defecation. If there is vaginal or rectal penetration by the assailant or with an object, there may be severe trauma to these areas and the colon including deep lacerations or perforations and subsequent peritonitis (Figure 12.2). Trace evidence of the object may be found. On postmortem exam, the entire rectum and anal canal can be removed and the examined separately and the contents collected for analysis.

In addition to the injuries found in the study by Munro and Thrusfield, findings may include vulva and vaginal edema, or bruising or abrasions in the perianal or perivulvar region, or along the vaginal mucosa, rectal mucosa, or cervix. Evidence of chronic sexual abuse may be seen such as nodules, due to chronic inflammation, or scar tissue due to prior trauma, which should be evaluated in context with the animal's medical history. Vaginal penetration can force the vulva inward, protecting the internal vaginal mucosa to a certain length. Bruising, abrasions, or laceration injuries may be seen on the vulva and cervix depending on the depth of penetration.

SUSPICIOUS EXAMINATION FINDINGS

Sexual abuse victims often go undetected by the veterinary community. In addition to the findings previously discussed, there are certain physical findings that should raise the index of suspicion for sexual abuse. These findings may be related to acute or chronic abuse. It is important to consider other causes and take appropriate samples for testing.

Vaginal

Penetrating vaginal assault can result in hemorrhage from the vulva due to vaginal lacerations. Vaginal strictures may be the result of previous sexual abuse. Recurrent vaginitis may be indicative of repeated sexual abuse. Vaginitis can occur in sexually intact or neutered bitches, but is rare in queens. It may be caused by bacterial or viral infections, immaturity of the reproductive tract, androgenic stimulation, chemical irritation as with urine, or mechanical irritation. This mechanical irritation may result from neoplasia, anatomical abnormalities of the vagina or vestibule, foreign bodies, or human sexual penetration. The vaginal discharge associated with vaginitis may be mucoid, mucopurulent, or purulent, and rarely contains blood. Cytological findings may be non-septic or septic inflammation without hemorrhage. The vaginitis causes mucosal inflammation, hyperemia, and edema. It is common to find a concurrent urinary tract infection but it does not cause vaginitis. In addition to vaginitis, other causes of vaginal discharge include vulvitis, pyometra, metritis, abortion, uterine stump granuloma or abscess, or retained foreign body. Vaginoscopy may be needed if anatomical abnormalities and other mechanical causes are suspected (Johnson 2003).

Vaginal prolapse rarely occurs in the bitch or the queen. When seen, it is normally due to tenesmus, dystocia, or forced extraction of the male during the genital tie (Purswell 1995). Vaginal prolapse may be seen in dogs with estrogen stimulation, as is seen in proestrus or estrus. It also may recur after parturition or even at the end of diestrus. Vaginal prolapse is primarily seen in young, intact, large breed dogs. The tissue becomes swollen because of marked edema. The presence of a vaginal prolapse in a spayed female or without other predisposing causes is highly suspect for sexual abuse.

Anorectal

There may be suspicious findings or injuries in the anus or rectum in sexual abuse victims. Anal tears can be caused by anal penetration or attempted penetration. Dilation of the anus can be indicative of spinal cord disease, spinal injury, or anal penetration and trauma. However, after death the anus relaxes and can be mistaken for traumatic stretching.

Proctitis is the inflammation of the rectum. This may be seen due to trauma from rectal penetration or retained foreign bodies in sexual abuse. Proctitis may be associated with recurrent rectal prolapses. Clinical signs of hematochezia, dyschezia, tenesmus, and pain may be seen with proctitis. Abdominal radiographs, proctoscopy, and colonoscopy should be considered for animals showing these signs. Rectal foreign bodies can cause rectal fistulas, perirectal abscesses, and peritonitis (Washabau and Brockman 1995). Rectal strictures may be caused by neoplasia or previous sexual abuse.

Sexual abuse should be considered as a possible cause for rectal prolapse. Appropriate swabs should be taken prior to treatment. It is important to evaluate the history for predisposing causes. Rectal prolapse is usually secondary to straining as a result of rectal irritation. This irritation can be secondary to several predisposing factors, including enteritis, diarrhea, colitis, rectal foreign bodies, or sexual abuse. Also, it may be seen due to a sudden increase in abdominal pressure such as with blunt force trauma. Rectal prolapse is generally uncommon in animals with long-standing tenesmus and dyschezia (Washabau and Brockman 1995). Rectal prolapse may be partial, involving the protrusion of the rectal mucosa through the anal orifice, or complete, with the protrusion of all layers of the rectum. It may or may not involve layers of the anal canal. The rectal mucosa exposed increases straining, which promotes further prolapse.

ZOONOTIC DISEASE

A consideration for any sexual abuse case is the possibility of zoonotic disease transmission during the assault. This pertains to any disease that is unique to the animal that could have been transferred to the assailant including bacterial or parasite infections of the genital, intestinal, or urinary tract. Any intestinal parasite that has zoonotic potential, such as roundworms, may be transmitted to the assailant through the fecal–oral route. Because there may be residual fecal material around the genitalia, this transmission may occur through any sexual contact with the animal. DNA typing of the human and animal parasite infections may be performed and compared to determine if the animal is the source of the human infection.

There are several bacteria that the animal may normally carry which may cause infections in the assailant. The aerobic bacteria normally found in the vagina have been isolated from fifty-nine healthy, breeding bitches. The bacteria, listed in descending order by percentage of isolates, are as follows: *Pasteurella multocida* (98%), β-hemolytic strepto-coccus, *E. coli*, unclassified gram-positive rods, unclassi-fied gram-negative rods, Mycoplasma, α-hemolytic and non-hemolytic streptococcus, Pasteurella, enterococci, *Proteus mirabilis*, *Staphylococcus intermedius*, corniforms, coagulase-negative staphylococcus, and *Pseudomonas* sp. (10%) (Nelson and Feldman 1996).

In addition, the animal may carry bacteria with zoonotic potential which can cause infection in the animal, assailant, or both. *Coxiella burnetii*, which causes Q fever, may be in a variety of animals including livestock, dogs, and cats. It is excreted through urine, feces, and milk, and infection occurs through direct contact or inhalation of the bacteria. *Leptospira* spp. can infect dogs and rarely cats. It can be transmitted to humans via urine from animals, usually by human contact with abraded skin or mucous membranes. *Brucella canis* is an infection of dogs that is spread between dogs primarily through venereal transmission. Humans can be infected by direct contact with vaginal or preputial discharges from the dog (Lappin 2003).

EVALUATION AND DIFFERENTIATION OF HUMAN AND CANINE SPERM AND SEMEN

In human sexual abuse cases, the presence of sperm is evidence of sexual contact within the past seventy-two hours. The motility and condition of the sperm can help establish timelines of the assault. In human rape cases, the sperm remains motile in live victims from one to six hours and less often up to twelve to twenty-four hours (Di Maio and Di Maio 2001). The mouth of humans is a hostile environment for sperm with improbable recovery of motile sperm (Platt, Spitz, and Spitz 2006). Sperm can survive longer in the cervical mucus than in the vaginal area. Typically the tail is lost after sixteen hours in the cervicov-aginal region and after six hours in the rectum (Platt, Spitz, and Spitz 2006), though non-motile sperm with tails have been recovered in the cervicovaginal region up to twenty-six hours in living rape victims (Di Maio and Di Maio 2001). Sperm heads may be recovered for forty-eight to seventy-two hours after sexual contact from the cervicovaginal area but positive samples have been reported up to ten days later (Platt, Spitz, and Spitz 2006). Anorectal smears may be positive for sperm for up to twelve hours, though sperm heads may be found in anal swabs up to forty-five hours later and up to sixty-five hours in rectal swabs (Di Maio and Di Maio 2001). Oral smears may be positive for sperm up to six hours (Platt, Spitz, and Spitz 2006).

The sperm survival in deceased victims is shorter as a result of destruction due to decomposition. In humans,

sperm may be identified for an average of twenty-three to thirty-eight hours postmortem in the vagina and for twelve to twenty-eight hours in the rectum (Platt, Spitz, and Spitz 2006), though it has been reported for up to two weeks in vaginal samples (Di Maio and Di Maio 2001). Dry specimens are stable from any site and sperm may be recovered for up to twelve months or longer (Platt, Spitz, and Spitz 2006).

Sperm may not be present in sexual abuse cases due to lack of ejaculation, condom use, aspermia resulting from a vasectomy or disease, sperm lysis, or drainage of the semen out of the area. For cases in which there are no visible sperm it may be possible to get male DNA from epithelial cells in the ejaculate or sperm lysis. The victim DNA can overwhelm the quantity of the assailant DNA, creating interpretation problems in mixed profile results. The use of Y-chromosome short tandem repeats (Y-STRs) may be helpful, especially in compromised sexual evidence (Johnson et al. 2005).

IFI Independent Forensics offers the Sperm Hy-Liter™ test; it is available through their laboratory service or avail-able for purchase by other laboratories. This test is a mono-clonal antibody-based test specific for human sperm heads. It produces fluorescence of the sperm heads without debris interference and has no cross reaction with animal sperm (dog, cat, horse, cow, sheep, goat, pig, and mouse were tested). The test also may be conducted on smear slides and stain extracts.

IFI Independent Forensics also created the first human semen confirmation test kit for use in the field or lab, called Rapid Stain Identification Semen (RSID™). This test detects semenogelin in humans and does not cross react to animal seminal fluid (dog, cow, goat, sheep, and pig were tested). It also does not cross react to blood, urine, saliva, menstrual blood, or vaginal secretions.

A specimen can be analyzed for acid phosphatase which is present in high quantities in human semen and low quan-tities in vaginal secretions. Acid phosphatase levels remain elevated for eight to twenty-four hours in the vagina, then begin to decrease, returning to normal within forty-eight hours. The average postmortem interval is thirty hours in the vagina, thirty-five hours in the rectum, and thirty-three hours in the mouth (Platt, Spitz, and Spitz 2006). Because sperm can be identified days later, this test can indicate the assault was more recent.

In humans, P30 is a semen-specific glycoprotein of pro-static origin which is only present in semen regardless of the presence of sperm. The P30 declines to undetectable levels within forty-eight hours; therefore, its presence indi-cates recent sexual contact. There have been cases in which

Table 12.1. Differentiation of canine and human sperm and semen.

Test	Canine	Human
Size and Shape	Head size approximately 7 × 4 µm, dimple on head posterior where human neck-piece would normally be located	Head size average 4.6 × 2.6 µm
Christmas tree stain	Acrosomal cap pale red, postacrosomal region red, with a colorless band between the two	Postacrosomal region dark red
H&E stain	Acrosomal cap pale purple fading to colorless at the tip, postacrosomal region pale purple and darker at the posterior	Acrosomal cap very pale purple, postacrosomal region dark purple, with a clear demarcation line between the two
Acid phosphatase	Negative	Positive
Anti–P30	Negative	Positive

Source: Schudel, D. 2001. Screening for Canine Spermatozoa. *Science and Justice.* 41(2):117–119.

the acid phosphatase was negative and the P30 was positive, confirming the sexual contact (Di Maio and Di Maio 2001).

In canine sexual abuse cases, it may be important to differentiate human sperm and semen from canine. Canine sperm and semen has distinct differences in size, shape, staining, and test results (Table 12.1). In a published report of an alleged male canine sexual assault on a human female, vaginal swabs (collected within a few hours of the assault) and bloodstained clothing, bedding, and mattress samples were tested. The canine sperm recovered from the vaginal area showed no evidence of tails on any of the cells. This may be due to the different environment of the human vaginal area vs. canine or a pre-existing abnormality of the suspect canine. The canine sperm head is larger and has a dimple on the head posterior where the human neck-piece would normally be located. The staining technique is important to highlight the differences between canine and human sperm. The Christmas tree stain, vs. the hemotoxylin and eosin stain (H&E), provides more distinct features with less background interference in bloodstained samples. The canine semen has been shown to test negative in the acid phosphatase and anti-P30 tests (Schudel 2001).

REFERENCES

Ascione, F.R. 2005. Bestiality: Petting, "Humane Rape," Sexual Assault, and the Enigma of Sexual Interactions between Humans and Non-Human Animals. In: *Bestiality and Zoophilia*, A.M. Beetz and A.L. Podberscek, eds. pp. 120–129. Ashland, OH: Purdue University Press.

Beetz, A.M. 2005a. Bestiality and Zoophilia: Associations with Violence and Sex Offending. In: *Bestiality and Zoophilia*, A.M. Beetz, and A.L. Podberscek, eds. pp. 46–70. Ashland, OH: Purdue University Press.

Beetz, A.M. 2005b. New Insights into Bestiality and Zoophilia. In: *Bestiality and Zoophilia*, A.M. Beetz and A.L. Podberscek, eds. pp. 98–119. Ashland, OH: Purdue University Press.

Di Maio, V.J. and D. Di Maio. 2001. *Forensic Pathology*, Second edition, Boca Raton, FL: CRC Press.

Johnson, C.A. 2003. Disorders of the Vagina and Uterus. In: *Small Animal Internal Medicine*, R.W. Nelson and C.G. Couto, eds. pp. 870–881. St. Louis: Mosby.

Johnson, C.L., R.C. Giles, J.H. Warren, J.I. Floyd, and R.W. Staub. 2005. Analysis of Non-Suspect Samples Lacking Visually Identifiable Sperm Using a Y-STR 10-Plex. *Journal of Forensic Science.* 50(5):1116–1118.

Kennedy, D.M. 2012. Microbial Analysis of Bitemarks by Sequence Comparison of Streptococcal DNA. Presented at the American Academy of Forensic Sciences, 20–25 February, Atlanta, Georgia.

Lappin, M.R. 2003. Zoonoses. In: *Small Animal Internal Medicine*, R.W. Nelson and C.G. Couto, eds. pp. 1307–1321. St. Louis: Mosby.

Munro, R. and H.M.C. Munro. 2008. Sexual Abuse of Animals. In: *Animal Abuse and Unlawful Killing: Forensic Veterinary Pathology*, pp. 94–96. Edinburgh: Elsevier.

Munro, H.M. and M.V. Thrusfield. 2001. Battered Pets: Sexual Abuse. *Journal of Small Animal Practice* 42:333–337.

Nelson, R.W. and E.C. Feldman. 1996. *Canine and Feline Endocrinology and Reproduction*, Second edition. Philadelphia: W.B. Saunders.

Parra, F. and L. Alfonso. 2012. Paraphilias Carried to the Limit—Child and Dog Victims of a Subject With Schizoid Personality Traits. Presented at the American Academy of Forensic Sciences Annual Scientific Meeting, 20–25 February, Atlanta, Georgia.

Platt, M.S., D.J. Spitz, and W.U. Spitz. 2006. Investigation of Deaths in Childhood, Part 2: The Abused Child and

Adolescent. In: *Spitz and Fisher's Medicolegal Investigation of Death: Guidelines for the Application of Pathology to Crime Investigation*, Fourth edition, W.U. Spitz and D.J. Spitz, eds. pp. 357–416. Springfield: Charles C. Thomas Publisher, Ltd.

Purswell, B.J. 1995. Vaginal Disorders. In: *Textbook of Veterinary Internal Medicine: Diseases of the Dog and Cat*, Vol. 2, Fourth edition, S.J. Ettinger and E.C. Feldman, eds. pp. 1642–1648. Philadelphia: W.B. Saunders.

Rao, V., E. Lew, and E. Matshes. 2005. Sexual Battery Investigation. In: *Forensic Pathology: Principles and Practice*, D. Dolinak, E. Matshes, E. Lew, eds. pp. 468–485. Oxford: Elsevier.

Schedel-Stupperich, A. 2002. [Criminal Acts Against Horses—Phenomenology and Psychosocial Construct] (Article in German). *Dtsch Tierärztl Wochenschr.* 109(3):116–9.

Schudel, D. 2001. Screening for Canine Spermatozoa. *Science and Justice.* 41(2):117–119.

Schulz, M.M., M.G.S. Buschner, R. Leidig, H.-D. Wehner, P. Fritz, K. Häbig, M. Bonin, M. Schütz, T. Shiozawa, and F. Wehner. 2010. A New Approach to the Investigation of Sexual Offenses—Cytoskeleton Analysis Reveals the Origin of Cells Found on Forensic Swabs. *Journal of Forensic Sciences.* 55(2):492–498.

Sinclair, L., M. Merck, and R. Lockwood. 2006. *Forensic Investigation of Animal Cruelty: A Guide for Veterinary and Law Enforcement Professionals*. Washington, DC: Humane Society Press.

Spitz, W.U. 2006. Selected Procedures at Autopsy. In: *Spitz and Fisher's Medicolegal Investigation of Death: Guidelines for the Application of Pathology to Crime Investigation*, Fourth edition, W.U. Spitz, ed. pp. 1243–1274. Springfield: Charles C. Thomas Publisher, Ltd.

Washabau, R.J. and D.J. Brockman. 1995. Recto-Anal Disease. In: *Textbook of Veterinary Internal Medicine: Diseases of the Dog and Cat*, Vol. 2, Fourth edition, S.J. Ettinger and E.C. Feldman, eds. pp. 1398–1409. Philadelphia: W.B. Saunders.

Zequi S.C., G.C. Guimarães, F.P. da Fonseca, U. Ferreira, W.E. de Matheus, L.O. Reis, G.A. Aita, S. Glina, V.S.S., Fanni, M.D.C. Perez, L.R.M. Guidoni, V. Ortiz, L. Nogueira, L.C.A. Rocha, G. Cuck, W.H. da Costa, R.R. Moniz, J.H. Dantas Jr., F.A. Soares, and A. Lopes. Sex with Animals (SWA): Behavioral Characteristics and Possible Association with Penile Cancer. A multicenter study. 2011. *Journal of Sexual Medicine*. Online publication October 24.

13
Animal Fighting

Melinda D. Merck

It's not the size of the dog in the fight, it's the size of the fight in the dog.

Mark Twain

OVERVIEW OF DOG FIGHTING

Dog fighting is a violent blood sport that is illegal in all 50 of the United States and is a felony in most states. Some states have felony laws for the spectators of dog fighting. In addition to animal cruelty, dog fighting is associated with illegal gambling, drugs, and firearms. Dog fighting investigations are typically a large scale response involving a large number of dogs and an intensive crime scene investigation, which requires proper planning (Chapter 4). It is important for the veterinarian to be familiar with all aspects and issues of dog fighting to recognize and interpret evidence found on the animal or at the scene.

THE FIGHTING DOG

Historically, a variety of breeds and types of dogs have been used for fighting including the Akita, Bully Kutta, Dogo Argentino, Dogue de Bordeaux, Fila Brasiliero, Presa Canario, Shar-Pei, and the Tosa Inu (McMillan and Reid 2009). However, it is the American Pit Bull Terrier (APBT) that is viewed as the most common fighting breed. A pit bull is actually a type of dog and not a specific breed. The term pit bull usually refers to the American Pit Bull Terrier, the American Staffordshire Terrier, and the Staffordshire Bull Terrier. The APBT is typically a moderate size dog, compact, densely muscled, weighing between 20 and 40 kg. Because there are large variations of physical characteristics within the pit bull breeds that overlap with other breeds, the identification can be extremely difficult. The inherent identification problem and the lack of unique genetic breed markers through DNA testing are critical issues for breed-specific legislation.

The original fighting dog from England appears to be the bulldog. The breed was ultimately cross-bred with terrier-type dogs selected for characteristics to make them better fighters, producing the Staffordshire Bull Terrier (named after the location of Staffordshire). Eventually, breeding took place outside of Staffordshire, England, and the breed's name was changed to pit bull terrier because the dog was bred primarily for the fighting pit. Once the dog came to America, there was a breed split by those who liked the breed as a pet and began selecting against undesirable traits (Dinnage, Bollen, and Giacoppo 2004).

The APBT has several behavioral traits that are desirable for superior fighting abilities. They are quickly aroused, highly trainable, and seem to have high tolerance for pain. They have strong social bonds with humans and are reported to be amiable and easy going with adults and children (McMillan and Reid 2009). For centuries breeding practices have selected for certain physical and behavioral traits for the exceptional fighting dog. These include compact body size, strength, agility, rapid arousal, altered response to social signals, "gameness", stoicism, fearlessness, increased pain tolerance, and strong social affinity for humans (McMillan and Reid 2009). Both males and

Veterinary Forensics: Animal Cruelty Investigations, Second Edition. Edited by Melinda D. Merck.
© 2013 John Wiley & Sons, Inc. Published 2013 by John Wiley & Sons, Inc.

females are used in dog fighting with the females often competing with other females.

Starting in the 1970s there has unfortunately been a negative shift in breeding by certain societal areas desiring more human aggression traits in the pit bull. This appears to be due to cultural influences desiring mean, frightening dogs as status symbols. The result is practices of indiscriminate cross-breeding APBT with other breeds to achieve exaggerated intimidating looks and behavior with the lack of selection against human-directed aggression (McMillan and Reid 2009). It is reported that the majority of reported dog bites and dog attacks attributed to pit bulls are actually the pit bull mixes. In actuality, the American Canine Temperament Testing Association reported in 2009 that between 1977 and 2008 the APBTs had a pass rate of 85.3% compared to all breeds at 81.9% (McMillan and Reid 2009).

The fighting pit bull needs to have excellent agility and athleticism to succeed in winning and avoid serious injuries. In addition to physical attributes, there are desirable behavioral and fighting style traits. During a fight the dogs try to target vulnerable areas on the opponent's body while protecting their own. The individual dog often has a preferred method of fighting, targeting specific body areas such as legs ("leg dogs"), chest ("chest dogs") or face ("face fighters" or "face crunchers"). They face each other to fight and may rear up on their hind legs to engage.

The majority of wounds and scarring related to fighting are located on the face and front legs. They also be found on the hindlegs but these are usually fewer. There may be injuries to the vulnerable areas such as the ventral body or groin area. These are typically seen in poor fighting dogs. They may rarely occur to a superior fighting dog if during the fight the dog failed to protect the vulnerable areas. However, injuries in these areas are significantly less in number when compared to the head, neck, chest, and legs. The bite style of grab, hold, puncture, shake, and tear is desired to inflict the maximum amount of tissue damage.

The most desired characteristic of fighting dogs is gameness—the animal's willingness to continue to fight regardless of the adversity, risk, injuries, pain, or suffering the dog endures. Game dogs will not quit and continue at their task regardless of the conditions or circumstances. The term "deep game" or "dead game" refers to a dog's willingness to fight until death or the opponent's death. Traditionally, if a dog quits, it is culled by the owner. This has led to intense selective pressure resulting in dogs that will fight until removed or are physically unable to fight (McMillan and Reid 2009). Fighting dogs seem to have increased pain tolerance as part of their gameness which

appears to be a general characteristic and not limited to the fighting environment.

Fighting dogs are selected for their courage or fearlessness and will repeatedly attack superior opponents. This appears to be separate from gameness. The APBTs have been reported to show courage in the fighting pit and normal or extreme fear responses in non-fighting circumstances (McMillan and Reid 2009). Pit bulls can become almost instantly behaviorally aroused. They have been selected not to show behavioral signals of an imminent attack, such as raising hackles or baring of teeth, displaying an unsignaled style of offensive aggression (McMillan and Reid 2009). In addition, these dogs show altered response to social signals. In normal agonistic encounters between individuals it ends when one displays cut-off or submissive signals. These include averted gaze, lowered body posture, ventral body exposure, and vocalizations such as whining or yelping. During a fight, the APBTs do not respond with inhibition to the opponent's cut-off signals and will continue to attack. It does appear that fighting dogs are capable of routine interactions with other dogs outside the fighting pit (McMillan and Reid 2009).

In other types of aggressive encounters within a social group or with unfamiliar dogs, such as competition for resources, their behavior is such to minimize risk of serious injury. Dogs assess the capabilities and motivations of their opponent through a series of postures, vocalizations, and threats to show their robustness. At this point there may be resolution without a physical fight if one dog signals defeat. If it escalates to fighting, the dogs target non-vulnerable areas of the body showing bite inhibition with bite and release, especially with members of the same social group. There is continual assessment of the likelihood of winning and at some point one will show cut-off signals, thus ending the fight (McMillan and Reid 2009). In the fighting dog there is no bite inhibition.

In predatory behavior there is usually stalking then attack with the bites directed toward vulnerable areas with the intent to kill. These may occur as slashing bites to limbs or abdomen, holding bites to the neck or back, and bite-hold-shake injuries. This may be followed by dissection and feeding, though not all dogs complete this act. With fighting dogs there is no stalking, dissecting, or feeding. Some pit bulls do not show dog aggression until two to three years of age at social maturity. The type of aggression in fighting dogs appears to be a combination of predatory and intraspecific social behavior system (McMillan and Reid 2009).

Another characteristic associated with fighting pit bulls is a dysfunctional sexual behavior system. The females often require muzzling or human or other types of restraint, such as the breeding (rape) strand, for mating to occur. Sometimes these restraints are used because the owner is unsure of the female's estrus status. The fighting male pit bull may be unable to respond in the normal conciliatory manner when the female displays normal courtship aggression (McMillan and Reid 2009).

The fighting dog has been selected to be highly aggressive toward other dogs but not humans. The APBT appears to have strong social affinity to humans. This is a crucial characteristic because these dogs must be handled safely before, during, and after the fight. These interactions include training, washing, handling within the fight pit, and medical care afterwards. This makes human-directed aggression an intolerable trait of the fighting dog. It has been stated that the APBT has been the only breed held to such an exacting standard (McMillan and Reid 2009).

FIGHTING CLASSIFICATIONS

There are three categories of fighting dog owners: the professional (organized), the hobbyist (midlevel), and the street fighter. The professional dog fighter travels around the county to participate in fight venues as fight referees, participants, organizers, or handlers for their own dogs. The owner invests a large amount of money in training, equipment, and purchasing dogs. Their fight venues are usually high-stakes matches featuring experienced fighting dogs with established bloodlines. Their dogs are often given performance-enhancing steroids and may be on chronic antibiotics for injury infections due to frequent fighting matches. The stud fees for their dogs are usually high (Dinnage, Bollen, and Giacoppo 2004).

The hobbyist fighters typically enjoy the local fighting circuit with a greater emphasis on the gambling and drug dealing. They tend to socialize together and set up fighting venues that are used on a regular basis. This group tends to live within a reasonable proximity of each other and they tend to know each other. They usually spend the minimal amount of time necessary on training and conditioning the dog and may steal neighborhood animals to use as "bait" animals. The main financial focus is gambling winnings to offset the owner's investment (Dinnage, Bollen, and Giacoppo 2004), though they breed winning animals and sell the offspring. The hobbyist may be involved with some of the front activities such as weight pulling and showing.

The street fighters use their dogs, which are often a mixed pit bull breed, for more than fighting purposes. They are often involved with gangs and other illegal activity and the dogs are used for protection. Illicit drugs may be hidden under the dog's collar, harness, or housing. If the dog is aggressive toward humans, it is the most likely fighting dog to cause a fatal dog attack (Dinnage, Bollen, and Giacoppo 2004). Impromptu matches may occur in public areas, abandoned property, or private residences with easy pedestrian access but limited vehicle access. These fights are not conducted under normal dog fighting rules and continue until one dog gives up or someone calls the match off. They do not typically engage in the formal training practices by serious dog fighters but may steal neighborhood animals to use for training. Generally, these dogs are kept in neglectful conditions and may have suffered physical abuse. The dogs may have been debarked and/or declawed to allow them to attack without audible warning.

THE FIGHT AND THE DOG FIGHTING PIT

In the typical dog fighting situation, there is initially an agreement between the individuals on the entry fee, wager, date, time, place, fighting rules, dogs to fight, and weight class. Approximately six to eight weeks before the fight date, the dog will be placed in "keep" which is the training period (see below). The fights are held in clandestine locations, making detection of dog fighting difficult for law enforcement. There are several versions of dog fighting rules which describe in detail the process of the fight (see Appendix 32 for Cajun Rules). Certain terminology is associated with dog fighting (Appendix 31). The dogs are weighed and if the dog exceeds the weight class the fight and any money is forfeited. The dogs are first washed before the fight, usually by the opponent's handler to ensure no irritating substances are on the coat. The handlers are in the pit in a corner with a "scratch line." They "face" their dogs, turning them around to face each other. Then they are released and they have to cross their respective scratch lines and engage. There are timed rounds, each beginning again with facing the dogs. The handlers have to disengage the dogs at the end of each round, often requiring break/bite sticks (see below). These sticks are also used if they get "fanged," i.e., when a tooth becomes embedded in tissue or skin and the dog cannot get it loose. The fights may go on for hours with severe loss of blood and injuries in the dogs. The fight ends if a dog refuses to scratch (cross the scratch line), is removed by the handler (possibly due to serious injury), or dies. Regardless of the outcome of the fight, most dogs that have been fought have injuries and may have problems related to blood loss, dehydration, pain, heat exhaustion, or shock. Dogs that refuse to scratch or perform poorly may be later culled by killing.

The dimensions and configuration of the pit vary. They may be 14–20 square feet with walls 2–3 feet high. The floor may be covered with canvas or carpet to improve traction for the dogs. Most pits are portable, with the walls made of wood or chain-link panels, or they may be made from hay bales. The scratch line is a diagonal line, drawn with tape or paint, in opposite corners for each dog to be held at before they are released to fight. They are usually 12–14 feet apart, depending on the fighting rules. Occasionally, there is a center line on the floor. Suspected blood stains may be tested (see Canine CODIS below and Chapter 2).

TRAINING AND FIGHTING PARAPHERNALIA

Several types of equipment are used to train and condition fighting dogs and during a fight. The training starts when the dogs are young. They are exercised daily and conditioned to be aggressive to other animals. They may be given small live animals to use as toys or the animal may be used to entice the puppies to jump up, grab, and hold on. As the animals get older or during the "keep" training period, bait animals may be used, such as cats, rabbits, small dogs, or wildlife. Neighborhood pets may be stolen and used as bait animals.

For conditioning, the pit bull dog may be forced to run on a treadmill for several hours a day. There are many types of treadmills that may be found such as a wooden slat mill or a converted human treadmill. They typically have wooden sides to act as blinders and a hook for a harness attachment to hold the dog on the treadmill. A jenny or cat mill may be used for conditioning. This resembles a miniature horse walker in which the dog is harnessed to a projecting spoke. A small bait animal may be attached to these training devices to entice the dog to exercise. Swimming conditioning is commonly used, often by suspending the dog in a harness in a pool of some kind, commonly an above-ground pool. A flirt pole, often a long bamboo pole with a toy or animal hide attached to the end, is used to entice the dog in any conditioning or exercise.

Weights are usually added to the chain tethers or collars for strength building. The dog may be removed from normal chain tie-out and chained to an elevated wire runner, usually with chain weights attached, to have continuous conditioning, especially when the ground is sloped.

The springpole is used to reinforce the desired bite characteristics for dog fighting. This device consists of suspending an object (hide, inner tube, tire, toy, punching bag), usually connected to a large spring, at a distance from the ground. The dog is trained to jump up, grab, shake, and hold onto the suspended material. This exercise builds up the jaw muscles and leg muscles from jumping.

A breeding stand, also called a rape stand, is used to strap a female in position to facilitate breeding and prevent her from fighting with the male dog (see above). It should be noted that this device is not used or required for routine dog breeding practices. These stands come in a variety of designs that may have been purchased or handmade. The stand is typically adjustable for different body lengths and heights with straps to immobilize the female, especially the head and/or neck.

A break stick is used during a fight when dogs need to be separated, such as when the dogs are engaged in a bite hold or are fanged. The stick is inserted in the side of the mouth and manipulated to pry apart the jaws. Break sticks are typically wedge shaped, usually made of wood or plastic, and may be handmade or purchased. Other items may be used to pry the mouth open such as tools, tool handles, or scraps of wood or sticks. Injuries to the buccal or gum mucosa may be caused by the use of a break stick.

All training and paraphernalia should be examined for evidence of use. The first consideration for any suspected blood stains is to conduct presumptive blood testing. This is to confirm the presence of blood and identify possible areas for DNA testing. Exclusionary presumptive blood testing may be considered (Chapter 3). Depending on the case, DNA testing may be desired for many reasons including to match biological samples to individual dogs and to submit samples to Canine CODIS (Chapter 4). In addition to the fighting pit, biological samples may be found on paraphernalia, used medical supplies, medical treatment areas, training areas, housing, and transport vehicles. The use of an alternate light source (ALS) or UV light can help detect biological and trace evidence (Chapter 2). Blood evidence protocols for the fighting pit are discussed in Chapter 2.

Common explanations offered by defendants regarding blood evidence associated with the pit include male-female fighting during attempted breeding, female estrus, or whelping. The bloodstain sample can be tested to identify male or female sources. To exclude whelping as a source of male DNA, the sample may be analyzed for testosterone levels to determine if the male DNA is from a sexually mature or immature male (fighting dogs are typically not neutered). This test usually needs to be conducted at human crime laboratories due to the nature of the sample (e.g. swab, carpet).

A variety of medical supplies, supplements, and equipment may be found which often include medications and supplies for critical care, infections, pain, and wound treatment (Appendix 35). Surgical supplies for injuries or ear cropping may be found. There is typically a large amount of medications and supplies which can indicate there was a high expectation of injury, infection, and/or life-threatening conditions for the animals. The use of androgenic and performance enhancing drugs and supplements may be used with fighting dogs. Diuretics may be used to decrease the dog's weight for the weigh-in prior to a fight. Any empty, used syringes may be tested to determine the substance that was inside the syringe/needle. DNA may be obtained from the needle to identify the species and individual animal that received the injection. The supplies may have been obtained from the Internet or through a veterinarian who may or may not have knowledge that their purpose was for use in dog fighting. Sometimes a veterinary professional (doctor, technician, staff, student) is involved with stealing or purchasing supplies for the dog fighter and providing veterinary care.

Other miscellaneous paraphernalia include dog fighting journals, manuals, and fight records. There may be training records including diet, supplements, and exercise regimens. There are often pedigree or breeding records, sometimes accompanied by photographs of the breeding or whelping. Videos of actual dog fights may be found embedded in other personal or commercial recordings.

CANINE CODIS: FIGHTING DOG COMBINED DNA INDEX SYSTEM

The Canine CODIS database, established at the Veterinary Genetics Laboratory at the University of California Davis, is the first forensic DNA database of dogs exclusively used for dog fighting (Appendix 37). It is similar to the FBI's human CODIS database used in criminal and missing person investigations. The Canine CODIS database contains individual DNA profiles from dogs that are seized during dog fighting investigations as well as profiles from unknown samples collected at suspected dog fighting venues. DNA can be used to identify relationships between dogs and thereby allow investigators to establish connections between those who breed and train dogs for fighting.

Upon seizure of live dogs in a dog fighting case, cheek swabs are collected and submitted to the laboratory for DNA testing. Appropriate DNA samples from deceased dogs also can be submitted. Items or DNA samples collected from dog fighting investigation crime scenes can be searched against the Canine CODIS database in an effort to identify the source. The DNA profile is then searched against the Canine CODIS database. In the event that the query returns a hit, the agency submitting the query sample and the agency that submitted the database sample are notified. The samples and results are owned by the submitting agency. Privacy is maintained and no information about either case is disclosed, with only contact information for the two agencies exchanged. The agencies may then discuss the value, if any, of the DNA connection for their investigation and prosecution. This exchange of information may help the agency and prosecutors to expand and strengthen dog fighting investigations and prosecutions.

The value of this database lies in the ability to build a searchable database for the investigator for his or her area and surrounding regions by continual submission of samples from the investigation. Samples may also be submitted without a search request and, upon approval by the lab, be placed in the database for a reduced fee. This database contains no breed-specific information and cannot be used for that purpose. It is established solely for prosecuting criminal dog fighting cases, and only law enforcement professionals engaged in investigating dog fighting casework can contribute samples.

EXAMINATION OF THE ANIMAL

General considerations

Fighting dogs may be male or female, adult or juveniles. These animals should be examined and photographed as soon as possible after seizure. Because of these dogs high arousal, it is imperative that proper restraint be used. Precautions should be taken to block visualization of other animals when handling the dog. It is preferable to have the same person handling the animal from removal from housing, during examination, and return to housing or transportation vehicle. This person will have a better sense of the dog and its reactions which can help prevent any behavior issues. Measurements of the dog may need to be taken for blood spatter analysis (Chapter 2). Buccal swabs should be taken from each dog seized for dog fighting for potential DNA testing. This may be for the case or in the event the dogs are stolen. Dogs seized from fighting investigations are at high risk for being stolen at the sheltering site and re-entering the fighting arena. Microchipping the seized dogs may be a consideration for the investigating and prosecuting agencies.

The dogs should be examined for injuries and a time estimate given for the injuries (Chapters 3 and 11). It should be noted that puppies from fighting dogs can exhibit fighting aggression at a young age, inflicting serious injuries to their littermates. Dogs that were recently fought may have blood loss from their injuries; therefore, the calculated loss should be estimated (Chapter 3). Each wound and scar should be documented and completely described (see below). It is not uncommon to find older, healed fractures. Radiography can provide documentation and detect hidden injuries. Detection of injuries on exam may be difficult because these dogs may not exhibit signs of pain that are easily recognizable.

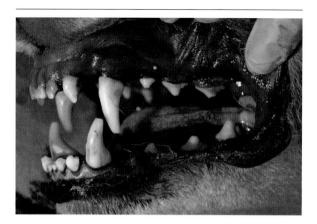

Figure 13.1 Wearing of the tips of canines and premolars.

The mouth should be examined for injuries. The buccal and gingival mucosa can be injured with the use of break sticks. There may be evidence of bite wounds inside the mouth, such as the hard palate, with or without corresponding wounds on the face. Historically, it has been said that dog fighters may file the teeth of their dogs. This may happen in lower level fighting but the appearance of filing is often due to the chronic chewing on chains and other objects (Figure 13.1). If filing is suspected, DNA from the tool used may confirm species or the individual dog it was used on.

Fighting dogs may or may not have their ears and/or tail cropped. Dogs use their body, especially the tail and ears, to communicate aggression or submission and to signal emotion or intention. Even though this communication is reduced through breeding selection and training, the removal of the ears or tails can further decrease this undesired behavior for fighting purposes. It should be noted that removal of the ears to the level of the ear opening is usually indicative of a dog that is not a good fighter (i.e., undesirable ear communication) and is being used for breeding due to desirable conformation characteristics. An additional benefit for ear cropping in fighting dogs is to reduce or eliminate an area the opponent can grab onto, shake, tear, or injure. Often, this surgery is performed by an unlicensed individual. Anesthesia, sedation, or perioperative pain control may or may not be used, or used inappropriately, and restraints may be required to perform the procedure. This can lead to additional charges of practicing veterinary medicine without a license and unlawful possession and use of controlled substances. Ear crop surgery performed without adequate hemostasis can result in life-threatening hemorrhage.

Anabolic steroids and mimetics are used to increase muscle mass and endurance and have been shown to increase aggression in animals (Williams et al. 2000). The chronic use of anabolic steroids or drugs with similar effects can cause physical changes and can adversely affect the cardiovascular, hepatic, and endocrine systems. Abnormally large muscle development may be seen, which may be more recognizable when compared to the younger adults. Cardiac changes such as hypertrophy and live damage may be seen. It also can result in abnormal psychoses-like behaviors including unpredictability, abnormal affect, and abnormal responses to the environment or stimuli. The chronic use of androgenic drugs can cause gynecomastia.

Examination often includes findings of neglect (Chapter 11). These dogs commonly have skin lesions or wounds related to their housing, including the areas over the bony prominences such as the pelvis region. A common finding is ventral neck alopecia and inflammation, sometimes with deep abrasion injuries and infection, which is the result of the dog repetitively pulling against the chain tether. This is also an indicator of longer term tethering.

Each dog should have a full blood work-up, including heartworm testing and a fecal exam. Heartworms, intestinal parasites, and anemia are common problems found. *Babesia gibsoni* is a common parasite found in fighting dogs. A study on dogs seized from dog fighting cases found that 33.8% were infected with *B. gibsoni* when compared to randomly selected shelter dogs with no known history of fighting (infection rate 0.5%). Furthermore, dogs with scars on the face, head, and forelimbs were 5.5 times more likely to be infected with *B. gibsoni* than dogs without scars. One dog was reported to be infected with the canine small *Babesia* "Spanish isolate" known as *Theileria annae* (Yeagley et al. 2009).

Pit bulls are predisposed to several health problems that are unrelated to fighting. They are highly susceptible to the parvovirus. They are also prone to demodectic mange, dermatophytosis, flea allergy dermatitis, acral lick granulomas, acute moist dermatitis, pressure calluses, false pregnancy, anterior cruciate ligament rupture, and hip dysplasia (Dinnage, Bollen, and Giacoppo 2004).

Dog fighting injuries and scar charts

Fighting dogs have characteristic scars and injuries related to their fighting behavior, as discussed above, that differ from other dog fight injuries commonly seen (Figure 13.2). Most dogs other than fighting dogs have good bite inhibition, rarely producing deep puncture wounds, and only act violently aggressive in extreme circumstances. They normally stop fighting when one of the dogs shows submission

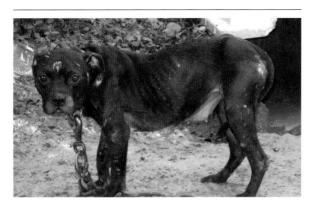

Figure 13.2 Scar pattern on fighting dog.

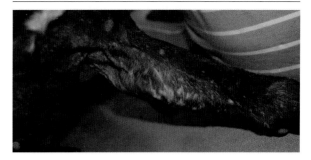

Figure 13.3 Medial leg scars and wounds.

(whining or rolling over) or withdraws. Bites injuries, which are often not present or are relatively minor, are normally found on the scruff of the neck, shoulders, or haunches. Fighting dogs have been selectively bred for decreased bite inhibition and to ignore normal displays of submission and to repeatedly attack.

Fighting dogs grab, hold, and shake their opponents, which can create deep tissue punctures, lacerations, and fractures. They repeatedly attack, causing multiple injuries. The goal is to wear out their opponent to the point that the dog will not get up or "scratch" for another round. This is accomplished through the infliction of injuries and blood loss, and outlasting the opponent to the point of physical exhaustion or death from injuries.

When examining a dog from suspected dog fighting there may be scars and wounds in various stages of healing. Bite wounds or scars on the leg may or may not have opposing teeth injuries (Figure 13.3). As with all dog bites, the teeth may or may not penetrate the skin of animals yet still cause deep tissue injury. Severe injuries to the leg may heal with severely constricting scars and present as ring injuries. Degloving of the distal extremities may be seen; this occurs when a dog bites down on the lower leg and pulls, creating a degloving injury partially or fully encircling the leg (Sinclair, Merck, and Lockwood 2006). Match dogs, or dogs ready for fighting, are usually twenty to twenty-four months old. Dogs younger than eighteen months often have not been fought and have little to no scars. Puppies may have injuries from intra-littermate or maternal aggression. Evidence of dog fighting may be found on skeletal remains (Chapter 3).

The pattern of scars and wounds related to dog fighting should be documented on a scar chart (Appendix 33). A separate diagram should be used for wounds or skin lesions that are not related to the actual fighting. The purpose of

the scar charting is not to show every injury but to show a generalized pattern of injury location and the stage of healing through the use of dots, dashes, and lines. A blue pen should be used for scars/healed wounds and a red pen for fresh/healing wounds. A black pen should not be used because it can be misinterpreted as a printing artifact. An estimate for the age of wounds can be noted on the scar chart using a number or letter that corresponds to a key that is created and recorded on the form. The analysis of the scar/wound patterns may be termed "consistent with staged dog fighting" to differentiate from other types of dog fighting. Unless the injuries resulted from a dog fight that was witnessed by someone (i.e., eyewitness statements, investigators, or veterinarians) the conclusion statement can only be "consistent with."

Several common defenses are offered to the scar and wound injury findings. Defendants may claim the injuries are a result of a yard incident, i.e., an accidental fight between two dogs. The presence of multiple injuries in different stages of healing is not supportive of this explanation, which at minimum may be explained by multiple "yard incidents" in which the owner still failed to take appropriate preventative action to protect the animals.

Another defense is that the injuries or scars are due to another type of animal such as wildlife. Raccoons and opossums have smaller canine teeth than dogs and usually only bite a few times in the muzzle or chest regions. Occasionally the owner will claim the injuries and/or scars are from using the dogs for hog or bear hunting. Hogs use their tusks for defense, moving their head side to side in slashing motions. The expected injuries are large lacerations or possibly large puncture wounds if the dog was impaled. Dogs used for hog hunting are traditionally fitted with protective vests to guard against traumatic injuries. Wounds associated with bear hunting may be due to bites or lacerations from claw swipes. The bite wounds are expected to have associated crushing injuries such as fractured bones. In bear hunting it is common for the hunted bear to "tree" to avoid the dog. When evaluating any explanation offered for scars or wounds, it is important to consider the expected defensive and aggressive behavior of the hunted animal.

Special tests

Consideration should be given for certain drug testing, especially in dogs that have obvious dog fighting injuries or physical changes consistent with drug use. Urine is the ideal source for the testing of anabolic steroids and mimetics, testosterone, other hormones, and diuretics. Hair and serum may be potentially used for testing. Part of the necropsy exam should include examination for injection sites. These can be removed *en bloc* for toxicology analysis. Any entomology evidence on the deceased animal may be analyzed for drugs (Chapter 15). A large quantity of urine may be needed to perform the test and samples should be collected as soon as possible due to the drug elimination periods. Oral forms may be found in the urine two to twenty-four days later; injectable anabolic steroids may last up to thirty days and nandrolone may last up to eight to twelve months. Studies have been conducted on the urine metabolites and time frames of excretion for testosterone, methyltestosterone, mibolerone, and boldenone in greyhound dogs. On average, the urine excretion of the metabolites were maximally excreted within two to eight hours of administration. There was a bi-modal excretion pattern at twenty-four hours post-administration, thought to be due to recirculation of the parent compound (Williams et al. 2000). The testing laboratory should be consulted regarding sample handling and submission.

Other performance-enhancing drugs may be used such as bronchodilators (e.g., albuterol) or epinephrine. The dogs may have been given or exposed to illegal drugs, such as methamphetamine or cocaine. The use of over-the-counter urine kits has been studied in dogs and found to be useful for barbiturates, opioids, benzodiazepams, and amphetamine/methamphetamine, but is not useful for testing for marijuana (tetrahydrocannabinol, also known THC). It is thought that fecal testing may provide better test results for THC (Chapter 10) (Teitler 2009). Clenbuterol is a sympathomimetic that has an anabolic steroid effect. It is a commonly abused drug by humans and may be used in horses and cattle. Irritants such as hot pepper and gunpowder have been reportedly fed to fighting dogs to increase their agitation. Gunpowder ingredients vary based on the manufacturer and type of gunpowder. The stomach contents and feces should be collected from deceased dogs for potential toxicological analysis.

COCKFIGHTING

Overview

Cockfighting is illegal in most of the United States, and is a felony in several of the states. The sport of cockfighting involves fighting that often results in death from injuries or by the owners.

The cocks are fitted with gaffs or knives on their legs to use during the fight (Figure 13.4). These come in a variety of styles and lengths. Heeling is the act of attaching the steel gaffs or knives to the roosters' legs. The stump where the natural spur has been cut off is wrapped in moleskin or tape and the gaff/knife is attached with leather straps and waxed string. Plastic spurs attached with superglue also may be used. The fighting ring or pit usually has a diameter of 15–20 feet with walls 3 feet high. The ring may be circular or rectangular and made of plywood, cement blocks, bales of hay, canvas, or Plexiglas®. There may be smaller pit arenas called drag pits.

Suspected blood stains may be tested (Chapter 2). There may be training paraphernalia used to test or enhance the bird's aggression such as moving devices with feathered targets attached. Miniature boxing gloves may be attached over the cut spur to use for training fights.

The housing of the gamecocks is not typical of a normal show breeding operation for purebred poultry. There are typically more roosters than hens, whereas breeders and exhibitors of purebred birds have more females and fewer breeding cocks, usually one male bird with one to fifteen

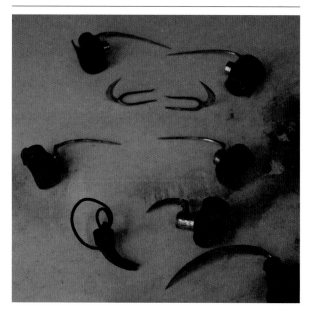

Figure 13.4 Cockfighting knives and gaffs.

females in a large coop or house. Typically purebred breeders only have a few breeder birds and show their offspring. The breeders may not be in top condition when they are in production.

In fighting operations a gamecock may be housed staked out by a tether attached to its leg with access to some type of housing, typically an A-frame type structure. This permits housing of large number of cocks in close proximity without risk of injury to each other. They also may be housed in separate cages. Legitimate breeding or exhibitor operations house breeding or show cocks in cages, i.e., not staked out, to keep the birds, especially their feathers, in the best possible condition.

It is not required to show the bird's pedigree or lineage for showing; therefore, most breeders do not keep records or they have a small amount of breeding records to reproduce show winners. In fighting operations there is a financial motivation to establish a game-winning line of gamecocks by profiting from the sale of the offspring. There are usually extensive records documenting wins and that prove pedigree and lineage.

The fighting gamecock

Gamecocks used in fighting are usually from two main varieties: Spanish gamecocks and Yankee gamecocks (Dinnage, Bollen, and Giacoppo 2004). The birds are often a hybrid of these varieties to maximize the aggressive traits. The fighting cocks have altered blood vessels with thicker tunic media and tunica adventitia of veins and much faster blood coagulation times than non-fighting cocks (McMillan and Reid 2009). The show standards for exhibition birds are distinct and they are required to be disease tested by the state and wear leg bands at all times (Dinnage, Bollen, and Giacoppo 2004). It is important to note that raising birds for exhibition vs. cockfighting is not mutually exclusive.

Often, the wattles, earlobes, and comb have been trimmed (dubbed) to prevent injury during a fight and reduce the bird's overall weight (Figure 13.5). The natural spur is removed leaving a sufficient stump to anchor the artificial spurs or gaffs (Figure 13.6). Some birds have their feathers shaved around the legs and over different body regions. Serious cockfighters put their birds through intensive training and conditioning, called a "keep," to improve the birds' strength and endurance prior to a fight and reduce their fight weight. They may use performance-enhancing drugs and sometimes illegal drugs, including drugs or supplements to increase the iron or RBCs. The labels should be examined for information pertaining to cockfighting. Some products state on the label that they are to be used before a fight.

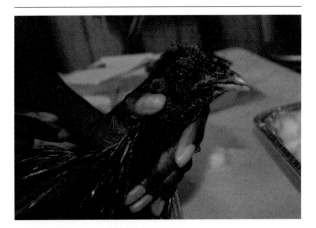

Figure 13.5 Fighting rooster with comb, wattles, and earlobes removed.

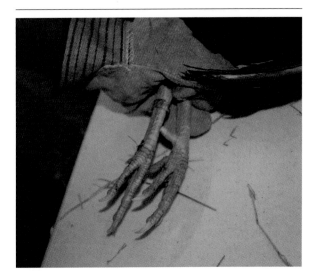

Figure 13.6 Cockfighting rooster with cut spur and leg band.

There is a Standard of Perfection for the showing of gamecocks. The physical alterations performed on fighting gamecocks are grounds for disqualification or are considered to be defects reducing the bird's chance of winning. These include the intentional removing of feathers; shortening or removal of spurs; and removal of the comb, wattles, or earlobes. There are show classes that allow dubbing but it has to be done per the standards for the class. The Old English Game types are dubbed with a hump on the back of the comb and the earlobes and wattles are removed. The Modern game class allows dubbing flat to the head but these birds do not have the right body shape and are not used in

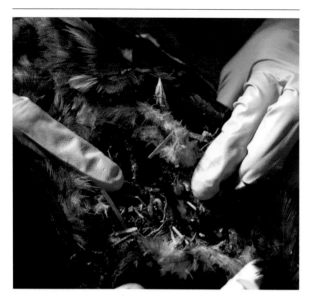

Figure 13.7 Sharp force injury caused by cockfighting knife.

fighting. Shaving of feathers is grounds for disqualification in shows because the color of the feathers cannot be viewed. Most fighting cocks do not fit the Standard of Perfection's color patterns or leg color and would be disqualified. The fighting bird's behavior is typically aggressive and in a show environment would prevent judging. Lack of bathing or grooming is also considered a defect.

As with fighting dogs, fighting gamecocks have been selected for "gameness" (see above). They do not display submission, they target their opponent's head, and are tenacious fighters that inflict maximum repeated injury. As with fighting dogs, certain fighting lines have particular fighting styles of pecking, kicking, or leaping. They are also easily and quickly aroused to fight even by a visual image of another rooster or sounds of other birds. They are rarely aggressive to their human handlers. Gamecocks are gentle with females during courtship, unlike the fighting dogs. The breeding hens are selected for non-aggression to care for their young and usually are housed together (McMillan and Reid 2009).

Examination of the animal

The birds usually have evidence of multiple injuries and defects in different stages of healing. These injuries (scars or wounds) and defects can be documented using on a chart similar to the dogfighting scar chart (Appendix 34). These birds have wounds that are primarily located on the head. The faces are usually swollen, especially around the

eyes, and the globe may be pierced which may be difficult to detect due to tissue swelling. The noses may be covered in blood, causing respiratory difficulty. There may be additional wounds to the body, punctured lungs, and fractures to the legs and wings (Figure 13.7). They may be suffering from neglect and have a poor body condition score (see Chapter 17 for poultry BCS scale). Evidence of cockfighting may be found on skeletal remains (Chapter 3).

The fighting gamecock often has been given drugs to enhance its performance, as seen with dog fighting, including hormones (testosterone), blood-clotting agents (vitamin K), and stimulants. Strychnine is a stimulant that is often used to increase the rooster's agitation and aggression (Dinnage, Bollen, and Giacoppo 2004). They may also be given digitalis as a heart stimulant. Additional drugs and supplements used in cockfighting are similar to those used in dog fighting, including antibiotics, caffeine, methamphetamines, dextrose capsules, vitamin B_{12}, and vitamin B_{15}.

Disease testing

For purebred shows, all poultry breeders must have documentation that the bird has been certified disease free by the United States Department of Agriculture (USDA). These diseases include *Salmonella pullorum* (typhoid), *Salmonella enteritidis*, Mycoplasma gallisepticum, Mycoplasma synoviae, *Mycoplasma meleagridis*, and avian influenza. Under the National Poultry Improvement Plan (NPIP) the USDA will visit the farm to test the birds and issue an NPIP number that is in effect for one year. All breeders and farms that have been issued the NPIP number are listed in the USDA NPIP book. There are federal and state regulations for international, interstate and intrastate shipping of birds. These regulations may vary regarding specific disease testing requirements. There is often illegal transportation of birds associated with cockfighting. This poses a substantial risk to the poultry industry in all regions of the world. Outbreaks of exotic Newcastle disease (END) in Mexico and the United States have been linked to the illegal smuggling of gamecocks for the purpose of cockfighting.

OTHER TYPES OF ANIMAL FIGHTING

Organized animal fighting may revolve around other species of animals including fish (beta or Chinese fighting fish), small birds, and horses.

Canary and finch fighting rings, in which male birds are paired against each other in a confined space and fought to the death, are based on territorial and mating aggression. When finches fight in the wild they are free to retreat and avoid fatal injuries. The cages have a small compartment in which to place a female bird to increase the male's arousal and a divider that is removed to allow the birds to fight. The bird's beak may be sharpened for fighting. Injuries may be seen on the body or legs including complete limb detachment. Saffron finches, native to South America, appear to be commonly used for fighting due to their extremely territorial and combative behavior. The advantages of using small birds for animal fighting include the ability to conceal and transport the birds, even in large numbers, and the small space required to fight. They are much less disruptive than dogs or roosters and are easy to breed, which allows flock growth without drawing attention.

Horse fighting has been outlawed throughout most of the world but may still be found in areas of southeast Asia. The basis for the fighting is the horse's natural battle for leadership. Dominant male horses, normally stallions, will fight until one concedes or retreats. In a confined fighting setting the horses bite, kick, and strike until one succumbs, flees, or is killed. The horses suffer a range of injuries from superficial to severe with some resulting in death.

Hog-dog fighting, also called hog-dogging or hog-dog rodeo, involves the use of a captured wild hog that is placed in an enclosed pen with one to two dogs, usually pit bulls. The dogs are released and timed for how quickly they can attack and pin the hog, whose tusks, the hog's only defense, have been cut off. The injuries to the hog can be fatal. In addition to animal cruelty, there may be additional applicable law violations concerning the illegal captivity of a wild animal. Some fighters may even have wild hog breeding operations in violation of state statues. Evidence of hog-dog fighting may be found on the skeletal remains of hogs (Chapter 3).

REFERENCES

Dinnage, J., K. Bollen, and S. Giacoppo. 2004. Animal Fighting. In: *Shelter Medicine for Veterinarians and Staff*, L. Miller and S. Zawistowski, eds. pp. 511–521. Ames, IA: Blackwell Publishing.

McMillan, F.D. and P.J. Reid. 2009. *Selective Breeding in Fighting Dogs: What Have We Created?* Presented at the UFAW International Symposium: Darwinian Selection, Selective Breeding and the Welfare of Animals, 22–23 June, University of Bristol, Bristol, UK.

Sinclair, L., M. Merck, and R. Lockwood. 2006. *Forensic Investigation of Animal Cruelty: A Guide for Veterinary and Law Enforcement Professionals*. Washington, DC: Humane Society Press.

Teitler, J.B. 2009. Evaluation of a Human On-site Urine Multidrug Test for Emergency Use With Dogs. *Journal of the American Animal Hospital Association.* 45(2):59–66.

Williams, T.M., A.J. Kind, W.G. Hyde, and D.W. Hill. 2000. Characterization of Urinary Metabolites of Testosterone, Methyltestosterone, Mibolerone and Boldenone in Greyhound Dogs. *Journal of Veterinary Pharmacology Therapy.* 23:121–29.

Yeagley, T.J., M.V. Reichard, J.E. Hempstead, K.E. Allen, L.M. Parsons, M.A. White, S.E. Little, and J.H. Meinkoth. 2009. Detection of *Babesia gibsoni* and the Canine Small Babesia "Spanish isolate" in Blood Samples Obtained from Dogs Confiscated from Dogfighting Operations. *Journal of the American Veterinary Medical Association.* 235(5):535–539.

14
Postmortem Changes and the Postmortem Interval

Melinda D. Merck and Doris M. Miller

Taceant colloquia. Effugiat risus. Hic locus est ubi mors gaudet succurrere vitae.
(Let conversation cease. Let laughter flee. This is the place where death delights to help the living.)
                                          Latin Proverb

OVERVIEW

Determining the postmortem interval (PMI) can be used to establish the time of death. The PMI may be used to support or refute investigation information such as suspect or witness statements. Another consideration is the possible time lapse from the fatal injury to the time of death, called the survival period, such that the time of death does not equal the time of the fatal injury.

The time of death and survival period may be used to determine criminal charges in animal cruelty cases. Several postmortem changes can provide valuable information in death investigations. Most of these changes are affected by environmental conditions. These conditions should be recorded to assist with the estimation of the postmortem interval as discussed in detail in Chapter 2.

The postmortem interval determination is usually an estimate unless the death was witnessed. As a general rule, the longer the PMI, the broader the time of death estimate. Forensic entomology has the greatest ability to provide an accurate time of death based on the arrival and succession of insects postmortem (Chapter 15). New methods are constantly being explored and researched in forensic science to determine the postmortem interval and the postmortem submersion interval in aquatic deaths. The window of time

for the PMI may be narrowed by using a variety of methods in conjunction with examination findings.

There are three sources to determine the time of death: anamnestic evidence (based on the deceased's habits, movements, and activities), environmental and associated evidence (present in the vicinity of the body), and corporal evidence (present in the body). All of these sources plus any witness or investigative findings, including when the animal was last seen alive, should be assessed prior to forming an opinion on time of death or injury.

EXAMINATION OF THE BODY

After an animal dies, the body undergoes a variety of changes. These postmortem changes include livor mortis, rigor mortis, algor mortis, and decomposition. The changes that are most consistent are more helpful with time of death determination. There are two methods for estimating time of death: rate and concurrence. The rate method refers to measuring change that occurs at a known rate and is either initiated or stopped by death. These changes include rigor mortis, algor mortis, and putrefaction. The concurrence method compares the occurrence of events that took place at known times around the time of death such as eating just prior to death.

Livor Mortis

Livor mortis, also referred to as hypostasis or lividity, is the pooling of blood due to gravitational forces in dependent body sites after the heart stops beating. Lividity is most useful in determining the body position at time of death and whether the body was moved. Lividity is not typically pronounced in companion animals and is primarily evident externally in light-colored skin, mucous membranes, and the sclera (Figure 14.1). It also may be found on the internal body surfaces and internal organs, where it is most noticeable on the surface of the lungs. Lividity on internal organs can be mistaken for congestion or injury. It does not affect scarred areas due to the lack of blood vessels (Perper 2006).

The color of lividity is usually reddish purple to violet due to continued oxygen dissociation after death (Pounder 2011), but it may vary due to blood oxygen content, environmental conditions, or certain poisonings (Table 14.1). A pink to cherry-red discoloration is associated with any condition causing increased oxygenated hemoglobin: carbon

monoxide (due to formation of carboxyhemoglobin), cyanide, and fluoroacetate poisoning; bodies recovered from water, covered with wet wrappings, or prolonged contact with wet surfaces where moisture prevents the escape of oxygen resulting in excess bright red oxyhemoglobin in the skin; and cold environmental temperatures at time of death (Perper 2006, Di Maio and Di Maio 2001). Postmortem refrigeration may cause purple lividity to turn pink due to the oxidation by air of reduced hemoglobin to oxyhemoglobin (Perper 2006; Pounder, 2011). In humans, brown-red lividity may be seen in deaths associated with methemoglobin formation such as potassium chlorate or nitrobenzene poisoning (Dix and Graham 2000). Green discoloration is seen with hydrogen sulfide poisoning (Perper 2006).

Pink teeth may be seen due to postmortem lividity. This is caused by the diffusion of hemoglobin from hemolyzed pulp blood, after autolysis or osmosis, into the dentinal tubules creating red discoloration of the teeth. It is more prominent on teeth with single roots than multiple roots (Figure 14.2). It is more common in victims in which sudden death occurred where the blood can remain liquid due to increased fibrinolytic activity. One of the most important requirements for this postmortem phenomenon is the existence of water or high concentrations of aqueous solution intimately surrounding the teeth (Campobasso et al. 2006). This includes burials where there is high moisture or water in the soil.

In humans, the blood becomes permanently incoagulable within thirty to sixty minutes after death regardless of cause of death. This blood change is due to the release of fibrinolysins, especially from small blood vessels and serous surfaces. Clots may persist if they are too large to be

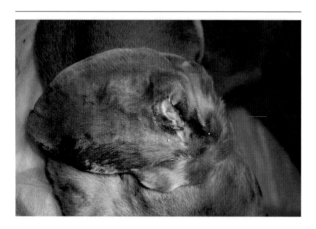

Figure 14.1 Lividity visible on light colored skin surface.

Table 14.1 Postmortem lividity discoloration.

Etiology	Livor color	Mechanism
Normal	Blue-purplish	Venous blood
Carbon monoxide	Pink, cherry-red	Carboxyhemoglobin
Cyanide	Pink, cherry-red	Excess oxygenated blood due to inhibition of cytochrome oxidase
Fluoroacetate (insecticide/rodenticide)	Pink, cherry-red	Inhibition of oxidative cellular metabolism
Refrigeration, hypothermia, immersion in water, contact with wet surfaces	Pink, cherry-red	Oxygen retention in cutaneous blood by cold air/water
Acetaminophen, sodium chlorate, nitrite, naphthalene, phenols, phenazopyridine, and skunk spray	Brown	Methemoglobin
Hydrogen sulfide	Green	Sulfhemoglobin

Source: Perper, J.A. 2006. Time of Death and Changes After Death, Part 1: Anatomical Considerations. In: *Medicolegal Investigation of Death*, Fourth edition, W.U. Spitz and D.J. Spitz, eds. pp. 87-127. Springfield: Charles C. Thomas Publisher.

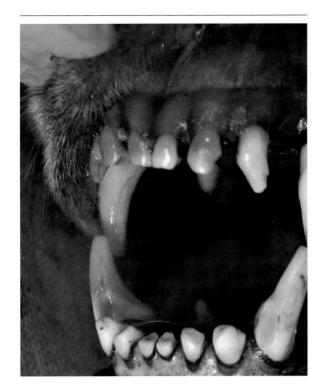

Figure 14.2 Pink teeth discoloration.

liquefied by the fibrinolysin. This may not occur in deaths associated with cachexia or septicemia. It is reported in asphyxia deaths, in which the blood remains liquid longer than normal (Pounder 2011).

In humans, lividity may be evident as early as twenty minutes to several hours after death, beginning as patches or blotches which deepen in intensity and coalesce over time, reaching maximum intensity at around twelve hours. Lividity may become fixed in eight to twelve hours. If the body is moved prior to the fixation, livor will shift, responding to gravity (Di Maio and Di Maio 2001), with slight discoloration from lividity in the new dependent areas. The pattern of primary lividity may fade if the body is moved within the first six hours after death. Lividity may be delayed or difficult to identify in cases associated with chronic anemia or massive hemorrhage (Pounder 2011). Livor mortis can speed up with accelerated decomposition or slow down with cool ambient temperatures, becoming fixed in twenty-four to thirty-six hours in humans (Di Maio and Di Maio 2001).

Lividity is considered fixed when blood shifting and drainage no longer occur as a result of blood leakage from the blood vessels due to hemolysis and breakdown of the blood vessel walls caused by decomposition. Fixation of lividity is determined by the lack of blanching when pressure is applied to the area. The presence of fixed lividity in non-dependent areas indicates the body was moved after death. Areas that were pressed against a firm surface do not have lividity, known as "contact pallor" or "pressure pallor," due to the compression of blood vessels preventing blood pooling. This allows determination of whether the body was moved and reconstruction of the body's position after death. This same pallor is seen with any constricting material or device on the body which may contain patterns related to the object used.

Lividity may be mistaken for bruising, which does not blanch with applied pressure. The area should be incised to differentiate between bruising and lividity. A bruised area has diffuse hemorrhage into the soft tissues, whereas lividity is characterized by blood confined within the blood vessels and may wiped or washed away (Di Maio and Di Maio 2001). Microscopic exam differentiates between the two. The presence and interpretation of lividity may be obscured by the color changes caused by decomposition. As decomposition progresses, the blood vessels break down and the blood hemolyzes, diffusing into the surrounding tissues (imbibition). It can also become difficult to distinguish between lividity and a putrefying area of bruising. The hemoglobin may undergo secondary changes such as sulphemoglobin formation (Pounder 2011).

Intense areas of lividity may have petechiae and be mistaken for antemortem hemorrhage. Gravity may cause pooling of the blood to rupture small vessels causing postmortem petechiae, called Tardieu spots, or larger purpura. This is most commonly seen in the subcutaneous tissue in animals associated with hanging or suspension of the body at the time of death. This false hemorrhage may be differentiated from antemortem petechiae based on location. Antemortem petechiae may extend beyond the areas of lividity or may be located in non-dependent areas on the body. In humans, this pseudo-hemorrhage can take eighteen to twenty-four hours and indicates rapidly approaching decomposition. It may occur in as little as two to four hours in cases in which the limbs are hanging over something or the body is suspended (Di Maio and Di Maio 2001).

Lividity in the region of the head can make evaluation of injuries difficult. As decomposition progresses, hemolyzed blood can leak from the blood vessels into the soft tissues of the scalp, which may be confused with the bruising from head trauma which can occur without abrasions or lacerations. This leakage of blood below the scalp can be difficult to distinguish from antemortem bruising (Di Maio and Di Maio 2001).

Leakage also can occur inside the brain into subarachnoid or subdural spaces, creating a very thin, localized blood film coating the surface. The brain should be examined closely for other signs of hemorrhage to eliminate postmortem changes.

Human drowning victims may show confusing postmortem "hemorrhage" on the scalp where the head was floating down. In addition, a small amount of blood seepage may be seen in the anterior soft tissues and muscles of the neck (Di Maio and Di Maio 2001). This pseudohemorrhage in the neck area may be microscopically indistinguishable from acute hemorrhages associated with contusions. Immunohistochemical analysis of platelet and endothelial cell activation may be useful to differentiate antemortem bleeding (see below and Chapter 3). In large areas of extravasated blood there may be sedimentation separation of neutrophils mimicking acute inflammation (Pollanen, Perera, and Clutterbuck 2009). It is important to evaluate the neck findings carefully and in the context of the body position after death.

Rigor Mortis

Rigor mortis is postmortem muscle contraction that immobilizes the joints of the body. Rigor mortis occurs because of the depletion of adenosine triphosphate (ATP), which causes the muscle proteins actin and myosin to stay locked together until decomposition breaks them down. ATP is a source of energy for muscle contractions that needs to be replenished. ATP is used faster with exercise or exertion, with the consumption of ATP continuing after death. Three metabolic systems supply ATP: the phosphagen system, glycogen–lactic acid system, and aerobic system (Di Maio and Di Maio 2001). Animal experiments have shown that a certain level of free calcium ions is required for rigor development and that calcium binding agents inhibit its formation (Perper 2006).

Two primary factors influence the onset and duration of rigor: environmental temperature and the degree of muscular activity prior to death. Rigor sets in faster, sometimes in minutes, if prior to death there was exercise (such as with chasing), violent struggle, convulsions, or high body temperature (as seen with sepsis). Rigor usually occurs in all muscles at the same time, but is noticeable in the smaller muscle groups first, primarily the jaw. It may first occur in muscles where there was higher exertion prior to death. It occurs in the involuntary muscles, such as the heart and eye, which can produce changes that are mistaken for antemortem conditions such as unequal pupil diameters or apparent cardiac hypertrophy (Perper 2006).

It is important to know how the body was handled and transported prior to examination. Rigor may be forcibly broken by stretching the limbs and will not reform if it was fully developed at the time. When rigor recurs it is with reduced stiffness. Once rigor has occurred, it then dissipates in the same apparent order of formation. In some cases rigor is almost instantaneous at the time of death; this is called cadaveric spasm. It is due to the depletion of ATP after rigorous exertion such as struggling or running just prior to death. In humans this is linked to violent deaths and cases of electrocution (Dix and Graham 2000). The body's position is frozen in rigidity which can help determine if the body was moved postmortem.

Many factors affect rigor. Rigor mortis disappears with decomposition, although it is possible for both decomposition and rigor to still be present in cold drowning cases (Di Maio and Di Maio 2001). In warmer climates the development of putrefaction may displace rigor within nine to twelve hours postmortem (Pounder 2011). Cold body or ambient temperatures reduce the rate and may stop the formation or dissipation of rigor. Rigor may be difficult to evaluate in cases in which the body was frozen in cold weather. Freezing arrests the process, but it resumes upon thawing. High temperatures speed up the formation of rigor.

Rigor may be delayed or be very mild in emaciated bodies (Di Maio and Di Maio 2001). In humans, the onset is more rapid in children and the elderly, or it may be poorly developed, especially if the person was debilitated (Perper 2006). In deaths from septicemia or cachexic diseases the onset is rapid and passes quickly. It is delayed in asphyxia deaths, especially carbon monoxide poisoning, and death associated with shock or severe hemorrhage (Pounder 2011). Exposure to intense heat results in heat stiffening due to coagulation of the muscle proteins (Chapter 11). This is associated with muscle shortening and can obscure rigor mortis.

There is great variability in the onset and duration of rigor mortis. In general if there is rapid onset the duration will be relatively short. Rigor should be assessed as complete, partial, or absent, noting the distribution by attempted flexion of the different joints. It should be established that there was no previous manipulation of the body by others. All factors that can affect the formation, duration, and dissipation of rigor should be considered.

In humans, rigor may appear two to four hours after death and reach full formation in six to twelve hours, depending on perimortem factors, cause of death, and temperature conditions. In general for humans, rigor starts to disappear approximately thirty-six to forty-eight hours after death in temperate climates (Pounder 2011) but may last up to six days. In hotter conditions, rigor may come and go in twenty-four hours or less (Di Maio and Di Maio 2001).

Algor Mortis

Algor mortis refers to the cooling of the body after death to reach the ambient temperature. The body temperature may increase if the ambient temperature is higher than the internal temperature at death or if the body is exposed to direct sunlight. Algor mortis is much more accurate in the first twenty-four hours after death but is affected by numerous variables, which can limit its usefulness in narrow, accurate time of death determination based on a single body temperature reading. These variables include external wrappings; nutritional state; contact with hot or cold objects; body temperature at death; and environmental temperature, wind, and relative humidity. To approximate time of death, the temperature at the time of death and rate of cooling must be estimated. It is important to keep in mind that "normal" body temperature is an average of that species. One must also consider that death does not always occur immediately following the precipitating injury or event along with the effects on body temperature at the time death. It is important to consider factors that would increase or reduce the body temperature at time of death including sepsis, physical exercise/exertion, brain trauma or disease, seizures, drugs, environmental exposure, shock, and diseases such as hyperthyroidism.

The process of heat loss is affected by conduction, which is the loss of heat through transfer to objects in contact with the body, convection, which is the movement of air over the body causing cooling, and radiation, which is the loss of heat from the body through infrared heat rays. In addition to ambient temperature, the rate of cooling is affected by the body condition score due to fat acting as an insulator and reducing heat loss. The position of the body can affect the rate of heat loss (e.g., a curled body position slows down heat loss). It is also affected by the type and temperature of the surface on which the body is laying, the presence of any covering, whether the body becomes wet, and the weather conditions (e.g., dry, humid, and windy). Smaller animals cool faster because they have a larger surface area compared with mass. The density of the haircoat as an insulator must be considered as well. To complicate matters further, the conditions found at the scene are most likely variable since the time of death, including fluctuating ambient temperatures, changing weather conditions, and the cover over the animal changing with sun movement.

The animal's temperature may be taken rectally, as deep as possible, provided that it is not a sexual assault investigation. A special thermometer that will register extremely high and low temperatures, found at evidence collection supply companies, is needed (Appendix 37). It is not recommended to take liver temperature due to the risk of iat-rogenic damage to the organ. One study of dogs showed close correlation of rectal and liver temperature postmortem (Proctor et al. 2009). Whenever possible, the animal's temperature should be taken at the scene. If sexual assault is suspected, rectal swabs should be taken prior to taking the temperature. Rectal temperatures may be taken hourly over a three- to six-hour period to establish the rate of cooling for the environmental conditions. Refrigeration of the body further alters the cooling, rendering algor mortis assessment irrelevant. The body temperature will keep cooling until it reaches ambient temperature or, if on a cooler surface, until it reaches the temperature of the surface on which it is laying.

Human studies show that the temperature cooling follows a sigmoid shape with a plateau at the beginning and end of the process. Under average environmental conditions, human bodies cool at a rate of 2°F–2.5°F/hour (1.1°C–1.3°C) for the first hours and then slow to an average of 1.5°F–2°F (0.8°C–1.1°C) during the first twelve hours and 1°F (0.6°C) for the next twelve to eighteen hours. The initial plateau is attributed to the heat generated by the residual metabolic process of the tissues and metabolic activity of intestinal bacteria; it rarely lasts longer than three to four hours (Perper 2006). It may also be due to the time required to establish a temperature gradient. Therefore, a plateau is more likely to occur if the environmental temperature is relatively high, there is body and/or surface insulation (which slows down conduction and convection heat loss), and/or the body is large with a greater amount of external body fat (Henssge et al. 1995).

One study in humans found that rectal temperature actually can elevate in the early postmortem period and return to normal in four hours, possibly a result of continued metabolic activity of bowel bacteria and the body (Di Maio and Di Maio 2001). The slowing of the cooling rate toward the end is due to the gradient reduction between the body and the ambient temperature (Perper 2006). In humans, the average rate of heat loss is 1.5°F (0.8°C) loss per hour under 70°F–75°F (21°C–24°C environmental temperatures:

$$\text{Time since death (hours)} = [\text{Normal body temp (°F)} - \text{rectal temp (°F)}] \div 1.5$$

A study was conducted on dogs indoors with still room air and an average ambient temperature of 70.7°F (21.5°C). The postmortem rate of cooling was 0.9°F (0.5°C), which is similar to what is reported in humans: 1°F–1.5°F (0.6°C–0.8°C). The study found the sex, body mass, and haircoat density had no effect on the rate of body temperature reduction. However, increased body weight and body volume decreased the rate of body temperature reduction (Proctor et al. 2009).

Another study of draft effect on body cooling found that moderate airflow did not significantly affect the rate; it also found that the air movement closest to the bodies was actually minimal (Kaliszan 2011).

A study of algor mortis was conducted on beagles. The dogs were all approximately the same size (median 12.1 kg) and in good (not overweight) body condition. They were placed uncovered in lateral recumbency on plastic trays. They were kept in an enclosed, well-ventilated room with still air at 34%–63% humidity and ambient temperatures from 10.9°C–16.8°C (52°F–62°F). The study found that during the first ten hours postmortem the rectal temperatures dropped steadily, without a plateau, and were easily distinguishable within two-hour intervals. After ten hours, the temperatures tended to overlap with less clear separation. At seventeen hours postmortem all rectal temperatures were below 19°C (66°F). All dogs had reached ambient temperature twenty-four to forty-eight hours after death (Erlandsson and Munro 2007).

Decomposition

Overview

Decomposition involves the two processes of putrefaction and autolysis. Autolysis is a chemical process by the intracellular enzymes that causes the breakdown of tissue and organs. Heat accelerates autolysis, whereas cold slows it down. Freezing can stop the process and in some cases significant heat can inactivate the intracellular enzymes. Organs that have higher enzymes, such as the liver and pancreas, undergo autolysis faster. Microscopic exam may reveal autolysis of the tissues with no immune or inflammatory reaction. However, the presence or absence of an inflammatory reaction to an area of injury can help determine a time interval between injury and death (Chapter 3).

Putrefaction involves bacteria and fermentation and is often used interchangeably with the term decomposition. After death, bacteria from the gastrointestinal (GI) tract spread throughout the body. The rate of decomposition of internal organs differs with the abdominal organs, especially the GI tract, decomposing at an accelerated rate due to their high bacterial content (Perper 2006). Putrefaction is accelerated in animals that are septic prior to death and may continue even with refrigeration of the body.

In addition to the body, the development of putrefaction depends on the environment. The optimal temperatures for putrefaction are between 70°F and 100°F (21° and 38°C) (Pounder 2011). In high temperatures the rate of decomposition is accelerated and the body can reach an advanced state of putrefaction within twenty-four hours (Di Maio and Di Maio 2001). High environmental humidity enhances putrefaction and extremely high temperatures (above 100°F or 38°C) slow it down. This is because intense heat produces heat fixation of tissues and inactivates autolytic enzymes, causing delay of onset and progression (Pounder 2011). The rate slows down in cold temperatures (below 50°F or 14°C), and may even stop in extreme cold. Even under refrigeration, a non-septic body may still continue to decompose.

If the body is constricted in any way decomposition may be delayed. If the animal is overweight, has a heavy fur coat, or is wrapped creating heat retention, putrefaction may be accelerated. It may be delayed with exsanguination deaths because blood provides the path for spread of the putrefying organisms. It may be delayed with dehydration and accelerated with tissue edema such as congestive heart failure. It is more rapid in children but slow in unfed newborn infants due to the lack of intestinal bacteria (Pounder 2011). With burned remains, decomposition in charred areas progresses at a faster rate than areas with very light levels of charring (Gruenthal, Moffatt, and Simmons 2012).

Decomposition may be asymmetrical, occurring more rapidly in areas of injury. Decomposition may progress to skeletonization in only one part of the body because of insect feeding in areas of injury (Dix and Calaluce 1999). The general rate of decomposition on non-buried remains may not be affected by trauma. Studies of knife and gunshot wounds on pig cadavers found that the rate was unaffected. The rate was found to be most affected by the presence or absence of insects. Furthermore, it was found that the Diptera did not show preferential oviposition to the trauma sites. The volatile gases released from the natural orifices of the head are the primary attractant (Chapter 15) (Cross and Simmons 2010).

Decomposition usually occurs in six to thirty-six hours, though the onset and rate of putrefaction is variable depending on the environmental conditions and body condition prior to death. The duration is usually shorter if there is rapid onset. In humans, under temperate climate conditions, the early putrefaction changes in the anterior abdominal wall occur between thirty-six and seventy-two hours after death, progressing to gas formation in approximately one week. If the body is maintained above 80°F (27°C) after death then the changes are seen within twenty-four hours with gas formation appearing in two to three days (Pounder 2011).

In buried and surface remains, it is the presence or absence of insects that affects the rate of decomposition;

their presence increases the rate and their absence decreases it. The body size is an influential factor when insects are present, with smaller bodies decomposing faster than larger bodies (Simmons, Adlam, and Moffatt 2010).

One study in rabbits found that the presence of feeding larvae increase the intra-abdominal temperatures to 5°C (9°F) above ambient. The increased rate of decomposition in smaller bodies is due to the increased heat distributed throughout a smaller body mass and because of the proportionally greater volume of dipteran larval mass relative to the smaller body size resulting in faster consumption (Simmons et al. 2010). Another study on buried rabbit remains with insect access prior to burial found an approximately 30% enhanced decomposition rate when compared to the remains without insect access. It also reported that the total body decomposition score was the most valid tool to use for the PMI estimation (Bachmann and Simmons 2010).

Because burials are often shallow, there is the potential for insect colonization of the remains. A study found that larvae from the families Sarcophagidae and Muscidae were the first to colonize buried remains, arriving at five days for one-foot burials and at seven days for two-feet burials (Pastula 2012).

The rate of decomposition in buried remains depends on the depth of the grave, the temperature of the soil, the water drainage, and the permeability of any wrapping or enclosure in which the body was placed. In deep burials, especially in clay soil, the decomposition is slowed due to the restriction of air. In humans buried in well-drained soil, the body will become skeletonized in about ten years; a child's body becomes skeletonized in about five years (Pounder 2011).

A general rule, assuming the same environmental temperature, is that one week of putrefaction in air is equivalent to two weeks in water which is equivalent to eight weeks buried in soil. Soil pH can affect rate of decomposition. In acidic soil the rate may increase up to three times greater than alkaline soil. Decomposition by-products affect the immediate soil environment, initially becoming more alkaline and then acidifying (Haslam and Tibbett 2009).

Immersion in sewage or similar contaminated water enhances putrefaction. Trauma appears to affect decomposition rates in buried remains. A study of pig carcasses with simulated blunt and sharp force trauma showed a faster rate of decomposition than the non-trauma control with sharp force trauma having the faster rate of all categories (Boyd, Sliwa, and Boyd 2010). In water environments, disposal of remains in plastic bags tends to result in more preservation due to bacterial inhibition and reduced oxygen levels (Pakosh and Rogers 2009).

A study of decomposition of small pigs was conducted in Virginia by the FBI's National Center for the Analysis of Violent Crime in 1998. Five small pigs, less than 30 pounds, were placed in different environments: surface deposit, no covering; surface deposit covered with tree branches and deadfall; enclosed in a roll of carpet; shallow grave of less than 1 foot; and suspended by a rope from a tree approximately 2.5 feet above the ground. The pigs were deposited in late May and monitored for seventy-five days with average temperatures from 60°F–90°F (16°C–32°C). Their observations found that pigs rapidly decompose. In all the pigs except the hanging pig, the soft tissue was almost completely consumed, leaving the skeletal components by day twelve. The hanging pig was more protected from scavenging and insect activity. It was most exposed to the sun and wind, causing rapid desiccation and mummification and preserving the skeletal elements. The majority of scavenged skeletal elements were recovered within fifteen feet of the original body location (Morton and Lord 2002).

Sequence of Decomposition Changes

The sequence of decomposition in humans begins with a greenish discoloration of the abdomen, usually in the first twenty-four to thirty-six hours. This discoloration then develops on the head, neck, and shoulders along with bacterial gas formation, causing bloating of the face. Marbling occurs in these areas because of hemolysis of the blood within the vessels and the hemoglobin reacting to hydrogen sulfide, developing a greenish-black discoloration along the blood vessels at the surface of the skin. In sixty- to seventy-two hours, the body develops generalized bloating in which the eyes may bulge and the tongue may protrude from the mouth. Bloating may cause healing surgical incisions or scars to dehisce, mimicking incised, stab, or gunshot wounds (Lew and Matshes 2005). This is followed by development of vesicles on the skin, skin and hair slippage, and the color of the body becoming pale green to green-black. The internal organs shrink and the weight decreases. A red-colored decomposition fluid, known as purge fluid, can drain from the mouth and nose and may be found in the body cavities. This may be mistaken as being secondary to an injury, but the amount of fluid is usually small inside the body cavities (Figure 14.3). There may be diffusion of bile pigments from the gall bladder to the adjacent tissues. In humans, the perforation of the stomach fundus or lower esophagus may occur within a few hours of death in cases of cerebral injuries or terminal pyrexias. This is known as neurogenic perforation of the esophagus or stomach and is a result of autolysis rather than putrefaction

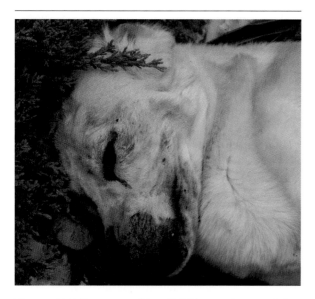

Figure 14.3 Decomposition fluid (purge) around the mouth and face which can be mistaken for hemorrhage.

(Pounder 2011). The postmortem leakage of duodenal contents into the stomach contributes to autodigestion and perforation of the gastric wall, i.e., gastromalacia. Both esophagomalacia and gastromalacia are devoid of vital reaction (Perper 2006).

The general indicators of antemortem hemorrhage vs. postmortem changes may be the size (focal or patterned vs. irregular, blotchy, or diffuse as with lividity), location of the discoloration (e.g., nondependent areas), and/or any associated injuries. Decomposition also causes hemolyzed blood to leak out of the broken down blood vessels into the surrounding tissue (imbibition), usually within twelve to twenty-four hours after death, which can be mistaken for antemortem bruising (see Lividity). Wound vitality may be evaluated even after there is hemolysis of the red blood cells in the associated hemorrhage through the detection of their components post-lysing. The hemoglobin chain is the most resistant to putrescence. One immune-histochemical method that has been used is the application of monoclonal antibody directed against hemoglobin alpha chain. This can also be used to determine postmortem wounds (Andrello and Basso 2012).

Changes in the eyes are difficult to interpret and depend on whether the eyes are open or closed. In humans with closed eyes, a white scummy deposit develops on the cornea, making it cloudy by twenty-four hours postmortem. The absence of intraocular fluid is consistent with a minimum

time of death of four days. If the eye is partially open and exposed to a dry environment a brown to black band may develop on the sclera, called *tache noire* (black spot), which is a result of drying and not an area of bruising (Perper 2006).

Following the wet decomposition the surface tissues begin to dry, collapse, and darken, developing a leathery texture. The organs and tissues become desiccated and shrink. Depending on the species and breed, an extremely thick hair mat could indicate a fall or winter coat vs. a thin hair mat which may indicate a summer coat, providing information regarding the season of death (Gonder 2009). Next, the body may become mummified or skeletonized. The time frame for skeletonization of the body depends on environmental conditions, insect activity, and scavengers (see Animal Forensic Osteology in Chapter 3). In humans, if the body is exposed to the elements and available to insects and scavengers, skeletonization can occur within nine to ten days. The last two organs to decompose are the uterus and prostate in humans (Di Maio and Di Maio 2001).

Mummification can occur in hot, dry conditions when the body rapidly dehydrates. The skin appears brown or black and leathery, and shrinkage may cause it to split, especially around the neck, axillae, and groin, mimicking injuries. Newborns, due to their size and lack of intestinal bacteria, often mummify (Pounder 2011). Decomposition continues with the internal organs turning blackish brown with a putty-like consistency (Di Maio and Di Maio 2001); the organs may dry and be preserved. Mummification can preserve tissues which assists with recognition of injuries and identification. The time for mummification varies but under ideal conditions it may be well advanced in a few weeks (Pounder 2011).

Adipocere is a grayish-white to brown, firm, wax-like material made up of the fatty acids oleic, palmitic, and stearic acids which inhibit putrefactive bacteria. Adipocere acts to preserve the body which can assist in the recognition of injuries and identification. It is found primarily in the subcutaneous tissue and other fatty deposit areas and gives off a sweetish rancid odor. It also may be seen in the viscera, though that is not a common finding.

Adipocere formation may occur when a body is found immersed in water or in a damp, warm, anaerobic environment. It may be seen also in bodies that have been placed in bags or other types of confinement in which the water content of the body is sufficient (Figure 14.4). In these warm, moist environments, fat undergoes hydrolysis by endogenous lipases and bacterial enzymes to free fatty acids. These are then converted to hydroxyl fatty acids by bacterial enzymes, primarily *Clostridium perfringens*. A study of

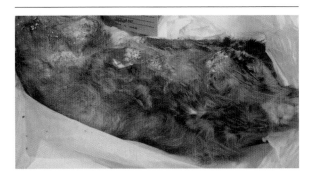

Figure 14.4 Hoarding case: presence of adipocere on a deceased cat found inside a plastic bag in the residence.

adipocere formation in animals found that it did not form in chicken or kangaroo, presumably due to the lack of sufficient fatty tissue, while it did form in the other species tested: pig, cattle, sheep, and rabbit (Forbes et al. 2005).

Adipocere formation can take weeks to several months to develop and is resistant to chemical bacterial destruction. In warm, damp conditions it may appear after three to four weeks. Normally it requires months with extensive adipocere seen after five to six months. In submersion cases it may be seen after a year, and with burials after three years (Pounder 2011). In general, adipocere indicates the postmortem interval is at minimum weeks to several months.

Using Decomposition Changes to Determine the Postmortem Interval

The estimation of the postmortem interval may be possible using gross, histologic, and immunohistochemistry findings. An indoor study was conducted on beagle dogs, all the same size and body condition, with necropsies performed at twenty-four hours, seventy-two hours, seven days, and twenty-three days (see Algor Mortis for the study conditions). Distinct gross changes were noted at different postmortem intervals. The study found the heart, liver, lungs, pancreas, tonsils, thyroid, and urinary bladder were the most useful organs for differential histologic findings. Differential staining of the B and T lymphocytes in the superficial cervical lymph nodes and tracheal bronchial nodes was reported. The combination of these gross, histologic, and immunohistochemistry findings provided a set of markers that are summarized in Table 14.2 (Erlandsson and Munro 2007).

An outdoor study of wolf carcass decomposition was conducted in Montana. The yearlong study documented decompositional changes associated with the postmortem

interval. The stages of decomposition were correlated with the seasons in that region, see Table 14.3 for a summary (Gonder 2009).

Decomposition scoring has been used to help estimate the postmortem interval with the combined use of accumulated degree days (ADDs). ADDs are an accumulated average of daily temperatures in degrees Celsius over the course of the decomposition cycle. The daily average is calculated as the average of the daily maximum and minimum air temperatures from the nearest weather station. There are usually some discrepancies between the weather station and the actual site temperatures which can affect calculation results either by under- or overestimation (Dabbs 2012). Multiple temperature readings may be collected directly from the site and compared to the weather station to estimate the discrepancies. For greater accuracy, a temperature data logger may be placed at the site to collect true high and low temperatures for comparison. Low cost data logger models are available such as the iButton Thermachron®. Because freezing temperatures severely inhibit biological processes associated with decomposition, temperatures below 0°C (32°F) are recorded as zero. This decomposition scoring system is based on visual classifications that ranked observations and allocated a score allowing decomposition to be quantified (Table 14.4). The body areas are scored separately because they do not necessarily display the same aspects of decomposition (Adlam and Simmons 2007).

Studies have shown the time to different states of decomposition can be correlated to ADDs. Using the decomposition scoring system as a total body score (TBS), the ADDs can be determined by plugging the TBS into the following formula (Megyesi, Nawrocki, and Haskell 2005):

$$ADD = 10^{(0.002*TBS*TBS+1.81)} \pm 776.32$$

The y^x key on a scientific calculator can be used for the final step: enter 10, press the (y^x) key, then enter the total for the (0.002*TBS*TBS + 1.81) to calculate the ADD. In this formula the error rate is doubled from 388.16 to 776.32 to achieve a 95% prediction interval for a given TBS (Megyesi, Nawrocki, and Haskell 2005).

Determining the Postmortem Submersion Interval (PMSI)

A human aquatic decomposition scoring system has been developed to determine the ADD (Table 14.5). By summing the score as the total aquatic decomposition score (TADS), it can be plugged into the following equation to determine ADD (Heaton et al. 2010):

Table 14.2 Differential gross, histologic, and immunohistochemistry findings associated with PMI in ten beagle dogs.

PMI	Findings
Less than 24 hours	Rigor mortis developing or present in most muscle groups
24 hours	Blue-green skin discoloration of caudal abdomen and flanks, variable degree
	Froth in trachea and main-stem bronchi
	Bile green/brown/yellow
	Urinary bladder: signs of fragility in transitional epithelium
	Thyroid: variable autolysis
48 hours	Lungs: limited loss of epithelium from terminal bronchioles
48–72 hours	Bile turning yellow/red
	Thyroid: variable autolysis
3 days	Rigor mortis present in jaw, elbow, and hindlimbs, variable elsewhere
	Drying of tip of tongue and lip
	Exposed eyes shrunken
	Froth in trachea and main-stem bronchi
	Lung: progressive loss of epithelium, clumps of epithelium separated by denuded areas
	Bile duct epithelium detachment
	Urinary bladder: detachment of transitional epithelium, leaving single layer of triangular and spike-shaped cells
	Thyroid: variable autolysis
	Pancreas: detachment of ductal epithelium
	Tonsil: variable detachment of outer layers of epithelium
	B-cell staining reduced; T-cell staining unaffected
7 days	Rigor mortis present in jaw and hindlimbs, not in elbow
	Skin discoloration of abdomen and flanks: moderate
	Exposed eyes collapsed
	Froth in trachea and main-stem bronchi
	Thoracic cavity: hemoglobin-stained fluid, majority on lower side
	Endocardium: light bluish discoloration
	Bile turning red-brown
	Lung: Complete loss of all bronchiole epithelium; bronchi lining present; alveolar septa thickened with loss of definition
	Liver: majority of hepatic nuclei autolyzed, bile duct epithelium detached
	Urinary bladder: only small areas of epithelium attached
	Thyroid: considerable disruption of normal architecture, detachment of majority of follicular epithelium
	Pancreas: detached clumps of epithelium in duct lumina
	Tonsil: only small areas of epithelium attached
	B-cell staining weak; T-cell staining unaffected
23 days	Skin discoloration of abdomen and flanks: marked
	Hypostatic congestion of ear pinnae turning green or dark
	Hair and superficial layers of the epidermis readily detached
	Skin of scrotum and foot pads dry and hard
	Rhinarium: loss of "fingerprint" pattern
	Peeling of tongue epithelium
	Mold/fungi on eyes
	Teeth: pink discoloration

Table 14.2 (*Cont'd*)

PMI	Findings
	Heart: epicardium discolored, surface remained shiny; blood-stained pericardial fluid; myocardial nuclear difficult to recognize, cross striations clearly visible
	Bile red-brown
	Lungs: irregular patches of bronchial epithelium; further loss of alveolar septa definition
	Liver: marked autolysis of hepatocytes
	Urinary bladder: complete loss of epithelium
	Pancreas: only outline of architecture remained
	Tonsil: complete loss of epithelium, lymphoid nodules indistinct
	B-cell staining very weak; T-cell staining remained strong

Source: Elandsson, M. and R. Munro. 2007. Estimation of the Post-Mortem Interval in Beagle Dogs. *Science and Justice*. 47:150–154.

Table 14.3 Decomposition stage and seasonal time of death field estimates for Lubrecht wolf carcasses in Montana.

Decomposition stage	Fall	Winter	Spring	Summer
Fresh	1–3 days (longer if late fall	1–100 days (if frozen)	1–25 days	1–3 days
Bloat	3–20 days	Unlikely active stage	20–30 days	3–10 days
Active decay	15–40 days	Unlikely stage, carcass under snow may have internal maggot activity	25–35 days (winter carcass can be at active stage in spring with dried foot/nose pads, hard/stiff ears)	10–20 days
Advanced decay	40–90 days	155–205 days (possibly unfrozen under snow)	35–95 days	20–90 days
Dry	90 days to 1 year or longer	90 days to 1 year or longer	90 days to 1 year or longer	90 days to 1 year or longer

Source: Gonder, C. 2009. Wildlife Decomposition Analysis for Time of Death Estimates. Wildlife Field Forensics.

$$ADD = 10^{([TADS-3.706]\div 7.778)}$$

The PMSI can be inferred by summing the average daily temperatures retrospectively from the date the body was recovered until the estimated ADD is reached. This can be used as the estimated time frame when the body entered the water. Adipocere formation preserves body tissues, delaying decomposition. Therefore, extreme care should be taken when applying this model to cases where adipocere is present (Heaton et al. 2010).

Diatoms are the dominant form of algae in the first stage of algal succession on bodies submerged in freshwater or marine environments. The analysis of diatoms may assist in the estimate of the postmortem submersion interval in addition to providing a geographic link between the aquatic crime scene and a suspect (Chapter 9). Studies have found a significant correlation between algal diversity as a function of time which may be used to estimate the PMSI (Zimmerman and Wallace 2008).

Flow Cytometry and DNA Degradation

Flow cytometry has been investigated as a possible instrument to determine time of death in the early postmortem period in humans. The test involves looking at the degradation of nuclear DNA using flow cytometry and comparing it to the degradation in known controls. The percentage of degradation is then correlated to the postmortem interval in hours. The spleen, peripheral blood, and liver have been looked at as possible sources for testing. Research has shown that hepatocyte degradation has a linear correlation with the time elapsed since death. The presence of hepatic neoplasia does not alter the findings. In addition, hepatic tissue is ideal because of the ease of obtaining samples through a biopsy needle (Di Nunno et al. 2002).

Table 14.4 Decomposition Scoring of Body Regions

Stage	Points	Description
Head and neck		
Fresh	1	Fresh, no discoloration
Early decomposition	2	No skin discoloration, maggots visible
	3	Some flesh relatively fresh, fur loss
	4	Discoloration, brownish, drying of nose and ears, and heavy maggot activity
	5	Purging of decompositional fluids, wet flesh
	6	Skin brown to black
Advanced decomposition	7	Caving in of flesh and tissues of eyes and throat
	8	Wet decomposition, bone exposure less than 50% scored area
	9	Desiccation, bone exposure less than 50% scored area
Skeletonization	10	Bone exposure greater than 50% scored area, wet tissue
	11	Bone exposure greater than 50% scored area, desiccated tissues, incisor loss, and disarticulation
Torso-thorax and abdomen		
Fresh	1	Fresh, no discoloration
Early decomposition	2	Skin appears fresh, fly eggs, few maggots
	3	Flesh appears red-brown, small amount fur loss (less than 30%)
	4	Bloating, purging of decompositional fluids, heavy maggot activity
	5	Bloat loss, severe fur loss (greater than 70%), heavy maggot activity
Advanced decomposition	6	Wet decay, abdominal collapse where internal structure is lost, flesh gray green
	7	Wet decay, bone exposure less than 50% scored area
	8	Surface mummification, bone exposure less than 50% scored area
Skeletonization	9	Black skin, bones greasy, body fluids occasionally present
	10	Bones with desiccated black skin less than 50% scored area
	11	Bones largely dry and white, mummified skin
	12	Bones beginning to weather
Limbs		
Fresh	1	Fresh, no discoloration
Early decomposition	2	Flesh appears fresh, some maggots
	3	Some flesh still fresh, fur loss
	4	Discoloration of skin to brown, drying of extremities
	5	Black skin, leathery appearance
Advanced decomposition	6	Wet decomposition, bone exposure less than 50% scored area
	7	Wet decomposition, some disarticulation
Skeletonization	8	Bone exposure greater than 50% scored area, dry papery skin
	9	Bones largely dry and disarticulating
	10	Bones dry and white

Source: Adlam, R.E. and T. Simmons. 2007. The Effect of Repeated Physical Disturbance on Soft Tissue Decomposition—Are Taphonomic Studies an Accurate Reflection of Decomposition? *Journal of Forensic Sciences* 52(5):1007–1014.

Vitreous Humor

Overview

The potassium concentration in the vitreous humor has been used in human forensics to aid in the determination of the postmortem interval. It is not affected by age, sex, cause of death, or season of death in humans. After death, autolysis starts when cell metabolism stops and subsequently the integrity of all tissues throughout the body are lost. Selective cell membrane permeability and the active cell membrane transport ceases. In turn, this causes ions to

Table 14.5 Aquatic decompositional scoring.

Facial score	Description
1	No visible changes.
2	Slight pink discoloration, darkened lips, goose pimpling.
3	Reddening of face and neck, marbling visible on face. Possible early signs of animal activity/predation, concentrated on the ears, nose, and lips.
4	Bloating of the face, green discoloration, skin beginning to slough off.
5	Head hair beginning to slough off, mostly on the front. Brain softening and becoming liquefied. Tissue becoming exposed on face and neck. Green/black discoloration.
6	Bone becoming exposed, concentrated over the orbital, frontal, and parietal regions. Some on the mandible and maxilla. Early adipocere formation.
7	More extensive skeletonization on the cranium. Disarticulation of the mandible.
8	Complete disarticulation of the skull from torso. Extensive adipocere formation.
Torso (body) score	
1	No visible changes.
2	Slight pink discoloration, goose pimpling.
3	Yellow/green discoloration of abdomen and upper chest. Marbling. Internal organs beginning to decompose/autolysis.
4	Dark green discoloration of abdomen, mild bloating of abdomen, initial skin slippage.
5	Green/purple discoloration, extensive abdominal bloating, tense to touch, swollen scrotum in males, exposure of underlying fat and tissues.
6	Black discoloration, bloating becoming softer, initial exposure of internal organs and bones.
7	Further loss of tissues and organs, more bone exposed, initial adipocere formation.
8	Complete skeletonization and disarticulation.
Limb Score	
1	No visible changes.
2	Mild wrinkling of skin on hands and/or feet. Possible goose pimpling.
3	Skin on palms of hands and/or soles of feet becoming white, wrinkled, and thickened. Slight pink discoloration of arms and legs.
4	Skin on palms of hands and/or soles of feet becoming soggy and loose. Marbling of the limbs, predominantly on upper arms and legs.
5	Skin on hands/feet starting to slough off. Yellow/green to green/black discoloration on arms and/or legs. Initial skin slippage on arms and/or legs.
6	Degloving of hands and/or feet, exposing large areas of underlying muscles and tendons. Patchy sloughing of skin on arms and/or legs.
7	Exposure of bones of hands and/or feet. Muscles, tendons, and small areas of bone exposed in lower arms and/or legs.
8	Bones of hands and/or feet beginning to disarticulate. Bones of upper arms and/or legs becoming exposed.
9	Complete skeletonization and disarticulation of limbs.

Source: Heaton, V., A. Lagden, C. Moffatt, and T. Simmons. Predicting the Postmortem Submersion Interval for Human Remains Recovered from U.K. Waterways. *Journal of Forensic Sciences.* 55(2):302–307.

diffuse across the membranes, depending on the gradients. The vitreous humor is more isolated than other structures in the body and more resistant to bacterial degradation resulting from decomposition. It is relatively more stable postmortem compared with blood or cerebrospinal fluid.

The potassium gradient reverses postmortem and diffuses from the lens and retinal blood vessels into the vitreous humor. There may be different levels in the anterior, central, and posterior layers of the vitreous until equilibrium has been reached. As much vitreous as possible should be removed to eliminate the problem of concentration variation in the layers (Henssge et al. 1995). Traditionally in large animals, the aqueous is sampled for electrolyte testing. The laboratory should be contacted regarding sample handling and submission.

The vitreous potassium is of more value after the first twenty-four hours after death because other measurements are accurate in that postmortem interval (Henssge et al. 1995). The vitreous potassium increases as postmortem time increases, but there is great variability, which increases the longer the postmortem interval. Potassium levels are controlled by the rate of decomposition, so anything that affects this rate also affects the rise in potassium levels (Di Maio and Di Maio 2001). Potassium levels in human burn cases have been found to be higher than in non-burn cases (Garg 2004).

Sampling and Testing

Sampling technique of the vitreous is important (Chapter 3). Any contamination of tissue will alter the results. A sample from each eye should be taken. In humans it is normal to have up to a 10% difference between the right and left eye, though some studies have found no statistical differences (Garg et al. 2004). A study in dogs found there were no appreciable differences between the right and left eyes (Proctor et al. 2009). Although there are differences between the individual eye measurements, the mean value does not change and the regression lines used for analysis are the same (Henssge et al. 1995).

A study on canine vitreous potassium levels found the average level of 6.0 mEq/L immediately after death, the same as antemortem levels (5.92 mEq/L). The normal canine serum potassium is 3.5–5.3 mEq/L. The study found the average increase in vitreous potassium was 0.5 mEq/L/hour, the same as what is reported in humans (Proctor et al. 2009). The relationship of potassium concentration and postmortem interval is linear up to 120 hours and has been shown to be more reliable after the first twenty-four hours postmortem than other chemical tests (Sturner 2006). In humans, the formula established by Henssge was found to provide reliable estimates except when environmental temperature has been close to refrigeration levels during the PMI:

$$PMI = 5.26 \times K + concentration - 30.9$$

The 95% confidence level of the formula is ±20 hours for the first 100 hours postmortem (Sturner 2006). The estimate for PMI may be undervalued by 0.3 hour, with a standard deviation of nineteen hours (Henssge et al. 1995). A study by James et al. on postmortem vitreous potassium

levels was conducted on 100 human bodies in which the PMI was known that came to the forensic center. The study showed similar results to the formula from Henssge (Ross, Hoadley, and Sampson 1997). A more recent study from 120 autopsy cases resulted in a new vitreous potassium formula to determine the PMI (Jashnani, Kale, and Rupani 2010):

$$PMI(hours) = 1.076(K^+) - 2.815$$

Intraocular Pressure

The measurement of the intraocular pressure using a tonometer as a postmortem indicator has been used in humans. In a study conducted on cadavers who had died at a hospital and were stored in refrigerated conditions at 4°C (39°F), the postmortem interval correlated with the intraocular pressure with 95% probability (Table 14.6) (Balci et al. 2010). The normal range for humans is 11–21 mmHg ± 2–6 mmHg. The normal range for dogs and cats is 15–30 mmgHg.

Gastrointestinal Evaluation

Gastric emptying time and the gastric contents are helpful in human cases to help narrow down the postmortem interval. In an animal, when it is known what and when it last ate, it may be possible to use that information. Gastric emptying time is affected by many factors, including solid or liquid food, the fat and caloric content of the food, water intake, volume of food ingested, and whether the animal was fed meals or free-choice. It can be affected by the age and size of the animal, although in cats increasing age does not slow down the gastric emptying time as it does in humans. The emptying time may be delayed with emo-

Table 14.6 Postmortem interval according to intraocular pressure.

Intraocular Pressure (mmHg)	Postmortem Interval
≥25	<30 minutes
20–25	30–120 minutes
15–20	120–240 minutes
10–15	240–360 minutes
5–10	360–480 minutes
<5	>480 minutes

Source: Balci, Y., H. Basmak, B.K. Kocaturk, A. Sahin, and K. Ozdamar. 2010. The Importance of Measuring Intraocular Pressure Using a Tonometer in Order to Estimate the Postmortem Interval. *The American Journal of Forensic Medicine and Pathology*. 31(2):151–155.

Table 14.7 Gastric emptying times.

Dogs	Solids 4.7–15 hours	Liquid 0.5–3.5 hours
Cats	Solids 4.7–12.5 hours	Liquid 1 hour
Average normal for dogs and cats: < 14 hours		

tional stress, shock, certain diseases, drugs (while some drugs increase it), and extreme cold or hot environmental conditions. It may be increased with moderate exercise and decreased with more exhaustive exercise (Perper 2006). Table 14.7 is a compilation of maximum and minimum reported times in dogs and cats. For any determination of the postmortem interval, gastric emptying time must be placed in context with all the other postmortem findings.

The evaluation of specific species of gut flora and the pattern of microbial changes as a function of the postmortem interval is an area of research in humans. This is based on the knowledge that specific microbes, identified with DNA, increase exponentially after death then decrease in later stages of composition (Hauther 2012).

Citrate Content of Bone

Citrate is present in living and animal cortical bone at a very uniform initial concentration of 2 ± 0.1 weight%. The concentration of bone citrate remains constant, buried or not, for the first four weeks postmortem, then linearly declines as a function of time. There may be variation if the body was inside a plastic body bag, with long bones a better site for sampling (Kanz, Reiter, and Risser 2012). The linear decline appears to be independent of rainfall and temperature except that it drops to zero for storage below $0°C$ ($32°F$). This temperature effect can be corrected to determine PMI by using the following equation where 'w' = number of months in each year when the temperature (T) < $0°C$ (Schwarcz, Agur, and Jantz 2010):

$$t^* = t\left(1 - \left[w/12\right]\right) \text{ in days}$$

This t* is then used in the following equation where t = t* for the PMI in days and C(t) is the residual citrate level at 't' (Schwarcz, Agur, and Jantz 2010):

$$C(t) = -0.661\log t + 20.99\, r^2 = 0.986$$

Nasal Mucociliary Motility

A new tool for estimating the postmortem interval may be the evaluation of nasal mucociliary motility. This motility is known to persist postmortem in humans. Scraping of the nasal mucosa is performed and the cells observed on a slide. A study was conducted in humans with a known time of death. The ciliary motility was measured as beat number/second and categorized as present (3–4/sec), hypovalid (1–2/sec), and absent. Except for cases of bacterial or fungal infections, motility was present in the majority of cases at four to six hours postmortem; it was hypo-valid in a higher percentage at ten to twelve hours postmortem; and absent at twenty-four hours postmortem (Solarino 2011).

DETERMINING THE PMI: EXAMINATION OF THE CRIME SCENE

Several types of evidence can be found at the crime scene, on the animal's body, or through investigation that can help determine the time of death. Investigators need to question neighbors to find out when the animal was last seen alive and its condition. The animal's environment and housing conditions can provide information regarding time intervals including entomology evidence and the presence and condition of feces (Chapters 11 and 15). All findings, including examination findings, must be analyzed together to reach the most accurate time of death.

It is possible to evaluate blood stain findings at the scene to assist in the estimation of time of death. Older blood stains can be analyzed to determine if the stain age is years older (Chapter 2). The blood may be fresh or clotted, and the serum separated or dried. It may be in a large pool, or there may be blood spatter. Blood can continue to seep from the body after death due to the effects of gravity. By recording the blood stain size, estimated blood loss, condition of the blood stains, and environmental factors, forensic scientists can help determine the postmortem interval. Using these findings, they can determine the blood stain volume and perform experiments to determine the length of time for that amount of blood to clot, the serum to separate, or the blood to dry on similar surfaces under similar environmental conditions.

Forensic botanists can analyze plant evidence found at the scene and on the body to help determine the postmortem interval, whether the body was moved, and the original location of the body (Chapter 4). The time frames for the postmortem interval are often months, years, or seasons. The plant specimens may include leaves, twigs, roots, pollen, fungi, and algae that can be analyzed. These plant specimens may be found on the body or in the gastric contents.

REFERENCES

Adlam, R.E. and T. Simmons. 2007. The Effect of Repeated Physical Disturbance on Soft Tissue Decomposition—Are Taphonomic Studies an Accurate Reflection on Decomposition? *Journal of Forensic Sciences.* 52(5):1007–1013.

Andrello, L. and P.R. Basso. 2012. Wounds Vitality Evaluation in Decomposed Corpse: The Application of Monoclonal Antibody Against Hemoglobin Alpha Chain. Presented at the Academy of Forensic Sciences Annual Scientific Meeting, 20–25 February, Atlanta, Georgia.

Bachmann, J. and T. Simmons. 2010. The Influence of Preburial Insect Access on the Decompositional Rate. *Journal of Forensic Sciences.* 55(4):893–900.

Balci, Y., H. Basmak, B.K. Kocaturk, A. Sahin, and K. Ozdamar. 2010. The Importance of Measuring Intraocular Pressure Using a Tonometer in Order to Estimate the Postmortem Interval. *The American Journal of Forensic Medicine and Pathology.* 31(2):151–155.

Boyd, D.C., L.N. Sliwa, and C.C. Boyd. 2010. Differential Decomposition of Non-Traumatized, Blunt Force, and Sharp Force-Traumatized Pig Carcasses. Presented at the American Academy of Forensic Sciences Annual Scientific Meeting, 22–27 February, Seattle, Washington.

Campobasso, C.P., G. Di Vella, A. De Donno, V. Santoro, G. Favia, and F. Introna. 2006. Pink Teeth in a Series of Bodies Recovered From a Single Shipwreck. *The American Journal of Forensic Medicine and Pathology.* 27(4):313–316.

Cross, P. and T. Simmons. 2010. The Influence of Penetrative Trauma on the Rate of Decomposition. *Journal of Forensic Sciences.* 55(2):295–301.

Dabbs, G.. 2012. A Comparison of Site-Specific Versus National Weather Service Temperature Data and its Applicability to Estimation of Postmortem Interval Using Accumulated Degree Days. Presented at the American Academy of Forensic Sciences Annual Scientific Meeting, 20–25 February, Atlanta, Georgia.

Di Maio, V.J. and D. Di Maio. 2001. *Forensic Pathology,* Second edition. Boca Raton, FL: CRC Press.

Di Nunno, N., F. Costantinides, S.J. Cina, C. Rizzardi, C. Di Nunno, and M. Melato. 2002. What Is the Best Sample for Determining the Early Postmortem Period by On-the-Spot Flow Cytometry Analysis? *The American Journal of Forensic Medicine and Pathology* 23(2):173–180.

Dix, J. and R. Calaluce. 1999. *Guide to Forensic Pathology.* Boca Raton, FL: CRC Press.

Dix, J. and M. Graham. 2000. *Time of Death, Decomposition and Identification: An Atlas.* Boca Raton, FL: CRC Press.

Elandsson, M. and R. Munro. 2007. Estimation of the Post-Mortem Interval in Beagle Dogs. *Science and Justice.* 47:150–154.

Forbes, S.L., B.H. Stuart, B.B. Dent, and S. Fenwick-Mulcahy. 2005. Characterization of Adipocere Formation in Animal Species. *Journal of Forensic Sciences.* 50(3):633–640.

Garg, V., S.S. Oberoi, R.K. Gorea, and Kiranjeet Kaur. 2004. Changes in the Levels of Vitreous Potassium with Increasing Time Since Death. *Journal of Indian Academy of Forensic Medicine.* 26(4):136–39.

Gonder, C.. 2009. Wildlife Decomposition Analysis for Time of Death Estimates. Wildlife Field Forensics.

Gruenthal, A., C. Moffatt, and T. Simmons. Differential Decomposition Patterns in Charred Versus Un-Charred Remains. *Journal of Forensic Sciences.* 57(1):12–18.

Haslam, T.C.F. and M. Tibbett. 2009. Soils of Contrasting pH Affect the Decomposition of Buried Mammalian (*Ovis aries*) Skeletal Muscle Tissue. *Journal of Forensic Sciences.* 54(4):900–904.

Hauther, K. 2012. Time Since Death Estimation From Gut Flora. Presented at the American Academy of Forensic Sciences Annual Scientific Meeting, 20–25 February, Atlanta, Georgia.

Heaton, V., A. Lagden, C. Moffatt, and T. Simmons. 2010. Predicting the Postmortem Submersion Interval for Human Remains Recovered from U.K. Waterways. *Journal of Forensic Sciences.* 55(2):302–307.

Henssge, C., B. Knight, T. Krompecher, B. Madea, and L. Nokes. 1995. *The Estimation of the Time Since Death in the Early Postmortem Period,* B. Knight, ed. New York: Oxford University Press.

Jashnani, K.D., S.A. Kale, and A.B. Rupani. 2010. Vitreous Humor: Biochemical Constituents in Estimation of Postmortem Interval. *Journal of Forensic Sciences.* 55(6):1523–1527.

Kaliszan, M. 2011. Does a Draft Really Influence Postmortem Body Cooling? *Journal of Forensic Sciences.* 56(5):1310–1314.

Kanz, F., C. Reiter, and Da.U. Risser. 2012. Citrate Content of Bone for Time-Since-Death Estimation: Results from Burials with Different Physical Characteristics (Wooden Coffins Versus Plastic Body Bags) With Known PMI. Presented at the American Academy of Forensic Sciences Annual Scientific Meeting, 20–25 February, Atlanta, Georgia.

Lew, E. and E. Matshes. 2005. Postmortem Changes. In: *Forensic Pathology: Principles and Practice*, pp. 527–554. Oxford: Elsevier.

Megyesi, M.S., S.P. Nawrocki, and N.H. Haskell. 2005. Using Accumulated Degree-Days to Estimate the Postmortem Interval from Decomposed Human Remains. *Journal of Forensic Sciences.* 50(3):618–626.

Morton, R.J. and W.D. Lord. 2002. Detection and Recovery of Abducted and Murdered Children: Behavioral and Taphonomic Influences. In: *Advances in Forensic Taphonomy*, W.D. Haglund and M.H. Sorg, eds. pp. 151–171. Boca Raton, FL: CRC Press.

Pakosh, C. and T.L. Rogers. 2009. Soft Tissue Decomposition of Submerged, Dismembered Pig Limbs Enclosed in Plastic Bags. *Journal of Forensic Sciences.* 54(6):1223–1228.

Pastula, E.C. 2012. Insect Timing and Succession on Buried Carrion. Presented at the American Academy of Forensic Sciences Annual Scientific Meeting, 20–25 February, Atlanta, Georgia.

Perper, J.A. 2006. Time of Death and Changes After Death, Part 1: Anatomical Considerations. In: *Spitz and Fisher's*

Medicolegal Investigation of Death: Guidelines for the Application of Pathology to Crime Investigation, Fourth edition, W.U. Spitz and D.J. Spitz, eds. pp. 87–127. Springfield: Charles C. Thomas Publisher, Ltd.

Pollanen, M.S., C. Perera, and D.J. Clutterbuck. 2009. Hemorrhagic Lividity of the Neck: Controlled Induction of Postmortem Hypostatic Hemorrhages. *The American Journal of Forensic Medicine and Pathology.* 30(4):322–326.

Pounder, D. 2011. Time of Death. Lecture notes for Forensic Medicine Course, Department of Forensic Medicine, University of Dundee, Dundee, Scotland. www.dundee.ac.uk/forensicmedicine.

Proctor, K., W.J. Kelch, and J. New. 2009. Estimating the Time of Death in Domestic Canines. *Journal of Forensic Sciences.* 54(6):1433–37.

Ross, J.A., P.A. Hoadley, and B.G. Sampson. 1997. Determination of Postmortem Interval by Sampling Vitreous Humour. *The American Journal of Forensic Medicine and Pathology* 18(2):158–162.

Schwarcz, H.P., K. Agur, and L.M. Jantz. 2010. A New Method for Determination of Postmortem Interval: Citrate Content of Bone. *Journal of Forensic Sciences.* 55(6):1516–1522.

Simmons, T., R.E. Adlam, and C. Moffatt. 2010a. Debugging Decomposition Data—Comparative Taphonomic Studies and the Influence of Insects and Carcass Size on Decomposition Rate. *Journal of Forensic Sciences.* 55(1):8–13.

Simmons, T., P.A. Cross, R.E. Adlam, and C. Moffatt. 2010b. The Influence of Insects on Decomposition Rate in Buried and Surface Remains. *Journal of Forensic Sciences.* 55(4):889–892.

Solarino, B. 2011. Nasal Mucociliary Motility: New Forensic Tool for Estimating Time Since Death. Presented at the 63rd Annual Scientific Meeting of the American Academy of Forensic Sciences, 21–26 February, Chicago, Illinois.

Zimmerman, K.A. and J.R. Wallace. 2008. The Potential to Determine a Postmortem Submersion Interval Based on Algal/Diatom Diversity on Decomposing Mammalian Carcasses in Brackish Ponds in Delaware. *Journal of Forensic Sciences.* 53(4):935–941.

15

Forensic Entomology: The Use of Insects in Animal Cruelty Cases

Gail S. Anderson

"Who saw him die?"
"I," said the fly
"With my little eye,
I saw him die."
                    Anonymous

INTRODUCTION

Insects are now commonly used in homicide investigations, but their use in animal cruelty cases is less well known. Forensic entomology is the study of insects related to legal matters. A subset of forensic entomology, medicolegal entomology, is broadly considered to be the study of insects associated with a dead body in order to understand as many features about the death as possible. The most notable of these features is the length of time that insects have been associated with the body to imply a minimum elapsed time since death. Medicolegal entomology has a very long history, dating back to the tenth century in China (Cheng 1890, Reprinted 1985, cited in Greenberg and Kunich 2002), and it has come into its own in the last few decades, commonly being used in homicide investigations. Several texts are devoted to this subject, for example Smith 1986, Greenberg and Kunich 2002, Gennard 2007, Haskell and Williams 2008, Magni et al. 2008, Amendt et al. 2010, and Byrd and Castner 2010.

Certain species of insects feed for all or part of their life cycle on dead organic material and so are intricately associated with a carcass. Such species are referred to as carrion or necrophagous insects. Other species of insects do not feed directly on the remains but instead are attracted to the carcass by the presence of the earlier carrion feeders;

hence, a complex ecological food web develops. Forensic entomologists use their understanding of carrion insect ecology and development to analyze the insects on the remains, giving death investigators information about the tenure of insects on the body as well as other taphonomic information.

Although medicolegal entomology is primarily used in human death investigations, carrion insects feed on dead organic matter and do not discriminate between the human, animal, or any other species. Therefore, the principles of medicolegal entomology apply equally well to animals and can be used to estimate the length of time insects have been present on a dead animal, thereby inferring minimum elapsed time since death in exactly the same manner as in a human death investigation (Anderson 1999). Although most medicolegal entomology questions pertain to minimum elapsed times since death, insects also can be used to determine whether a carcass has been moved from the original site of death or has been disturbed after death, the presence and position of wounds, and whether the animal has been poisoned.

Although primarily involved in death investigations, many carrion insects colonize necrotic tissue in living victims and medicolegal entomology has been very useful in estimating length of time of neglect, or time since injury in human neglect cases, particularly in infants and the elderly (Goff et al. 1991, Benecke 2004, Benecke 2010). Fortunately, such human cases are relatively rare, but these cases are featured more commonly in animal investigations and may be of much greater value in cruelty cases (Anderson and Huitson 2004).

Veterinary Forensics: Animal Cruelty Investigations, Second Edition. Edited by Melinda D. Merck.
© 2013 John Wiley & Sons, Inc. Published 2013 by John Wiley & Sons, Inc.

There are, therefore, three main arenas in which medico-legal entomology can be of value in an animal cruelty investigation: when an animal is found dead inside a residence, when an animal is found dead outdoors, and when a live animal is found to have been colonized by insects.

PRINCIPLES OF MEDICOLEGAL ENTOMOLOGY

Insects are invariably the first witnesses to a death, arriving at the remains almost immediately afterward, assuming appropriate conditions exist such as exposure, season, weather, and time of day. They often arrive within minutes in the presence of blood (Anderson and VanLaerhoven 1996). In medicolegal entomology insect colonization of remains is usually divided into two periods based on the manner that an entomologist analyzes the entomological evidence, although in reality the two are actually part of a continuum.

Initial fly colonization and development

The first method in medicolegal entomology involves analyzing the predictable insect life cycle on a carcass. The first insects to arrive on a body are flies or Diptera in the family Calliphoridae, commonly called blow flies or blue or green bottle flies. In some regions of the world flies in the family Sarcophagidae or flesh flies are also early arrivals.

Female blow flies are not attracted to the body to feed themselves but instead are searching for a suitable medium on which to lay their eggs. The female will walk over the substrate, "tasting" with taste receptors on her tarsi or "feet" to ensure that the substrate is a suitable medium for larval development and then she will lay or oviposit her eggs in batches of approximately 200. These eggs hatch after a predictable period of time into first instar or first stage larvae (maggots). These larvae require a protein meal but are very delicate and cannot usually break adult human skin. Therefore, the female, in her only attempt at maternal care, ensures that the eggs are laid in or close to a wound or natural orifice allowing the newly enclosed larvae to feed in liquid protein, either as blood or in the moist mucosal tissue (Figure 15.1). Hence, blow flies are extremely adept at locating wounds and can even locate a venapuncture (Figure 15.2).

Larvae feed by first externally digesting the tissue using rasping mouthparts and secreting proteolytic enzymes, and then imbibing the resultant liquid protein (Erzinclioglu 1996). The larvae feed voraciously and molt into second and then third instar larvae. The third instar larvae in particular remove a large amount of tissue and also frequently aggregate in masses which generate heat from friction and metabolic activity. After a period of time the third instar undergoes a behavioral and physiological change, although

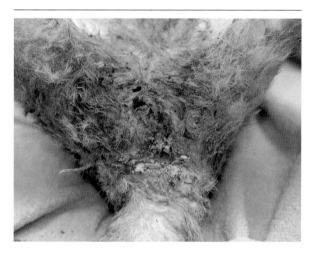

Figure 15.1 Fly eggs on perineum.

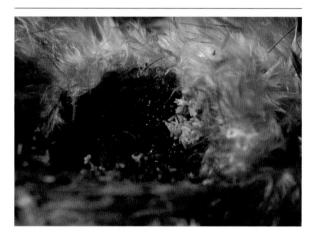

Figure 15.2 Fly eggs deposited on the margin of a fighting wound in a deceased gamecock.

it does not molt. At this stage it enters a wandering or dispersal stage, leaving the food source in search of a dry protected area in which to pupate. After a period of dispersal, the insect pupates or forms a hard outer cocoon inside which the insect metamorphoses into the adult fly. Once metamorphosis is complete, the adult fly breaks off the operculum of the pupal case and emerges, leaving behind the empty pupal case and operculum, now broken into two ecdysial caps, as physical forensic evidence that the cycle has been completed.

Insect development is temperature dependent, that is, the rate of development increases as temperature increases and vice versa. This relationship is relatively linear at optimum temperatures, making it predictable. This predictable relationship is what allows a forensic entomologist to analyze the insects on the remains to estimate the length of time that the insects have been feeding on the carcass and in so doing, infer the minimum elapsed time since death. The entomologist requires four pieces of information to estimate the length of time that the insects have been feeding on the body:

- The oldest stage of insects on the remains. In other words, how far through the life cycle have the oldest insects progressed. This is determined by a physical, microscopic examination of the insects and by raising the insects collected from the remains to determine how much longer is required to reach adulthood under controlled conditions.
- The species of insect. Every species develops at a different rate so it is imperative to correctly identify the insects down to species. This is done using morphological features and published entomological keys. Adult insects are relatively easy to identify morphologically. This is why it is best to ensure that some collected insects are kept alive to be raised to adulthood, greatly facilitating identification. If only preserved larvae are available, these can be identified using morphological features in the mouthparts, but this is more difficult, especially in the early instars. DNA can be used to identify species in cases in which very young instars are present or only damaged insects are available (Wells and Stevens 2010).
- The temperature to which the insects were exposed. Ambient temperature is usually determined based on official weather station data such as that collected by the U.S. Department of Agriculture (USDA) or Environment Canada, and is often supplemented by the placement of a datalogger at the scene to ensure that the weather station is appropriate for the area. This is particularly important in cases indoors, where indoor temperature may be very different from outside temperatures (Appendix 37).
- Known developmental records. It is imperative to have known, published, regional developmental records for the insect species in question.

With the above information, the simple question is "How long does it take *this* insect species to reach the oldest stage on the remains, under *these* given conditions?" The answer might be that the oldest insects on the carcass are third instar Calliphoridae, identified as *Calliphora vicina* (Robineau-Desvoidy) and the mean temperature at the crime scene was 23°C. Published data state that *C. vicina* takes a minimum of seventy-seven hours or just over three days to reach the beginning of the third instar at a mean

temperature of 23.3°C (Anderson 2000). Therefore, the oldest insects are at least three days old, meaning that they have been feeding on the remains for at least three days. One can then infer that the carcass has been dead for at least three days. This is a minimum because the insects are already in this stage so death could have occurred earlier but not later. Therefore, the entomologist can stand in court and state that the carcass has definitely been dead for at least three days; it could be longer but could not be less.

Insect succession

Blow flies and sometimes flesh flies are the first colonizers of fresh remains and they will continue to oviposit, or in the case of flesh flies, larviposit (lay live larvae) on the remains as long as there is fresh tissue available. Once the first arrivals have completed their life cycle and emerged as adult flies, a minimum elapsed time can be given based on the completed life cycle, but entomologists must then turn to the second method for analyzing insects, examining the insect succession and ecological relationships of insects on the carcass.

As an animal carcass decomposes it goes through a predictable range of biological, chemical, and physical changes. At first, when fresh, it is attractive to the flies that prefer fresh tissue. As these insects feed they change the carcass so that it becomes no longer attractive to these insects, but more attractive to other insects. Over the decomposition process, as the nutritional contents of the tissues change, different species are attracted and repelled over time. The species of insects that colonize the remains over time are predictable, arriving in a sequential manner. Therefore, an entomologist can analyze the insects present on the remains and give a window of time in which death must have taken place, based on the insects present at the time of recovery as well as the remains of insects that previously colonized the remains.

Caution must be taken when using this method because unlike blow fly development, which is primarily dependent on temperature, the sequence of insects that colonize remains over time depends on many variables including geographic region, season, and habitat which can have a major impact on which species will colonize, their arrival times, and tenure (Anderson 2010). It is therefore imperative that local and regional data are available to interpret such information. It is not possible to extrapolate data from one area to another without such localized and regional information. This second method usually gives a broader range of estimated time of colonization, for instance: the animal has been colonized for at least six months; therefore, it has been dead six months or more.

Case history example

On September 28 in a large metropolitan Canadian city neighbors contacted police to report a fluid leaking out from underneath a garage door in a home from which they had heard a great deal of barking then whining some weeks earlier. The garage contained the remains of a large dog as well as many bags of feces in a cardboard box and a slurry-like substance in a dog bowl. This scene contained three major sites of insect infestation.

The first was the carcass itself. Larval blow flies were collected from the oral and nasal cavities of the deceased dog. These ranged in larval stage from second to third instar *Lucilia sericata* (Meigen), with one or two specimens just beginning to enter the prepupal or wandering, non-feeding stage of the third instar. The second site was at a thick slurry-like material found in a bowl. Again, third instar and a single prepupal third instar *L. sericata* were collected. The final site was approximately 30 cm away from the dog carcass close to a number of blue plastic bags and a cardboard box. These bags contained what appeared to be feces. Empty puparia of *Fannia* species (Diptera: Fanniidae) were collected from this area, indicating that *Fannia* had completed its' entire life cycle in the area. Fanniidae are commonly attracted to fecal material. Species could not be determined because only empty puparia were present.

The garage temperature appeared to be similar to the outdoor ambient temperatures with a mean temperature of around 15°C. *Lucilia illustris* (Meigen) has been shown to take a minimum of 135.7 hours or 5.7 days to reach the beginning of the third instar and 233.7 hours or 9.7 days to reach the beginning of the prepupal or wandering stage of the third instar at a mean temperature of 15.8°C (Anderson 2000). The actual species of *Fannia* present is unknown but *F. cannicularis* (L), a common species, has been shown to take thirty-six days to complete development from egg to adulthood at a mean constant temperature of 15°C (Meyer and Mullens 1988).

In order to estimate the most accurate development rate at the scene temperatures, the data generated at other temperatures can be converted to thermal units or degree days. Degree day calculations are most accurate when developed from data closest to that in question (Anderson 2000). Based on the known developmental data, *L. sericata* requires a minimum of 89.3 accumulated degree days (ADD) to reach the beginning of the third instar and 153.9 ADD to reach the beginning of the prepupal stage of the third instar. Using temperature data from a nearby Environment Canada weather station, 89.3 ADD would have been accumulated between September 23 and 24 and 153.9 ADD by September 19. The insects were well into the third instar so the carcass must have been colonized before September 23 and possibly as early as September 18.

The dog carcass was not heavily colonized, suggesting only one or two flies may have been responsible for the eggs laid on the remains. In many cases large maggot masses form on remains, generating their own heat and increasing the temperature to which the insects are exposed. However, in this case, the low numbers of maggots were insufficient to affect carcass temperature. Furthermore, the actual temperature inside the garage was not known; it could only be implied from the outdoor weather data.

The larvae in the bowl were of a similar age, suggesting that the material in the bowl was colonized at the same time as the dog. Empty puparia of *Fannia* species associated with the bags of feces showed that at least one generation of this fly had completed its life cycle. A single generation would require 540 ADD, based on the development data noted above. These would have been accumulated between August 25 and 26, indicating that this species had been present for at least that time. However, because the puparia were empty, it is only possible to say that the insects had been there since at least August 25 to 26, but they but could have been there for considerably longer because several generations could have colonized over time.

The insects on the dog and slurry indicated that colonization had occurred by at least September 23 or 24 and most probably before September 18. Because the remains were inside a garage, it is probable that colonization was delayed until the odor could attract insects from outside. In experiments inside a house in Alberta, insects were delayed by five days before they entered and colonized pig carcasses, so a similar delay also may have occurred (Anderson 2011). The insects on the fecal material suggested that the feces had been present for more than a month and could have been present for much longer.

In addition, the insects indicated that the dog had been deceased for at least five days and more probably for at least ten days. Due to the possible delay in colonization, it is entirely possible that the dog had died fifteen or more days prior to discovery, but had certainly been deceased for at least five days.

CUTANEOUS MYIASIS: THE INSECT COLONIZATION OF LIVE ANIMALS

Many of the insects that are normally found on dead animals also feed on living animals, either on the necrotic tissue of a wound or on hotspots or on living tissue. The colonization of a living animal (or human) by dipteran (fly) larvae is called myiasis. The analysis of insects on a living animal can help estimate elapsed time since colonization, which can indicate the length of time of neglect or timing of an injury. The most common Diptera or true flies found causing myiasis include blow flies (Calliphoridae), flesh flies (Sarcophagidae), house flies (Muscidae), and scuttle flies (Phoridae) (McIntosh et al. 2011).

There are three categories of myiasis:

- Accidental, when larvae are accidentally eaten or licked from a wound
- Facultative, when larvae are normally free-living on carrion or feces but occasionally infest living animals. They usually feed on necrotic tissue but sometimes also feed on healthy tissue
- Obligatory, when larvae live exclusively on or in the host, consuming live tissue

Obligatory parasites have evolved to co-exist with the host so they are usually not as damaging as facultative parasites because such an existence is not normal in their life cycle. Also, many more larvae are involved in facultative parasitism, with the area becoming more and more attractive as it becomes further colonized, so it can result in massive infestations. There are three levels of myiasis: primary, secondary, and tertiary. Primary myiasis is caused by obligate parasites which initiate a wound in healthy tissue and colonize unbroken skin. Secondary myiasis is caused by facultative larvae which cannot break healthy skin so they colonize at a wound site or natural orifice. These are the usual insects found on dead animals. Primary myiasis agents also may be present because they may have caused the original wound. Tertiary myiasis is caused by facultative larvae when the animal is close to death.

Facultative myiasis, wherein carrion insects colonize a wound or damaged tissue such as a hotspot or scoured area, are of the most interest in animal cruelty cases. Colonization occurs after the wound is formed or when a neglected pet develops necrotic tissue; therefore, the tenure of insect colonization gives a minimum elapsed time since the animal was ill-treated or neglected. This is perhaps best illustrated in the fly-strike seen in domestic animals, particularly sheep, where infestation can become so extensive that the entire skin of the animal may slough off. Sheep fly-strike can cause losses in the hundreds of millions of dollars in areas where sheep are extensively raised such as Australia and Britain. Ironically, in many cases, the insects keep the wound clean, removing necrotic tissue. Maggot debridement therapy, the use of insects to debride wounds, has been used for centuries and is still commonly used in human medicine (Sherman et al. 2000). Its use in veterinary medicine is just now being explored (Sherman et al. 2007).

It is quite possible that an animal that was colonized while alive may later die. This can cause problems because it might be erroneously assumed that the animal was only colonized after death, giving an incorrect estimation of elapsed time since death. When a colonized carcass is discovered several methods can be used to determine whether it is likely that the animal suffered from myiasis prior to death rather than just postmortem colonization.

First, the condition of the remains may suggest that myiasis was probable, such as extensive signs of scouring or large hotspots. Second, the actual location of the larval masses might suggest that the animal was colonized in life. For example, in the case of an abandoned baby in Hawaii, insects were first attracted to fecal material in the diaper and then laid eggs in areas of diaper rash. The toddler was found alive but had she not been found until after death, it is possible that the evidence could have been misinterpreted (Goff et al. 1991). If insects had been collected and submitted to the entomologist without information about collection site, the entomologist would have simply aged the insects. However, because the entomologist was present and collected the insects himself he noted the collection site and knew that this is not a usual first colonization site, because it was covered and protected, as opposed to the uncovered facial orifices. Had the child been found dead, the entomologist would still have been able to suggest that the child was probably colonized in life due to the unusual colonization pattern. This highlights the importance of documenting where insects are collected and the value of having an entomologist present at a scene and autopsy/necropsy (Goff et al. 1991). Finally, some species of obligate parasites can continue their development after the host has died. Therefore, the presence of obligate parasites such as the primary screw-worm, *Cochliomyia hominivorax* (Coq), on a dead animal would indicate that it was first colonized in life.

The factors that increase the risk of myiasis in an animal include neglect or lack of regular care, a primarily outdoor life, an unnoticed injury, a long, ungroomed coat which increases proliferation of mats, feces and/or urine in the coat and causes hot spots or sores, and age of the animal, with older animals more likely to be colonized (Anderson and Huitson 2004).

The presence of larvae on a live animal is considered to be extremely repugnant and this can make a myiasis case appear much worse than it is. In many cases of facultative myiasis, the insects are cleaning the wound and not actually causing damage. Of course, this does not mean they should not be removed, but their actual presence is not as repugnant as it may seem. This is particularly important to remember when the larvae are in the wandering, non-feeding stage of the third instar when it can appear that the entire animal is writhing with maggots and completely infested. In reality, there is usually one small feeding area, while the majority of the observed maggots are not feeding but simply dispersing from the feeding site. A simple combing or bath will remove them.

A further problem with live animal infestations is that while the animal is alive and mobile, the wandering, non-feeding third instar larvae may drop off anywhere as the animal moves around. In a carcass, these larvae can predictably be recovered from the nearby ground surface and top surface layer of substrate, but when the animal is mobile they could have dropped anywhere and may therefore often be missed (Anderson and Huitson 2004).

The presence of larvae on living animals is repugnant to most people and hence evidence of myiasis in neglect or abuse cases can be extremely probative in court. Such evidence can be common in puppy mill situations where large numbers of animals are kept in close quarters, often with little attention or care, and where fighting, scouring due to feces, or urine soaking of the coat can easily lead to extensive myiasis. Although most cases of myiasis may be due to neglect, it may also occur when a wound is unattended, so may be very pertinent in an act of deliberate cruelty.

OTHER USES FOR INSECTS IN ANIMAL CRUELTY INVESTIGATIONS

Although forensic entomologists are mostly called on to estimate the length of time that insects have been present on an animal and so infer a minimum elapsed time since death or injury, insects can tell the entomologist much more than this. In neglect cases with unsanitary environments, such as hoarding, insects may feed on pet food or animal waste (Figure 15.3). Entomologists can provide time frame information from this evidence that is important to the investigation.

Wound site

Blow flies are first attracted to wound sites if they are present, because they provide a liquid protein meal for their offspring. This is a survival strategy, so blow flies have evolved to be extremely efficient at locating wounds. In the absence of a wound, blow flies usually are first attracted to natural orifices. Once decomposition has advanced and insect activity is extensive, it may be very difficult for the

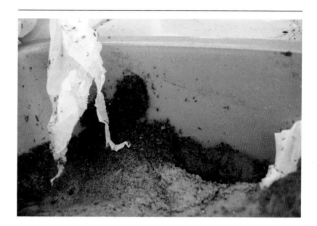

Figure 15.3 Visible insect evidence in litter box from a hoarding case.

veterinarian to discern whether the animal sustained a wound. However, an irregular pattern of insect activity suggests the presence of a wound or hotspot. It is not up to the entomologist to identify a wound site, but rather it is the veterinarian who identifies the wound and possibly indicates the weapon that caused it. The entomologist can assist in indicating whether the colonization pattern is normal and whether the potential wound site was colonized before the orifices, based on larval age. This can be very valuable in determining whether or not the death was natural. Extensive colonization of an area other than the orifices also may suggest myiasis prior to death due to neglect or injury.

Poisoning

Decomposed remains are often too degraded for normal toxicological analyses; however, larval insects feeding on an animal carcass will accidentally ingest any foreign materials in the animal such as poisons or pesticides. Therefore, insects from the body can be used as toxicological specimens when animal tissue is no longer viable. A great deal of research has been conducted on using insects as toxicological specimens in human cases and animal studies. They have invariably shown that insects are excellent indicators of the presence or absence of a particular toxin, but they cannot be used consistently to quantify the toxin (Goff and Lord 2009).

Larvae bioaccumulate the toxin throughout their larval lifetime, sequestering the toxin in the larval cuticle which later becomes part of the sclerotized puparium or pupal case. Therefore, the toxins can be recovered from the larva, pupa, and empty pupal case (Bourel et al. 2001), making them valuable toxicological specimens. It also has been shown that not only do the primary colonizers, the Diptera larvae, accumulate the toxins, but so do secondary insect species feeding on the larvae (Nuorteva and Nuorteva 1982), and the toxins can still be recovered from their puparia and exuviae (Miller et al. 1994). Empty Diptera puparia and Coleoptera exuviae have been recovered decades after death (Gilbert and Bass 1967), meaning that such specimens could be very valuable in determining possible cause of death years after the animal died. Human studies concentrate on illegal and therapeutic drug levels, but the same principles apply to more common substances found in animals such as poisons or pesticides.

Insects also have been shown to indicate the presence of other materials on or in the carcass, such as gunshot residue (Roeterdink et al. 2004, LaGoo et al. 2010). This could be extremely valuable in proving that a wound was due to a gunshot even if the projectile is not recovered.

It should be noted that illicit and therapeutic drugs as well as toxins can impact insect development (Goff and Lord 2009) so it is imperative that the entomologist is informed of any toxicological results when he or she is asked to make an assessment of elapsed time since death.

Relocation of remains

Insects can be used in some cases to determine if an animal has been relocated from the original death site and point investigators to the original scene. If the carcass is left at the original site for any length of time, for instance in the home or outside in a shed, insects will colonize the remains, assuming conditions are appropriate. If the offender eventually disposes of the animal in a different habitat, then further insects will colonize at the second site. If the two sites are different, it is possible that different species of insects will prevail in each area. For instance, some species of blow fly live primarily in rural areas, living on normally occurring dead animals, whereas other species have adapted to live close to human habitation (synanthropic), feeding primarily on garbage. If an animal is found in a rural area with older, urban insects present, it suggests that the carcass has been relocated after death.

DNA

In some cases an animal may have decomposed at a particular site but the perpetrator, perhaps alerted to a potential investigation, has disposed of the carcass. If maggots and pupae are still present at the scene, these can be analyzed to determine the identity of the DNA within the gut system. Blow fly larvae have a large food storage area called a crop within the foregut portion of the digestive system. In feeding larvae, this can be clearly seen through

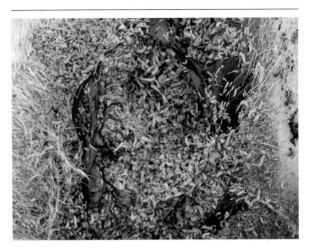

Figure 15.4 Maggot mass with visible dark red crops. (Photo courtesy of Dr. Gail Anderson.)

the translucent cuticle as a large, oval, red or brown area (Figure 15.4). It has been shown that the host DNA can be recovered and identified to species and, if pre-mortem DNA samples from the suspected deceased animal can be located, the DNA could be used to individualize the host on which the insects fed (Wells et al. 2001, Linville et al. 2004). This would prove first that the insects located at the scene had fed on, for example, a cat, rather than the garbage as claimed by the perpetrator, but could also individualize the actual animal. Even if insects have moved to a secondary food source, the original host DNA can be recovered for up to twelve hours (Stuyt et al. 2010).

COLLECTION OF INSECT EVIDENCE

As with any evidentiary material, entomological evidence is only of value if it is collected properly. There are many references available describing appropriate collection techniques (Anderson and Cervenka 2001, Amendt et al. 2007, Haskell and Williams 2008). A brief description is presented here. There are some differences between collecting insects from a live animal than from a carcass, although the principles are the same.

If possible it is best if a forensic entomologist can attend the scene and necropsy to perform the collection themselves. Failing that, an animal cruelty investigator or veterinarian can collect the evidence and then courier it to a forensic entomologist. The collection can be divided into two main types: collecting blow fly evidence and collecting the later successional species.

Samples of insects of all stages should be collected from different areas of the body and from the ground, including soil or carpeting, etc. Insects often congregate in wounds and in and around natural orifices. The two main insect groups on bodies are flies (Diptera) and beetles (Coleoptera). Both types of insect look very different at different stages of their lives. See Appendix 36 for a collection checklist for animal cases.

Collection of blow fly evidence from a deceased animal

Blow flies can be found as eggs, larvae or maggots, pupae, empty pupal cases, and adults.

Eggs

Eggs are very tiny, but are laid in clumps or masses, and are usually found in or very near a wound or natural orifice. They can be collected with a child's paint brush dipped in water or with forceps. Half should be preserved in 75%–95% alcohol or 50% isopropyl alcohol. The rest should be placed in a vial on top of a little damp tissue paper to prevent dehydration. If it will be more than a few hours before the entomologist receives them, they should also be given a small piece ($2-3\,cm^3$) of beef liver. Make sure there is tissue or sawdust present if liver is added to prevent drowning. Insects are air breathers and require ventilation. Newly emerged maggots can escape through tiny holes; therefore, the tradition of poking holes in the lid is not effective. A double layer of paper towel held over the top of the vial with a rubber band makes an excellent and secure lid, as long as the vial stays upright. No lid other than the paper towel is needed.

If the *only* insect evidence on the animal is eggs, then these are extremely important and can age the death or colonization time to a matter of hours. In such a case, however, the time of eclosion or hatch of the eggs is very important. The collector should therefore observe the live eggs periodically (every one to two hours) for evidence of hatch. This is easy to see with the naked eye because although the newly eclosed larvae are almost as small as the eggs, they are more translucent and are mobile. The observer should rate the hatch as zero hatch, 5% hatch, 30% hatch, etc. If the eggs are not observed and simply shipped to an entomologist, they will hatch in transit and most of useful data will be lost.

If larvae or maggots are present on the animal then the larvae will be older than the eggs and it is much less imperative to collect and observe the eggs. If the eggs are of a different species than the larvae, they may still be valuable because they may have a longer eclosion time. However, once the animal is well colonized with larger larvae present, there is no need to collect eggs.

Larvae or maggots

Maggots are found in large aggregations or masses on the animal or crawling on or near the remains. The maggot masses generate a lot of heat which speeds up development. Therefore, it is important for collectors to note the site and temperature of each maggot mass. Digital thermometers can be acquired very cheaply at drug stores or in the cooking section of grocery stores. Caution must be used when taking the temperature because it is important not to create artifacts in the animal with the thermometer. Instead of thrusting the probe into the mass, the thermometer should be rested gently on top, while putting a little pressure on the probe from a finger. The roiling motion of the maggots will roll the thermometer to the center with less chance of tissue damage. If no thermometer is available, then the observer should estimate the size of the mass, such as size of a golf ball, baseball, football, etc.

Large maggots are usually older and are the most important, but smaller maggots may belong to a different species. Therefore, both large and smaller maggots should be collected, with the emphasis on larger maggots. Samples should be collected from different areas of the carcass and the surrounding area, keeping each sample separate. Older larvae in one area may suggest the presence of a wound or myiasis.

When collecting maggots, it is always important to search for the oldest. Therefore, once the animal itself has been examined and insects collected from the body, the next question is, have any of the larvae begun to move from the body? A search must then be made of the surrounding area so that a further collection can be made. If these wandering insects are missed, the entomologist will underestimate the length of time of colonization by up to several days.

As discussed, third instar larvae eventually leave the food source to find a suitable area in which to pupate (Figure 15.5). They may wander some distance from the carcass so the soil for a meter or two around the carcass should be carefully sifted. Some may burrow down into leaf litter, so the soil below and surrounding the carcass should be checked to a depth of several centimeters. If the remains were on a slope, the body fluids will seep downhill and insects will be found here, feeding on the fluids. This means that a very intensive search of the carcass and the surrounding area must be made to get the entire picture. If indoors, the carpet or flooring should be searched, with particular attention paid to areas underneath furniture, rugs or appliances, and edges of walls.

Maggots are prey for birds and vertebrate scavengers so in the larval stage, they naturally move away from the light

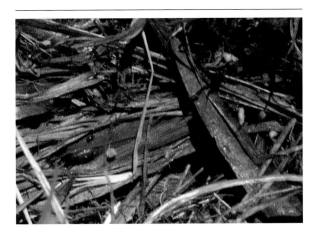

Figure 15.5 Migrating larvae (right aspect) and single puparium (left).

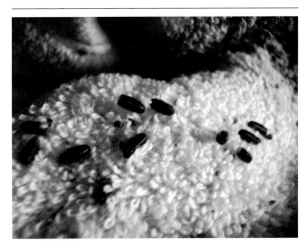

Figure 15.6 Pupae, pupa casings, and ecdysial caps.

(negatively phototropic). Hence, if they have already left the remains, they will usually be found under some form of protective covering and this must be considered when searching for prepupal larvae. The distance migrating larvae will travel before pupating depends on many biotic and abiotic factors, but it is particularly governed by species and substrate type (Greenberg 1990, Kocarek 2001, de Andrade et al. 2002, Anderson 2011). Even in a species that would normally pupate close to the carrion, if the substrate is not suitable, such as concrete or linoleum, they will continue to move until they reach a more protective substrate such as soil or under a rug.

When each exhibit is collected, a proportion of the larvae should be preserved immediately for two reasons. The first reason is to show the entomologist, if he or she is not present at the scene, what stage the larvae were at when collected, because if they are kept alive they will continue to develop, giving a misleading impression to the entomologist when they are examined. Secondly, preserving these insects allows them to be presented in court as an exhibit or given to another entomologist for a second opinion if requested by opposing counsel.

In most cases, approximately half of each exhibit should be preserved. The specimens should be preserved by first immersing them in very hot but not boiling water to destroy their internal enzymes, then draining and placing them in 70%–95% alcohol. If hot water is not available, then they should be immediately placed in alcohol, but without the hot water immersion they do not preserve as well. Formaldehyde or formalin should be avoided due to poor preservation and health risks (Amendt et al. 2007). A good sample from each site should contain approximately 100 maggots. If only very few maggots are available, then at least 10% should be preserved.

The other half of each sample must be kept alive so that they can be raised to adulthood for ease of identification and also to indicate the length of time needed to complete development in controlled conditions. The living specimens should be placed in a vial, with air and food, as for eggs. Plastic urinalysis vials are best because they do not break in transit or at a scene, are lightweight and sterile, and many come with an attached label. A damp piece of paper towel should be placed in the bottom to allow some moisture, and to wick away damp body fluids from the maggots that could otherwise drown them. This also provides topography to increase surface area of the vial, allowing more maggots to survive. There should be only enough maggots to cover the bottom of the vial. Too many in one vial will drown.

The live larvae need to be fed so a small piece (approximately 2–3 cm^3) of meat such as beef liver should be added to each vial. The larvae also need air, so discard the supplied lid and instead cover the vial with two layers of dry paper towel secured with an elastic band. This prevents escape but allows adequate ventilation.

Pupae and pupal cases

Pupae and empty puparia or pupal cases are extremely important and are easy to miss. They are often found in fur or in the soil or bedding near the carcass (Figure 15.6). They may be in or under carpet or other material in the home or kennel. When larvae are searching for a good location to pupate, they look for dry, secure areas away from the wet food source (the animal) in which to pupate. They range from 10–20 mm, and are oval, like a football.

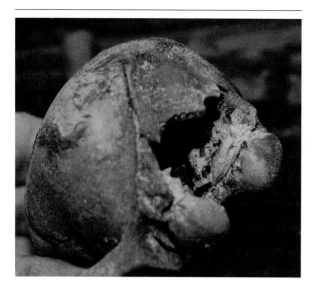

Figure 15.7 Insect evidence inside a dog skull.

They are pale and whitish when first beginning to pupate but are dark brown when completely tanned.

Once the insect has metamorphosed into an adult fly, it breaks open the end of the hardened case using a hemolymph or blood-filled sac to push off the tip of the puparium (Erzinclioglu 1996). It then emerges and moves away to expand and then dry and harden its out covering or cuticle. This is much the same as is seen in butterflies when they emerge from the chrysalis. The empty puparia or pupal case is left behind as evidence that the entire blow fly life cycle has taken place and is valuable evidence in estimating the minimum length of tenure of insects on the carcass. The puparia are made of heavy chitin so they are extremely durable and can be found years, decades, and longer after the fly has emerged (Figure 15.7) (Teskey and Turnbull 1979).

When insects are collected in the pupal stage it is very simple to allow the flies to emerge naturally as long as they are kept alive, and then the adult is easy to identify morphologically. Therefore, all pupae should be kept alive. This is different than with maggots because if some maggots are not preserved, they will change during transit to the entomologist. However, although pupae may change in transit by emerging as adult flies in the vial, the development can still be shown because both adult fly and empty puparium are present. Therefore, it is best not to preserve pupae because it makes them extremely difficult to identify, since pupae have very few distinguishing features.

Pupae may be found anywhere in the area surrounding the carcass and in the same areas as wandering or non-feeding third instar larvae. Therefore, the substrate should be searched all around the carcass, paying particular attention to soil and the underside of carpets, furniture, bedding, etc. Pupae should be collected and placed in a urinalysis vial with some damp paper towel. They are extremely fragile so this will help protect them during transit. They do not need food but do require air, so again, the vial should be covered with two layers of paper towel and secured with an elastic band. If a pupa is found when it is still a pale color, it is just entering pupation, so such specimens should be kept separate, photographed, and labeled as pale colored, because they will darken in a few hours. Such a specimen can be aged to a matter of hours.

An empty pupal case appears very similar to a live pupa in its puparium but is open at one end, where the adult fly has emerged. Although pupal cases are difficult to identify in most cases, when the operculum or tip of the case is broken off by the emerging fly, it breaks into two small parts called ecdysial caps. Just about the only pieces of the larva which are not reincorporated into the adult fly are the previously hardened areas such as the spiracular slits which are still seen in the empty pupal case, the anterior respiratory horn, and the mouthparts of the larva. The mouthparts are found attached to one of the ecdysial caps and the anterior respiratory horn on the other. The mouthparts in particular can be very helpful in identifying the species so these tiny bits of chitin should be searched for very close to, or sometimes still attached to, the empty puparia.

Empty pupal cases are not alive but are still extremely valuable in interpreting time frame. They should be collected as for pupae, with some paper towel to cushion them, but no air is required and the original screw lid can be applied.

Adult blow flies

Adult blow flies are extremely difficult to catch but fortunately have very little forensic value because there are equal chances that they have just emerged from the remains or just flown in. Therefore, when large adult, flying, metallic flies are seen buzzing around the carcass, they have little value and can be ignored because an entomologist cannot associate them with the carcass. However, if the flies have just emerged, they are of value because they cannot yet fly and therefore are intricately associated with the scene. Such flies are referred to as teneral and they appear crumpled, small, damp, and khaki colored and they make rapid scuttling movements. They often perch on nearby vegetation or furniture in an effort to dry their wings and bodies. Such flies should be collected and kept alive in a vial. The lid can be screwed on or paper towel used. The air

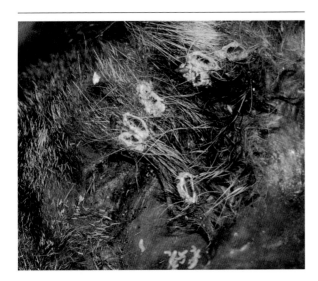

Figure 15.8 Multiple species and life cycle stages on a deceased animal.

in the vial is enough for them to continue to dry. Once dry they can be identified and can indicate minimum development times on the remains.

Collection of insects other than blow flies

If the animal has been dead for a few weeks, later successional species will also be found. Other insects found on or near the remains include larvae, pupae, puparia, and adults of other species of Diptera or true flies; and larvae (or grubs), cast larval skins, pupae, puparia and adult Coleoptera or beetles (Figure 15.8). In these cases, it is the presence or absence of each species and whether it is an adult or immature insect that is most important rather, than the very specific developmental cycle of the blow fly. Therefore, immature and adult specimens of other Diptera and of Coleoptera can be placed directly into alcohol. If desired, some immature Diptera can be kept alive on damp paper towel in a vial as for blow flies but they are much harder to feed because they require the material to be at a certain level of decomposition, as opposed to blow flies which require only fresh food. A small portion of tissue from the carcass can be used for this.

Any pupae of either flies or beetles should be kept alive as described for blow flies to allow emergence. Both adult flies and beetles are valuable. Living beetles should not be kept together or with other evidence because many are predators and will eat other evidence. Small adult flies can be picked up using a small paintbrush dipped in alcohol and just touching the fly. The brush will pick it up so it can be placed in alcohol in a vial.

It is simplest to prepare a vial of alcohol and simply drop any beetle evidence into it rather than collecting each insect separately. Beetles are found under and around a carcass and move quickly, so the investigator must be prepared to catch them when the carcass is moved.

Collection of blow fly evidence from a live animal

Although the evidence collected from a live animal is the same as that described above, the actual collection needs to be quite different for the health of the animal. If only eggs are present, these can be easily collected by simply combing them out of the animal's coat. However, if maggots are present they should be collected by a veterinarian because if a maggot is accidentally broken while still in the wound, it can result in anaphylaxis or protein shock and even death. Therefore, only a trained professional should carefully flush the maggots out for collection.

When insects on a living animal reach the non-feeding stage of the third instar, they wander away from the actual feeding site, often making it appear as if the animal is literally dripping with maggots and in much worse condition than a full appraisal will show. Caution should be exercised to ensure the living animal is fully examined to determine the actual extent of the colonization. The wandering behavior also means that the insect evidence could be lost anywhere as the animal moves around. To recover these wandering third instar larvae and subsequent developmental stages such as pupae, the best area to search is the place where the animal sleeps because larvae may have left the animal during this time frame. Thus, a careful search of bedding is warranted.

Photographs and videography

Photographs and/or a video of the scene, the carcass *in situ*, and the site after removal of the carcass are extremely useful.

Labeling

In all cases, each vial must be carefully labeled using a pencil or alcohol-proof permanent pen with the time and date of collection, file number, name of collector, area of carcass or scene, and the stage collected.

Handling

Most specimens are fairly fragile and are best picked up with gloved fingers or forceps. Very tiny or delicate specimens can be picked up using an artist's brush dipped in water or alcohol depending on what the investigator is about to do with them. Make sure all the vials are very well sealed.

Packaging

The insects should be taken to the entomologist as soon as possible. It is important to contact the entomologist first so he or she is expecting the case. The insects should be couriered or hand delivered to maintain continuity of evidence. They should be packaged in a cardboard box because it provides lots of air. Each vial can be taped so that it remains upright. The whole box must remain upright throughout transit.

Other samples

Soil and leaf litter samples are also useful. About a coffee can size of soil from under or very near the carcass is valuable. If the soil below the carcass is extremely wet, it is better to collect the soil from near the remains. The can should only be half-full of soil to allow room for air. The entomologist can examine this more carefully in the lab for smaller insects.

Other required information

The entomologist will want to know many things about the animal and the scene. Useful information about the remains includes:

- Was the carcass wrapped, buried, or covered? If so with what, and how deep?
- What is the cause of death?
- Are wounds present? In particular, is there blood at the scene?
- Are poisons or pesticides suspected to be involved? If so, a toxicology report should be submitted to the entomologist when complete.
- What position is the carcass in?
- What were the animal's living conditions?
- What is the state of decomposition?
- Are there maggot masses present? How many and how big?
- What is the temperature of the center of the maggot mass(es)?
- Is there any other meat or carrion around that might also attract insects?
- Is there a possibility that death did not occur at the present site?

Useful information about the scene includes:

- Were the remains found inside a residence or structure or outside? Describe the scene. If inside, describe the house, provide photos.
- If outside, is the scene forested, open grassland?
- What types of vegetation are present? Are there trees, grass, bushes, shrubs?
- Is the soil type rocky, sandy, muddy?

- What was the weather like at the time of collection? Sunny, cloudy?
- What were the temperature and possibly humidity at collection time?
- What are the elevation and map coordinates of the death site?
- Is the site in shade or direct sunlight?
- Finally, mention anything unusual, such as whether it is possible that the carcass may have been submerged at any time.

SUMMARY

Insects can provide valuable evidence in an animal cruelty investigation, just as they currently do in homicide investigations. As in human cases, their primary value lies in indicating a minimum elapsed time since death which can help support or refute a suspect's alibi and assist investigators in determining a timeline. In addition, insect evidence can be used as toxicological specimens, to indicate the presence of a wound site, to suggest whether a carcass has been relocated, and to identify the animal used as a substrate using DNA. Their collection is very straightforward and is likely to only add a few minutes to the investigation time, but may provide very powerful evidence in court.

REFERENCES

Amendt, J., C.P. Campobasso, E. Gaudry, C. Reiter, H.N. LeBlanc and M.J. Hall. 2007. Best Practice in Forensic Entomology—Standards and Guidelines. *International Journal of Legal Medicine.* 121(2):90–104.

Amendt, J., M.L. Goff. 2010. *Current Concepts in Forensic Entomology*, C.P. Campobasso and M. Grassberger, eds. Dordrecht: Springer.

Anderson, G.S. 1999. Wildlife Forensic Entomology: Determining Time of Death in Two Illegally Killed Black Bear Cubs, a Case Report. *Journal of Forensic Sciences.* 44(4):856–859.

Anderson, G.S. 2000. Minimum and Maximum Developmental Rates of Some Forensically Significant Calliphoridae (Diptera). *Journal of Forensic Sciences.* 45(4):824–832.

Anderson, G.S. 2010. Factors That Influence Insect Succession on Carrion. In: *Forensic Entomology: The Utility Of Arthropods In Legal Investigations*, Second edition, J. Byrd and E. Castner, eds. pp 201–250. Boca Raton: CRC Press.

Anderson, G.S. 2011. Comparison of Decomposition Rates and Faunal Colonization of Carrion in Indoor and Outdoor Environments. *Journal of Forensic Sciences.* 56(1):136–142.

Anderson, G.S. and V.J. Cervenka. 2001. Insects Associated with the Body: Their Use and Analyses. In: *Advances in Forensic Taphonomy. Methods, Theory and Archeological Perspectives*, W. Haglund and M. Sorg, eds. pp. 174–200. Boca Raton: CRC Press.

Anderson, G.S. and N.R. Huitson. 2004. Myiasis in Pet Animals in British Columbia: The Potential of Forensic Entomology for Determining Duration of Possible Neglect. *Canadian Veterinary. Journal.* 45(12):993–998.

Anderson, G.S. and S.L. VanLaerhoven. 1996. Initial Studies on Insect Succession on Carrion in Southwestern British Columbia. *Journal of Forensic Sciences.* 41(4):617–625.

Benecke, M. 2004. Neglect of the Elderly: Forensic Entomology Cases and Considerations. *Forensic Sciences International.* 146:195–199.

Benecke, M. 2010. Cases of Neglect Involving Entomological Evidence. In: *Forensic Entomology: The Utility of Arthropods in Legal Investigations*, Second edition, J.H. Byrd and J.L. Castner, eds. pp. 627–635. Boca Raton: CRC Press.

Bourel, B., L. Fleurisse, V. Hédouin, J.C. Cailliez, C. Creusy, M.L. Goff, and D. Gosset. 2001. Immunohistochemical Contribution to the Study of Morphine Metabolism in Calliphoridae Larvae and Implications in Forensic Entomotoxicology. *Journal of Forensic Sciences.* 46(3):596–599.

Byrd, J.H. and J.L. Castner. 2010. *Forensic Entomology: The Utility of Arthropods in Legal Investigations.* Boca Raton: CRC Press.

Cheng, K. 1890, Reprinted 1985, cited in Greenberg and Kunich 2002. *Zhe yu gui jian bu [Additional Cases in the History of Chinese Trials] (English Translation).* Beijing: Chung-hua Shu Chu.

de Andrade, J.B., F.A. Rocha, P. Rodrigues, G.S. Rosa, L.D.B. Faria, C.J. Von Zuben, M.N. Rossi, and W.A.C. Godoy. 2002. Larval Dispersal and Predation in Experimental Populations of *Chrysomya albiceps* and *Cochliomyia macellaria* (Diptera: Calliphoridae). Memórias do Instituto *Oswaldo Cruz.* 97:1137–1140.

Erzinclioglu, Z. 1996. *Blowflies.* p. 71 Slough: Richmond Publishing Co. Ltd.

Gennard, D.E. 2007. *Forensic Entomology: An Introduction.* p. 224. Chichester: John Wiley and Sons Ltd.

Gilbert, B.M. and W.M. Bass. 1967. Seasonal Dating of Burials From the Presence of Fly Pupae. *American Antiquity.* 32(4):534–535.

Goff, M.L., S. Charbonneau, and W. Sullivan. 1991. Presence of Fecal Matter in Diapers as Potential Source of Error in Estimations of Postmortem Intervals Using Arthropod Development Patterns. *Journal of Forensic Sciences.* 36(5):1603–1606.

Goff, M.L. and W.D. Lord. 2009. Entomotoxicology. Insects as Toxicological Indicators and the Impact of Drugs and Toxins on Insect Development. In: *Forensic Entomology: The Utility of Arthropods In Legal Investigations*, J.H. Byrd and J.L. Castner, eds. pp. 427–436. Boca Raton: CRC Press.

Greenberg, B. 1990. Behaviour of Postfeeding Larvae of Some Calliphoridae and a Muscid (Diptera). *Annals of the Entomological Society of America.* 83(6):1210–1214.

Greenberg, B. and J.C. Kunich. 2002. *Entomology and the Law: Flies as Forensic Indicators.* p. 306. Cambridge: University Press.

Haskell, N.H. and R.E. Williams. 2008. *Entomology and Death: A Procedural Guide.* p. 216. Clemson: East Park Printing.

Kocarek, P. 2001. Diurnal Patterns of Postfeeding Larval Dispersal in Carrion Blowflies (Diptera: Calliphoridae). *European Journal of Entomology.* 98:117–119.

LaGoo, L., L.S. Schaeffer, D.W. Szymanski, and R.W. Smith. 2010. Detection of Gunshot Residue in Blowfly Larvae and Decomposing Porcine Tissue Using Inductively Coupled Plasma Mass Spectrometry (ICP-MS). *Journal of Forensic Sciences.* 55(3):624–632.

Linville, J.G., J. Hayes, and J.D. Wells. 2004. Mitochondrial DNA and STR Analyses of Maggot Crop Contents: Effect of Specimen Preservation Technique. *Journal of Forensic Sciences.* 49(2):341–344.

Magni, P., M. Massinelli, R. Messina, P. Mazzuco, and E. Di Luise. 2008. *Entomologia Forense: Gli insettis nelle indagini giudiziarie e medcio-legali.* Torino: Edizioni Minerva Medica.

McIntosh, M.D., R.W. Merritt, R.E. Kolar, and R.K. Kimbirauskas. 2011. Effectiveness of Wound Cleansing Treatments on Maggot (Diptera, Calliphoridae) Mortality. *Forensic Science International.* 210(1–3):12–15.

Meyer, J.A. and B.A. Mullens. 1988. Development of Immature *Fannia* spp. (Diptera: Muscidae) at Constant Laboratory Temperatures. *Journal of Medical Entomology.* 25(3):165–177.

Miller, M.L., W.D. Lord, M.L. Goff, B. Donnelly, E.T. McDonough, and J.C. Alexis. 1994. Isolation of Amitriptyline and Nortriptyline from Fly Puparia (Phoridae) and Beetle Exuviae (Dermestidae) Associated with Mummified Remains. *Journal of Forensic Sciences.* 39(5):1305–1313.

Nuorteva, P. and S.L. Nuorteva. 1982. The Fate of Mercury in Sarcosapropahgous Flies and in Insects Eating Them. *Ambio.* 11(1): 34–37.

Roeterdink, E.M., I.R. Dadour, and R.J. Watling. 2004. Extraction of Gunshot Residues from the Larvae of the Forensically Important Blowfly *Calliphora dubia* (Macquart) (Diptera: Calliphoridae). *International Journal of Legal Medicine.* 118(2):63–70.

Sherman, R.A., M.J.R. Hall, and S. Thomas. 2000. Medicinal Maggots: an Ancient Remedy for Some Contemporary Afflictions. *Annual Review of Entomology.* 45:55–81.

Sherman, R.A., H. Stevens, D. Ng, and E. Iversen. 2007. Treating Wounds in Small Animals with Maggot Debridement therapy: A Survey of Practitioners. *Veterinary Journal.* 173:140–145.

Smith, K.G.V. 1986. *A Manual of Forensic Entomology.* p. 205. London: Trustees of The British Museum (Nat. Hist.) and Cornell University Press.

Stuyt, M., R. Ursic-Bedoya, D. Cooper, N. Huitson, G.S. Anderson, and C. Lowenberger. 2010. Identification of Host Material from Crops and Whole Bodies of *Protophormia terraenovae* (R-D) (Diptera) Larvae, Pupae, and Adults, and the Implications for Forensic Studies. *Canadian Society of Forensic Society Journal.* 43(3):97–110.

Teskey, H.H. and C. Turnbull. 1979. Diptera puparia from Pre-Historic Graves. *Canadian Entomology.* 111:527–528.

Wells, J.D., F.G. Introna, G. Di Vella, C.P. Campobasso, J. Hayes, and F.A.H. Sperling. 2001. Human and Insect Mitochondrial DNA Analysis from Maggots. *Journal of Forensic Sciences.* 46(3): 685–687.

Wells, J.D. and J. Stevens. 2010. Molecular Methods for Forensic Entomology. In: *Forensic Entomology: The Utility of Arthropods In Legal Investigations*, J.H. Byrd and J.L. Castner, eds. pp. 437–452. Boca Raton: CRC Press.

16
Large Animal Cruelty

Dana M. Miller and Melinda D. Merck

I keep six honest serving men
(They taught me all I knew);
Their names are What and Why and When
And How and Where and Who
                Rudyard Kipling (1865–1936)

INTRODUCTION

As with the investigation of any allegation of animal cruelty, it is necessary to be familiar with both the species and the alleged crime being investigated. Livestock species may present particular challenges for investigators for many reasons. Most animal control agencies focus on companion animals resulting in a significant disparity of knowledge between species groups. As a result, complaints regarding livestock are often at least initially investigated by officers who have little training specific to the species involved. Unfortunately, the individuals making the initial determination of the presence or absence of an offense may have a limited understanding of the requirements for a particular species or for what constitutes normal.

The investigation of cruelty involving livestock species is further complicated by the animal cruelty laws themselves. Nearly every state has an exemption in their animal cruelty statute for either "accepted" or "customary" agricultural practices. This exemption places an increased burden on investigators requiring they not only be familiar with the species but also with those practices that would be considered customary or accepted. Some U.S. states, such as Iowa (§717.1 to §717.7) and Virginia (§3.2-6503.1), have entirely different code sections for cruelty or neglect toward companion animals and those considered livestock

species. Still other states, such as Louisiana (§102.1) and South Carolina (§47-1-40(C)), exempt particular species (those described as "fowl") from their animal cruelty laws, leaving these animals with little protection under the law.

The initial screening of complaints is typically conducted by non-veterinary personnel such as animal control officers, humane investigators, or law enforcement officers. However, because of the complexity of investigating livestock cruelty cases, officers, especially those not familiar with livestock, are encouraged to work with an experienced veterinarian before forming a conclusion of whether cruelty is present and how it should be charged. Other times, veterinarians may be called to properties at which clear indicators of animal cruelty exist (either due to a recent visit to the client by animal control or for other reasons). In these cases, the veterinarian may have either an ethical or legal obligation to report such cruelty (Chapter 1). The initial "investigator" then may be either a humane law enforcement officer or a veterinarian. To be most effective, the investigator is more aptly an investigatory team with multiple members contributing information from their area of focus and expertise. Ideally, this team is comprised of a humane law enforcement officer, an experienced veterinarian, and additional appropriate members such as a qualified farrier, nutritionist, extension agent, entomologist, etc.

ASSESSING PAIN AND SUFFERING

The ability to assess pain and suffering is of critical importance to veterinary forensic medicine. Nearly every state's animal cruelty statutes include a provision wherein the infliction of pain or suffering directly constitutes

Veterinary Forensics: Animal Cruelty Investigations, Second Edition. Edited by Melinda D. Merck.
© 2013 John Wiley & Sons, Inc. Published 2013 by John Wiley & Sons, Inc.

Table 16.1 Indicators of pain.

Positive behavioral signs	Negative behavioral signs	Physiological responses
Kicking (at painful areas or in response to manipulation)	Social isolation from flock or herd	Increased heart rate
Pawing/foot stamping	Depression/dull appearance	Increased respiratory rate
Biting/chewing	Reluctance to move	Increased blood pressure
Tail flicking/tail clamping	Passive immobility (poultry)	Sweating
Lameness/abnormal gait	Inappetance/weight loss	Decreased production
Bruxism (tooth grinding)		Pupillary dilation
Vocalization (bawling, pleating, grunting, etc.)		Increase in rectal temperature
Head pressing		Changes in gastric sounds (horse)
Restlessness/agitation		
Changes in facial expression		
Aggression		

animal cruelty. Often, the determination of pain and suffering in livestock species is complicated by the individual investigator or the court's perception of the ability of livestock to experience pain.

The lack of an animal's ability to experience pain is a frequently asserted defense to animal cruelty, particularly in cases involving livestock victims. This assertion is not consistent with the scientific literature or accepted standards within veterinary medicine (Chapter 4). Defendants or defense counsel often make analogies to surgical procedures that are performed during the course of production for which analgesics are not regularly provided, claiming that it demonstrates a lack of pain perception. Despite the American Veterinary Medical Association's (AVMA) position that pain and suffering are clinically important conditions (AVMA 2011) and the policy that animals "should be cared for in ways that minimize fear, pain, stress, and suffering" (AVMA 2006), analgesic use in livestock for pain management remains underutilized.

Numerous studies have been conducted documenting pain which results from routine surgical procedures used in livestock; yet a recent survey of Canadian veterinarians found disparate use of analgesics for known painful procedures performed on cattle, pigs, and horses (Hewson et al. 2007). The use of analgesics by veterinarians in that study varied significantly based on both the species and age of the animal undergoing the procedure. Interestingly, when the degree of pain experienced by the animal during a particular procedure was rated by responding veterinarians, the numeric scoring remained relatively consistent among all species rated (Hewson et al. 2007). That study concluded that the differences in the use of analgesics during surgical procedures between species groups were

more likely related to other factors in the particular industry segment such as the economic value of the animals, drug cost, and availability of drugs rather than the degree of pain experienced by the animal.

It is important to recognize that the lack of use of analgesics in a particular species group for veterinary procedures should not be construed as evidence of a lack of pain experienced by those animals, when numerous studies have consistently found that they do experience pain. Rather, studies such as these can be useful in determining whether specific practices should be considered customary or accepted husbandry practices. From an evolutionary perspective, the exhibition of any physiologic dysfunction by animals can have a significant disadvantage for survival, especially for prey species. As a result, most of our common agriculture species have adapted to conceal pain associated with any type of dysfunction, making it difficult to recognize pain.

Pain can be difficult to recognize in many agricultural species though with training there are many behavioral and physiological indicators of both acute and chronic pain (Underwood 2002). While the signs of pain vary between species and individuals within a species there are many commonalities between livestock species (Table 16.1).

INVESTIGATION OF CRUELTY

Like animal cruelty involving companion animals, cruelty toward livestock can take many forms and can either be acts of commission or omission. While heinous cruelty through acts of commission are often more likely to be prosecuted, acts of omission, such as neglect, occur far more frequently. Often neglect arises when well-intentioned people obtain animals without the adequate knowledge or finances to care for them properly. The specific husbandry requirements of livestock make this even more likely to occur with these species. Despite an individual's intentions and regardless of the species involved, neglect can result in profound suffering.

The most frequent victims of animal cruelty resulting from neglect are those that are being kept for non-commercial purposes. As a generalization, animals kept for their production value are less likely to be the victims of criminal neglect. This is partially due to the legal exemption for customary agricultural practices and partially due to financial motivation because prolonged neglect results in a decline in production.

Neglect of livestock can result from failure to provide appropriate feed, water, shelter, routine foot care, dental care, or other veterinary care. As with companion animals, embedded halters or neck collars can result when these items are placed on growing animals and then left for prolonged periods of time without adjustment. In all cases of neglect, it is important to document what would have been obvious to an owner and in what ways that level of care deviates from accepted husbandry standards. Specifically, one should note at what point an owner should have taken action and continued to fail to do so.

STARVATION

Starvation is one of the most prevalent types of cruelty resulting from neglect. Anecdotally horses and small ruminates (sheep and goats) appear to be the most common livestock victims of starvation. This is likely related to their desirability as pets rather than being kept solely for their economic benefit.

Regardless of the species, it is important to completely document environmental findings as they relate to husbandry assessment. The examination of the property should include the entire environment accessible to the animal(s) with particular attention paid to the type, quantity, and condition of feed material, and the presentation or availability to all the animals. Because most domestic livestock are herbivorous, particular attention should be paid to the species and condition of plants present. Starvation events in livestock can occur at any time of year, although there is often a seasonality associated with this type of cruelty based on the availability of forage material. Depending on the climate, plant growth can be greatly reduced either in the winter, summer, or both. During these periods it is important that owners of livestock supply supplemental forage (the plant material that makes up the bulk of the diet of herbivorous species). In cases in which animals are confined in a manner that prevents typical grazing or browsing behaviors, it becomes the responsibility of the owner to provide all the necessary feed required to maintain animals in a manner that promotes health.

In its simplest form, feed for large animals can be broken into the following types.

Forage

Forage is the common term for plant material consumed by grazing animals. It is commonly used to refer to growing plants or may be used as a broader term for all plant material consumed (including hay, silage, haylage, etc).

Hay

Hay is plant material that has been preserved for use as feed through drying. Generally, hay is fed to livestock during periods when there is inadequate live forage available in a pastured setting or when livestock is confined, preventing grazing. There is significant variability in the nutritional value of hay depending on the species, age, and handling of the plants during the preservation process.

Straw

Similar to hay, straw is plant material that has been preserved through drying. Generally, straw consists of the more fibrous stems of the plants once the seed heads have been removed for grain production. Straw has relatively low nutritional value and therefore has more limited usefulness as feed. Under certain circumstances, straw can be fed to increase the roughage in livestock diets without significantly increasing the energy content (as may be indicated for obese animals). Within the United States straw is also commonly used as bedding material.

Silage/haylage

Silage is a type of fermented forage containing a relatively high moisture content that is commonly fed to ruminant species (predominately cattle). Numerous plants can be used to make silage, and depending on the plants used, it may be either referred to as silage, haylage, or other names. Generally, the entire plant is chopped and then anaerobically fermented. During the fermentation process it takes on a characteristic odor that is often unpleasant to people not familiar with the product. Note: silage and haylage are rarely fed to horses in the United States.

Concentrates

Grains and pelleted feed comprise what are commonly considered concentrated feed for livestock due to the increased nutritional density compared to forage. The necessity and amount of concentrated feed varies based on the species and function of the animal. Concentrates are used in feeding programs in which animals require higher amounts of energy. In general, intensive livestock systems often incorporate higher amounts of concentrated feeds than less intensive pastured systems.

There is significant variation in the forage requirements of different species of livestock. Ruminants (such as cattle, sheep, and goats) have microorganisms in their gastrointestinal tract which aid them in the digestion of plants that have relatively high cellulose content. This enables them to derive energy from plants that non-ruminants cannot. Equines, which are hindgut fermenting species, have a more limited ability to derive energy from fully mature plants that are high in cellulose. As a result, plants that are suitable feed for cattle or goats are often not appropriate for horses. Because of these differences the investigator must be familiar with the plants and the dietary requirements of the particular animal species.

If the investigator is not familiar with forage identification, samples of all forage (common pasture plants, hay, and silage) should be collected at the time of investigation so that the quality and suitability as feed can be assessed later. Large animal veterinarians and agricultural extension agents can be helpful in identifying these plants and determining their suitability as food for the livestock species present. Forage samples should be preserved in paper bags rather than plastic or glass containers because the moisture content can cause the plant material to mold or rot.

While laboratory analysis of feed (especially hay and silage) is an integral part of optimizing feed plans for high-end production, it can unnecessarily complicate relatively straightforward starvation cases. If samples can be evaluated by someone with sufficient experience (such as a veterinarian, livestock nutritionist, or extension agent), they can be generally quantified as excellent, good, moderate, or poor quality forage without the additional expense of laboratory analysis. Forage that is wet, moldy, or otherwise spoiled can be classified as unsuitable for consumption. Where multiple bales of hay are present, samples should be taken from several bales whenever possible because there can be significant variation in quality between bales. Sampling hay from the center of bales, rather than just the outside, is more representative. Hay probes (a metallic coring device) can be useful to obtain samples from the center of the bale although hand sampling is generally considered acceptable. In cases where the plants themselves are not collected, numerous photographs should be taken of both the pasture plants and hay to be used later for identification.

Feeding methods

Specific husbandry systems dictate whether animals are being fed in a portion-controlled manner or ad libitum (with feed present at all times). Typically, agriculture systems in which animals are being prepared for humane slaughter and therefore in a rapid phase of growth, such as a feed lot, finisher operation, or broiler chicken production, are more likely to provide animals access to free choice feed. Other less intensive feeding operations, such as cow-calf operations or pasture-reared poultry, provide animals with the opportunity to forage for food over comparatively large areas. In these cases an increased emphasis is placed on the food that animals find growing naturally and supplemental feed may only be provided as necessary during periods in which natural food sources are scarce. There are many circumstances in which animals are maintained in management structures which do not involve access to free choice feed at all times. For example, the majority of horses are maintained in settings where concentrated feed is provided on a portion-controlled basis once or twice daily.

Forage can either be provided ad libitum in addition to concentrates or also in portion-controlled allotments.

Necropsy findings

The necropsy procedures for large animals are covered in Chapter 3. The findings of starvation are similar in both large and small animals (Chapter 11). The rumen normally accounts for approximately 25% of a healthy ruminant's live weight while in an underweight animal it may be higher. In sheep, the presence of moderate fluid in the rumen, which is normally relatively dry, is an indicator of starvation and not recent ingestion of water. The presence of food in the rumen of animals is not necessarily an indicator of adequate feeding and should be analyzed for nutritional value. Due to the slow digestion and passage of fibrous material in the rumen and intestines, wet, semi-solid digesta may be found in starved animals (Munro and Munro 2008a).

BODY CONDITION SCORING

Because of the large variety of production systems, the absence of food alone should not be construed to indicate that feed is not being offered. The use of body condition scoring provides an accepted scientific way to assess the nutritional status of individual animals and by extension, the historical provision of feed over a longer period of time.

All body condition scoring systems provide a mechanism for evaluation of the amount of fat and muscle present in the animal being assessed. Each system is specific to the species of animal being evaluated, although there are many commonalities to all systems. Each scoring system provides a numerical score that represents the physical condition of the animal. These are most commonly provided on a basis of either 1–5 or 1–9 where 1 is emaciated and 5 or 9 represents an obese animal. (The most notable difference to this is the Tufts Animal Care and Condition score frequently used for dogs, in which 1 represents an animal deemed in adequate condition and 5 represents an emaciated animal.) By matter of convention, within the United States horses and beef cattle are scored on a 9-point scale whereas dairy cattle, sheep, goats, and swine are scored on a 5-point scale (see Chapter 17 for poultry and Appendix 37 for large animal resources).

The majority of body condition scoring systems were developed for the production setting where they provide producers an objective means to evaluate their nutritional programs. In true production settings there is a significant emphasis in keeping animals at a specific body condition appropriate for their production purposes. For example, the ideal condition at the time of breeding is generally lower than the ideal condition just before parturition (giving birth). Animals that are either over conditioned (too fat) or under conditioned (too thin) have reduced productivity (reduced conception rates, more difficulty giving birth, or reduced lactation). Therefore, familiarity with body condition scoring and the reported production goals can provide the investigator with valuable information about the producer not only in terms of evaluating their feeding program, but also with regard to their adherence to accepted husbandry standards.

There are a limited number of explanations for animals found to be in poor (emaciated) body condition. Either the animals have not been provided with adequate feed (because of the quality, quantity, or presentation of such feed) or a medical condition exists which has prevented the utilization of such feed or is causing inappetance. In starvation, the atrophy of muscle masses begins at twenty-four hours for monogastric animals, slightly longer in calves and lambs, and for adult ruminants it can be delayed for three days (Munro and Munro 2008a). The role of the investigator, usually along with the veterinarian, is then to determine which of those possible causes is responsible for the condition.

Animals that are found to be in poor body condition should receive feed with increased frequency to promote weight gain. When owners notice a decline in body condition despite increased feeding attempts, they have a responsibility to seek veterinary advice to determine the cause of the malnutrition. Johnes disease, bovine leukosis, advanced neoplasia, severe dental disease, and many other causes can all lead to emaciation. Investigators should look both for evidence of veterinary care as well as attempts to feed for weight gain, i.e., with more access to feed than would be observed during a maintenance period.

EVALUATION OF WATER

A good source of fresh, clean water is important for any animal, including all livestock species. Dirty or contaminated water can discourage animals from drinking adequate amounts as well as pose a significant hazard to the health of the animals drinking it. While natural sources of water are often used for livestock they pose significant challenges for the producer. Temperature extremes can make the provision of fresh water through natural sources more difficult; however, this seasonal variation is to be expected and prepared for rather than used as an excuse for failure to provide potable water during the winter or during droughts.

An evaluation of the water source should always be made during any investigation of neglect. The water should be evaluated for its cleanliness and potability. Any obvious sources of contamination should be recorded including excessive manure, deceased animals, and trash. In addition, excessive algae, mud, or other debris also should be recorded because they can impact the suitability of water. The investigator should measure or at least estimate the distance between feed sources, shelter, and water. Long distances between these necessary elements of care can increase metabolic demands on animals. When animals have to range over long distances to meet their basic care requirements, it increases the caloric needs of the animal and can reduce the feed intake during excessively hot or cold periods. Therefore, the distance between the primary water source, feed, and shelter should be recorded as part of any investigation of neglect.

Finally, in cases where automatic watering systems are present, their functionality should always be assessed. If samples are being taken to evaluate for bacterial contamination, it is important to chill or refrigerate samples for transport and get them to the laboratory for analysis as quickly as possible.

HOOF CARE

The significance of hoof care varies with species, and while hoof care is most important for horses and small ruminants, it cannot be neglected without consequence in any livestock species. The hoof is a functional modification which forms the foot of the animal. It is comprised of a tough keratinized outer wall and a somewhat softer sole. Essentially, the hoof is a functional modification of the toenail/fingernail which has been adapted to form the weight-bearing surface.

Equids (including horses, donkeys, and mules) have a single digit or hoof on each leg. Even-toed ungulates (cattle, sheep, goats, and pigs) each have two weight-bearing hooves on each leg, commonly referred to as claws, with two smaller non-weight-bearing digits, referred to as dewclaws. Like the nails on humans, the hoof is a living structure comprised of both sensitive and insensitive tissues. The outermost keratinized layer, called the hoof capsule, grows continuously downward, originating from the point of attachment to the leg; this is known as the coronary band. The hoof capsule attaches to the deeper more sensitive structures through a series of interdigitating laminae. In the center of each hoof or claw is the terminal bone of the limb known as the "distal phalanx," "P3," or "coffin bone." The sensitive and insensitive laminae interlock similar to interlacing fingers and provide the mechanism for which force is transmitted to the bony column and up the limb. Because of this mechanism, changes in the shape of the outer hoof can be felt by the animal even though the keratinized hoof is insensitive. Ultimately, the force that is transmitted can affect the bones upwards in the limb.

Hoof care in horses

Horse hooves are commonly accepted to grow at a rate of approximately 1 cm (or 3/8 inch) per month. As a result, a typical domestic horse requires hoof trimming on a regular basis to maintain proper alignment of the hoof and leg. The actual rate of growth for a particular horse is highly dependent on many factors including individual genetics, nutrition, and season. Therefore, while average horses require trimming of their hooves approximately every six weeks some horses may require trimming every four to ten weeks.

Maintaining proper balance of the hoof and equine leg through trimming and, when necessary, shoeing is typically done by a person known as a farrier. This profession requires a specialized skill set with knowledge of equine anatomy, physiology, and medicine. Additionally, a qualified farrier also requires knowledge of metal working (to fabricate, adjust, and apply shoes as needed) and physics (to understand the effect of various forces applied to the limb).

In the United Kingdom there is generally a greater recognition of the suffering that can result from unskilled persons attempting to shoe horses and as a result there are laws that prevent non-registered persons from practicing farriery. Unfortunately, in the United States there is no such specialized training required to practice farriery. There are, however, multiple professional organizations of farriers within the United States designed to provide a standard of professional competence. The largest such organization is the American Farrier's Association which

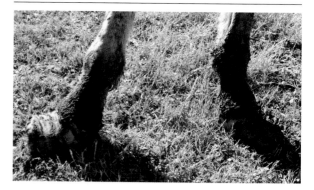

Figure 16.1 Severely overgrown rear hooves of a horse demonstrating the impact that this condition has on the angles of the joints upward in the limb. Prolonged neglect of necessary hoof trimming has caused both hooves to deviate laterally (to the outside) resulting in the horse walking on the medial hoof wall. Although this horse received proper farrier care following seizure, it continued to have chronic lameness issues, achieving only pasture soundness.

provides multiple levels of certification. Whenever possible, cases involving equine neglect of the feet should include not only a veterinarian but also a qualified farrier, preferably a certified farrier, for the evaluation, treatment, and court testimony.

When hoof care is neglected for prolonged periods of time, the overgrowth of the hoof capsule places an increased amount of strain on the laminae and transmits the forces upwards in the limb. Frequently severe overgrowth is combined with chronic laminitis (inflammation of the laminae) and can result in an "elf-shoe" appearance of the hoof. Depending on the conformation of an individual animal, the overgrowth of the hoof capsule can twist the limb in any direction (Figures 16.1, 16.2a, and 16.2b). In some circumstances, the hoof capsule can curve inward rather than flaring outward. When this occurs it may only be visible if the foot is picked up and viewed from the bottom (Figures 16.3a and 16.3b). Eventually, if hoof overgrowth or imbalance are allowed to continue, the upward transmission of force can cause repetitive microtrauma to the articular surfaces of the joints. This then leads to the development of osteoarthritis or degenerative joint disease which is ultimately irreversible and painful.

Unfortunately, overgrowth of the hoof wall is not always apparent without picking up the foot. It is important for the investigator to remember that husbandry conditions such as mud or tall grass can obscure visualization of even

(a)

(b)

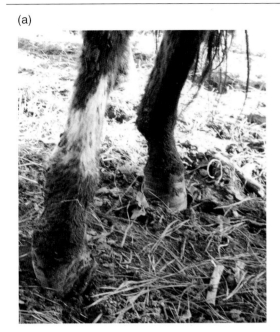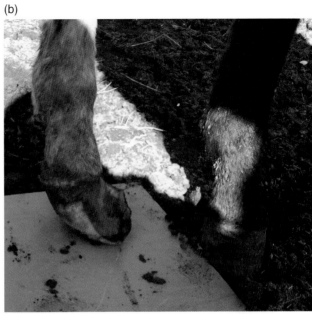

Figure 16.2 Severely neglected rear hooves shown without (a) and with (b) the aid of a plywood board. Note that in this case the hoof was deviated medially (to the inside).

significant abnormalities. When these conditions are present, animals should be removed from their enclosures and carefully evaluated. Small sections of quarter- or half-inch plywood can easily be painted a medium blue tone to provide a cheap portable surface that horses can be made to stand on to make photographic documentation of these conditions more obvious (Figures 16.2a and b and 16.3a and b). When present, both osteoarthritis and laminitis should always be considered significantly painful and animals should receive appropriate analgesics as part of their treatment course. Studies have concluded that the inability to alleviate the "unrelenting and severe pain" associated with these diseases is the leading cause of euthanasia in the laminitic horse (Collins et al. 2010).

Hoof care in ruminants

Although ruminants generally require less frequent trimming of the hooves, proper hoof care remains important. When cattle walk, the lateral (outside) claw is most prone to damage and irritation. This damage stimulates growth of the keratinized horny layer which shifts an increased portion of weight to the inner claw. If the feet are left untrimmed, this ultimately results in lameness and pain. As a result, 92% of lameness in cattle involves the rear feet and of those, 68% affects the outside claw (Stull 2004).

The foundation of good foot care begins with appropriate shelter. Avoiding unnecessary exposure of animals to sharp rocks or trash, muddy ground, and broken concrete can help to reduce the occurrence of foot abnormalities. Additionally, the regular use of properly maintained footbaths can help prevent many infectious causes of hoof disease. Within the dairy industry, good production standards dictate that cows should be observed regularly for lameness and gait abnormalities. These abnormalities have been shown to decrease cow productivity because of reduced feed intake, milk production, and fertility (Green et al. 2002). Several scoring systems have been developed for the use in cattle to look at factors such as back posture while standing and moving, head bobbing, symmetry of gait, and reluctance to bear weight (Appendix 37). It is recommended that cattle be observed regularly and that thorough examination and trimming be provided when cows show early signs of lameness (such as arched back posture) to prevent more serious and painful conditions (Stull 2004).

Hoof care in small ruminants

Small ruminants such as sheep and goats typically wear their hooves naturally if they are ranging over abrasive surfaces. If these animals are kept on soft ground, however, they generally require trimming of their hooves every few months. The outer hoof wall should be trimmed to prevent

(a)   (b)

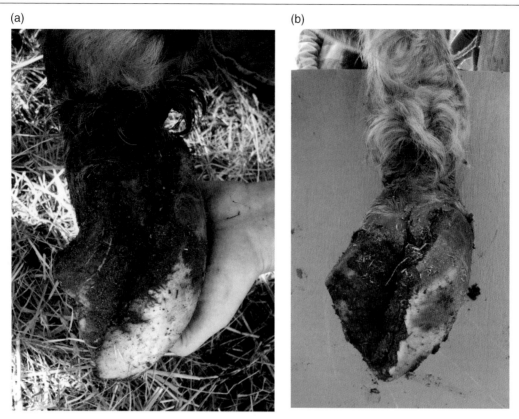

Figure 16.3 Severely neglected hooves shown without (a) and with (b) the aid of a plywood board. Note these are the same hooves in Figure 16.2; however, viewing them from the underside provides a much more complete picture of the abnormalities.

it from extending past the sole of the foot to prevent it from forming a flap which can trap moisture and bacterial and fungal organisms which can lead to disease.

DENTAL CARE

One of the most significant differences between domestic livestock species and companion animals (and humans) is that of dental structure. As an adaptation to their relatively fibrous diet, equines and ruminants both have developed teeth referred to as hypsodont or high crowned. Unlike the brachyodont (or low crowned teeth) that primates, carnivores, and pigs have, the hypsodont teeth erupt continuously throughout the animals' life. As a result of this continuous growth, the occlusion of equine and ruminant teeth changes throughout their lives. Failure to provide appropriate dental care is an important cause of starvation and malnutrition, particularly in horses.

In the horse, the maxilla (upper jaw) is slightly wider than the mandible (lower jaw), resulting in slightly uneven

wear of the teeth even under normal circumstances. Generally the buccal surface (outer edge) of the upper cheek teeth and the lingual surface (inner edge) of the lower cheek teeth will develop sharp points over time. A veterinarian or equine dentist files these sharp points as needed to keep the occlusive surface flat in a procedure called "floating" the teeth. Typically equine veterinarians recommend dental examination as part of an annual physical examination starting shortly after birth, with floating recommended as needed to keep the teeth in good condition. In the normal horse, these exams should take place annually up to the age of about fifteen years and every six months thereafter; however, floating is not generally recommended at every examination.

Even in the clinically normal horse, when teeth are not floated regularly, they can develop significant enamel points that can cause laceration or ulceration of the cheeks and tongue. In addition to the pain that results from that condition, many other abnormalities can occur that reduce

(a)

(b)

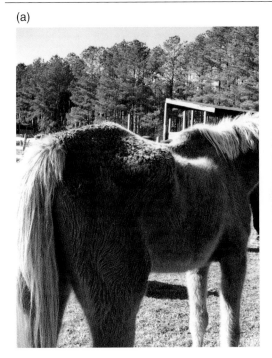
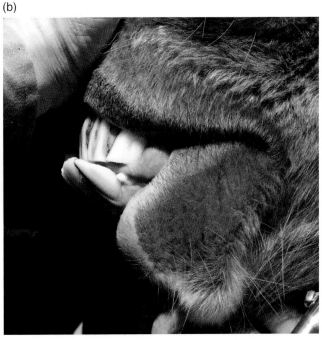

Figure 16.4 (a and b). Incisor malocclusion which has resulted in profound emaciation. Although grass was present on this property, because of this dental abnormality it was inadequate to provide sufficient nourishment for this horse. In this case the owner failed to provide *appropriate* feed material given the dental condition of the horse. Additionally, the owner failed to provide veterinary care (dental care) necessary to prevent or alleviate suffering.

the horses' efficiency at masticating feed material, ultimately reducing its feed efficiency. Step defects, wave mouths, ramps, and incisor abnormalities are all common findings in the emaciated horse. Incisor abnormalities can prevent the prehension of forage by preventing the clipping off of grasses by the teeth (Figures 16.4a and 16.4b). Cheek tooth abnormalities can reduce the efficiency of grinding concentrated or forage based feed. Often, when these abnormalities are present, a horse will drop feed, a behavior known as quidding. Quidding can result from pain associated with chewing and the mechanical abnormalities present. During the investigation of equine starvation, the investigator should look for evidence of quids which often take the form of "balls" of chewed hay or grasses that are mixed with saliva. These can be helpful in determining if any feed is being provided to the horses in question.

Dental abnormalities are most frequently a contributory cause of starvation, although they can be the primary cause. For example, in circumstances where horses are provided with only a forage based diet despite severe dental

abnormalities, starvation can occur in the presence of feed material. In those cases, rather than a straightforward case of failing to provide any feed, the owner may have failed to provide feed that is appropriate for the individual animal's condition (i.e., soaked grain rather than forage). Following the seizure of horses due to severe cases of starvation, horses are frequently re-fed prior to correcting dental abnormalities because floating teeth usually requires sedation. In cases of severe abnormality, re-feeding efforts may require the modification of feed material (such as providing soaked grain); however, when appropriate feed is provided these horses have been shown to gain weight. Although anecdotal, this evidence shows that when suitable quantities of *appropriate* feed are provided, horses can be maintained at an appropriate body condition despite dental abnormality. This example illustrates why a dental examination is indicated during the investigation of starvation, especially in cases in which some of the animals are in good or fair body condition and others are in poor condition.

SHELTER

The provision of appropriate shelter to animals is a nearly universal legal requirement. Failure to provide shelter often constitutes animal cruelty; however, there is significant variation in the legal definition of what constitutes shelter for a particular state. Some states have lengthy legal definitions of "shelter," attempting to encompass all aspects of the word, while many states have no legal definition to the term.

Nearly all animal cruelty laws leave a degree of subjectivity regarding the "adequacy" or "suitability" of shelter. While this can be frustrating to many investigators, it also provides a degree of ambiguity which is necessary given the huge degree of variability in requirements for shelter for individual animals. Legal definitions which leave a large degree of latitude may require an expert witness to assist the court in determining the adequacy of shelter for a particular case.

In narrow terms, shelter can be described as something that offers protection from adverse weather conditions. In broader terms, adequate shelter can encompass far more. When evaluating the adequacy of shelter, investigators should include an animal's entire enclosure and assess its suitability for the species, age, size, physical condition, type, and purpose of each animal. Adequate shelter should include not only that which protects an animal from the adverse effects of weather (rain, snow, sleet, hail, temperature extremes, and direct sun) but also should prevent animals from physical injury and adverse effects to their health from disease (Figures 16.5, 16.6a, and 16.6b).

To truly be appropriate shelter, an animal's environment must provide adequate space for the animal to promote both physiological and behavioral health. It should allow the animal to express a range of movements and behaviors appropriate for the species. Whenever possible, suitable shelter should allow for safe interaction with other animals of the same species. Additionally, shelter should be maintained in a sanitary manner so as not to unnecessarily expose the animal(s) to potentially harmful pathogens. Because of the large number of factors encompassed in the term "shelter" it is nearly impossible to construct a concrete definition that would be universally applicable to all species, life stages, and varying degrees of physical condition. Additionally, in commercial production settings there is often a balance between an individual animal's needs and overall production goals.

While livestock are often believed to have lower requirements for shelter than other species of domestic animals, their needs may often be underestimated by both producers and investigators. For example, donkeys are

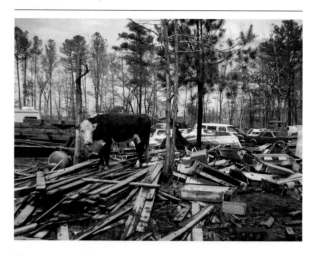

Figure 16.5 Appropriate shelter encompasses more than just shelter from the elements. Animals must also be provided with safe enclosures in which normal behaviors can be exhibited. Failure to provide a safe enclosure can result in charges of animal cruelty, as was the case with the owner of this Herford cow.

commonly maintained throughout the United States and Canada as guardians of other types of livestock against predators. These animals are generally provided with shelter similar to the stock that they guard despite their origins in northern Africa and the Mediterranean. A retrospective study of hypothermia cases in donkeys in western Canada has shown that without adequate shelter for this species, hypothermia can result in winter months without any other underlying disease process (Stephen, Baptiste, and Townsend 2000).

Additionally, the number of animals is a consideration in determining the needs for shelter. Beef cattle are often maintained in large herds in the western United States with limited access to physical shelter. However, the size of their herd can reduce their need for a physical structure on the basis of their herding behavior. The animals on the outer edge can provide a wind break for those on the interior of the herd. The constant motion of the herd allows for shifting positions so that the animals on the outside can rotate position with those on the interior, preventing animals from becoming hypothermic even in adverse weather conditions. Additionally, their ability to range over large areas allows them to use the topography to find naturally occurring sheltered areas. While herding behavior may provide protection from the elements it does not inherently indicate that cattle have lower requirements for shelter than other livestock species. Indeed, where the herd size is limited or animals

(a)

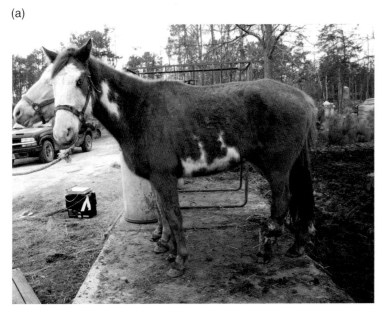

(b)

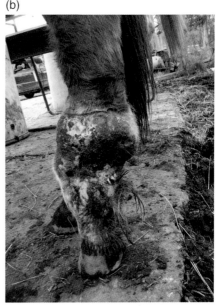

Figure 16.6 (a and b) Animal cruelty often results from many causes, as was the case with this horse. The horse first injured herself on unsafe material present in the pasture. The owner then failed to provide necessary veterinary care to alleviate suffering. Note the indicators of chronic pain shown, including reluctance to bear weight on the affected limb resulting in alteration of the hoof conformation when compared to the opposite limb and marginal body condition. Obvious abnormalities in locomotion and guarding of the affected area were also demonstrated on examination.

are kept singly, they lack the protection from the elements that may be provided by larger herds, thus significantly increasing their requirements for additional shelter. In the latter case it is important to weigh the needs of the animal(s) relative to the actual conditions present rather than to make assumptions about their needs based on conditions that may be present under other management systems.

Likewise, physical condition (including body condition score and medical conditions) also affects the type of shelter necessary. A horse in good body condition requires a lower degree of shelter during the winter while the same horse in poor (e.g., emaciated) body condition clearly has a higher requirement for shelter from adverse weather to reduce the energy requirements necessary to thermoregulate.

ACCIDENTAL AND NON-ACCIDENTAL INJURIES

The assessment of injuries to determine non-accidental vs. accidental causes should include environmental and animal behavior factors. The large animal forensic necropsy procedures and general considerations for all necropsies are discussed in Chapter 3. Accidental injuries can occur due to animal interaction or environmental hazards such as

with shelter or fencing. The investigation should include a thorough examination of the environment the animal had access to and any co-housed animals, and evaluation of husbandry practices. Animals may be at risk to suffer from undetected injures and an unsafe environment if husbandry practices do not include routine inspection for environmental hazards or animal injuries. Acceptable husbandry standards for production animals include a protocol for continual assessment of animal interactions and adjustments made to prevent stress and injuries. Failure to provide timely and appropriate medical care for injuries can result in cruelty charges. Untreated injuries can lead to more severe illness or result in irreversible damage, often requiring euthanasia.

Non-accidental injuries can result from a variety of causes that are discussed throughout this textbook. Common causes seen in large animals include blunt force trauma, sharp force trauma, gunshot, asphyxia, poisoning, horse fighting, and sexual abuse. The aging of bruising by gross appearance and histologic changes has been established for sheep and cattle (Tables 16.2 and 16.3). The use of incorrect and abusive training methods can lead to injuries from blunt

Table 16.2 Macroscopic aging of bruising in sheep and cattle.

Color	Approximate age
Red, hemorrhagic	0–10 hours
Dark	24 hours
Watery consistency	24–38 hours
Rusty orange, soapy texture	More than 72 hours

Source: Munro, R. and H. Munro. 2008. Wounds and Injuries. In: *Animal Abuse and Unlawful Killing: Forensic Veterinary Pathology*, pp. 30–47. Edinburgh: Elsevier.

Table 16.3 Histologic aging of bruising in lambs and calves.

Histologic findings	Age
Small numbers of neutrophils and macrophages present in extravasated blood found in tissues	Immediately before death
Greater hemorrhage, recognizable fibrin strands, many neutrophils, few macrophages	8 hours
Increase in macrophages resulting in equal ratio of neutrophils and macrophages	By 24 hours
Macrophages greatly outnumber neutrophils; capillaries with plump endothelium can be seen invading damaged tissues	By 48 hours

Source: Munro, R. and H. Munro. 2008. Wounds and Injuries. In: *Animal Abuse and Unlawful Killing: Forensic Veterinary Pathology*, pp. 30–47. Edinburgh: Elsevier.

force trauma, cosmetic alterations, and techniques used to achieve desired gaiting and head and tail carriage.

Within equine competitive and commercial industries there can be practices that cause inhumane treatment, injuries, and death. These include rodeos, carriage horses, shows, racing, mule/horse diving, and donkey basketball (Cheever 2004).

The cause and manner of death in cases involving insurance fraud can be difficult to determine based on the perpetrator's goal to avoid detection by striving for the appearance of the death to be due to natural or accidental causes. In horses, one method that has been used is to obstruct the nares with ping-pong balls in an attempt to avoid causing physical damage. The balls are then removed after the horse asphyxiates, eliminating physical evidence. In addition to postmortem findings found with asphyxia (Chapter 9), close examination of the nares and nasal passages can reveal evidence of injury to the mucous membranes such as capillary hemorrhage.

REFERENCES

AVMA. 2011. Pain in Animals. American Veterinary Medical Association Policy Statement. http://www.avma.org/issues/policy/animal_welfare/pain.asp.

AVMA. 2006. AVMA Animal Welfare Principles. American Veterinary Medical Association Policy Statement. http://www.avma.org/issues/policy/animal_welfare/principles.asp.

Cheever, H. 2004. Recognizing and Investigating Equine Abuse. In: *Shelter Medicine for Veterinarians and Staff*, pp. 499–510. Ames: Blackwell Publishing.

Collins, S.N., C. Pollitt, C.E. Wylie, and K. Matiesek. 2010. Laminitic Pain: Parallels with Pain States in Humans and other species. *Veterinary Clinics of North America Equine Practice*. 26(2010):643–671.

Green, L.E., V.J. Hedges, Y.H. Schukken, R.W. Blowey, and A.J. Packington. 2002. The Impact of Clinical Lameness on the Milk Yield of Dairy Cattle. *Journal of Dairy Science*. 85:2250–2256.

Hewson, Ca.J., I.R. Dohoo, K.A. Lemke, and H.W. Barkema. 2007. Canadian Veterinarians' Use of Analgesics in Cattle, Pigs, and Horses in 2004 and 2005. *Canadian Veterinarian Journal*. 48:155–164.

Munro, R. and H. Munro. 2008a. Neglect. In: *Animal Abuse and Unlawful Killing: Forensic Veterinary Pathology*, pp. 16–29. Edinburgh: Elsevier.

Munro, R. and H. Munro. 2008b. Wounds and Injuries. In: *Animal Abuse and Unlawful Killing: Forensic Veterinary Pathology*, pp. 30–47. Edinburgh: Elsevier.

Stephen, J.O., K.E. Baptiste, and H.G.G. Townsend. 2000. Clinical and Pathologic Findings in Donkeys with Hypothermia: 10 Cases (1988-1998). *Journal of the American Veterinary Medical Association*. 216(5):725–729.

Stull, C.L. 2004. *Dairy Welfare Evaluation Guide*. University of California Davis, Cooperative Extension.

Underwood, W.J. 2002. Pain and Distress in Agricultural Animals. *Journal of the American Veterinary Medical Association*. 221(2):208–211.

17
Avian Cruelty

Don J. Harris, Melinda D. Merck, and Dana M. Miller

It will never be possible to eliminate all chance of error or misjudgment, but the forensic science service strives to do the greatest good for the greatest number, for the greatest part of time.
    Professor Michael Green, University of Sheffield

PET BIRD CRUELTY

For decades, animal cruelty has been documented on many levels with frequent media displays of abuse involving dogs, cats, horses, livestock, and wildlife. Avian abuse has unique aspects based on the avian species including their physiology and behavior. Avian cruelty includes physical abuse and neglect. Birds such as poultry, canaries, and finches may be used for animal fighting (Chapter 13). Birds also may be victims of sexual abuse and poisoning (Chapters 10 and 12). Notably, birds have been abused or killed in association with acts of domestic violence.

Only recently has much attention been given to the mistreatment of pet birds. An often cited and the most obvious example of cruelty to pet birds is the confinement in small cages of creatures that, through flight, represent freedom. Keeping a macaw in a 9-foot^3 cage is a bit like keeping a killer whale in a swimming pool. In reality, this is the proverbial tip of the iceberg.

Pet birds are abused by individuals who are naively unaware of the birds' true needs, those who intentionally seek to disturb or harm them, and veterinarians who are oblivious to the unique biological, psychological, and medical needs of avian patients. Pet birds have not been domesticated as have dogs and cats. They are still essentially wild creatures and it is only in the past few decades that they have been raised extensively in the presence of humans. They have been taught to coexist with people, but they have not lost the instincts that evolved in the wild. We have only recently begun to realize what avian species truly require to thrive and as we discover these needs we realize how extensively they have been deprived and abused in the past.

AVIAN ABUSE DEFINED

Any time a pet bird receives care that is insufficient or harmful to the animal's physical and/or mental health the treatment may be considered abusive. Birds possess two characteristics that make them especially vulnerable to abuse. Many species of pet birds are extraordinarily intelligent. On the other hand, some pets, such as goldfish, perhaps, need minimal mental stimulation. Certain species of birds, however, benefit from and to some degree require the same kinds of environmental enrichment as do young children. In her book Irene Pepperberg describes how Alex, an African grey parrot, demonstrates thought processes that are sometimes comparable to those of four- to five-year-old children (Pepperberg 1999). It is this high level of cerebral functioning that makes birds especially vulnerable to psychological abuse. It also makes them one of the best and worst specimens to be kept as pets (AWC 2011b).

Unlike other pets, some birds have the ability to verbally communicate needs, wishes, and emotions. While other pets signal their feelings by wagging tails or purring, the verbal communication offered by birds is possibly easier for owners to understand and relate to. This is what contributes to the tremendous bond described by many bird

Veterinary Forensics: Animal Cruelty Investigations, Second Edition. Edited by Melinda D. Merck.
© 2013 John Wiley & Sons, Inc. Published 2013 by John Wiley & Sons, Inc.

owners. Unfortunately, the same level of mental functioning that gives birds these special qualities also creates needs that often go unsatisfied. Neglect, innocent or otherwise, can become a form of psychological abuse.

From a physical perspective, birds in the wild spend countless hours and expend immeasurable energy flying, foraging, and socializing. While a lack of sufficient socialization could be considered psychological abuse, the deprivation of normal levels of activity and exercise becomes a form of physical abuse (AWC 2011a). Obesity and poor body condition are common findings in caged birds.

When birds fail to receive appropriate mental and physical exercise, they often develop behavioral disorders ranging from weaving to excessive screaming to self-mutilation. This can cause anxiety and frustration in the owners. The owners may attempt to discipline the birds, sometimes to an abusive degree, which begins a vicious cycle.

With appropriate interaction and enrichment, birds can be fascinating and endearing pets. When treated improperly, the degree to which they can suffer physical and especially mental anguish can be profound. Ultimately, the physical and mental stimulation from normal ranging and flock dynamics might be difficult to reproduce in captivity.

INTENTIONAL ABUSE

Intentional abuse of pet birds includes forms of maltreatment that occur with the understanding that the bird is being harmed, even though the abuser may claim justification for his or her actions. One of the most common examples is the scenario in which a pet bird screams excessively, albeit normally, causing its owner to strike the cage. The rationalization is distraction and discipline to gain control of the screaming. The reality is usually increased fear on the part of the bird, frustration on the part of the owner, and an outcome of abuse with the potential for perpetuation and exacerbation of the problem. The end result is often the opposite of that which is desired. The bird may become so frightened of the abusive individual that even the approach of that person causes vocalization which turns to terrified screaming and ultimately escalates the problem.

A less obvious example of overt abuse is when an individual knowingly keeps a pet bird in a cage intended for much smaller species and never provides freedom from the cage. In addition to keeping an animal that normally has unlimited space in which to fly, the cages are sometimes placed in secluded areas. This arrangement can be considered abusive on three levels: the bird is spatially confined, it is denied socialization typical of the species, and the secluded area may not receive the required amount of fresh air and lighting . It is not unusual to find birds relocated to remote corners of a garage or basement in an attempt to remove the source of noise. This becomes exponentially abusive through not only what the bird is denied, but also from the noxious substances the bird might be exposed to, such as mold, chemicals, and carbon monoxide.

While screaming birds are sometimes relocated in an attempt to buffer the noise they can produce, some are subjected to physical abuse as a means of discipline. As described earlier, most often the bird's cage will be struck in an attempt to distract the bird from screaming. Occasionally, the bird itself will be struck. Injuries from direct and indirect blunt force trauma such as fractured limbs, broken beaks, and lacerations are common findings. Striking the bird directly is often the result of the bird biting the individual handling it. Birds bite their owners for various reasons; for instance, in response to someone else being in close proximity. Whether this is the result of territorial, possessive, or fearful perceptions is not always clear. However, this is one reason that the practice of allowing birds to perch on their owners' shoulders is strongly discouraged. Injuries such as pierced ears, eyebrows, lips, and even tongues may result from a pet bird biting its owner. In most cases, the bird is ultimately punished or abused because the owner allowed the bird to be placed in a position of risk to the bird and owner.

Spraying birds with jets of water from a spray bottle or water pistol to stop them from screaming is a practice that has been widely adopted. While this does not usually cause the physical injury seen with physical striking, it may cause the pet birds to become fearful of showers, which are important to their well-being.

A more malicious form of abuse is frequently seen when pet birds are maintained in outdoor habitats. Being caged outdoors allows the noise produced by the birds to be heard for great distances. Unfortunately, this increases the potential for the birds to annoy others. Even the normal talking mimicry which is sometimes manifested as incessant vocalization can be irritating to some people. Birds in these situations may suffer injury or death from gunshot wounds inflicted by neighbors who can no longer tolerate the noise. Occasionally these birds are simply the victims of vandalism for no reason other than the fact that they are easy targets. This is a manifestation of the familiar phrase "shooting fish in a barrel." There is an additional issue of safety because birds kept in outdoor habitats are also vulnerable to attack by other predatory animals such as cats, rats, raccoons, owls, and hawks.

Many owners do not realize the seriousness of their decisions. By far, the most common form of abuse through mismanagement is the decision to feed deficient diets. The

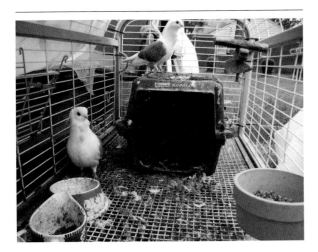

Figure 17.1. Severely contaminated bowls, improper shelter, and unsanitary environment.

author (Harris) has experienced countless situations in which an owner has been fully informed of what constitutes a proper diet for a particular species of pet bird, only to have the owner resort to feeding a diet that is clearly and grossly deficient. The most classic example of this is when a bird is fed a diet of pure sunflower seeds, usually with the explanation that "that's all he'll eat." The true reason for the bird's refusal to eat other foods is usually nothing more than unwillingness on the part of the owner to put forth the effort necessary to maintain a healthy diet.

Contrary to popular opinion, birds in captivity do not naturally select the correct assortment of foods to provide balanced nutrition when offered a variety of foods. Like children, they eat things that they like. Getting a pet bird to eat a balanced diet requires starting at a young age and providing a high quality commercial (usually pelleted) diet that contains as close to balanced nutrition as current veterinary knowledge provides. If a bird was weaned onto a poor quality diet, such as a seed mix, it will be necessary for the owner to go through a transition process to get it to consume a healthier diet. Many owners either give up too early or decide from the beginning that it's not worth the trouble. In either case, the owner is making the decision to feed a deficient diet.

Another form of intentional abuse is when an owner chooses to allow a bird's habitat to go without cleaning and maintenance for an unreasonable length of time. Unfortunately, it is common to find accumulated feces, moldy food, and algae growth in water bowls inside birds' cages. Owners may choose simply to add food and water to the containers in the cage when they appear empty, rather

that removing the containers and cleaning them on a regular basis. Failure to maintain a clean environment exposes the animal to pathogenic organisms and disease (Figure 17.1). Cleaning should occur frequently enough to prevent the development of unsanitary conditions.

UNINTENTIONAL ABUSE

Unintentional abuse is as damaging, physically and mentally, as intentional abuse. However, it may be easier to address and correct when it is due to ignorance. Feeding an inadequate diet is probably one of the most common forms of abuse that results from a simple lack of knowledge. Commercial seed-only preparations are grossly deficient (Harrison 2009), yet many are marketed as "complete and balanced" diets. Food labels implying that seed-only diets are nutritionally complete harm the pet by providing inadequate nutrition and the manufacturer may be held accountable.

Insufficient housing, including cage size and appropriate environmental enrichment, is a common problem for birds. It is generally accepted that the width of the cage should be at least 1.5 times the wingspan of the bird, the depth equal to the wingspan, and the height two to three times the height of the bird from the top of the head or crest to the tip of the tail. Unfortunately, these recommendations do not provide the bird with enough space for normal exercise. Disputes rage on over the appropriateness of keeping a bird in a cage, especially in one in which it is unable to fly. Some claim that if the birds are conditioned appropriately they are content in enclosed spaces; others argue that no animal can be happy if it is not able to behave the way it does in nature. Several publications discuss the husbandry for captive birds including the physical and mental health issues resulting from inappropriate environments (Young 2003, Seibert 2005).

Environmental enrichment is another key component to appropriate housing. Many birds are confined to cages with only the perch and food and water bowls. This type of environment lacks appropriate mental stimulation (HMC 2011). A barren enclosure, i.e., solitary confinement, could be considered a form of torture. On the other hand, it is possible to overwhelm a pet bird by crowding the cage with random, sometimes pointless toys. Ideally the cage should be used the same way a person uses a bedroom: the bird should be brought out for exercise, play, and mental stimulation. However, some may argue that ideally birds should not be kept as pets at all.

Most of the above problems may be the result of owners not understanding what birds truly require, such as owners only feeding sunflower seeds. In other cases, problems sometimes result from excessive attention as opposed to insufficient attention. Pet birds are often harmed by excessive pampering, or "spoiling." Psychological damage is often caused by the naive desire to do the right thing. There is a large amount of published information regarding the development of "psychological disorders" when birds do not get enough attention. In the author's (Harris) experience, the reverse is more often true. When young birds are pampered and nurtured around the clock, they become dependent on that degree of attention and can become extremely distressed, manifesting severe behaviors when the attention is withdrawn. Some of the worst cases of feather picking and self-mutilation are the result of birds being pampered to an extreme degree and then abandoned.

Inconsistencies by the owner can be psychologically damaging to pet birds. An owner may be affectionate and playful for a period of time, later becoming physically abusive or, at the very least, inattentive. Anthropomorphizing in these cases is not inappropriate. Understandably, the pet becomes confused and extremely anxious. In many cases, the bird may become self-destructive and therefore self-abusive.

VETERINARY ABUSE

It is notable that one form of abuse is the handling of avian patients by veterinarians who are not adequately prepared to do so. All veterinarians took an oath at the beginning of their careers stating, "above all, do no harm." Cases of veterinary abuse range from injuries resulting from improper wing trims to fatalities following the administration of unnecessary medications in inappropriate doses, sometimes for diseases that did not exist.

There are numerous ways in which veterinarians can harm or abuse pet birds. The most common form of veterinary abuse of avian species is the medical diagnosis and treatment of patients for which the practitioner is inadequately trained. Avian species are very different from dogs, cats, horses, and other domestic species. The anatomy, physiology, and metabolism of medications in birds are unique in many ways. It is not appropriate to extrapolate the care of avian patients from other species by simply scaling based on size. Drug doses on a mg/kg basis vary from other species. In addition, there are biochemical differences in birds that cause the interpretation of laboratory data to be different from other species. Anatomic differences between birds and mammals make the interpretation of avian radiographs different from those of mammals. In most situations, specialized knowledge and experience with birds is required for the safe and appropriate practice of veterinary medicine in this species.

The simplest form of veterinary maltreatment of avian species involves grooming, including the routine trimming of the nails, wings, and beak. Improper or unwarranted trimming can result in great harm to the patient. Veterinarians often perform beak trimming either because they believe it to be necessary or at the request of the owner. In most cases, a bird's beak never needs to be trimmed. Proper occlusion and normal abrasive surfaces within an appropriately designed habitat allow the bird to maintain normal shape and length of the beak. There are certainly cases in which a problem exists and trimming is necessary but it is not required of all pet birds.

Nail trimming is commonly performed on avian pets but often it is for the comfort of the owner, not for the health of the bird. Nail overgrowth does occur and trimming can be required. However, overgrowth of a pet bird's nails is usually the result of a deficiency in husbandry.

Wing trimming is a widely accepted practice used to prevent birds from flying. Some argue that denying a bird flight is abusive in itself. This is an issue that must be considered on a case-by-case basis. There is, however, a degree of trimming that is abusive. Birds with trimmed wings will continue to attempt to fly. In doing so, they will leap from high places. Proper wing trimming leaves enough lift in the wings to allow the bird to descend to the floor slowly and under some degree of control. If the wings are over-trimmed, the bird will fall hard enough to injure itself.

There are four common injuries are associated with excessive wing trimming:

- The tip of the beak may fracture into the quick, resulting in extreme pain and hemorrhage
- The skin over the bird's sternum, the keel, may split open, leaving a longitudinal open wound
- The bird may land tail-first, causing the pygostyle to hyperextend and tearing the skin horizontally along the entire base of the tail
- The fleshy tips of the bird's wings may become traumatized from flapping against perches or other surfaces without the protection of the normally protruding feathers

In some cases all four injuries may be seen due to the severity of the wing clipping. Ultimately, while wing trimming may be desirable in some pets, it should be done in a manner that reduces the ability of the bird to fly without rendering it vulnerable to injury. There is not a particular pattern of trimming that can be used on every patient. Experience and familiarity with various trimming patterns dictate what is appropriate for each patient.

Another practice that can be abusive is the manner in which some birds are restrained during physical exam and/or grooming. Some well-socialized birds may be restrained with relative ease, whereas many experience fear or panic when manually held down for a procedure. Unrelenting fighting and screaming are common when avian patients are physically restrained. The struggling can become so intense that the bird may spontaneously eviscerate. The use of isoflurane is strongly recommended for even the simplest of procedures involving avian patients during which the patient might be severely stressed. This is a safe method to handle these animals when performed by experienced avian practitioners.

The manner in which a patient will tolerate handling may be suggested from the initial encounter. If the bird is apprehensive about being approached, or if the approach lacks finesse, the stress of restraint may prove to be excessive. The unskilled, awkward approach to the initial capture and restraint of an avian patient may be considered another form of abuse.

Probably the most common examples of veterinary mismanagement of avian cases are those in which a sick patient is presented, no diagnostics are performed, and the patient is randomly placed on medication. While this approach may sometimes actually prove to be beneficial, the patient may not respond because the medication was inappropriate. In other cases the patient's condition will actually worsen due to an ill effect of the medication. At the very least, this approach does not constitute sound veterinary practice. In many cases, the use of even basic diagnostics will direct an appropriate course of action.

One more scenario that can be abusive is when the veterinarian is unfamiliar with the proper husbandry of avian species and fails to recommend proper care to the owners. Although the license to practice veterinary medicine covers all animal species, the generalized lack of knowledge for a particular species and failure to consult with a species expert may result in unnecessary harm to the animal. The resolution of veterinary abuse of avian patients requires one of two directions: practitioners can choose to dedicate themselves to furthering their knowledge of not just avian medicine, but of avian biology and behavior, or refer to someone who is more qualified to handle a particular situation.

Case examples of veterinary abuse

Case 1: An African grey parrot was presented weak and marginally responsive. A review of records from the previous veterinarian revealed that the bird had been diagnosed with hypothyroidism and placed on a thyroid supplement. Both the history and the laboratory data failed to support the diagnosis. The dose of thyroid medication administered was 1,000 times the recommended dose. The bird could not be saved.

Case 2: A 57-year-old macaw with a distended abdomen was presented "in the terminal stages of heart disease" to see if anything else could be done for the cardiac problem. The bird had been on medication for the "heart failure" for nine months. No diagnostics whatsoever had been performed by the clinic that originally saw the bird. Diagnostics and radiographs taken revealed that the bird was suffering from a retained egg. No evidence of heart disease was detected. Surgery successfully resolved the problem.

Case 3: An African grey parrot was presented with all four of the injuries seen when the wings are overclipped. There were no flight feathers present on either wing. The owner had already filed a complaint with the Board of Veterinary Medicine and initiated a lawsuit. The court found in favor of the owner.

POULTRY CRUELTY

With the ever increasing popularity of poultry as pets investigators of animal cruelty are encountering chickens, ducks, geese, and other "farm" birds with more frequency than ever before. Much like livestock, these birds can present particular challenges to the investigators of cruelty complaints because of issues with familiarity with the species involved and exemptions in the existing cruelty laws. Some states, such as Louisiana (§102.1) and South Carolina (§47-1-40(C)), exempt particular species (those described as "fowl") from their animal cruelty laws leaving these animals with little legal protection.

Within the United States chickens have become the most popular species of backyard poultry which is likely due to their compact size, inquisitive nature, and usefulness in egg production. While the incredible variations in breeds of chickens make this species desirable to poultry owners it also presents an additional challenge to investigators. Different breeds of chickens can have enormously different physical appearances and identification of the breed or breed mix can be helpful in determining if certain physical characteristics are within normal for the breed.

For example, the chicken shown in Figure 17.2 was a common source of complaints in one neighborhood due to the lack of feathers in the bird's neck and concerns over the bird's welfare. Evaluation of this bird by an experienced poultry veterinarian showed that the bird had several physical characteristics similar to that of a Turken or Naked Necked chicken (a breed recognized by the American Poultry Association). The characteristic lack of feathers on the neck in this crossbred chicken therefore was within

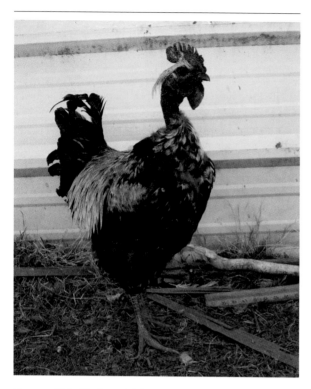

Figure 17.2. Turken chicken.

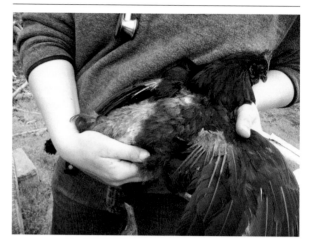

Figure 17.3. Characteristic pattern of feather loss due to excessive mounting of roosters.

normal for that breed mix and the case was easily resolved by educating the nearby neighbors about the breed's physical characteristics.

Conversely, the chicken shown in Figure 17.3 was present on a property already under investigation for neglect of the other animals. Animal control officers ensured that each animal, including all of the birds present, were evaluated by someone with the experience in that species. This hen showed a characteristic pattern of feather damage over the back and proximal wings that was consistent with trauma from excessive mounting by the roosters on the property. Left to continue, this excessive mounting can result in significant wounds over the dorsum, lateral body walls, and back of the head. If left untreated, these wounds can result in deaths of the hen. Ensuring an appropriate ratio of hens to roosters or separating overzealous roosters is the responsibility of the poultry owner. In both cases, proper identification of the sex and breeds present was an important component in determining if animal cruelty was present and how to remedy the problem.

Evaluation of housing and husbandry

As with all birds, the evaluation of housing requires knowledge of the husbandry requirements for the species

involved. Chickens, particularly bantam or small breeds, may be comfortably housed in relatively small areas whereas turkeys, ducks, geese, and swans require larger enclosures to exhibit a range of normal behaviors. Small commercial poultry producers or non-commercial poultry owners often have a high degree of variability in the housing provided to birds. Whether birds are confined or allowed to free-range, it is still important to ensure that they have adequate shelter, clean water and food. Failure to provide suitable housing and feed/water systems can result in significant suffering. Ulcerative pododermatitis (bumblefoot), necrotic keel lesions, frostbite, severe coccidiosis, and traumatic injuries to the wings and head are all common findings in poultry kept in unsanitary or unsafe conditions (Figures 17.4–17.8).

Modern commercial production systems for poultry often involve a high degree of confinement. Whether these involve confined egg-layers, floor-raised layers, broilers, broiler-breeders, or turkeys, all have considerable costs to the welfare of the birds. These systems are designed to maximize production while minimizing economic losses from predation, intestinal parasitism, cannibalism, broken eggs, etc. Regardless of an individual's personal beliefs involving humane concerns, these systems generally fall within accepted industry standards and therefore are exempted under most animal cruelty laws. It is unfair and often dangerous, however, to simply "scale back" the principles of these systems (such as space per bird) to an individual bird or small number of birds kept in a non-commercial setting. Sadly, this is frequently the defense offered to circumstances involving significant neglect.

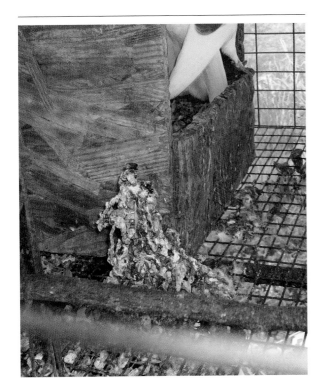

Figure 17.4. Severe feces contamination in pigeon cage.

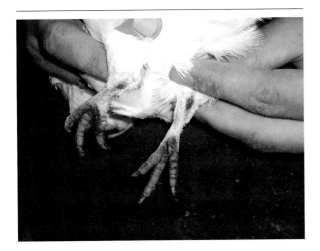

Figure 17.5. Hock lesions on pigeon from that cage.

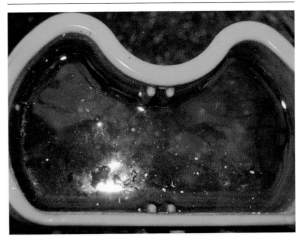

Figure 17.6. Pigeon cage: contaminated water.

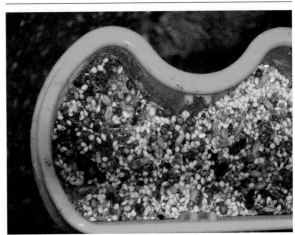

Figure 17.7. Pigeon cage: moldy seed in bowl.

Although modern poultry production systems involve a high degree of confinement, they also incorporate a high degree of control over other important factors such as temperature , lighting, air quality, litter management, parasite control, and careful nutritional management. When abusers of poultry put forth a defense of "accepted husbandry standards" it is important to evaluate all of these management factors that can contribute to the acceptability of their practices, not just the one factor that they are claiming is accepted.

Figure 17.9 illustrates one such case in which a rooster was continually confined to a wire dog kennel type crate despite educational efforts aimed at improving husbandry. Although the defense claimed that it is accepted to confine poultry with limited space, this method of confinement failed to provide the other necessary elements that are essential in intensively reared poultry situations. No care was provided with respect to temperature control or shelter from freezing rain and snow. There was neither separation from fecal material nor attempts to minimize exposure to parasites. In addition, the food was thrown on the ground directly

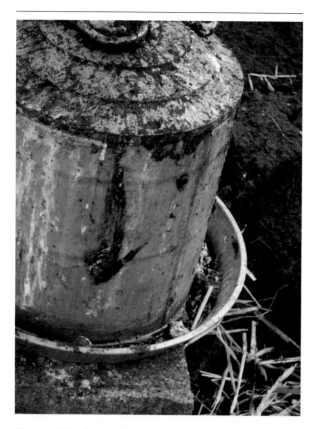

Figure 17.8. Severely contaminated chicken waterer.

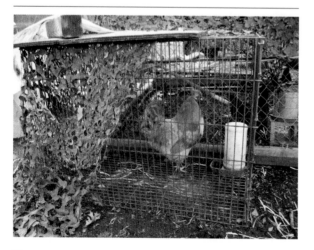

Figure 17.9. Inadequate caging and continual confinement.

onto the feces and the water was regularly contaminated with feces. As a result, the bird in question had multiple early lesions likely to develop into ulcerative pododermatitis

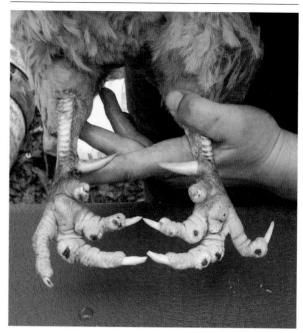

Figure 17.10. Multiple bumbles.

(bumbles) and had frostbite on the comb (Figure 17.10). Ultimately, this owner was convicted of animal cruelty for this failure to provide the necessary elements of care despite the assertion that confinement was "accepted."

Euthanasia and humane slaughter

In nearly every state animal cruelty laws prohibit the "unnecessary" or "cruel" killing of animals. With companion animals the determination of whether a death is unnecessary or cruel is relatively easy compared to that of animals for which humane slaughter and culling are routine. Within the United States, and with regard to companion animals, there is a near universally accepted standard that, regardless of reason, if an owner no longer wishes to continue custody of their animal(s) they have a responsibility to relinquish the animal to a shelter, re-home it through other methods, or have it humanely euthanized by a veterinarian. With regard to poultry, for which much of the slaughter and euthanasia are frequently conducted by non-veterinary personnel, the determination of whether a death is necessary or humane becomes an important component of cruelty investigation.

Culling flocks, the elective euthanasia of poultry, is a commonly accepted practice among commercial flocks and some small flock owners. This culling commonly occurs as the result of birds developing medical abnormalities or an excess number of unwanted males. Additionally, when birds are reared for the purpose of home slaughter, it is the responsibility of the owner to ensure that the slaughter is humane.

Most poultry euthanasia conducted by non-veterinary personnel is conducted through the use of physical methods such as cervical dislocation or decapitation. When properly performed these are recognized by the American Veterinary Medical Association (AVMA) as humane methods (AVMA 2007); however, if improperly applied they can result in significant pain and suffering. Properly applied cervical dislocation of poultry is conducted by firmly grasping the bird's body in one arm against the person's body (similar to a football) while grasping the bird's head just behind the skull. The bird's neck is then stretched while pressure is applied to the C1/C2 cervical vertebrae in a quick oblique fashion resulting in dislocation. This results in the dislocation of the cervical vertebrae high enough to paralyze respiratory muscles and quickly cause death with a minimum of consciousness. This procedure requires a high degree of training and individual competence to be humane. There are realistic constraints for the proper use of these methods based on the physical limitations (strength or arm span) in the human performing these techniques. In older, mature birds, large species, or certain varieties of birds, conducting cervical dislocation humanely may not be possible.

Unfortunately, in both the commercial and non-commercial sector, when people who commonly perform these techniques are poorly trained or become insensitive to the bird's condition, they may take shortcuts that cause unnecessary suffering and inhumane death. One such common shortcut involves simply grasping the bird anywhere along the neck and quickly flinging its body in a circular motion. While this will result in death, it occurs by causing multiple cervical fractures anywhere along the length of the neck rather than by cervical dislocation (Figure 17.11). Death from this method is significantly prolonged (when compared to true cervical dislocation) and should not be considered humane.

GENERAL EXAM FINDINGS IN PET BIRD AND POULTRY CRUELTY

The exam findings in birds associated with different types of abuse are similar to those of other animals as documented throughout this textbook. The avian forensic necropsy procedures and general forensic necropsy considerations are discussed in Chapter 3. In some cases, it may be obvious that a pet bird is being abused, although clinical signs alone may not provide evidence of abuse. Unfortunately, pet birds are highly prone to physical injury. The ability to

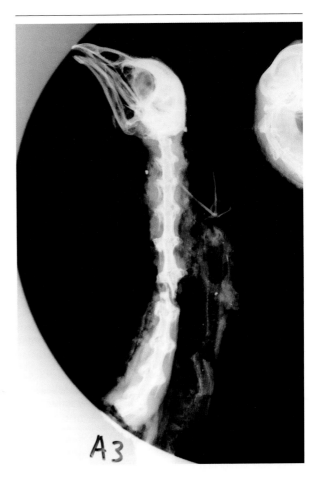

Figure 17.11. Cervical fracture in a fighting rooster.

distinguish between accidental and non-accidental injury can be difficult and is often determined when the clinical history or husbandry does not match the exam findings. The examination for birds should follow the same protocols as outlined in Chapter 3 with consideration of forensic evidence identification, collection, and analysis. A complete history should be obtained including the husbandry, environment, scene findings, medical records, and any photographs or video from investigators. For large scale bird cases, the rapid bird exam record and the basic small pet bird care in temporary shelters may be useful (Appendices 25 and 28). The body condition should be assessed and an appropriate score may be assigned (Table 17.1). Diagnostic procedures may be performed to document obvious and hidden injuries or medical conditions.

Evidence of blunt force trauma (Chapter 5) may be seen in abused birds. Abrasions to the head or wings could be the result of being struck or flying into a wall. Contusions

Table 17.1. Body condition scoring for poultry.

Score	Description
0	Protruding keel bone and depressed contour of breast muscles (concavity)
1	Prominent keel bone with poorly developed breast muscles (flat)
2	Less prominent keel bone and moderate breast development (slightly convex)
3	Plump breast muscles which provide a smooth contour with the keel

Source: Gregory, N.G. and J.K. Robins. 1998. A Body Condition Scoring System for Layer Hens. *New Zealand Journal of Agricultural Research*. 41:555–559.

Table 17.2. Bruising color changes in poultry.

Time elapsed since injury	Bruising coloration
2 minutes	Red
12 hours	Dark red-purple
24 hours	Light green-purple
36 hours	Yellow-green-purple
48 hours	Yellow-green
72 hours	Yellow-orange
96 hours	Slightly yellow
120 hours	No skin discoloration

Source: Munro, R. Munro, H.M.C. Munro. 2008d. Wounds and Injuries. In: *Animal Abuse and Unlawful Killing: Forensic Veterinary Pathology*, pp. 30–47. Edinburgh: Elsevier.

may be obscured by feathers, and plucking or shaving can reveal the extent of the bruising (Munro and Munro 2008d). The color of bruising changes over time and has been recorded in poultry (Table 17.2). A fractured leg is a common sequela to being flung from the hand of a person holding a bird. This may be due to the rotational forces at the initiation of the event or caused by surface impact. Fractured legs also may result from accidental falls. It is not uncommon to discover an old, healed fracture of a wing or leg during a physical exam. Aging of the injury may provide evidence of when the injury occurred and further investigation may be necessary to determine if the injury was accidental or non-accidental. The behavior of the owner may be a greater indication of possible abuse than the appearance of the injury.

Physical trauma is not always reflected in the findings of the physical exam. Blunt trauma that is not apparent externally is sometimes revealed in laboratory data. The most common findings in a patient who has experienced blunt trauma are an elevated creatine kinase (CK) and aspartate aminotransferase (AST). While these findings can be due to other causes, elevations of these analytes in a suspected abuse case are supportive evidence of trauma.

Gunshot injuries may be seen in pet birds and poultry and are discussed in detail in this textbook (Chapter 8). The small size of birds may result in exit wounds that are the same size as the entrance wounds due to the short projectile path. Radiographs may reveal metal fragments in the wound track and help determine trajectory. Both entrance and exit wounds may have bruising around the wound margins, though the exit wound often has more associated hemorrhage. Bone injuries, especially to the skull, may show signs indicating the direction of travel.

Air-powered weapons have limited kinetic energy that is sufficient to cause fatal injury (Munro and Munro 2008b).

Injuries to the eyes are common with these weapons. Radiographs may reveal evidence of prior shooting injuries. On postmortem exam these older projectiles may be partially or fully encapsulated with fibrous tissue without evidence of hemorrhage (Munro and Munro 2008b).

In shotgun injuries, the pellets may pass around the body making it impossible to estimate the gunshot range. This distribution of pellets within the body, wide distribution vs. a mass of pellets in close contact, can help determine the gunshot range (Munro and Munro 2008b). Powder tattooing of the skin from gunpowder may be inhibited by the feather density.

Rifle injuries from low velocity .22 bullets may travel along the fascial planes in the skeletal muscle or track within the subcutaneous layer in large birds without penetrating the deeper tissues (Munro and Munro 2008b).

Animal attack injuries may be seen in birds. The type of injuries seen depends on the species and breed of the attacking animal (Table 17.3) The severity of injuries may be masked by the feathers. The types of injuries seen are similar to those from other predator attacks (Chapter 6). Bone fractures are more common in medium to small birds due to their light structure (Munro and Munro 2008a).

Sexual abuse of birds, especially poultry, may be seen. The injuries to birds are often fatal due to severe damage through the urogenital opening. Injuries associated with restraint may be seen on the body, legs, feet, wings, and/or neck. Neck injuries associated with strangulation, including fractures, may be seen (Chapter 9).

Thermal related injuries may be seen in birds. Frostbite is commonly seen, primarily in the feet, although it may present as distal wing necrosis. While frostbite is uncommon in free-ranging chickens that are able to seek shelter, it can occur when chickens are improperly confined in caging that fails to suitably protect them from the elements.

Table 17.3. Comparison of dog and large cat attacks on domestic geese.

	Dog attack	Large cat attack
Weight of goose	4.3 kg	5.9 kg
Neck injuries	None	Multiple bites (12 left, 10 right), massive hemorrhage, spinal cord severed
Back injuries	Four skin puncture wounds (2–6 mm diameter), subcutaneous hemorrhage, muscle lacerations (4–30 mm in length)	None
Chest	Four puncture wounds (right) with extensive hemorrhage, muscle lacerations, rib fractures, extensive hemorrhage within thoracic cavity, right lung laceration	Five puncture wounds (claw marks) of right ventral chest, five puncture wounds and slit wounds in pectoral muscles deep to skin wounds, three fractured ribs (left), ruptured liver
Cause of death	Crushing of chest, chest hemorrhage, lung laceration	Neck trauma with severance of spinal cord

Source: Munro, R., H.M.C. Munro. 2008a. Bite Injuries. In: *Animal Abuse and Unlawful Killing: Forensic Veterinary Pathology*, pp. 82–87. Edinburgh: Elsevier.

The damage from frostbite can be seen in these birds, particularly along the combs and waddles. Edema appears in the legs and/or feet in twenty-four hours. Skin blistering seen in mammals does not occur in birds. It may take three to six weeks for clear demarcation of dead and viable tissue. Predisposing factors for frostbite include lack of acclimation, malnutrition, metal leg bands, over-tight bandaging, previous injury, unseasonable weather, and wire cages (Munro and Munro 2008c). Electrothermal burns may be seen in birds that have contact with high-voltage cables. The skin edges may be carbonized with the surrounding skin and feathers covered with soft, brown crumbly material which is from heated blood and tissue (Munro and Munro 2008c).

The physical presentation of a pet bird in an advanced stage of illness may be suggestive of neglect due to failure to provide care. While it is true that avian species can mask signs of illness, there is almost always some change in a pet bird's behavior that signals a change in condition. This change may be subtle and difficult to detect by individuals unfamiliar with the particular bird's routines and behavior expressions. Unfortunately, many owners may acknowledge awareness of these changes but fail to realize their significance. While the neglect may have been unintentional, the bird still suffers the consequences of delayed medical intervention and care.

A bird's behavior when approached may sometimes be evidence that abuse is occurring. An examiner may find a bird in perfect physical condition in a spotless carrying cage, only to discover a near panic response when the bird is approached. This response was discussed in the section on veterinary abuse, but the response is frequently evidence that the patient is being abused in the home. Well-socialized pet birds can be apprehensive, but in most cases they are cooperative and even overtly friendly. They usually step up onto the hand of the examiner and accept placement on exam perches and scales. Birds that have been physically abused are almost always on the defensive from the very beginning of the exam. Some begin to posture and vocalize from the moment the practitioner enters the exam room. Defensive posturing includes crouching, weaving in place, spreading of the wings, open mouth with or without vocalizing, etc. If not contained, patients will occasionally launch themselves from their position, such as a table top perch, the top of a cage, or the owner's shoulder, into the wall of the exam room. It is for this reason that it is recommended for all pet birds to be kept in their carrying cages in the exam room until their removal is approved. It is not unusual for birds to experience these same responses in the absence of a history of abuse. The reality is that these fractious pets may have experienced the abuse of improper socialization, as described earlier. In the end, it is also possible that a particular pet bird simply has a fractious personality, with no history of abuse whatsoever. Thus, the ultimate problem posed to practitioners is determining which patients have been abused and which have not based on these behavioral clues.

REFERENCES

American Veterinary Medical Association (AVMA). 2007. *AVMA Guidelines on Euthanasia.* http://www.avma.org/issues/animal_welfare/euthanasia.pdf.

Avian Welfare Coalition (AWC). 2011a. *Animal Welfare Issues: From Extinction to Euthanasia.* http://www.avianwelfare.org/issues/pets/htm.

Avian Welfare Coalition (AWC). 2011b. *Keeping Parrots as Pets.* http://www.avianwelfare.org/issues/pets/htm.

Harrison, G. 2009. *Handbook for a Healthier Bird.* Brentwood, TN: HBD International.

Hartz Mountain Corporation (HMC). 2011. *Keeping Your Bird Entertained.* http://www.hartz.com/Birds/Habitats/Keeping_Your_Bird_Entertained.aspx.

Munro, R. and H.M.C. Munro. 2008a. Bite Injuries. In: *Animal Abuse and Unlawful Killing: Forensic Veterinary Pathology*, pp. 82–87. Edinburgh: Elsevier.

Munro, R. and H.M.C. Munro. 2008b. Firearms Injuries. In: *Animal Abuse and Unlawful Killing: Forensic Veterinary Pathology*, pp. 55–64. Edinburgh: Elsevier.

Munro, R. and H.M.C. Munro. 2008c. Injuries Associated with Physical Agents. In: *Animal Abuse and Unlawful Killing: Forensic Veterinary Pathology*, pp. 70–74. Edinburgh: Elsevier.

Munro, R. and H.M.C. Munro. 2008d. Wounds and Injuries. In: *Animal Abuse and Unlawful Killing: Forensic Veterinary Pathology*, pp. 30–47. Edinburgh: Elsevier.

Pepperberg, I.M. 1999. *The Alex Studies: Cognitive and Communicative Abilities of Grey Parrots.* Harvard University Press.

Seibert, L. 2005. Mental Health Issues in Captive Birds. In: *Mental Health and Well-Being in Animals*, pp. 285–294. Ames: Blackwell Publishing.

Young, R.J. 2003. *Environmental Enrichment for Captive Animals, UFAW Animal Welfare Series.* Oxford: Blackwell Publishing.

Appendix 1
Colorado Veterinary Medical Association Protocol for Mandatory Reporting of Animal Cruelty and Animal Fighting

December 2007

Dear Colorado veterinarian,

On July 1, 2007, it became mandatory for Colorado veterinarians to report animal cruelty and animal fighting. The new law states that if a veterinarian suspects that he or she is treating an animal that has been subjected to cruelty or animal fighting, it must be reported to the appropriate authority. In addition, the veterinarian is protected under the law if he or she reports the incident in good faith.

The Colorado Veterinary Medical Association, the Colorado Association of Certified Veterinary Technicians, the Denver District Attorney's Office and the Animal Assistance Foundation came together to facilitate understanding and implementation of this new law. We have developed supporting material to assist you with the spirit and the letter of this law. Please share this information with your practice team so everyone is aware of this new requirement and how to comply.

Identifying animal abuse and even human abuse can sometimes be difficult. A number of resources are available to assist you. In this packet you'll find:

• Pertinent definitions from the cruelty statutes, and relevant sections of the new provisions for reporting contained in the veterinary practice act

• Sample protocol for the veterinary professional
• Suggestions for recording information in the patient's medical record
• Chart on patterns of non-accidental injury
• Magnet for recording and displaying contact information
• Primer on finding the contact numbers for the magnet

Additional resources are located on the Colorado Veterinary Medical Association Website (www.colovma.org):

• Reporting forms, available through a link to the Colorado Department of Agriculture Web site (colorado.gov/ag/animals) Bureau of Animal Protection section
• Resources compiled by the Canadian Veterinary Medical Association on its Web site (canadianveterinarians.net/animal.aspx) that include recognizing animal abuse, reporting animal abuse, collecting evidence and other areas
• Links to other Web sites with supplemental information

Please share this packet of information with your entire team—after all, it will be a group effort to recognize, report, and record suspected animal cruelty. Please contact any of the supporting partners if you have any questions or comments Thank you for being watchful for suspected cruelty to animals.

Veterinary Forensics: Animal Cruelty Investigations, Second Edition. Edited by Melinda D. Merck.
© 2013 John Wiley & Sons, Inc. Published 2013 by John Wiley & Sons, Inc.

CRUELTY LAW AND DEFINITIONS

General

You and your entire staff should become familiar with cruelty laws:

- At a minimum, familiarize yourself with the statutory definitions of "animal," "cruelty," "animal fighting," and "dangerous animal." Within each statute there may be additional critical definitions such as "mistreatment" and the various forms of criminal intent. These can be found at www.state.co.us (look for Colorado Revised Statutes). Cruelty to Animals may be found at § 18-9-02, Animal Fighting may be found at § 18-9-204, and the new mandatory reporting law may be found at § 12-62.121.
- Update your cruelty law files on a yearly basis.
- Know the mandatory reporting laws as well as any immunity provisions. This would also include being aware of any privilege or confidentiality exceptions.

Statutory definitions

Colorado Revised Statutes: §18-9-201 Definitions

- "Animal" means any living dumb creature.
- "Mistreatment" means every act or omission that causes or unreasonably permits the continuation of unnecessary or unjustifiable pain or suffering.
- "Neglect" means failure to provide food, water, protection from the elements, or other care generally considered to be normal, usual, and accepted for an animal's health and wellbeing consistent with the species, breed, and type of animal.
- "Sexual act with an animal" means an act between a person and an animal involving direct physical contact between the genitals of one and the mouth, anus, or genitals of the other. A sexual act with an animal may be proven without allegation or proof of penetration. Nothing in this subsection shall be construed to prohibit accepted animal husbandry practices.

Cruelty to animals

Colorado Revised Statutes: §18-9-202: *Cruelty to animals, aggravated cruelty to animals, neglect of animals*

1. (a) A person commits cruelty to animals if he or she knowingly, recklessly, or with criminal negligence overdrives, overloads, overworks, torments, deprives of necessary sustenance, unnecessarily or cruelly beats, allows to be housed in a manner that results in chronic or repeated serious physical harm, carries or confines in or upon any vehicles in a cruel or reckless manner, engages in a sexual act with an animal, or otherwise mistreats or neglects any animal, or causes or procures it to be done, or, having the charge or custody of any animal, fails to provide it with proper food, drink, or protection from the weather consistent with the species, breed, and type of animal involved, or abandons an animal.

    (b) Any person who intentionally abandons a dog or cat commits the offense of cruelty to animals.

1.5. (a) A person commits cruelty to animals if he or she recklessly or with criminal negligence tortures, needlessly mutilates, or needlessly kills an animal.

    (b) A person commits aggravated cruelty to animals if he or she knowingly tortures, needlessly mutilates, or needlessly kills an animal.

1.6. (a) "Serious physical harm" means any of the following:

    (i) Any physical harm that carries a substantial risk of death;

    (ii) Any physical harm that causes permanent maiming or that involves some temporary, substantial maiming; or

    (iii) Any physical harm that causes acute pain of a duration that results in substantial suffering.

1.8. A peace officer having authority to act under this section may take possession of and impound an animal that the peace officer has probable cause to believe is a victim of cruelty to animals or animal fighting and as a result is endangered if it remains with the owner or custodian. If, in the opinion of a licensed veterinarian, an animal impounded pursuant to this subsection is experiencing extreme pain or suffering, or is severely injured past recovery, severely disabled past recovery, or severely diseased past recovery, the animal may be euthanized without a court order.

Animal fighting

Colorado Revised Statutes: §18-9-204.

1. (a) No person shall cause, sponsor, arrange, hold, or encourage a fight between animals for the purpose of monetary gain or entertainment.

    (b) For the purposes of this section, a person encourages a fight between animals for the purpose of monetary gain or entertainment if he or she:

    (i) Is knowingly present at or wagers on such a fight;

(ii) Owns, trains, transports, possesses, breeds, sells, transfers, or equips an animal with the intent that such animal will be engaged in such a fight;

(iii) Knowingly allows any such fight to occur on any property owned or controlled by him;

(iv) Knowingly allows any animal used for such a fight to be kept, boarded, housed, or trained on, or transported in, any property owned or controlled by him;

(v) Knowingly uses any means of communication for the purpose of promoting such a fight; or

(vi) Knowingly possesses any animal used for such a fight or any device intended to enhance the animal's fighting ability.

3. Nothing in this section shall prohibit normal hunting practices as approved by the division of wildlife.

4. Nothing in this section shall be construed to prohibit the training of animals or the use of equipment in the training of animals for any purpose not prohibited by law.

Mandatory reporting

Colorado Revised Statutes: §12-64-121. Reporting requirements—immunity for reporting—veterinary-patient-client privilege inapplicable

1. A licensed veterinarian who, during the course of attending or treating an animal, has reasonable cause to know or suspect that the animal has been subjected to cruelty in violation of section 18-9-202, C.R.S., or subjected to animal fighting in violation of section 18-9-204, C.R.S., shall report or cause a report to be made of the animal cruelty or animal fighting to a local law enforcement agency or the bureau of animal protection.

2. A licensed veterinarian shall not knowingly make a false report of animal cruelty or animal fighting to a local law enforcement agency or to the bureau of animal protection.

3. A licensed veterinarian who willfully violates the provisions of subsection (1) or (2) of this section commits a class 1 petty offense, punishable as provided in section 18-1.3-503, C.R.S.

4. A licensed veterinarian who in good faith reports a suspected incident of animal cruelty or animal fighting to the proper authorities in accordance with subsection (1) of this section shall be immune from liability in any civil or criminal action brought against the veterinarian for reporting the incident. In any civil or criminal proceeding in which the liability of a veterinarian for reporting an incident described in subsection (1) of this section is at issue, the good faith of the veterinarian shall be presumed.

5. The veterinary-patient-client privilege described in section 24-72-204 (3) (a) (XIV), C.R.S., may not be asserted for the purpose of excluding or refusing evidence or testimony in a prosecution for an act of animal cruelty under section 18-9-202, C.R.S., or for an act of animal fighting under section 18-9-204, C.R.S.

SAMPLE PROTOCOL FOR THE VETERINARY PROFESSIONAL

If you are suspicious

1. **Dial 911** if you are concerned for the safety of yourself, your staff, or others.

2. **Do NOT compromise the timely treatment of the animal**.

3. Remember that everything you do, write, and say is likely to be disclosed to law enforcement authorities and to the accused (who may be your client). If you are called to testify under oath or to give a statement, you may be asked about anything you have documented. Be objective, honest, and thorough.

4. If possible, have another veterinarian (or witness) document their observations and assessments. They may support or contradict your findings—either way, it is beneficial and will lead to a well-documented objective conclusion.

5. Document what the client tells you when explaining the animal's condition.

   (a) Note the relationship between the client and the animal (owner, pet-sitter, neighbor, "good Samaritan," etc.).

   (b) What is the client's behavior? Concerned? Apathetic?

   (c) Your client may admit incriminating conduct. It is essential to try to write down exactly what is said whether or not it seems truthful, embellished or not truthful.

   (d) Note if the client's account changes.

   (e) Note if one client's account is inconsistent with another person's account.

   (f) Is the client an established client? Do you have a treatment history for the animal?

   (g) A client whose history includes consistently having new or young animals could also be an indicator.

   (h) You may be confronted with instances in which a very young child (under 10 years) is responsible for the act(s). You must intervene and report. A parent or guardian may minimize or deny the existence of a problem. If the circumstance allows, try to communicate your concerns to the child's parent or guardian.

6. Conduct a thorough examination of the animal and note its condition in the veterinary record (see Reporting in the Medical Record below).

7. Report your suspicions to law enforcement or agency with jurisdiction to handle these types of crimes (see Primer for Reporting, below, for suggestions).

    (a) In most instances, you should report the suspected violation to your local law enforcement agency.

    (b) It is not realistic for you to expect to remain anonymous.

    (c) You will be asked to provide your name, phone number, and a detailed description of the issue, which includes the species of the animal(s), location, owner, etc., so that authorities can follow up on the case.

    (d) You will not be expected to "investigate" the case. Peace officers (for example: police, sheriff, district attorney investigators, authorized employees of the Bureau of Animal Protection and authorized animal control officers) will conduct the investigation. They will ultimately determine whether or not cruelty or neglect charges will be filed, and, if so, which charges against which individual(s).

    (e) Officers cannot comment on a case until the investigation is completed, especially if there is a possibility of pending litigation.

8. Document to whom you reported and when.

9. Additional guidance after reporting:

    (a) You should not discuss the matter with members of the media.

    (b) Upon request, you should provide copies of veterinary medical records to law enforcement officials and turn over any relevant physical evidence.

    (c) Complete a written (or tape-recorded) statement. The more thorough, at or near the time of the event, the better able you will be to refresh your memory in the future.

    (d) It is important that you know who you are talking to and who they represent. Additionally, it is advisable to refresh your memory about the case (by reviewing your records and statements) prior to any discussions with others. You have the right to speak or not to speak to anyone regarding the matter.

    (e) If you are concerned about safety issues, the police or prosecuting attorney can assist with a restraining order.

    (f) If you testify in court, whoever subpoenas you should be able to work with you and make it as convenient as possible. Simply tell the truth to the best of your ability.

Related family violence concerns

1. Familiarize yourself with related family violence issues and know your state statutes regarding the veterinarian's legal responsibilities regarding reporting child abuse or domestic violence. Links to supporting Web sites can be found at www.colovma.org.

2. If you are able to do so, offer space at your clinic or kennel as a "safe haven" for pets.

Signalment

- Date and time of exam
- Animal's name, species, gender and reproductive status, age, color, identification or unusual markings, tattoos, microchip, etc.
- You might want to consider asking how long the owner has had the animal, if you don't know
- Name of owner, contact information
- Note all veterinary staff members involved with exam

Verbal account of injury

- Reason for bringing in the animal and chief complaint (by client)
- Any documentation concerning what the client tells you when explaining the animal's condition including relationship, behavior, conduct concerning the animal's injury, any changes/inconsistencies of the account, age of suspected abuser (adult, child, etc.)

Reporting in the medical record

- Your client may make a statement to you regarding what happened. It is essential to try to write down exactly what is said.
- Document the timeliness of seeking veterinary care.

Photography

Attach any pictures of the animal. Remember to take "before and after" pictures, and full body shots as well as close-ups. Document that all photos came from the same animal. Remember that fur and feathers may conceal injury, so you may consider shaving the animal. Be sure the photos are "in context"—take full body shots and close-ups. Video recording could be used to document an animal's gait or other behavior, if applicable. Do not delete any photographs even if they are out of focus.

Physical findings

Perform a complete physical exam noting any abnormalities or unusual findings. You can add a physical sticker to indicate the location of the injuries on the body. Note if these are new or old injuries. A wound diagram using a silhouette drawing for that species may be helpful.

Also include:

- How animal was brought in (walked in on own, limping, carried, etc.)
- Note whether the animal was in pain or was suffering
- Weight (if first time seeing the animal, ask if the animal's weight has changed)
- Body condition (be specific as to what score scale you use, or be very descriptive)
- Coat condition (note any unusual patterns, suspected parasites, or foreign material)
- Dental condition
- Behavior of animal (nervous, shy, apathetic, pain, suffering, etc.)
- Any physical evidence (embedded collar, bullet fragment, burned fur/feathers, etc.)

Diagnostic tests

- Document all laboratory tests performed (be sure findings and diagnosis are in the medical record).
- Additional research may be warranted if the case is unusual or peculiar, such as unique issues related to certain types of poison.
- If taking radiographs, include a full body radiograph, or obtain several radiographs that cover the entire body. There may be additional injuries that aren't immediately apparent upon initial exam.
- Try to keep concern about expenses a non-issue. The money spent on exams and tests may corroborate or negate your findings, which may serve to be priceless in the long run. Also, if the individual responsible for the abuse is convicted, it is likely he/she will be ordered to reimburse you through a restitution order. There may be other forms of financial restitution as well.

Euthanasia

- If the animal is euthanized, note the reasons why. A reason might be "extreme pain and suffering," or "injured past recovery."
- If the animal is dead or must be euthanized, store the body until the body can be transported for a forensic necropsy. The forensic pathologist (or possibly animal control) will tell you whether to refrigerate or freeze. Note the date, time, who, and what agency when you release the body.

DO NOT return the animal (dead or alive) to the client. Remember to call law enforcement to assist if you anticipate any type of conflict with the client or if you feel your safety or the safety of others (human or animals) is at risk.

Releasing evidence (either physical evidence or the body)

Understand chain of custody. Identify physical evidence by labeling the envelope or box with date, patient name, your initials, etc. Put evidence in a safe place or refrigerate if there are perishable items. If you turn the evidence over to law enforcement, note date, time, who you gave it to, and the person's agency. Remember that the body of an animal, dead or alive, is evidence.

PRIMER FOR REPORTING (AKA: HELP! HOW DO I GET STARTED?)

This process can be beneficial beyond simply reporting animal cruelty. It is about building relationships with people in a parallel field. Establish a contact before you need them. It is easier now to find the correct contacts than when you are in the middle of a suspected cruelty situation and need advice quickly. It's good to know people involved in your local law enforcement, animal control, humane societies and others whom you may someday encounter.

AREAS ON THE MAGNET

In an emergency

Never compromise the safety of humans or animals. If there is a feeling of risk or harm, calling 911 is the quickest method of reaching authorities.

1) Local law enforcement

- It's the fastest and the best way to contact someone
- They know the law and can assist you with understanding the law
- Contact them when you suspect abuse; remember: you only report—not investigate—the incident
- Contact them if you are concerned that you, your staff, or your clinic needs protection
- Have more than one contact if possible; anticipate the need for an after-hours or emergency contact
- Use the internet and put in the name of the city or county you are in and search for "Police Department"

Here's a suggested script for requesting the correct contact:

PATTERNS OF NON-ACCIDENTAL INJURY

Head Trauma	Asymmetry from contusions or fractures Petechiae Ruptured tympanic membranes	Radiographs Inner ear exam
Abrasions or Bruising	Evidence of healing bruises or cuts (indicative of repetitive abuse) Embedded debris in skin or fur that can indicate dragging or throwing Fractured bones or ribs, including evidence of past injuries	Radiographs note location, size and shape to connect to potential weapon
Feet Injuries	Frayed nails Torn pads Debris caught between pads and fur, or within frayed nail	Swipe feet across paper to preserve trace evidence; in deceased animals, remove nail DNA
Burns	Smell wound for accelerants, oils or chemicals	Swab the wound before and after treatment for analysis of chemical Photograph burn patterns
Starvation	Evidence of pica Gastric ulcers Occult fecal blood Melena	Bone marrow fat analysis Routine profile Examine stomach content and feces
Embedded Collar	Visible signs of trauma Foul odor from infection and necrosis	Take pictures before and after shaving Measure width and depth of wound Save the collar
Dog Fighting	Characteristic puncture wounds on face, neck and front legs Evidence of starvation and beatings Evidence of heavy chain used as collar	Test for use of steroids, analgesics, hormones or diuretics
Gunshot Wounds	Fur forced in or out at entrance and exit wounds Singed fur or coat Abrasion rings Gunshot residue on or inside the wound	Remove bullets with fingers or cotton-wrapped forceps Photograph each wound before and after cleaning Shave and note powder patterns
Ligature Injuries	Crushing injury to skin, blood vessels and tissue Surrounding tissue may be inflamed and infected	Characteristic bruising pattern Trace evidence
Knife Wounds	Length and type of blade Note tapers on one or both ends of wound	Measure external wounds Measure wound depth Swab for DNA, both human and animal

Source: Melinda Merck, DVM. Reprinted with permission from The American Society for Prevention of Cruelty to Animals (ASPCA)

"Hello, my name is _____ and I'm a _____ (e.g., veterinarian, veterinary technician, receptionist) at _____ clinic. There is a new law that requires us to report animal cruelty. Who should I call within your agency, or do I need a different agency? We'd also like you to be aware of our clinic. Thank you."

2) Local animal care agency

This may be a humane society, animal control agency, or other organization that will deal directly with animal cruelty cases. Other examples include: shelters and rescues, including horse rescue that are available to law enforcement to house impounded animals (law enforcement may ask for some assistance as well). The brand inspector can also be a source of information regarding livestock laws.

3) Bureau of animal protection

Depending on the information gathered at the local level, state officials of the Bureau of Animal Protection may become involved upon the request of local law enforcement authorities. All cases involve local authorities as the investigators. Only law enforcement and district attorneys can file criminal cruelty and/or neglect charges against an individual.

ADDITIONAL CONTACTS

There may be more than one agency with jurisdiction in your area.

- District, county, and city attorney
- Animal control
- Humane society.

Appendix 2
Case Status Form

AGENCY/CASE #: _____

ANIMAL ID #: _____

OFFICER: _____

PERSON(S) CHARGED: _____

PROSECUTOR: _____

DEFENSE COUNSEL: _____

CHARGES:_____

COURT DATE:_____TIME:_____PLACE:_____

JUDGE:_____

OUTCOME: _____

NOTES:_____

UPDATES

DATE: _____

DATE: _____

DATE: _____

DATE: _____

DATE: _____

DATE: _____

DATE: _____

DATE: _____

DATE: _____

Veterinary Forensics: Animal Cruelty Investigations, Second Edition. Edited by Melinda D. Merck.
© 2013 John Wiley & Sons, Inc. Published 2013 by John Wiley & Sons, Inc.

Appendix 3
Evidence Log/Chain of Custody Form

Agency:_____

Case Number: _____

Evidence Holding Location: _____

Item ID	Evidence Description	Date	Initials	Purpose for Removal/Tests Performed

Veterinary Forensics: Animal Cruelty Investigations, Second Edition. Edited by Melinda D. Merck.
© 2013 John Wiley & Sons, Inc. Published 2013 by John Wiley & Sons, Inc.

Item ID____ Removal Date_____   Receipt Date_____

By_____   By_____

Release Sign_____   Receipt Sign:_____

Item ID____ Removal Date_____   Receipt Date_____

By_____   By_____

Release Sign_____   Receipt Sign:_____

Item ID____ Removal Date_____   Receipt Date_____

By_____   By_____

Release Sign_____   Receipt Sign:_____

Item ID____ Removal Date_____   Receipt Date_____

By_____   By_____

Release Sign_____   Receipt Sign:_____

Item ID____ Removal Date_____   Receipt Date_____

By_____   By_____

Release Sign_____   Receipt Sign:_____

Appendix 4
Photo Log

Agency: _____

Case Number: _____

Date of Incident/Exam: _____

Photographer: _____   Assisted By: _____

Digital CD Copies: _____ Provided to:_____

Photo #(s)	Notes

Appendix 5
Animal Cruelty Forensic Supplies

GENERAL

Animal Cruelty Investigation Kit, available from Tri-Tech, Inc. (see Webliography)

Privacy screens, tents, portable enclosures

Exam tables

Refrigeration or cooling unit

Calculator

Ammonia detector

EVIDENCE IDENTIFICATION, COLLECTION, AND PACKAGING

Evidence bags, various sizes: paper, plastic

Evidence containers: boxes, glass/plastic jars, arson/metal paint cans

Evidence envelopes: various sizes

Evidence tags

Evidence tape/labels

Clipboard, preferably with holding compartment

Forms: Evidence/chain of custody log, entomology, botany

Permanent markers, ink pens, pencils

PPE: masks, gloves, booties, Tyvek suit, gown

Presumptive blood test kits

Hidden blood detection supplies

ALS or UV light and UV spectacles

Flashlight (oblique lighting)

Scissors, knives

Forceps/tweezers: metal, plastic

Water, soap, disinfectant, alcohol, paper towels to clean and sanitize instruments

Tongue depressors to collect samples

Sterile swabs

Sterile water/distilled water

Swab boxes

Slides and slide mailers

Trace evidence lifters/clear tape

White paper/pharmaceutical folds for trace evidence

Magnifying glass

Mikrosil casting putty kit: brown

Trajectory rods

Rape kit

Large plastic bags

Zip-ties for body bags, tags

White sheets to wrap bodies

Bagging kit or paper bags

Rubber bands

Environmental thermometers

Entomology collection supplies

Botany collection supplies

Metal detector

SCENE DOCUMENTATION: MAPPING, PHOTOGRAPHY

Digital camera

Video camera

Camera tripod

Photo scales (ABFO no.2, others), photo markers

Evidence markers

Forms: Photo log, evidence/chain of custody

Graph paper

Measuring tapes: metal, vinyl

Permanent markers, dry erase markers, ink pens (variety of colors), pencils

Dry erase board

Crime scene barrier tape

Scene lighting, flashlights, extension cords

Veterinary Forensics: Animal Cruelty Investigations, Second Edition. Edited by Melinda D. Merck.
© 2013 John Wiley & Sons, Inc. Published 2013 by John Wiley & Sons, Inc.

GRAVE EXCAVATION/SURFACE REMAINS

In addition to above supplies:

GPS unit

Compass

Wooden stakes and hammer

Rebar/steel stakes

String

Crime scene tape

Line level

Plumb bob

Wooden measuring stick

Shovels

Axe

Metal detector

Hand trowels, variety of sizes

Paint brushes, hand brushes, tongue depressors

Dust pans

Buckets

T-square

Garden clippers, loppers

Heavy duty gloves

Tarps

Sifters, saw horses

Wheel barrow

Forms: Skeletal inventory, entomology, botany

Portable tables, chairs, tent

ENTOMOLOGY COLLECTION

Plastic spoon, soft forceps

Paint brush, water

Hand towel

Sweep net

Vials, pharmacy bottles, urine specimen bottles

Paper towels and rubber bands

70%–80% Ethyl alcohol

Killing jar or large zip lock bag, cotton balls, 100% acetone
   for killing adult insects

Vermiculite or sawdust

Beef liver

Petri dish or small container for live rearing

Larger plastic containers to hold live samples

Fine mesh to tape on cut-out plastic lids for live samples

Mailing labels and white paper to create labels, pencils

Forms: entomology

Appendix 6
Clandestine Burial Crime Scene Checklist

1. Conduct a strip/line (or appropriate type) search of the area. Flag the following items:
   a. Surface physical evidence
   b. Indicators of possible burial
   c. Indicators of human disturbance
2. Once the gravesite has been identified tape-off and secure the scene
3. Make assignment of duties for crime scene processing
4. Photograph the scene before processing
5. Survey site with a metal detector
   a. Flag all metal detector hits (do not remove at this time)
6. Examine scene for surface evidence and use evidence markers
   a. Biological evidence (tissue, bone, hair, teeth, nails, botany, and entomology)
   b. Physical evidence
7. Establish an area for equipment and work space
   a. Equipment
   b. Sifting
   c. Location for cleared material
8. Begin initial note taking and filling out worksheets with times, dates, locations, etc.
9. Select a datum point—something that is as permanent as possible that can be identified in the future (a large tree or some type of landmark); map/grid will be located from this datum point
10. Obtain a GPS coordinate at the datum point
11. Establish grid
12. Determine the size of the grid that is desired with burial site in center
13. Establish the grid on a north/south and east/west axis
14. Select one corner of the grid to be the reference point, called the subdatum, at the southwest corner
15. Ensure that the subdatum is the highest corner
16. Obtain a GPS coordinate at the subdatum to serve as a reference point and measurements to datum point
17. If unable to get GPS reading, take measurements from two different fixed locations to establish location of subdatum
18. Construct grid
19. Start by placing one wooden stake in the ground at the subdatum, flat side facing interior
20. From the subdatum, measure along a north axis (length determined by grid size) and place a second stake in the ground; this is the N/S axis
21. The stake should be placed diagonally from the second stake and east of the subdatum to create a right angle triangle; this establishes the E/W axis
22. To calculate the placement of the third stake, the Pythagorean theorem may be used to create a triangle with 90° at the subdatum
23. Pythagorean Theorem $A^2 + B^2 = C^2$

$$10^2 + 10^2 = C^2 \quad \rightarrow \quad 100 + 100 = C^2 \quad \rightarrow$$
$$200 = C^2 \quad \rightarrow \quad C = 14.14 \text{ feet}$$

$$8^2 + 8^2 = C^2 \quad \rightarrow \quad 64 + 64 = C^2 \quad \rightarrow$$
$$128 = C^2 \quad \rightarrow \quad C = 11.31 \text{ feet}$$

24. With a N/S axis wall of 10 feet, the third stake should be placed 14 feet diagonally from the second pin (or stake) and 10 feet from the subdatum on the E/W axis

Veterinary Forensics: Animal Cruelty Investigations, Second Edition. Edited by Melinda D. Merck.
© 2013 John Wiley & Sons, Inc. Published 2013 by John Wiley & Sons, Inc.

25. You should now connect the with survey string to form a 90° triangle with the intersections of the north/south and east/west lines at the subdatum

26. This method ensures that your grid is square and you have reference points of 90°

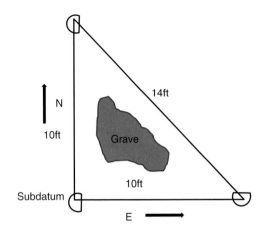

27. A string from the subdatum stake is tied at a measured point above the surface and a line level attached to take depth measurements within the grid

28. Now that the grid is in place, all items of evidence within and outside the grid can be measured

29. All measurements must be taken perpendicular to the grid wall for the most accuracy

30. Depth measurements should be taken for each item within the burial

31. All items outside the grid can be measured by extending the grid in the appropriate direction (south and west) and recording both the direction and the measurement

32. Photograph the completed grid

33. Consider collection of special evidence prior to removal of surface leaf litter or foliage
   a. Botany evidence
   b. Entomology evidence

34. Leaf litter on the surface can be removed by hand or light raking
   a. All material removed from the surface of the grid must be thoroughly searched
   b. All material removed should be placed aside in a designated area

35. Once all the loose material has been removed from within the grid, cut grass and roots with clippers down to the surface of the dirt, do not pull any materials out of the ground, clip them at the surface

36. Mark any evidence that is on the surface; log any evidence collected

37. Photographs should be taken periodically and especially prior to excavation

38. Begin to remove small amounts of soil from the top surface with a shovel to uncover the grave outline (called shining), looking for areas where the soil changes color

39. All soil that is removed from the area must be sifted and searched for evidence

40. Once the grave outline is identified you can begin to remove soil from gravesite with trowels, removing 1–2 cm at a time, keeping the surface level

41. Remember to move the trowels from the center of the grave toward the side walls

42. Take the soil down evenly over the surface of the grave

43. Do not scrape the trowel up the surface of the grave walls

44. When close to the remains it may be necessary to switch to smaller tools, such as brushes and tongue depressors

45. The goal is to completely expose the remains and dig them out on a pedestal if possible

46. Small loose bones or evidence may be documented and removed to prevent loss during excavation

47. Continue note taking, including the orientation, position, and description of the remains inside the grave or any other important details

48. Metal detecting should be conducted periodically throughout the digging processes until all of the metal detector hits are identified and cleared or collected

49. When the remains have become completely uncovered and they are pedestaled, the remains should be documented by:
   a. Sketches with measurements
   b. Photographs
   c. Notes

50. Once all the documentation is complete the remains are removed from the grave

51. Place the remains out on a tarp and conduct a detailed inventory

52. Take photographs of the bottom of the grave

53. Search the bottom of the grave with the metal detector

54. Continue to excavate until you confirm you have reached the bottom of the grave

55. Complete any remaining paper work

56. Package any evidence and remains.

Appendix 7
Veterinarian Crime Scene Checklist

- ☐ Lead agency name, address, contact numbers
- ☐ Case number
- ☐ Full street address of scene
- ☐ Name/contact info of person who authorized you to the scene
- ☐ Date and time of arrival
- ☐ Date and time of departure
- ☐ Exchange contact info with person in charge of the case
- ☐ Exchange contact info with person in charge of the scene
- ☐ Exchange contact info with PIO
- ☐ Obtain/exchange contact info with prosecutor (if assigned or present)
- ☐ Record all known info of alleged crime from lead officer
- ☐ Record search warrant information, verify what is covered and restricted in the warrant, name of person who obtained search warrant
- ☐ Identify person responsible for processing seized evidence
- ☐ Verify your role and responsibilities at the scene
- ☐ Name/contact info of person in charge of mapping scene
- ☐ Name of person responsible for overall photography and videography
- ☐ Obtain permission to take photographs
- ☐ Verify scene is secure and identify boundaries, location of any media
- ☐ Identify established entrance/exit for authorized personnel
- ☐ Conduct walk-through and document initial findings
- ☐ Determine team composition, equipment needs, issues to address
- ☐ Prioritize collection of evidence to prevent loss, destruction, or contamination
- ☐ Continuous note taking and photography/videography
- ☐ Record general observations
- ☐ Record weather information (outdoor scenes)
- ☐ Describe area
- ☐ Record HVAC settings and temperature (indoor scenes)
- ☐ Record number of live and deceased animals including names

- ☐ Housing conditions including food and water
- ☐ Record brand, expiration date and codes on food
- ☐ Presence and condition of urine and feces
- ☐ Record husbandry evidence
- ☐ Record medications and supplies including full Rx info, expiration dates
- ☐ Paraphernalia associated with crime
- ☐ Weapons
- ☐ Gunshot evidence
- ☐ Restraints
- ☐ Blood evidence
- ☐ Other biological evidence
- ☐ Trace evidence
- ☐ Botany evidence
- ☐ Impression evidence
- ☐ What is missing that should be here?
- ☐ What should not be here?
- ☐ Evidence log
- ☐ Photo log
- ☐ Assist/review law enforcement with evidence receipt
- ☐ Final scene walk through

DEATH SCENES

- ☐ Record general observations
- ☐ Record any obvious injury
- ☐ Record position of body
- ☐ Record rigor
- ☐ Record any noted lividity
- ☐ Record decomposition
- ☐ Record rectal temperature(s)
- ☐ Bag feet
- ☐ Wrap/bag body
- ☐ Arrange for transport/holding
- ☐ Entomology collection and documentation
- ☐ Botany collection and documentation
- ☐ Water temperature and samples (body found in water)

Veterinary Forensics: Animal Cruelty Investigations, Second Edition. Edited by Melinda D. Merck.
© 2013 John Wiley & Sons, Inc. Published 2013 by John Wiley & Sons, Inc.

Appendix 8
Deceased Animal Intake Questionnaire

Officer's name _____ Contact info _____

Agency _____ Date and time of arrival _____

Animal ID/name _____ Species _____ Breed _____ Sex_____

Status (circle):   Stray   Abandoned   Seized (owned)   Seized (relinquished)

Describe cruelty suspected: _____

Current investigation findings including any statements (attach officer's report): _____

_____

_____

_____

_____

Photos/videos: Copies provided___ To be provided_____ Chain of Custody Form signed_____

Date and location animal removed from/found: _____

Prior body holding: Refrig__ Freezer__ Rm Temp__ Date/time of holding_____

If animal was initially alive, describe observations, demeanor, exams, medical history:_____

_____

_____

ENVIRONMENT DESCRIPTION:

Indoor/outdoor _____ Weather/temperature conditions _____

Food _____ Water _____ Feces/Urine _____

Describe housing conditions, cleanliness, type of shelter, confinement _____

_____

Other animals _____

Scene description/findings (include physical, biological evidence, weapons, blood stains):

_____

_____

_____

_____

_____

Veterinary Forensics: Animal Cruelty Investigations, Second Edition. Edited by Melinda D. Merck.
© 2013 John Wiley & Sons, Inc. Published 2013 by John Wiley & Sons, Inc.

Appendix 9
Live Animal Intake Questionnaire

Officer's name _____ Contact info _____

Agency _____ Date and time of arrival _____

Animal ID/name _____ Species_____ Breed _____ Sex_____

Status (circle):   Stray   Abandoned   Seized (owned)   Seized (relinquished)

Describe cruelty suspected: _____

Current investigation findings including any statements (attach officer's report): _____

_____

_____

_____

_____

Medical history info: _____

Photos/videos: Copies provided_____ To be provided_____ Chain of Custody Form signed_____

Date and location animal removed from/found: _____

Animal demeanor at scene and any changes: _____

ENVIRONMENT DESCRIPTION:

Indoor/outdoor _____ Weather/temperature conditions _____

Food _____ Water _____ Feces/Urine _____

Describe housing conditions, type of shelter, confinement _____

_____

Cleanliness _____

Other animals _____

Scene description/findings (include physical, biological evidence, weapons, blood stains):

_____

_____

_____

_____

_____

Veterinary Forensics: Animal Cruelty Investigations, Second Edition. Edited by Melinda D. Merck.
© 2013 John Wiley & Sons, Inc. Published 2013 by John Wiley & Sons, Inc.

Appendix 10
Live Exam Form

Agency:

Officer:

Case #:

Examining veterinarian:

Date of exam: Time: Start Finish

SUBJECT OF EXAM:

METHOD OF ARRIVAL:

MATERIALS PROVIDED/REVIEWED:

CRIME SCENE/FORENSIC FINDINGS:

EXAMINATION FINDINGS:

Weight: T: MM/CRT: HYDRATION:

Coat Condition: Parasites:

BCS: (1) Emaciated (2) Very thin (3) Thin (4) Underweight 5) Ideal (6) Overweight (7) Heavy (8) Obese (9) Grossly obese

EENM (eyes, ears, nose, mouth):

Ausc/Abd Palp:

Perineal:

Musculoskeletal:

Additional findings:

Evidence of Medical/Surgical Intervention –

Radiographic Interpretation –

Evidence/Samples Collected and Testing:

Veterinary Forensics: Animal Cruelty Investigations, Second Edition. Edited by Melinda D. Merck.
© 2013 John Wiley & Sons, Inc. Published 2013 by John Wiley & Sons, Inc.

Appendix 11
Necropsy Exam Form

Agency:

Officer:

Case #:

Examining veterinarian:

Date of exam: Time: Start   Finish

SUBJECT OF EXAM:

ROUTE OF DELIVERY:

DESCRIPTION OF PACKAGING:

MATERIALS PROVIDED/REVIEWED:

CRIME SCENE/FORENSIC FINDINGS:

EXAMINATION FINDINGS:

External exam:

Decomposition score:

Rigor:

Lividity:

Rectal Temp:

Entomological Evidence:

BCS: (1) Emaciated   (2) Very thin   (3) Thin   (4) Underweight   (5) Ideal   (6) Overweight
(7) Heavy   (8) Obese   (9) Grossly obese

Veterinary Forensics: Animal Cruelty Investigations, Second Edition. Edited by Melinda D. Merck.
© 2013 John Wiley & Sons, Inc. Published 2013 by John Wiley & Sons, Inc.

Weight:

Coat condition:

Ectoparasites:

Head:

Chest:

Abdomen:

Perineum:

Legs:

Feet:

Tail:

Evidence of medical/surgical intervention:

Radiographic interpretation:

Internal exam:

Skin reflection findings:

Head:

Thoracic Cavity:

Abdominal Cavity:

Neck:

Respiratory Tract:

Cardiovascular System:

Gastrointestinal Tract:

Biliary Tract:

Pancreas:

Spleen:

Adrenals:

Urinary Tract:

Reproductive Tract:

Musculoskeletal System:

Samples Collected:

Additional Comments:

Appendix 12
Fixed Tissue List for Histopathology

Agency:

Animal ID:

Date:

Case #:

Lab Submission:

Veterinarian:

1. Preserve the tissues in 10% buffered formalin at a ratio of 1 part tissue to 10 parts formalin.
2. Samples should be no more than 0.5 cm to 1 cm thick and 3×4 cm (length and width) to fix properly. The exceptions are brain, spinal cord, and eye. The ratio of tissue to formalin is 1:10 in the wide mouth containers.
3. Tissues collected should be based on case information, medical history, and necropsy findings including lesions, wounds, and evidence of injury or disease.
   - ☐ Salivary gland
   - ☐ Oral/pharyngeal mucosa and tonsil
   - ☐ Tongue: cross section near tip including both mucosal surfaces
   - ☐ Lung: sections from several lobes including a major bronchus
   - ☐ Trachea
   - ☐ Thyroid/parathyroid
   - ☐ Lymph nodes: cervical, mediastinal, bronchial, mesenteric and lumbar; cut transversely
   - ☐ Thymus
   - ☐ Heart: sections from both sides including valves
   - ☐ Liver: sections from three different areas including gall bladder
   - ☐ Spleen: cross sections including capsule

GI Tract: 3-cm long sections of

   - ☐ Esophagus
   - ☐ Stomach: multiple sections from all regions of the lining
   - ☐ Intestines: multiple sections from different areas
   - ☐ Omentum: 3-cm square
   - ☐ Pancreas: sections from two areas
   - ☐ Adrenal: entire gland with transverse incision
   - ☐ Kidney: cortex and medulla from each kidney
   - ☐ Urinary bladder, ureters, urethra: cross section of bladder and 2-cm sections of ureter and urethra
   - ☐ Reproductive tract: entire uterus and ovaries with longitudinal cuts into lumens of uterine horns; both testes (transversely cut) with epididymis; entire prostate transversely cut
   - ☐ Eye
   - ☐ Brain: cut longitudinally along midline
   - ☐ Spinal cord: sections from cervical, thoracic, and lumbar cord
   - ☐ Diaphragm and skeletal muscle: cross section of thigh muscles
   - ☐ Opened rib or longitudinally sectioned femur: marrow must be exposed for proper fixation
   - ☐ Skin: full thickness of abdominal skin, lip, and ear pinna
   - ☐ Neonates: umbilical stump; include surrounding tissues

Veterinary Forensics: Animal Cruelty Investigations, Second Edition. Edited by Melinda D. Merck.
© 2013 John Wiley & Sons, Inc. Published 2013 by John Wiley & Sons, Inc.

Appendix 13
Canine Body Condition Score
for 1–9 and 1–5 Scales

(1/1) **Emaciated**: Ribs, lumbar vertebrae, pelvic bones, and all bony prominences evident from a distance. No discernible body fat. Obvious loss of muscle mass.

(2/1.5) **Very thin**: Ribs, lumbar vertebrae, and pelvic bones easily visible. No palpable fat. Some evidence of other bony prominence. Minimal loss of muscle mass.

(3/2) **Thin**: Ribs easily palpated and may be visible with no palpable fat. Tops of lumbar vertebrae visible. Pelvic bones becoming prominent. Obvious waist and abdominal tuck.

(4/2.5) **Underweight**: Ribs easily palpable with minimal fat covering. Waist easily noted when viewed from above. Abdominal tuck evident.

(5/3) **Ideal**: Ribs palpable without excess fat covering. Waist observed behind ribs when viewed from above. Abdomen tucked up when viewed from the side.

(6/3.5) **Overweight**: Ribs palpable with slight excess fat covering. Waist is discernible viewed from above but is not prominent. Abdominal tuck apparent.

(7/4) **Heavy**: Ribs palpable with difficulty; heavy fat cover. Noticeable fat deposits over lumbar area and base of tail. Waist absent or barely visible. Abdominal tuck may be present.

(8/4.5) **Obese**: Ribs not palpable under very heavy fat cover, or palpable only with significant pressure. Heavy fat deposits over lumbar area and base of tail. Waist absent. No abdominal tuck. Obvious abdominal distension may be present.

(9/5) **Grossly obese**: Massive fat deposits over thorax, spine, and base of tail. Waist and abdominal tuck absent. Fat deposits on neck and limbs. Obvious abdominal distention.

REFERENCES

www.aahanet.org/PublicDocuments/NutritionalAssessment Guidelines.pdf.
www.purina.com.

Veterinary Forensics: Animal Cruelty Investigations, Second Edition. Edited by Melinda D. Merck.
© 2013 John Wiley & Sons, Inc. Published 2013 by John Wiley & Sons, Inc.

Appendix 14
Feline Body Condition Score for 1–9 and 1–5 Scales

(1/1) Emaciated: Ribs visible on shorthaired cats, no palpable fat, severe abdominal tuck, lumbar vertebrae and wings of ilia easily palpated.

(2/1.5) Very thin: Ribs easily visible on shorthaired cats, lumbar vertebrae obvious with minimal muscle mass, pronounced abdominal tuck, no palpable fat.

(3/2) Thin: Ribs easily palpable with minimal fat covering, lumbar vertebrae obvious, obvious waist behind ribs, minimal abdominal fat.

(4/2.5) Underweight: Ribs palpable with minimal fat covering, noticeable waist behind ribs, slight abdominal tuck, abdominal fat pad absent.

(5/3) Ideal: Well-proportioned, observe waist behind ribs, ribs palpable with slight fat covering, abdominal fat pad minimal.

(6/3.5) Overweight: Ribs palpable with slight excess fat covering, waist and abdominal fat pad distinguishable but not obvious, abdominal tuck absent.

(7/4) Heavy: Ribs not easily palpated with moderate fat covering, waist poorly discernible, obvious rounding of abdomen, moderate abdominal fat pad.

(8/4.5) Obese: Ribs not palpable with excess fat covering, waist absent, obvious rounding of abdomen with prominent abdominal fat pad, fat deposits present over lumbar area.

(9/5) Grossly obese: Ribs not palpable under heavy fat cover; heavy fat deposits over lumbar area, face and limbs; distention of abdomen with no waist; extensive abdominal fat deposits.

REFERENCES

www.aahanet.org/PublicDocuments/NutritionalAssessment Guidelines.pdf.
www.purina.com.

Veterinary Forensics: Animal Cruelty Investigations, Second Edition. Edited by Melinda D. Merck.
© 2013 John Wiley & Sons, Inc. Published 2013 by John Wiley & Sons, Inc.

Appendix 15
Dog Diagram: Condition of Skin, Haircoat, and Nails Form

Date_____ Investigating Agency_____

Case#_____ Officer_____ Veterinarian_____

Animal ID_____ Breed_____ Color_____ Male_____ Female_____

Physical Care Scale: Haircoat and Nails (1) (2) (3) (4) (5)
Record skin lesions or wounds. Describe on diagram or comments section.

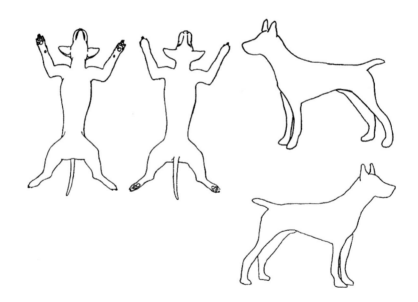

COMMENTS:

Veterinary Forensics: Animal Cruelty Investigations, Second Edition. Edited by Melinda D. Merck.
© 2013 John Wiley & Sons, Inc. Published 2013 by John Wiley & Sons, Inc.

PHYSICAL CARE SCALE

1. Adequate: clean, hair can be easily brushed or combed; nails ok
2. Lapsed: haircoat may be somewhat dirty or have a few mats present that are easily removed; remainder of coat can be easily brushed or combed; nails need a trim
3. Borderline: numerous mats but can still be groomed without a total clip down; no significant fecal or urine soiling; nails overgrown which may alter gait
4. Poor: substantial matting of haircoat; large sections of hair matted together; occasional foreign material embedded in mats; much of the hair will need to be clipped; fecal and urine soiling of hind end and legs; long nails that interfere with normal gait
5. Terrible: haircoat is single mat that prevents normal movement and interferes with vision; soiling of hind end and legs with trapped urine and feces; complete clipdown required; nails extremely overgrown into circles and may be penetrating pads causing pain and infection; nails interfering with normal gait

REFERENCE

www.tufts.edu/vet/hoarding/pubs/tacc.pdf

Appendix 16
Cat Diagram: Condition of Skin, Haircoat, and Nails Form

Date_____Investigating Agency_____

Case#_____Officer_____ Veterinarian_____

Animal ID_____Breed_____ Color_____ Male_____ Female_____

Physical Care Scale: Haircoat and Nails (1) (2) (3) (4) (5)
Record skin lesions or wounds. Describe on diagram or comments section.

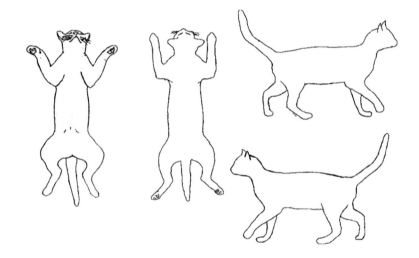

COMMENTS:

Veterinary Forensics: Animal Cruelty Investigations, Second Edition. Edited by Melinda D. Merck.
© 2013 John Wiley & Sons, Inc. Published 2013 by John Wiley & Sons, Inc.

PHYSICAL CARE SCALE

1. Adequate: clean, hair can be easily brushed or combed; nails ok
2. Lapsed: haircoat may be somewhat dirty or have a few mats present that are easily removed; remainder of coat can be easily brushed or combed; nails need a trim
3. Borderline: numerous mats but can still be groomed without a total clip down; no significant fecal or urine soiling; nails overgrown which may alter gait
4. Poor: substantial matting of haircoat; large sections of hair matted together; occasional foreign material embedded in mats; much of the hair will need to be clipped; fecal and urine soiling of hind end and legs; long nails that interfere with normal gait

Terrible: haircoat is single mat that prevents normal movement and interferes with vision; soiling of hind end and legs with trapped urine and feces; complete clipdown required; nails extremely overgrown into circles and may be penetrating pads causing pain and infection; nails interfering with normal gait

REFERENCE

(www.tufts.edu/vet/hoarding/pubs/tacc.pdf)

Appendix 17
Cat Skeleton Lesions Form

<table>
<tr><td colspan="2" align="center">SKELETAL LESIONS</td></tr>
<tr><td colspan="2">Date_____Investigating Agency_____</td></tr>
<tr><td colspan="2">Case#_____Officer_____Veterinarian_____</td></tr>
<tr><td colspan="2">Animal ID_____Breed_____Color_____Male_____Female_____</td></tr>
<tr><td colspan="2">Record injuries or abnormalities to skeleton. Describe on diagram or comments section.</td></tr>
</table>

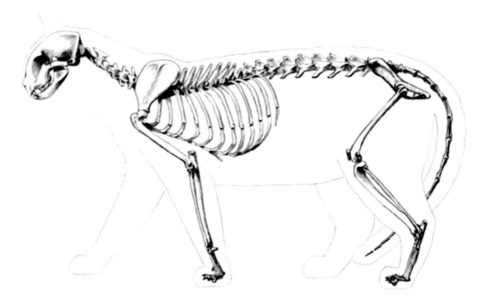

COMMENTS:

Veterinary Forensics: Animal Cruelty Investigations, Second Edition. Edited by Melinda D. Merck.
© 2013 John Wiley & Sons, Inc. Published 2013 by John Wiley & Sons, Inc.

Appendix 18
Dog Skeleton Lesions Form

<table>
<tr><td colspan="4" align="center">SKELETAL LESIONS</td></tr>
<tr><td>Date_____Investigating Agency_____</td></tr>
<tr><td>Case#_____Officer_____Veterinarian_____</td></tr>
<tr><td>Animal ID_____Breed_____Color_____Male_____Female_____</td></tr>
<tr><td>Record injuries or abnormalities to skeleton. Describe on diagram or comments section.</td></tr>
</table>

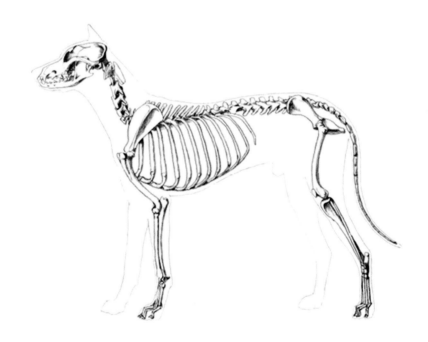

COMMENTS:

Veterinary Forensics: Animal Cruelty Investigations, Second Edition. Edited by Melinda D. Merck.
© 2013 John Wiley & Sons, Inc. Published 2013 by John Wiley & Sons, Inc.

Appendix 19
Cat and Dog Skeletal Inventory Form

Date_____ Case #_____ Animal ID:_____

Skull __ (Dentition: Dog I 1-3, C 1, P 1-4, M 1-2; Cat I 1-3, C 1, P 2-4, M 1)

Mandible __ (Dentition: Dog I 1-3, C 1, P 1-4, M 1-3; Cat I 1-3, C 1, P 3-4, M 1)

Notes:

Hyoid __
Notes:

Clavicle __
Notes:

Cervical vertebra (7) __
Notes:

Thoracic vertebra (13) __
Notes:

Lumbar vertebra (7) __
Notes:

Sacrum __
Notes:

Coccygeal vertebra __
Notes:

Pelvis __
Notes:

Ribs (13) __ Costal cartilage (13) __
Notes:

Sternum __
Notes:

Scapula__
Notes:

Humerus __
Notes:

Veterinary Forensics: Animal Cruelty Investigations, Second Edition. Edited by Melinda D. Merck.
© 2013 John Wiley & Sons, Inc. Published 2013 by John Wiley & Sons, Inc.

Case:_____ Animal ID:_____

Ulna __
Notes:

Radius __
Notes:

Carpals __
Notes:

Metacarpals __
Notes:

Phalanges (front) __
Notes:

Sesamoids __
Notes:

Femur __
Notes:

Patella __
Notes:

Tibia __
Notes:

Fibula __
Notes:

Tarsals __
Notes:

Metatarsals __
Notes:

Phalanges (hind) __
Notes:

Sesamoids __
Notes:

Additional bones:

Appendix 20
Live Exam Report Template

Agency:

Officer:

Case #:

Examining Veterinarian:

Date of Exam:

SUBJECT OF EXAM:

REASON FOR EXAM:

METHOD OF ARRIVAL:

CRIME SCENE/FORENSIC FINDINGS:

MEDICAL HISTORY:

ABBREVIATIONS: mm=mucous membranes; HLA=heart, lung auscultation; A=abdomen palpation; UR=unremarkable; BCS=body condition score

DEFINITIONS:

Body condition scale (Purina): (1) Emaciated (2) Very thin (3) Thin (4) Underweight (5) Ideal (6) Overweight (7) Heavy (8) Obese (9) Grossly Obese

EXAMINATION FINDINGS:

Evidence of Injury:

PROCEDURES AND RESULTS:

ENTOMOLOGY FINDINGS:

SUMMARY OF FINDINGS:

TIME OF INJURY:

MECHANISM OF INJURY:

CAUSE OF INJURY:

CONTRIBUTORY CAUSE:

MANNER OF INJURY:

CONCLUSIONS:

[NAME]   DATE:

[SIGNATURE]

Veterinary Forensics: Animal Cruelty Investigations, Second Edition. Edited by Melinda D. Merck.
© 2013 John Wiley & Sons, Inc. Published 2013 by John Wiley & Sons, Inc.

Appendix 21
Necropsy Report Template

Agency:

Investigator:

Case #:

Examining veterinarian:

Date of Exam:

SUBJECT OF EXAM:

REASON FOR EXAM:

METHOD OF ARRIVAL:

DESCRIPTION OF PACKAGING:

MATERIALS PROVIDED/REVIEWED:

CRIME SCENE/FORENSIC FINDINGS:

MEDICAL HISTORY:

ABBREVIATIONS: mm=mucous membranes; HLA=heart, lung auscultation; A=abdomen palpation; UR=unremarkable; BCS=body condition score

DEFINITIONS:

Body condition scale (Purina): (1) Emaciated (2) Very thin (3) Thin (4) Underweight (5) Ideal (6) Overweight (7) Heavy (8) Obese (9) Grossly obese

EXAMINATION FINDINGS:

External exam –

Rigor:

Decomposition:

Entomological evidence:

Body condition score:

Veterinary Forensics: Animal Cruelty Investigations, Second Edition. Edited by Melinda D. Merck.
© 2013 John Wiley & Sons, Inc. Published 2013 by John Wiley & Sons, Inc.

Weight:

Coat condition:

Ectoparasites:

Head:

Chest:

Abdomen:

Perineum:

Legs:

Feet:

Tail:

Evidence of medical/surgical intervention:

Radiographic interpretation:

Internal Exam:

Skin reflection:

Head:

Thoracic cavity:

Abdominal cavity:

Neck:

Respiratory tract:

Cardiovascular system:

Gastrointestinal tract:

Biliary tract:

Pancreas:

Spleen:

Adrenals:

Urinary tract:

Reproductive tract:

Musculoskeletal system:

Evidence of injury:

PROCEDURES AND RESULTS:

ENTOMOLOGY FINDINGS:

SUMMARY OF FINDINGS:

SURVIVAL PERIOD:

TIME OF DEATH:

CAUSE OF INJURY:

MANNER OF INJURY:

MECHANISM OF DEATH:

CAUSE OF DEATH:

CONTRIBUTORY CAUSE:

MANNER OF DEATH:

CONCLUSIONS:

[NAME]   DATE:

[SIGNATURE]

Appendix 22
Forensic Medical Protocol for Large Scale Cases

GENERAL

The animal evidence chief (AEC) has the final authority in all matters related to the animals and crime scene investigation. No changes in protocol may be done without AEC approval.

VETERINARY TEAMS

- Provide all veterinarians with contact info: cell phone number, email, office for questions that may arise at the scene and at the holding facility for the follow-up care.
- Provide all hospital locations (maps from scene and holding facility to their locations) and contact info where animals may need to be transported to.
- A forensic exam team leader should be at the receiving shelter site.
- The avian and equine vet should have or create similar records and protocol that is below for dogs/cats that is appropriate for those species.

SCENE ASSESSMENT

- The initial walk-through team which is comprised of the animal forensics chief and additional veterinarians depending on the size of the scene, should identify any critical animals and flag them with pre-determined markers. The walk-through team will brief the medical teams on the estimated number of animals, observed health conditions and any animals that are critical whose removal and assessment must be prioritized.

- Grave excavation/surface body dump: Any scene of grave excavation or surface body dump will be processed by a team determined and approved by the AEC.

EXAMINATIONS

Live Animals

Physical examination is to be conducted on all animals regardless of species. Examinations may be conducted by any state licensed veterinarian. Veterinarians that are licensed in other states but not the hosting state must comply with the practice act of the host state regarding examination, diagnosis, treatment, and drawing blood. The AEC will go over forms, photography, documentation, chain of custody, definition of evidence, and overall protocol with the forensic exam teams (FET) on the day of staging.

Issues to address:

- Prosecutor assigned to the case may need to request the non-state licensed veterinarians that are assisting as experts for this case
- Provide appropriate cameras for documentation by each medical team on and off-site
- Provide live animal exam forms for all vets to use (in triplicate)
- Protocol for animal ID, transfer of paperwork and lab specimens with animal to holding facility (chain of custody and continuity of animal care)

Veterinary Forensics: Animal Cruelty Investigations, Second Edition. Edited by Melinda D. Merck.
© 2013 John Wiley & Sons, Inc. Published 2013 by John Wiley & Sons, Inc.

Medical Record

An individual medical record must be made and maintained for each animal. These must be maintained where the animal is housed. This will consist of:

- Live exam form copy
- Daily care form
- Weight change form
- Copies of any lab results
- Any treatment or other care forms or recordings

Forensic Reports

- Overall: Reports will be prepared for the lead investigator and prosecutor. All exam forms, lab forms, and any animal health-related form will be given to the AEC. These forms are to be saved and organized by animal ID and location at each examination center by each team documenter.
- Live exams: All reports on dogs/cats examined will be written by the AEC and/or by a veterinarian approved by the AEC. All reports on other species will be written by the examining veterinarian for that animal.
- Deceased exams: All necropsy reports for dogs/cats will be written by the AEC and/or by a veterinarian approved by the AEC. All necropsy reports on other species will be written by the examining veterinarian for that animal.

Photography

All exams must be photographed using the proper forensic protocol and documentation. A general photo of the animal with the animal ID, case number, location, and date should be included in the first photo. Photos should be taken of the face, sides, rear, and top of the body as well as close-ups of any significant finding. When the digital card is full, the photos are to be downloaded on the appropriate computer or as directed by the AEC.

Examinations

Use the live exam forms provided. Forms are in carbonless triplicate. The bottom copy goes with the medical record. The original and second copy stay. The lab test request copy should be stapled together and kept in order by animal ID. They should be given to AEC.

Triage

All sick or critical animals at the scene will be assessed by the on-scene medical teams who will make the determination for euthanasia or treatment and where the animals are to be transported (hospital, ER, sheltering facility). All non-critical animals, determined by a veterinarian on-scene, will go to the holding facility for their initial examination and treatments by the shelter FE teams. It is critical to the animal's health and for the legal case that a veterinarian be continuously involved with this on-scene assessment. (Licensure issues as per the hosting state veterinary practice act.)

Diagnostic Testing

The purpose of diagnostic testing is to document overt and underlying health conditions. Laboratory and pathology submissions should include the following:

- Lab name and account
- Responsible party for payment
- The codes below should be used unless approved by the AEC.

Note that a template lab form will be provided to each medical holding team at the holding facility and on scene. Testing protocol lab codes
Considerations for dogs and cats

- Profile, CBC, fecal, UA
- Dogs only: HW, parvo
- Cats only: Felv/FIV
- Horses: by large animal vet
- Livestock: by large animal vet
- Birds: by avian vet

Test protocol (Example):

- Full blood work (which includes UA, Hw for dogs, Felv/FIV for cats in the panels) on all adult animals (6 months and older) regardless of health status determination
- Full blood work on all sick/thin animals regardless of age, unless exam findings determine blood work unnecessary
- Separated juvenile (less than 6 months) kittens, not sick/thin: Felv test only
- Diarrhea: fecal test
- Canines sick with diarrhea: parvo test

Additional diagnostics:

- To be determined by FE team veterinarian (state or non-state licensed as per state veterinary practice act) based on physical exam findings
- Payment for costs of additional diagnostics is:

Forensic Testing

- There may be evidence collected from the live animal that needs special forensic testing. This decision will be authorized by the AEC.
- Payment for costs of any forensics testing:
- Forensic evidence for dog fighting cases:

  A buccal DNA swab for each dog
  A separate scar/wound chart shall be completed for each dog and photographs of all scars/wounds

Treatments

Treatments may be performed by an appropriately licensed veterinarian or a veterinary aide/assistant/tech under the direction of such veterinarian (per the hosting state veterinary practice act). Basic treatments can be administered at the holding facility to reduce the workload of the on-scene medical teams.

- Organization responsible for medical supplies and cost:
- Treatments protocol (Example below: should always include parasite, vaccination protocol, and can be adjusted based on the legal nature of the case or available resources)

  Vaccinations
  Ectoparasite tx
  Deworming
  Minor wound treatment
  Antibiotics
  Eye medications
  SQ fluids
  Shaving (matted fur, medical reasons)
  Ear cleaning/tx
  Bathing (medical reasons)

Advanced/Emergency Treatments

Animals that require hospitalization, surgery or further diagnostics will be transported to a hospital or ER as determined by the veterinarian.

Post-Scene Animal Care

- The holding facility will need to be staffed with host state licensed veterinarians and supportive personnel as appropriate per the state veterinary practice act since the majority of treatments will be performed there. Also, it may be that the majority of animals are initially examined there.
- The holding facility will follow the live animal exam form for any initial exam (if not conducted on scene).

- The holding facility will follow the lab testing and treatment protocol as outlined by the above.
- All animals' follow-up care will be documented as per protocol: (establish sheltering protocol)
- Once the crime scene has been fully processed, all available and qualified personnel will move to the holding facility to provide support to the shelter and medical staff.
- All animals removed from the holding facility to go to foster/adoption/hospital site must have a summary status report. This report is to outline the animal's response to treatment, outcome, weight gain/loss, and any developing medical conditions.

Euthanasia Decisions

The determination to treat or euthanize is based on veterinarian assessment which must be approved by the animal evidence chief (veterinarian) or, if unavailable, his/her designated lead veterinarian in charge. The final decision for euthanasia will be made by the lead law enforcement agent and AEC or his/her designee which must be an authorized individual as per the hosting state veterinary practice act of 1967. Euthanasia can only be performed by the appropriate person as per the state veterinary practice act.

  Protocol for criteria to euthanize:

Deceased Animals

All euthanized and deceased animals will be held for necropsy. The AEC will determine how, where, and when a necropsy will be performed. The AEC must be notified if any animals are found dead at the scene, or die at the scene or after removal from the scene. All skeletonized remains will be examined by the AEC and/or other expert approved by animal forensics chief.

  Dogs/cats by:
  Horses by:
  Livestock by:
  Birds by:
  Issues to address:

- Where bodies can be held under REFRIGERATION ONLY until necropsies can be performed (temporary morgue)

MEDICAL SUPPLIES AND EQUIPMENT CONSIDERATIONS

- See general supply list to customize for each case
- Staff equipment: Vets to bring own stethoscope; consider bringing a digital camera, thermometer, oto/opthalmoscope if possible
- Spray bottles for cleaning cages/tables

- Veterinary grade disinfectant for spraying/cleaning cages and tables
- Paper towels
- Towels for handling, bedding
- Bowls
- Canned and dry food for dogs and cats
- Any extra microscopes for skin scrapings, fecal, UAs, etc.
- Medicated shampoos for dogs (Malaseb or something similar that is antibacterial/antifungal)
- Container for alcohol cotton balls, chlorhexadine solution with gauze
- Hand soap
- Fecal loops
- Exam gowns for contagious (PPE)
- Trash bags for bodies and evidence tags for body bags
- Euthanasia solution
- Handling equipment for Holding facility (no catch-poles for cats! Towels and bite buster sleeves work best), leashes, muzzles, etc.

Appendix 23
Large Scale Medical Supply List

Veterinary Forensics: Animal Cruelty Investigations, Second Edition. Edited by Melinda D. Merck.
© 2013 John Wiley & Sons, Inc. Published 2013 by John Wiley & Sons, Inc.

Medical Supplies

Exams	Quantity	Check	Animal First Aid	Quantity	Check	Crash Cart List	Quantity	Check	Needles and Syringes	Quantity	Check
Alcohol			22-g, 25-g, 18-g catheters			22-g, 25-g, 18-g butterflies			18-g needles		
Animal glucometer			Blade holder			Allergic reaction medications			1-cc 25-g		
Animal shampoo			Burn relief gel pack			Cardiac arrest medications			1-ml syringes		
Antibiotics injectable			Chlorhexidine scrub			Endotracheal tubes			22-g needles		
Antibiotics ophthalmic			Chlorhexidine solution			Laryngoscope			25-ml syringes		
Antibiotics oral			Cotton roll			Nutri-Cal$R$			3-cc 22-g		
Antibiotics topical			Dextrose 50% injectable			Shock medications			3-cc 25-g		
Bandage scissors			Forceps						3-cc oral syringes		
Bathmats for exam table surface			Hemostats						3-ml syringes		
Bite buster sleeves			Hydrogen peroxide						6-ml syringes		
Blood collection tubes: lavender top			Non-adhesive pads								
Blood collection tubes: SST			Porous tape								
Blood/urine/fecal tube centrifuge			Scissors								
Canine nail trimmers			Sutures								
Canned food			VetrapTM								
Clipper cleaner, cooling spray			Vitamin B injectable								
Controlled drug log											
Cordless clippers											
Corneal stain											
Cotton balls											
Cotton tip applicators											
Cover slips											
Dewormer (rounds, hooks, tapes, coccidia, giardia)											
Digital thermometers											

(continued)

Medical Supplies

Exams	Quantity	Check	Animal First Aid	Quantity	Check	Crash Cart List	Quantity	Check	Needles and Syringes	Quantity	Check
Ear cleaner											
Euthanasia solution											
Exam forms and diagram											
Exam gowns											
Eye solution											
Fecal loops											
Fecal sample cups											
Fecal solution											
Fecal tubes w/plastic caps for centrifuge											
Feliway$R$ spray											
Flea treatment: oral (Capstar$R$)											
Flea treatment: topical											
Fluids: 1 L											
Frosted microscope slides											
Gloves: large, nitrile only											
Gloves: medium, nitrile only											
Gloves: small, nitrile only											
Grooming tools: dematting comb, brush, flea comb											
Heating pads											
Hematocrit machine, tubes, clay, reader											
Immersion oil											
IV catheters											
IV lines (72-in lines) for sq fluids 10 to 15 drops/ml											
K-YR jelly											
Lab forms											
Lab test log											
Microscope											
Necropsy equipment											

Ophthalmoscope and
    otoscope
Pediatric milk
Rabies certificates
Scales
Sedative and reversals
SNAPR tests
Stethoscopes
Surgical blades (skin
    scraping)
Towels
Universal Microchip
    scanner
Urine multistix
Urine tubes
Vaccines
Whites nail trimmers
    (feline)

Appendix 24
Large Scale Live Animal Exam Form

AGENCY: Animal ID #_____

CASE #:   MICROCHIP: Y N #_____

DATE: DOCTOR: TIME:Start   Finish

BREED: COLOR: SEX: AGE EST:

TEMPERAMENT: WT (LBS):

BCS:(1) Emaciated   (2) Very thin   (3) Thin   (4) Lean   (5) Ideal   (6) Mildly overweight   (7) Overweight   (8) Obese
(9) Morbidly obese

T: MM/CRT: HYD:

EENM (eyes, ears, nose, mouth):

H/L:

ABD/PERINEUM:

U/G:

M/S:

SKIN:

FEET:

PARASITES:

APPETITE:

Veterinary Forensics: Animal Cruelty Investigations, Second Edition. Edited by Melinda D. Merck.
© 2013 John Wiley & Sons, Inc. Published 2013 by John Wiley & Sons, Inc.

COMMENTS:

SAMPLES TAKEN: ON-SCENE TESTS:

PARASITE TX: VACCS:

OTHER DIAGNOSTICS REQUIRED:

EUTH: Y N REASON: APPVD BY:

TX INSTRUCTIONS:

Appendix 25
Rapid Bird Exam Form

ID number: _____ **Date**_____

Type of bird: Budgie   Canary   Chicken   Cockatiel   Dove   Duck   Finch
Guinea   Peafowl   Pheasant   Pigeon   Quail   Turkey   Other _____

Age if known: Young   Adolescent   Adult   **Sex if known**:   Male   Female

Attitude: Aggressive   Active   Quiet   Depressed   Comatose   Died   in   Transit

Body Condition: _____/5 (1 Emaciated   2 Thin   3 Average   4 Heavy   5 Obese)

Abnormal Findings (circle): Posture   Respiration   Feathering   Eyes   Ears
Nostrils   Beak   Oral   Cavity   Head   Neck   Torso   Abdomen   Vent   Wings
Legs   Feet   Toes   Nails   Heart/Lungs   Other _____
Describe Abnormal Findings:

Plan: Regular Shelter Observation Cage Heated Brooder Quarantine
Further Exam Testing Treatment Euthanize Necropsy Other
Notes:

Dr. _____

Used with permission of Dr. Julie Burge

Veterinary Forensics: Animal Cruelty Investigations, Second Edition. Edited by Melinda D. Merck.
© 2013 John Wiley & Sons, Inc. Published 2013 by John Wiley & Sons, Inc.

Appendix 26
Botany Field Report

DATE: _____ AGENCY: _____ CASE NO: _____

LOCATION OF BOTANY COLLECTION SITE:

GENERAL DESCRIPTION OF SITE INCLUDING BOTANY (PHOTOS):

DESCRIPTION OF ANY SIGNS OF DISTURBANCE AT OR TO THE SITE (PHOTOS):

BOTANY COLLECTION

Type	Number of Samples	Location (site, object)	Collection Method

Veterinary Forensics: Animal Cruelty Investigations, Second Edition. Edited by Melinda D. Merck.
© 2013 John Wiley & Sons, Inc. Published 2013 by John Wiley & Sons, Inc.

Appendix 27
Dog Bite Investigation Worksheet

Agency

Case number

Bite level classification

Date   Time

Location of attack

Number of dogs involved in the attack

Nature of location (inside, outside, etc.)

Lighting

Weather at the time of the attack

Dog name

Breed

Sex   Age

Color, markings

Height

Weight

Owner name, address

Owner Race   Sex

Veterinary Forensics: Animal Cruelty Investigations, Second Edition. Edited by Melinda D. Merck.
© 2013 John Wiley & Sons, Inc. Published 2013 by John Wiley & Sons, Inc.

Disposition of dog

(Euthanized? Date, time, by whom. Euthanasia chemical used. Authorization of euthanization?)
(Returned to owners? Date, time, by whom, authorization)
(Destroyed at scene? By whom? Circumstances? Body retained for analysis?)

Source of dog-name/address

Type of source (breeder, pet store, etc.)

Number of previous homes

Parents known? Y/N

Parents owners-full info (supplementary case numbers)

Parents available for exam/interview? Y/N

Parents source-name/address

Parents source type

Siblings known? Y/N

Sibling owners name/address of each

Siblings available for exam/interview? Y/N
(supplementary case numbers)

Reproductive status of dog

Ever bred? Y/N

If female, is dog in estrus/recently been in/expected to be in soon? Y/N

Identity/location of progeny

Illness/injury? Y/N
Describe if yes

Vaccine history

Is dog currently on any medication? Y/N
If yes describe

Hearing?

Eyesight?

Hip conditions?

Blood tests

Samples taken-Date: Time:

By whom?

Fresh or post mortem?

    Chem/CBC
    Thyroid
    Steroids
    Testosterone
    Amphetamines/stimulants
    Hormones

Body condition/musculoskeletal

Parasites

Brain:

    Harvested?

    Date, time, by whom

    Freshly postmortem or delayed?

    Gross exam

    Rabies tested Y/N

    How preserved

Training/socialization

    Has dog had training? Y/N

    By whom, when, where, type

    Any earned titles? Y/N

    If yes list:

Used as:

    Guard dog Y/N
    Military dog Y/N
    Police dog Y/N
    Schutzhund Y/N

Has dog ever been fought? Y/N

Living conditions

> (Type of neighborhood-rural, suburbs, urban
> Type of residence-apartment, town home/patio home/duplex, single family home, property over 1 ac, other
> Containment: Fence, chain, tether, pen, indoor, none
> Primarily kept indoors or outdoors
> Sleeping arrangements)

> Diet

> Fed by

> Where, how often

Who disciplines dog

Usual method

Who has most frequent interaction with dog

Does dog have regular contact with other dogs? Y/N
Type, duration, frequency, location

Has dog shown aggression toward other dogs/animals? Y/N
Describe fully

Family:
> Type/ family makeup-adults/children/infants

> Basic dynamics

Quantity of contact with human family/quality

Aggression toward family members? Y/N

Contact with other humans:

> How often?

> Where?

> Adults, children, infants?

> Differing races?

> Disabled persons?

Aggression towards other humans:

> Adults Y/N
> Children or infants? Y/N
> Races Y/N
> Disabilities? Y/N
> Males vs. females?

Bite incident victim information:

Name

Address

Sex   Race   Height   Weight

If female, was victim menstruating at the time of the attack. Y/N

Relationship of victim to owner:

Relationship to dog

Was victim disabled or ill? Y/N
Under treatment for mental disability? Y/N
Any unusual physical attributes? Y/N Describe
Does victim have a history of seizures?
Does victim have a history of heart disease?
Victim dress at the time of the attack?

Victim's actions immediately before the attack.

Was victim known to the dog? Y/N
Did victim have contact with the dog prior to this incident? Y/N
Prior aggressive contact? Y/N

Witnesses to the incident?

Name

Address

Telephone

Details of the actual attack-sequence of events, response of victim, dog, and witnesses.

Exact injuries to victim. Order of injuries if established.

Details of any injuries to the dog, including when in the course of the attack injuries occurred.

Was the attack on dog's home territory or in a place familiar to the dog?

Were there other animals present or involved in the attack?

Full information and actions of each one.

Relationship of other dogs to the victim and to the primary dog.

Behavioral evaluation of dog:

    Date, time, location of evaluation-location type

    Physical demeanor of dog at initial contact

Responses of dog to stimuli (if available):

GR-growl
BT-bare teeth
LU-lunge/charge
SB-snap/bite-engage and release
BF-full bite

RR-retreat/run away
SR-submissive roll or urination
AG-evacuate anal gland
PR-Positive reaction
NR-No reaction
NA-Not available

Approach dog		Bend over dog/demand down	
Pet dog		Enter or leave room	
Hug dog		Reach toward dog w/o leash	
Approach on furniture		Reach toward dog w/leash	
Call off furniture		Put on/take off leash	
Push/pull off furniture		Put on/take off collar	
Disturb while resting/sleeping		Place in crate/pen	
Approach while chewing/playing		Remove from crate/pen	
Approach while eating		Leash restraint	
Touch while eating		Collar restraint	
Take dog food away		Bathe/groom dog	
Take human food away		Trim nails	
Take toy/chewy/bone		Response to obedience command	
Verbally correct		Veterinary clinic visit	
Physically punish		Strange adult enter house/yard	
Stare at dog		Strange child enter house/yard	
Response to familiar dog on leash		Familiar adult enter house/yard	
Response to strange dog on leash		Familiar child enter house/yard	
Response to familiar dog off leash		Stranger sudden approach	
Response to strange dog off leash		Familiar person sudden approach	

Used with permission of Jim Crosby.

Appendix 28
Basic Small Pet Bird Care
in Temporary Shelters

DIET

Most small birds will not eat unfamiliar foods. Try to find out what they are used to eating since brands may vary in appearance; try to gradually mix new food with old.

- Finches, canaries, small doves, and budgies can't open sunflower seeds. Give a seed mix made for their species if you can. Few know how to eat pelleted diets.
- In an emergency, you can use a seed mix made for other small species, or you can sift or pick out the larger seeds from parrot seed or wild bird seed with mostly millet.
- Check dishes twice daily if possible. A layer of empty seed hulls may cover the unopened seeds deeper in the dish, so blow or scrape away the opened shells.
- Birds may not eat every seed type in the mix. Watch droppings as described below.
- Give one food dish for each two birds and one water dish for each four birds. Most don't know how to drink from a bottle. Position dishes so they are in front of a perch.
- Grit is not necessary in a temporary shelter. Budgies and cockatiels never need grit.

HOUSING

Minimum temperature 60 degrees, maximum 85 degrees. A bird that is too cold will fluff out the feathers. Covering the cage isn't adequate; move to warm shelter.

- Panting is a sign of distress and overheating. Cool with water and fans immediately.
- Cage bars should not allow the head to push thru. Zip-tie cage to secure for moving.
- Some species may become aggressive when starved or overcrowded.

- Reduce stress with covers or barricades around two or three sides of the cage.
- Use newspaper or paper towels in the cage bottom and change daily.
- Place perches where the tail will not hit the cage bars, and not directly above other perches or dishes. The foot should wrap one-half to three-fourths of the way around the perch.

RESTRAINT

Never work on a flighted bird outdoors; move indoors or into a vehicle.

- Capture with a hand towel or paper towel if needed. A darkened room may make capture easier. Corner the bird in the bottom of the cage and wrap the towel around it.
- Gently encircle the neck with the thumb and forefinger to elongate the neck between the head and shoulders. Your fingertips should be touching under the lower beak through the towel. The weight of the towel will help keep the wings at the bird's side. Support the body in the palm of the hand. Never restrict breathing by compressing the chest.
- Do not trim the wings of finches, canaries, or small doves unless essential for safety.

COMMON MEDICAL PROBLEMS

Bacterial infections are very common. Keep cage and dishes clean; wash hands before handling; do not share food from your mouth.

- Over-the-counter antibiotics and those used in dogs are often ineffective in birds.

Veterinary Forensics: Animal Cruelty Investigations, Second Edition. Edited by Melinda D. Merck.
© 2013 John Wiley & Sons, Inc. Published 2013 by John Wiley & Sons, Inc.

- Birds are extremely sensitive to toxic fumes. Never use aerosols near birds; be cautious with disinfectant fumes or exhaust from vehicles when rescuing.
- Birds will hide symptoms of illness as long as possible. Report any subtle changes in sleeping, eating, breathing, droppings, or activity level immediately. A finch may die in twenty-four hours if not eating or drinking.

OTHER

There should be white urates and green/brown feces in each dropping. Watch for change in color or consistency. Birds that aren't eating pass only urates or fluid.

- Sick or injured birds may be picked on by cage mates. Remove immediately.
- Small birds greatly benefit from extra heat when sick. Warm to 80 or 85 degrees.

Used with permission of Dr. Julie Burge.

Appendix 29
Tuft's Animal Care and Condition Scale for Dogs

Veterinary Forensics: Animal Cruelty Investigations, Second Edition. Edited by Melinda D. Merck.
© 2013 John Wiley & Sons, Inc. Published 2013 by John Wiley & Sons, Inc.

Tufts Animal Care and Condition* (TACC) scales for assessing body condition, weather and environmental safety, and physical care in dogs

*A tool developed for veterinarians, animal control officers, police, and cruelty investigators by Tufts Center for Animals and Public Policy. Published in: Patronek, GJ. Recognizing and reporting animal abuse ~ a veterinarian's guide. Denver, CO:American Humane Association,1997.

I. Body condition scale (Palpation essential for long-haired dogs; each dog's condition should be interpreted in light of the typical appearance of the breed)

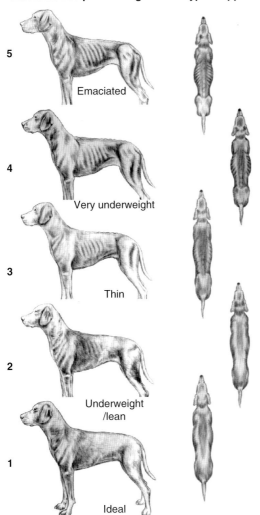

5 Emaciated

- All bony prominences evident from a distance
- No discernible body fat
- Obvious loss of muscle mass
- Severe abdominal tuck and extreme hourglass shape

4 Very underweight

- Ribs, lumbar vertebrae, and pelvic bones easily visible
- No palpable body fat
- Some loss of muscle mass
- Prominent abdominal tuck and hourglass shape to torso

3 Thin

- Tops of lumbar vertebrae visible, pelvic bones becoming prominent.
- Ribs easily palpated and may be visible with no palpable fat
- Obvious waist and abdominal tuck
- Minimal loss of muscle mass

2 Underweight /lean

- Ribs easily palpable with minimal SQ fat
- Abdominal tuck evident
- Waist clearly visible from above
- No muscle loss
- May be normal for lean breeds such as sighthounds

1 Ideal

- Ribs palpable without excess SQ fat
- Abdomen tucked slightly when viewed from the side
- Waist visible from above, just behind ribs

Body condition scale adapted from Laflamme, DP. Proc.N.A. Vet Conf 1993, 290–91; and Armstrong, PJ., Lund, EM. Vet Clin Nutr 3:83–87; 1996. Artwork by Erik Petersen.

Appendix 30
Tufts Animal Care and Condition Scale for the Environment

Tufts Animal Care and Condition* (TACC) scales for assessing body condition, weather and environmental safety, and physical care in dogs

*A tool developed for veterinarians, animal control officers, police, and cruelty investigators by Tufts Center for Animals and Public Policy. Published in: Patronek, GJ. Recognizing and reporting animal abuse ~ a veterinarian's guide. Denver, CO:American Humane Association,1997.

II . Weather safety scale

Read score off diagonal bars, by dog size:

In warm or hot weather:
- Subtract 1 pt. if water is available
- Subtract 1 pt. if dog is in a shaded area protected from full sun
- Add 1 pt. if dog is brachycephalic
- Add 1 pt. if dog is obese

In cool or cold weather:
- Add 1 pt. if toy dog
- Add 2 pts. if dog out in rain / sleet
- Subtract 1 pt. if dog is a northern or heavy-coated breed
- Subtract 1 pt. if dog has good shelter and bedding available
- Subtract 1 pt. if dog has been acclimated to cold temperatures

In all weather conditions:
- Add 1 pt. if dog is < 6 months of age or elderly

V. Large / Giant
Medium / Large
Small

Axes indicate temperature dog is exposed to, in °F

To determine score, draw a line up from the current temperature and parallel to the dotted lines, and read score on bars. Common sense must be used to take into account the duration of exposure to any given temperature when assessing risk; even brief periods of high heat can be very dangerous, whereas a similar duration of exposure to cold temperatures would not be life-threatening.

Interpretation of the TACC score from scales I - IV:

The Tufts Animal Condition and Care (TACC) score is assessed from the number of points read off either the **Body Condition Weather Safety, Environmental Health**, or **Physical Care** Scale. When multiple scales are evaluated, the highest score on any scale should be used to determine the risk of neglect. Multiple high scores are indicative of greater neglect, risk, or inhumane treatment than a single high score.

Score	Body condition, physical care, environ. health scales	Weather safety scale
≥5	Severe neglect and inhumane treatment. An urgent situation that justifies an assertive response to protect the animal.	Potentially life-threatening risk present. Immediate intervention to decrease threat to the animal required (provide water, shelter).
4	Clear evidence of serious neglect and / or inhumane treatment (unless there is a medical explanation for the animal's condition). Prompt improvement required.	Dangerous situation developing. Prompt intervention required to decrease risk (e.g. provide water, shade, shelter, or bring indoors). Warn owner of risk and shelter requirements.
3	Indicators of neglect present. Timely assessment; correction of problems and/or monitoring of situation may be required.	Indicators of a <u>potentially</u> unsafe situation, depending on breed, time outdoors. Inform owner of risk and proper shelter requirements.
2	A lapse in care or discomfort may be present. Evaluate, and discuss concerns with owner. Recommend changes in animal husbandry practices, if needed.	Risk unlikely, but evaluate the situation, and if warranted, discuss your concerns and requirements for proper shelter with the owner.
≤1	No evidence of neglect based on scale (s) used	No evidence of risk

Disclaimer: The TACC score is intended to be a simple screening device for determining when neglect may be present, for prioritizing the investigation of reported animal cruelty cases, and as a system for investigative agencies to use to summarize their case experience. The TACC score is not intended to replace definitive assessment of any animal by a veterinarian or law enforcement agent. A low TACC score does not preclude a diagnosis of abuse, neglect, or a dog requiring veterinary care upon more careful examination of an animal and its living situation.

III. Environmental health scale

5 **Filthy** - many days to weeks of accumulation of feces and / or urine. Overwhelming odor, air may be difficult to breathe. Large amount of trash, garbage, or debris present; inhibits comfortable rest, normal postures, or movement and / or poses a danger to the animal. Very difficult or impossible for animal to escape contact with feces, urine, mud, or standing water. Food and / or drinking water contaminated.

4 **Very unsanitary** - many days of accumulation of feces and / or urine. Difficult for animal to avoid contact with waste matter. Moderate amount of trash, garbage, or clutter present that may inhibit comfortable rest and / or movement of the animal. Potential injury from sharp edges or glass. Significant odor makes breathing unpleasant. Standing water or mud difficult to avoid.

3 **Unsanitary** - several days accumulation of feces and urine in animal's environment. Animal is able to avoid contact with waste matter. Moderate odor present. Trash, garbage, and other debris cluttering animal's environment but does not prohibit comfortable rest or normal posture. Clutter may interfere with normal movement or allow dog to become entangled, but no sharp edges or broken glass that could injure dog. Dog able to avoid mud or water if present.

2 **Marginal** - As in #1, except may be somewhat less sanitary. No more than 1-2 day's accumulation of feces and urine in animal's environment. Slight clutter may be present.

1 **Acceptable** - Environment is dry and free of accumulated feces. No contamination of food or water. No debris or garbage present to clutter environment and inhibit comfortable rest, normal posture and range of movement or pose a danger to or entangle the animal.

"Environment" refers to the kennel, pen, yard, cage, barn, room, tie-out or other enclosure or area where the animal is confined or spends the majority of its time. All of the listed conditions do not need to be present in order to include a dog in a specific category. The user should determine which category best describes a particular dog's condition.

IV. Physical care scale

5 **Terrible** - extremely matted haircoat, prevents normal motion, interferes with vision, perineal areas irritated from soiling with trapped urine and feces. Hair coat essentially a single mat. Dog cannot be groomed without complete clipdown. Foreign material trapped in matted hair. Nails extremely overgrown into circles, may be penetrating pads, causing abnormal position of feet and make normal walking very difficult or uncomfortable. Collar or chain, if present, may be imbedded in dog's neck.

4 **Poor** - substantial matting in haircoat, large chunks of hair matted together that cannot be separated with a comb or brush. Occasional foreign material embedded in mats. Much of the hair will need to be clipped to remove mats. Long nails force feet into abnormal position and interfere with normal gait. Perineal soiling or irritation likely. Collar or chain, if present, may be extremely tight, abrading skin.

3 **Borderline** - numerous mats present in hair, but dog can still be groomed without a total clip down. No significant perineal soiling or irritation from waste caught in matted hair. Nails are overdue for a trim and long enough to cause dog to alter gait when it walks. Collar or chain, if present, may be snug and rubbing off neck hair.

2 **Lapsed** - haircoat may be somewhat dirty or have a few mats present that are easily removed. Remainder of coat can easily be brushed or combed. Nails in need of a trim. Collar or chain, if present, fits comfortably.

1 **Adequate** - dog clean, hair of normal length for the breed, and hair can easily be brushed or combed. Nails do not touch the floor, or barely contact the floor. Collar or chain, if present, fits comfortably.

All of the listed conditions do not need to be present in order to include a dog in a specific category. The user should determine which category best describes a particular dog's condition. This scale is not meant for assessment of medical conditions, e.g., a broken limb, that clearly indicate a need for veterinary attention.

Appendix 31
Dogfighting Terminology

Break stick (breaking stick, bite stick): a wedge-shaped stick used to "break" the hold of a pit bull

Catchweight: a heavyweight, any dog over 52 pounds pit weight

Catmill (Jenny): a conditioning device consisting of one or more spokes projecting from a rotating central shaft in the ground. A dog is harnessed to one spoke or other fixture in front of the dog so that the dog will run in circles, attempting to catch the lure. Weights are frequently attached to ancillary spokes or a drag may be added to increase resistance

Chain weight: the regular weight of a dog kept on the yard

Champion: rank conferred by various pit dog publications on dogs that have won three contract matches

Cur: any dog that is not game; that shows signs and/or gives up or stops; cries, tail between the legs; may initially rear up and soon curr out

Curr out: to quit or give up

Down-dog: the dog receiving the most punishment during a match, usually down on the carpet

Fanged: when a dog inadvertently pierces his or her own lip with a canine tooth while attempting a bite hold on an opponent

Fast-mouthed: in combat, a dog that makes numerous bite holds in rapid succession

Flirtpole: an exercise device consisting of a pole, often bamboo, with a lure (often animal hide) attached; the dog chases the lure, which is guided by the trainer holding the pole

Game (Gameness): 1. The sport of dog-fighting; 2. The combined qualities of courage, aggression, and tenacity in the face of utter exhaustion and possible death.

Game test: to determine a dog's gameness by rolling until completely exhausted, then having the dog prove gameness by scratching to a fresh dog

Grand Champion: rank that can be conferred on a dog who has won five contract matches without any losses

Handle: the act of handling a dog and lifting him or her away from the opponent

Keep: A rigorous diet and exercise program designed to prepare and condition a dog for a contract match, usually four to six weeks prior to the fight; except for exercise periods, a dog in keep is usually isolated from other dogs

Match: a contracted dogfight

Match dog: a dog that is used or intended for use in a contracted match

Pick-up: occurs when a handler concedes a match by picking up his dog

Pit: arena where fights are conducted; a typical pit is constructed of plywood walls measuring 24 to 36 inches high and approximately 14 to 20 feet square, although concrete, sheets of metal, and bales of hay have been used to construct a pit; the floor of the pit is usually covered with carpet or canvas to allow increased traction; many pits are designed to be disassembled so as to be portable

Pit weight (match weight): when a dog is brought down from his usual weight and is ready to match

Veterinary Forensics: Animal Cruelty Investigations, Second Edition. Edited by Melinda D. Merck.
© 2013 John Wiley & Sons, Inc. Published 2013 by John Wiley & Sons, Inc.

Producer of Record (POR): a list of dogs established and maintained in the dog fighting journals; a sire and dam are given one point for each win of their immediate offspring; a male must have fifteen points and a female must have ten points to make the list; champion offspring will net the sire and dam of such one extra point; Grand Champion offspring will net two extra points for the sire and dam

Register of Merit (ROM): a list of dogs established and maintained by the Sporting Dog Journal; each dog is credited with one point for each champion produced and one additional point for each one of these champions who goes on to win a grand championship; a male dog must be the sire of at least four champions to get on the list and a female must be the dam of at least three champions

Roll/bump (schooling): a practice or training match

Scratch: a method by which a dog must demonstrate gameness in a pit contest; the act of rushing across the pit and taking hold of an opponent within a specified count, which can vary according to the rules of the fight; scratches are made from behind diagonal lines in opposite corners of the pit; the first scratch is a simultaneous release; subsequent scratches are alternating

Scratch lines: lines drawn diagonally across opposite corners of the pit from behind which the dogs are set down and released and the dog has to cross, or scratch, after being released

Spring pole: a device used for exercising a pit bull

Treadmill: a device for running a dog in place

Turn: a pit term that refers to a dog turning his head and shoulders away from his opponent; various rules are set for this because it can be mistaken for a maneuver or tactic of the dog

Turn-table: a device used to run a dog in place

Appendix 32
Cajun Rules for Dogfighting

Please note: All spelling and grammatical errors are included as in the original booklet entitled "Combat Rules"

CAJUN RULES

1. Size of pit optional; to be square with sides 2 feet high, scratch line 14 feet apart.
2. Referee to be chosen before the dogs are weighed in or washed and referee to conduct the contest according to these rules and his decision to be final.
3. Referee to see the dogs weighed at time agreed on and if either dog is over top weight agreed he loses forfeit money.
4. Parties to toss coin to see who shall wash first, each party to furnish two clean towels and a blanket.
5. If requested to do so the referee shall search the person named to wash the dog and then have him bare his arm to the elbow and wash both dogs in the same warm water and rinse them each in his half of the warm clean water provided for that purpose.
6. As the dogs are washed clean and dried they shall be turned over to their handlers and at once taken to their corners of the pit as designated by the referee, and the referee must search handlers for means of foul play and see that he hares his arms to the elbow before he receives his dog and must keep him arm bare in such a manner during the contest.
7. The dogs' owner or his representative shall be allowed at all times to be near his dog and watch to see that no harm is done him, and each owner shall be allowed to name a man or himself to watch over his opponent's dog and handler at all times to see he is given no unfair advantage.
8. Either dogs owner, handler or watcher if he sees anything wrong must at once appeal to the referee and get his decision. And if any handler, watcher or owner violates any of these rules and thereby favours either dog the dog so favoured must at once be declared the loser.
9. The interested parties shall choose a timekeeper at the pit side.
10. The dogs are placed in their corners of the pit, opposite corners, faces turned from each other, and only the dogs and their handlers inside the pit. Then the referee shall say "Face your dogs" each handler must always show his dogs full head and shoulders between his legs. The referee says "Let Go", but the handler must never push or shove their dogs, and handlers shall not leave their corners until the dogs are together.
11. Now when one of the dogs turns his head and shoulders away from his opponent after the fight is on it is a turn whether they are in holds are free, and the handler must claim the turn and the referee must the claim if he believes it is a turn or the referee must call the first fair turn he sees whether the handler claims it or not and when the referee calls a turn he shall say "Handle your dogs when they are free of holds" and each handler must pick up his dog as soon as he can without breaking a hold. Handlers carry their dogs to their respective corners immediately on picking them up, keeping the dogs face turned away from the center of the pit. The dog that turned first must scratch first. In five seconds more the referee shall say "Let Go", then the dog that made the first turn must he turned loose by his handler and this dog must go across and mouthe the other dog. If when he is turned loose he refuses to start at once or if he stops on the way over, or if he fails to reach his

Veterinary Forensics: Animal Cruelty Investigations, Second Edition. Edited by Melinda D. Merck.

opponent he has lost the fight and the referee must declare his opponent the winner. A handler is allowed to release his dog at any time he sees fit after the dog whose turn it is to cross has started over. He must turn loose when the dogs touch each other.

12. (a) If neither dog has made a turn and they cease to fight after 60 seconds of no action, the down dog is to scratch first, if he makes his scratch the fight is one and they shall scratch in turns until the contest is decided.

    (b) If the down dog fails to scratch the other dog is to scratch to win. If he fails to scratch to win. If he fails to scratch the contest shall be declared a draw by the referee.

    (c) No handler is to handle his dog until ordered by the referee if he does, it shall he declared a foul by the referee, and he is to forfeit the contest to his opponent.

    (d) No flash pictures or hitting on pit side shall be allowed unless agreed upon by the two contestants.

13. After the dogs are together this time either handler is to pick up his dog when they are not in holds, if ordered by the referee. If he catches his dog up free both handlers must handle their dogs at once, take their dogs to their corners and proceed same as the first turn, except this time the dog which went across before is allowed to remain in his corner while his opponent makes his scratch, or goes across, and they alternate or take it in turn about this matter until one of them is declared the winner under these rules.

The referee pays no attention to the turn after the first scratch.

14. If one of the dogs fangs himself, that is if he gets his teeth hung in his own lip, his handler is allowed to unfang him. If the dog have to be separated for this they are turned loose again both at the same time within two feet of each other in the center of the pit.

15. No sponging shall be allowed, and no towels or anything else taken into the pit by the handlers except a bottle of drink for his dog and a fan to cool him with. The handlers must taste their dogs drink before the referee to show that it contains no poison.

16. If the handler of either dog is seen to take anything from anyone on the outside of the pit he is to lose the battle. Each party shall have the opportunity to put a man near his opponents corner to watch the handler. Should he see the handler put anything on his dog he may appear to the referee, and if the referee finds anything on the dog he is to lose the battle.

17. Should either handler leave the pit with his dog before the referee renders his decision he is to lose the battle.

18. The handlers shall be allowed to encourage their dogs by voice or hand-clapping or snapping of their fingers, but must not touch their dog or use foul, dirty methods by saving their dogs from hard falls or keeping the other handler away from his dog, or in any way act unfairly. The referee must decide the battle against the one who does so.

19. Should the police interfere the referee to name the next meeting place.

Appendix 33
Dogfighting Scar and Injury Chart

Date_____Investigating Agency_____

Case#_____Officer_____ Veterinarian_____

Dog ID_____Breed_____ Color_____ Male_____ Female_____

Distinguishing marks_____ Chart created/verified by_____

CHART KEY: **Red**=fresh, healing **Blue**=healed, scars

Wound Age Estimate (assigned by veterinarian)

A =_____ B =_____ C =_____ D =_____ E =_____

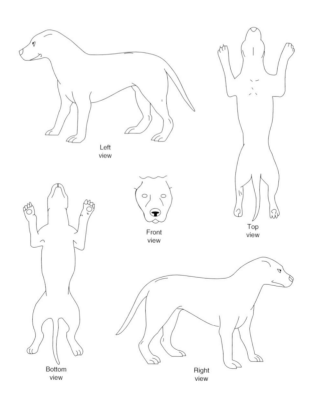

Left view

Front view

Top view

Bottom view

Right view

Appendix 34
Cockfighting Scar and Injury Chart

Date_____ Investigating Agency_____

Case#_____ Officer_____ Veterinarian_____

Animal ID_____ Band Info _____ Chart verified by_____

Spurs: Partially removed __ Sharpened__ Freshly cut__ Evidence of regrowth__

Combs: Complete removed__ Partially removed__ Fresh__ Recent__ Scarred__

Earlobes: Complete removed__ Partially removed__ Fresh__ Recent__ Scarred__

Wattles: Complete removed__ Partially removed__ Fresh__ Recent__ Scarred__

CHART KEY: **Red**=fresh, healing **Blue**=healed, scars

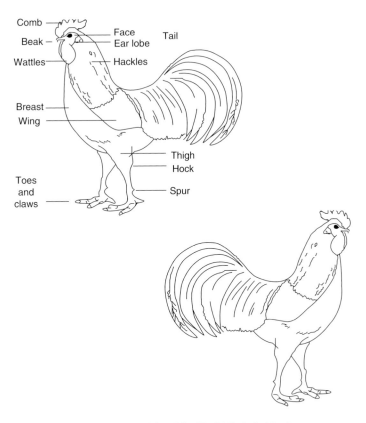

Veterinary Forensics: Animal Cruelty Investigations, Second Edition. Edited by Melinda D. Merck.
© 2013 John Wiley & Sons, Inc. Published 2013 by John Wiley & Sons, Inc.

Appendix 35
Examples of Vitamins, Drugs, and Medical Supplies Used in Dogfighting

Although many of the following vitamins, drugs, and veterinary supplies have legitimate uses, they are commonly found in connection with illegal dogfighting operations.

VITAMINS AND SUPPLEMENTS

The primary focus is on performance enhancement

- Magnum® supplements (source of seven different vitamins and minerals)
- Provim powder (dog condition and stress supplement)
- Vitamin B$_{12}$ (injectable)
- Liver and iron extract (used with injectable B$_{12}$ to increase red blood cell level, which increases the ability of blood to carry more oxygen)
- Canine red cell (vitamin and iron supplement)
- Clovite® conditioner (vitamins A, D, and B$_{12}$ supplement)
- Stress-Dex® (oral electrolyte with vitamins)
- Vitamin B$_{15}$ (acts as a catalyst to allow red blood to carry approximately 25% more oxygen and decreases lactic acid in muscle)
- Energy-Plus (used as a booster for dogs not reaching a peak performance level)

DRUGS

Categories include antibiotics; anti-inflammatories; analgesics; and surgery, critical care, weight loss, and performance enhancement (illicit drugs, androgenic/anabolic steroids) drugs

- Speed (amphetamine pills, capsules, or injectable solution for stimulating a tired dog)
- Illegal drugs (cocaine, methamphetamine)
- Dexamethasone (an anti-inflammatory agent that reduces swelling, delays shock, and relieves muscle pain and soreness)
- Hormones and androgenic steroids (testosterone derivatives used to build muscle mass and increase aggression).
- Anabolic steroid mimetics, e.g., clenbuterol
- Epinephrine
- Furosemide (injectable diuretic) for weight loss
- Painkillers (human and animal drugs)
- Antibiotics and combiotics (injectable, tablets, and capsules)
- Nitrofurazone topical antibiotic
- Prednisone (anti-inflammatory agent)
- Lidocaine

MEDICAL SUPPLIES

Categories include wound treatment, surgical, and critical care supplies

- IV kit, syringes, and needles in various sizes
- Lactated Ringers (intravenous solution for treatment of hypovolemic shock)
- Pad-Kote™ (topical ointment for foot pads)
- Sutures, suture needles, and needle holders
- Forceps, scalpel, and surgical scissors
- Alcohol prep pads and cotton-tipped applicators
- Sponges
- Dressing for wounds
- Blood hemoglobin test kits

Veterinary Forensics: Animal Cruelty Investigations, Second Edition. Edited by Melinda D. Merck.
© 2013 John Wiley & Sons, Inc. Published 2013 by John Wiley & Sons, Inc.

The following substances and methods (performance enhancing) are typically prohibited in professional sports and have been found associated with dog fighting activities.

ANABOLIC AGENTS (EXAMPLES)

- Androstenediol
- Androstenedione
- 1-Androstenedione
- Bolasterone
- Boldenone undecylenate
- Calusterone
- Clostebol
- Danazol
- Dehydrochloromethyltestosterone
- Dehydroepiandrosterone
- Desoxymethyltestosterone
- Dihydrotestosterone
- Dromostanolone
- Ethylestrenol
- Fluoxymesterone
- Formebolone
- Furazabol
- Gestrinone
- 17-Hydroxypregnenedione
- 17-Hydroxyprogesterone
- Hydroxytestosterone
- Mestanolone
- Mesterolone
- Methandienone
- Methandriol
- Methandrostenolone
- Methenolone
- Methyltestosterone
- Mibolerone
- 19-Norandrostenediol
- 19-Norandrostenedione
- Norbolethone
- Norclostebol
- Norethandrolone
- Normethandrolone
- 19-Nortestosterone
- Oxandrolone
- 6-Oxoandrosterone
- Oxymesterone
- Oxymetholone
- Progesterone
- Stanozolol
- Stenbolone
- Testosterone
- 1-Testosterone
- Tetrahydrogestrinone
- Trenbolone
- Related substances

PEPTIDE HORMONES (EXAMPLES)

- Human growth hormone (hGH): Saizen®, Humatrope®, Nutropin AQ®
- Animal growth hormones
- Human chorionic gonadotropin (hCG): Novarel®, menotropins
- Beta-2-agonists (clenbuterol, etc.)
- Anti-estrogenic agents (clomiphene, cyclofenil, tamoxifen)

MASKING AGENTS

- Epitestosterone
- Probenecid

MASKING AGENTS: DIURETICS (EXAMPLES)

- Acetazolamide
- Amiloride
- Bendroflumethiazide
- Benzthiazide
- Bumetanide
- Chlorothiazide
- Cyclothiazide
- Ethacrynic Acid
- Flumethiazide
- Furosemide
- Hydrochlorothiazide
- Hydroflumethiazide
- Methyclothiazide
- Metolazone
- Polythiazide
- Probenecid
- Quinethazone
- Spironolactone
- Triamterene
- Trichlormethiazide
- Related substances

CERTAIN STIMULANTS (EXAMPLES)

- Amphetamine
- Ephedrine
- Fenfluramine
- Methamphetamine
- Methylephedrine
- Modafinil
- Norfenfluramine
- Pseudoephedrine
- Phentermine
- Synephrine
- Aurantium

Appendix 36
Entomology Form for Animal Cases

COLLECION OF INSECT EVIDENCE FROM ANIMAL CARCASS

File number _____ **Agency** _____

Date of Collection _____ Time of Collection _____

Date found _____ Time found _____

Location found _____

_____

Officer in Charge _____ tel. _____ Email _____

Collecting officer _____ tel. _____ Email _____

Weather conditions at collection time (rain and temp.) _____

DESCRIPTION OF DEATH SCENE

Inside Residence/Building/Outbuilding?

House _____ Garage _____ Kennel _____ Barn _____ Other (describe) _____

Is building heated? If so what is indoor temperature? _____

Please describe location _____

_____

_____

Outdoors?

Garden _____ Field _____ Forest _____ Bush _____ Ditch _____ (Water? How much _____)

Please describe location _____

_____

Is the carcass in sun or shade _____?

If shade, describe vegetation, height, amount of shade over length of day _____

_____

Veterinary Forensics: Animal Cruelty Investigations, Second Edition. Edited by Melinda D. Merck.
© 2013 John Wiley & Sons, Inc. Published 2013 by John Wiley & Sons, Inc.

Exposure

Full sunshine _____ Partial sunshine _____ How long/day? _____ Shade? _____ How long/day? _____

In Water?

Pond _____ Lake _____ Creek _____ River _____ Ditch _____ Submergence level _____

Surface Carcass Resting On

Carpet _____ Tile _____ Linoleum _____ Hard wood _____ Furniture _____ Soil _____ Grass

Other (describe) _____

Are remains exposed .... or wrapped? .... If wrapped, describe wrapping, amount of coverage_____

_____

DESCRIPTION OF REMAINS

Species _____ Breed _____ Coat length/type _____

Approx. size/weight _____ Adult or immature? _____ No. of carcasses at site _____

Carcass position _____

Is carcass buried? _____ How deep? _____ What is the covering? _____

Are there wounds? _____ Type (gunshot, knife?) _____

Wound site (s) _____

_____

Stage of decomposition (fresh, active, advanced, skeletonized) _____

Describe decomposition _____

TAKE PHOTOGRAPHS OF:

General scene _____ Habitat surrounding body _____ Carcass _____ Wounds _____

Maggot mass(s) _____ Insect activity _____ Ground beneath body after removal _____

INSECT EVIDENCE

Are there any maggot masses (very large number of maggots all together in a mass)?

If so, how big _____, **where** _____, **temp. of center** _____

_____

_____

Description of insect evidence - e.g. maggots, pupae, adult beetles, larval beetles etc. _____

_____

_____

_____

COLLECTION

Collect from the carcass itself, and from the ground below and around the carcass. Use plastic urinalysis vials as specimen jars and collect with forceps or a teaspoon.

Eggs – collect samples from each area. Divide each sample into two. Half should be kept **ALIVE** in a vial which contains a small piece of paper towel and (within a few hours) a piece of meat. Cover the vial with two layers of paper towel held in place with an elastic band. Observe every 1-2 hours to note time of hatch. Other half should be **PRESERVED** by placing in a vial of alcohol (75-90% ethanol). **NOTE – eggs are only of value if no older insects present.**

Maggots – Collect samples from each area of maggots (e.g. mouth and wound). Divide each sample into two. Half should be kept **ALIVE** and placed in vial with paper towel and piece of meat as for eggs. Cover vial with two layers of paper towel. Observation not required. Do not put too many maggots in a vial—no more than one layer thick. Other half of sample must be **PRESERVED**. If possible, kill by pouring very hot water on sample for 5 minutes then placing in alcohol. If no hot water available, preserve directly in alcohol. Screw lid onto vial.

Once maggots have ceased feeding, they will leave the remains. If the carcass is on soil, loose material, thick carpet, or bedding, the insects may be several centimeters into the soil/carpet. If the carcass is on a hard surface such as cement, linoleum, or hard wood, they may have crawled away and will search for any shelter such as clothing, appliances, furniture, baseboards, or brush/hay. Search these areas and collect as above.

Maggots will pupate in similar areas **away** from the carcass as above depending on substrate or may pupate in coat if long. Pupae are football shaped and range in color from pale to dark brown (5 mm–1 cm long).

It is very important to search for pupae or, once the fly has emerged, the empty pupal cases. Search under and around the carcass for these. They are quite delicate—do not preserve them. Collect pupae and empty pupal cases separately and place in vials. Put paper towel in vials to cushion them. Air is required for pupae (paper towel lid) but not for empty pupal cases.

All other insects (beetles, other flies) can be placed in separate vials of alcohol. Label all exhibits with place and time of collection.

COLLECT SAMPLES FROM (for example):

Wounds _____ Head _____ Genitals _____ General carcass area _____ Under carcass _____ Where carcass meets ground _____ Soil/substrate around carcass _____ Soil/substrate when body removed _____

Exhibit no.	Site collected from i.e. area of carcass or soil	type e.g. maggots, beetle larvae, flies, beetles	approx. number maggots preserved— DO NOT KILL PUPAE!

Keep maggots and beetles (adult or larvae) separate. Keep samples from different sites separate.

Signature of Collector _____

Appendix 37
Webliography

AVIAN

Avian Welfare Coalition: information about avian welfare
www.avianwelfare.org

Handbook for a Healthier Bird
www.harrisonsbirdfoods.com/learningcenter/index.html

Keeping Your Bird Entertained
www.hartz.com/Birds/Habitat/Keeping_Your_Bird_
Entertained.aspx

CONSULTATION SERVICES

American Association of Forensic Science: contact lists of
forensic specialists
www.aafs.org

AZ Forensic Associates: provides consultation services for
blood stain pattern analysis
http://www.bloodstainevidence.com/

Canine Behavior and Aggression Consulting: also provides
consulting services for dog bite and dog attack
investigations
http://dogconsulting.org

Dr. Melinda Merck's Veterinary Forensics: Website offering training, consultation services, and case response for
animal cases; also contains forms and information on
veterinary forensic science
www.veterinaryforensics.com

Forensic Pieces: training and consultations offered in a
broad range of forensic sciences
www.forensicpieces.com

HAIRbase™: website containing a database of various
animal hairs to support forensic analysis
http://web.me.com/kwpmiller/HAIRbase/Welcome.html

U.S. Fish and Wildlife Service: crime lab responsible for
investigating federal fish and wildlife crimes
http://www.lab.fws.gov/

EQUIPMENT

Arrowhead Forensics: crime investigation and forensic
supply company
www.crime-scene.com

Entomology supplies and collection information
www.texasento.net/equip.htm
www.bioquip.com

Evident Crime Scene: crime scene and evidence collection
products
www.evidentcrimescene.com

Fitzco, Inc.: crime scene and evidence collection products
www.fitzcoinc.com

Hobo data loggers
www.onsetcomp.com

Law Enforcement Training and Resource Group: offers
new POCKET CSI™, a suite of applications for smart
phones for crime scene responders
www.letrg.com

Lynn Peavey: crime scene and evidence collection products
www.lynnpeavey.com

Sirchie: crime scene and evidence collection products
www.sirchie.com

Tri-tech USA: crime scene and evidence collection
products with veterinary forensic kit
www.tritechusa.com

Veterinary Forensics: Animal Cruelty Investigations, Second Edition. Edited by Melinda D. Merck.
© 2013 John Wiley & Sons, Inc. Published 2013 by John Wiley & Sons, Inc.

FORENSIC TESTING

American Association of Veterinary Laboratory Diagnosticians: access to the full list of accredited laboratories in the USA
www.aavld.org

Diagnostic Center for Population and Animal Health: bone marrow fat analysis and animal toxicology testing
www.dcpah.msu.edu

U.S. Fish and Wildlife Service—National Fish and Wildlife Forensics Laboratory
www.lab.fws.gov

Forensic toxicology
www.abarbour.net

Humane Society of the United States: has an entire department of highly experienced consultants for animal fighting investigations who can provide assistance as well as up-to-date general information about animal fighting
www.humanesociety.org

Independent Forensics: laboratory testing and products sold for field testing
www.ifi-test.com

Microtrace, LLC: private independent laboratory specializing in the characterization and identification of single, small particles and small quantities of unknown materials including animal hair
http://www.microtracescientific.com/

Purdue University Animal Disease Diagnostic Laboratory: bone marrow fat analysis
www.addl.purdue.edu/

Shelterwood Laboratories (DNA Diagnostics): animal DNA testing
www.dnadiagnostics.com

Therion DNA: animal DNA testing
www.therionDNA.com

Veterinary Genetics Laboratory of UC-Davis: features forensic animal DNA testing.
www.vgl.ucdavis.edu

Veterinary Genetics Laboratory Canine CODIS Dog Fighting database: the site for information on the Canine CODIS database
www.vgl.ucdavis.edu/forensics/CANINECODIS

Zoogen: animal DNA testing
http://zoogendna.com/

GENERAL INFORMATION

American Humane Association: offers training in disaster/temporary sheltering
http://www.americanhumane.org/animals/professional-resources/training/disaster-sheltering.html

Battered Pet Syndrome: Non-Accidental Physical Injuries That Occur In Dogs And Cats by Helen Munro
http://canadianveterinarians.net/pdfs/Munro_NonAccidentalInjuries.pdf

A Bibliography Related to Crime Scene Interpretation with Emphases in Forensic Geotaphonomic and Forensic Archaeological Field Techniques as a downloadable PDF
http://mai.mercyhurst.edu/research/research-materials/reference-guides/a-bibliography-related-to-crime-scene-interpretation/

Blood stain tutorial
www.bloodspatter.com

Canadian veterinary website with section on animal abuse
http://canadianveterinarians.net/animal-abuse.aspx

Crime & Clues: Website with information for crime scene investigation and forensic science
www.crimeandclues.com

Crime Scene Investigations: information by retired Sgt. Hayden B. Baldwin
www.feinc.net/cs-inv-p.htm

CSI Gizmos: site has templates for creating your own evidence markers, scales, and arrows. There are innovative investigation gadgets from the products page
www.csigizmos.com

Crime Scene Investigator Network: site has links to forensic articles and information
www.crime-scene-investigator.net

Diatom home page for Indiana University
www.indiana.edu/~diatom/diatom.html

Dr. Zeno's Forensic site: contains forensic information about several disciplines
www.geradts.com

FBI Forensic Science Communications
http://www.fbi.gov/about-us/lab/forensic-science-communications

Firearms ID: site includes information on ammunition identification, gunshot residue, shotgun pattern testing, etc.
www.firearmsid.com

Forensic Evidence: Website of information on forensic science, law, and public policy
www.forensic-evidence.com

Forensic Magazine: full issues, articles, products, and services and recent court rulings
www.forensicmag.com

Forensic Science Resources
http://www.tncrimlaw.com/forensic

Forensic science resources on the Internet: Website updated and maintained by The Gelman Library at George Washington University
www.istl.org/03-spring/internet.html

The Hoarding of Animals Research Consortium: contains the Tufts Animal Care and Condition Score
http://vet.tufts.edu/hoarding/

Incident Command System: information on the ICS system and links to the online independent study courses
http://www.fema.gov/emergency/nims/IncidentCommandSystem.shtm#item7

International Association for Identification: Scientific Working Group on Imaging Technologies (SWGIT)
http://www.theiai.org/guidelines/swgit/index.php

National Clearinghouse for Science, Technology, and the Law, a program of the National Institute of Justice: searchable database
www.ncstl.org

National Institute of Justice—A Guide for General Crime Scene Investigation: Processing the Scene
http://www.nij.gov/nij/topics/law-enforcement/investigations/crime-scene/guides/general-scenes/process.htm#collect

Necropsy Procedures for Wild Animals
http://www.vetmed.ucdavis.edu/whc/pdfs/necropsy.pdf

NetVet: Veterinary and Animal Government and Law Resources
http://netvet.wustl.edu/law.htm

Pet Abuse: this site contains a searchable animal abuse database
www.pet-abuse.com

Purina BCS: site for information on Purina body condition scale for dogs and cats
www.purina.com

Reddy's Forensic Page: Website listing forensic books and journals
www.forensicpage.com/new04.htm

Weather Data
www.wrh.noaa.gov
www.ncdc.noaa.gov
www.wcc.nrcs.usda.gov/snow

LARGE ANIMAL

BCS system: cattle
http://cdqa.org/docs/Appendix7.pdf

BCS (Henneke system): equine
http://www.trfinc.org/mc_images/category/4/eqfeb09bodyconditionscore.pdf

Dairy Welfare Guide
http://cdqa.org/info_dl.asp

Lameness/locomotion guide
http://cdqa.org/docs/Appendix3.pdf

UC-Davis Veterinary Medicine Extension Animal Welfare: this site has numerous welfare guides for multiple species of livestock and provides excellent resources for establishing what constitutes acceptable management practices
http://www.vetmed.ucdavis.edu/vetext/animalwelfare

LEGAL

Animal Legal Defense Fund: offers investigation and prosecution support for animal cruelty cases; site has resources including animal law info and foster agreement forms for animals in legal cases
www.aldf.org

Federal Animal Welfare Act
http://www.nal.usda.gov/awic/legislat/usdaleg1.htm

Georgia Legal Professionals for Animals
www.georgialpa.org

Gonzaga University: a selected bibliography and research guide for animal law
http://www.law.gonzaga.edu/Library-and-Technology/Files/Reference-and-Research/Research-Guides/AnimalLaw.pdf

Lewis and Clark Law School Center for Animal Law: site offers resources in animal law
http://www.lclark.edu/law/centers/animal_law_studies/

Michigan State University-Detroit College of Law: a searchable Website for animal cruelty laws and veterinary practice acts in the U.S. and internationally
www.animallaw.info

USDA Animal Welfare Page, including pdf and Word versions of the Animal Welfare Act
http://www.aphis.usda.gov/animal_welfare/publications_and_reports.shtml

ORGANIZATIONS

American Association of Forensic Science: source of the Journal of Forensic Science
www.aafs.org

American College of Forensic Examiners: source for the Forensic Examiner journal
www.acfei.com

Association of Shelter Veterinarians: site has guidelines for standard of care in animal shelter and the Five Freedoms
www.sheltervet.org

International Veterinary Forensic Sciences Association
www.ivfsa.org

National Association of Medical Examiners: source of The American Journal of Forensic Medicine and Pathology
www.thename.org

Index